E-learning and Digital Training in Healthcare Education: Current Trends and New Challenges

E-learning and Digital Training in Healthcare Education: Current Trends and New Challenges

Editors

Luís Proença
José João Mendes
João Botelho
Vanessa Machado

MDPI • Basel • Beijing • Wuhan • Barcelona • Belgrade • Manchester • Tokyo • Cluj • Tianjin

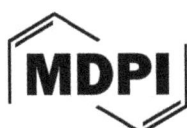

Editors

Luís Proença
Centro de Investigação
Interdisciplinar Egas Moniz
(CiiEM), Egas Moniz -
Cooperativa de Ensino
Superior
Portugal

José João Mendes
Centro de Investigação
Interdisciplinar Egas Moniz
(CiiEM), Egas Moniz -
Cooperativa de Ensino
Superior
Portugal

João Botelho
Centro de Investigação
Interdisciplinar Egas Moniz
(CiiEM), Egas Moniz -
Cooperativa de Ensino
Superior
Portugal

Vanessa Machado
Centro de Investigação
Interdisciplinar Egas Moniz
(CiiEM), Egas Moniz -
Cooperativa de Ensino
Superior
Portugal

Editorial Office
MDPI
St. Alban-Anlage 66
4052 Basel, Switzerland

This is a reprint of articles from the Topical Collection published online in the open access journal *Healthcare* (ISSN 2227-9032) (available at: https://www.mdpi.com/journal/healthcare/topical_collections/E-learning_Digital_Training_Healthcare_Education).

For citation purposes, cite each article independently as indicated on the article page online and as indicated below:

LastName, A.A.; LastName, B.B.; LastName, C.C. Article Title. *Journal Name* **Year**, *Volume Number*, Page Range.

ISBN 978-3-0365-4513-4 (Hbk)
ISBN 978-3-0365-4514-1 (PDF)

© 2022 by the authors. Articles in this book are Open Access and distributed under the Creative Commons Attribution (CC BY) license, which allows users to download, copy and build upon published articles, as long as the author and publisher are properly credited, which ensures maximum dissemination and a wider impact of our publications.

The book as a whole is distributed by MDPI under the terms and conditions of the Creative Commons license CC BY-NC-ND.

Contents

About the Editors ix

Preface to "E-learning and Digital Training in Healthcare Education: Current Trends and
New Challenges" xi

Tinggui Chen, Lijuan Peng, Xiaohua Yin, Jingtao Rong, Jianjun Yang and Guodong Cong
Analysis of User Satisfaction with Online Education Platforms in China during the
COVID-19 Pandemic
Reprinted from: *Healthcare* **2020**, *8*, 200, doi:10.3390/healthcare8030200 1

Mariana Morgado, José João Mendes and Luís Proença
Online Problem-Based Learning in Clinical Dental Education: Students' Self-Perception
and Motivation
Reprinted from: *Healthcare* **2021**, *9*, 420, doi:10.3390/healthcare9040420 27

Javier Ruiz-Labarta, Ana Martínez Martín, Pilar Pintado Recarte, Blanca González Garzón,
Juan Manuel Pina Moreno, Mercedes Sánchez Rodríguez, África Vallejo Gea, Luis Sordo,
Melchor Álvarez-Mon, Miguel A. Ortega, Coral Bravo Arribas and Juan A. De León-Luis
Workshop on Blood Loss Quantification in Obstetrics: Improving Medical Student Learning
through Clinical Simulation
Reprinted from: *Healthcare* **2022**, *10*, 399, doi:10.3390/healthcare10020399 39

Laura Orsolini, Silvia Bellagamba, Virginia Marchetti, Giulia Menculini,
Silvia Tempia Valenta, Virginio Salvi and Umberto Volpe
A Preliminary Italian Cross-Sectional Study on the Level of Digital Psychiatry Training,
Knowledge, Beliefs and Experiences among Medical Students, Psychiatry Trainees
and Professionals
Reprinted from: *Healthcare* **2022**, *10*, 390, doi:10.3390/healthcare10020390 53

Vivienne Mak, Sunanthiny Krishnan and Sara Chuang
Students' and Examiners' Experiences of Their First Virtual Pharmacy Objective Structured
Clinical Examination (OSCE) in Australia during the COVID-19 Pandemic
Reprinted from: *Healthcare* **2022**, *10*, 328, doi:10.3390/healthcare10020328 69

Vivienne Mak, Daniel Malone, Nilushi Karunaratne, Wendy Yao, Lauren Randell and
Thao Vu
A Video-Based Reflective Design to Prepare First Year Pharmacy Students for Their First
Objective Structured Clinical Examination (OSCE)
Reprinted from: *Healthcare* **2022**, *10*, 280, doi:10.3390/healthcare10020280 85

Osama Khattak, Kiran Kumar Ganji, Azhar Iqbal, Meshal Alonazi, Hmoud Algarni and
Thani Alsharari
Educational Videos as an Adjunct Learning Tool in Pre-Clinical Operative Dentistry—A
Randomized Control Trial
Reprinted from: *Healthcare* **2022**, *10*, 178, doi:10.3390/healthcare10020178 99

Henriette K. Helland, Thorkild Tylleskär, Monika Kvernenes and Håkon Reikvam
An Abrupt Transition to Digital Teaching—Norwegian Medical Students and Their Experiences
of Learning Output during the Initial Phase of the COVID-19 Lockdown
Reprinted from: *Healthcare* **2022**, *10*, 170, doi:10.3390/healthcare10010170 109

Reham AlJasser, Lina Alolyet, Daniyah Alsuhaibani, Sarah Albalawi, Md. Dilshad Manzar and Abdulrhman Albougami
Perception of E-Resources on the Learning Process among Students in the College of Health Sciences in King Saud University, Saudi Arabia, during the (COVID-19) Outbreak
Reprinted from: Healthcare 2022, 10, 40, doi:10.3390/healthcare10010040 121

Diana Jiménez-Rodríguez, Mercedes Pérez-Heredia, María del Mar Molero Jurado, María del Carmen Pérez-Fuentes and Oscar Arrogante
Improving Humanization Skills through Simulation-Based Computers Using Simulated Nursing Video Consultations
Reprinted from: Healthcare 2022, 10, 37, doi:10.3390/healthcare10010037 131

Rohit Kunnath Menon and Liang Lin Seow
Development of an Online Asynchronous Clinical Learning Resource ("Ask the Expert") in Dental Education to Promote Personalized Learning
Reprinted from: Healthcare 2021, 9, 1420, doi:10.3390/healthcare9111420 141

Eswara Uma, Pentti Nieminen, Shani Ann Mani, Jacob John, Emilia Haapanen, Marja-Liisa Laitala, Olli-Pekka Lappalainen, Eby Varghase, Ankita Arora and Kanwardeep Kaur
Social Media Usage among Dental Undergraduate Students—A Comparative Study
Reprinted from: Healthcare 2021, 9, 1408, doi:10.3390/healthcare9111408 153

Luyao Liu, Suzanne Caliph, Claire Simpson, Ruohern Zoe Khoo, Geenath Neviles, Sithira Muthumuni and Kayley M. Lyons
Pharmacy Student Challenges and Strategies towards Initial COVID-19 Curriculum Changes
Reprinted from: Healthcare 2021, 9, 1322, doi:10.3390/healthcare9101322 171

Dennis M. Hedderich, Matthias Keicher, Benedikt Wiestler, Martin J. Gruber, Hendrik Burwinkel, Florian Hinterwimmer, Tobias Czempiel, Judith E. Spiro, Daniel Pinto dos Santos, Dominik Heim, Claus Zimmer, Daniel Rückert, Jan S. Kirschke and Nassir Navab
AI for Doctors—A Course to Educate Medical Professionals in Artificial Intelligence for Medical Imaging
Reprinted from: Healthcare 2021, 9, 1278, doi:10.3390/healthcare9101278 183

Muhammad Azeem Ashraf, Muhammad Naeem Khan, Sohail Raza Chohan, Maqbool Khan, Wajid Rafique, Muhammad Fahad Farid and Asad Ullah Khan
Social Media Improves Students' Academic Performance: Exploring the Role of Social Media Adoption in the Open Learning Environment among International Medical Students in China
Reprinted from: Healthcare 2021, 9, 1272, doi:10.3390/healthcare9101272 193

Magdalena Roszak, Bartosz Sawik, Jacek Stańdo and Ewa Baum
E-Learning as a Factor Optimizing the Amount of Work Time Devoted to Preparing an Exam for Medical Program Students during the COVID-19 Epidemic Situation
Reprinted from: Healthcare 2021, 9, 1147, doi:10.3390/healthcare9091147 211

Rosita Rupa, Mirza Pojskic, Christopher Nimsky and Benjamin Voellger
Lessons Learned from Developing Digital Teaching Modules for Medical Student Education in Neurosurgery during the COVID-19 Pandemic
Reprinted from: Healthcare 2021, 9, 1141, doi:10.3390/healthcare9091141 229

Ann-Mari Fagerdahl, Eva Torbjörnsson and Anders Sondén
An Interprofessional E-Learning Resource to Prepare Students for Clinical Practice in the Operating Room—A Mixed Method Study from the Students' Perspective
Reprinted from: Healthcare 2021, 9, 1028, doi:10.3390/healthcare9081028 237

Lucija Gosak, Nino Fijačko, Carolina Chabrera, Esther Cabrera and Gregor Štiglic
Perception of the Online Learning Environment of Nursing Students in Slovenia: Validation of the DREEM Questionnaire
Reprinted from: *Healthcare* **2021**, *9*, 998, doi:10.3390/healthcare9080998 249

Lana A. Shaiba, Mahdi A. Alnamnakani, Mohamad-Hani Temsah, Nurah Alamro, Fahad Alsohime, Abdulkarim Alrabiaah, Shahad N. Alanazi, Khalid Alhasan, Adi Alherbish, Khalid F. Mobaireek, Fahad A. Bashiri and Yazed AlRuthia
Medical Faculty's and Students' Perceptions toward Pediatric Electronic OSCE during the COVID-19 Pandemic in Saudi Arabia
Reprinted from: *Healthcare* **2021**, *9*, 950, doi:10.3390/healthcare9080950 265

Juan Francisco Ortega-Morán, Blas Pagador, Juan Maestre-Antequera, Javier Sánchez-Fernández, Antonio Arco, Francisco Monteiro and Francisco M. Sánchez-Margallo
Lapnurse—A Blended Learning Course for Nursing Education in Minimally Invasive Surgery: Design and Experts' Preliminary Validation of Its Online Theoretical Module
Reprinted from: *Healthcare* **2021**, *9*, 951, doi:10.3390/healthcare9080951 279

Po-Yu Chen, Ying-Xiu Dai, Ya-Chuan Hsu and Tzeng-Ji Chen
Analysis of the Content and Comprehensiveness of Dermatology Residency Training Websites in Taiwan
Reprinted from: *Healthcare* **2021**, *9*, 773, doi:10.3390/healthcare9060773 293

Jitendra Singh and Barbara Matthees
Facilitating Interprofessional Education in an Online Environment during the COVID-19 Pandemic: A Mixed Method Study
Reprinted from: *Healthcare* **2021**, *9*, 567, doi:10.3390/healthcare9050567 303

Jung Hee Park, Woo Sok Han, Jinkyung Kim and Hyunjung Lee
Experiences of Pathology Course among Hospital Management Graduates
Reprinted from: *Healthcare* **2021**, *9*, 347, doi:10.3390/healthcare9030347 313

Jaeho Cho, Gi-Won Seo, Jeong Seok Lee, Hyung Ki Cho, Eun Myeong Kang, Jahyung Kim, Dong-Il Chun, Young Yi and Sung Hun Won
The Usefulness of the QR Code in Orthotic Applications after Orthopedic Surgery
Reprinted from: *Healthcare* **2021**, *9*, 298, doi:10.3390/healthcare9030298 327

Jingfang Liu, Xin Zhang, Jun Kong and Liangyu Wu
The Impact of Teammates' Online Reputations on Physicians' Online Appointment Numbers: A Social Interdependency Perspective
Reprinted from: *Healthcare* **2020**, *8*, 509, doi:10.3390/healthcare8040509 335

Yu-Ting Hsiao, Hsuan-Yin Liu and Chih-Cheng Hsiao
Development of a Novel Interactive Multimedia E-Learning Model to Enhance Clinical Competency Training and Quality of Care among Medical Students
Reprinted from: *Healthcare* **2020**, *8*, 500, doi:10.3390/healthcare8040500 351

Fang-Suey Lin and Hong-Chun Shi
To Develop Health Education Tools for Nasogastric Tube Home Caring Through Participatory Action Research
Reprinted from: *Healthcare* **2020**, *8*, 261, doi:10.3390/healthcare8030261 365

Fang-Suey Lin, Hong-Chun Shi and Kwo-Ting Fang
Exploring Pictorial Health Education Tools for Long-Term Home Care: A Qualitative Perspective
Reprinted from: *Healthcare* **2020**, *8*, 205, doi:10.3390/healthcare8030205 385

Avinash Koka, Mélanie Suppan, Emmanuel Carrera, Paula Fraga-Freijeiro, Kiril Massuk,
Marie-Eve Imbeault, Nathalie Missilier Perruzzo, Sophia Achab, Alexander Salerno,
Davide Strambo, Patrik Michel, Loric Stuby and Laurent Suppan
Knowledge Retention of the NIH Stroke Scale among Stroke Unit Health Care Workers Using Video vs. E-Learning: Protocol for a Web-Based, Randomized Controlled Trial
Reprinted from: *Healthcare* **2021**, *9*, 1460, doi:10.3390/healthcare9111460 403

About the Editors

Luís Proença

Luís Proença (Prof. Dr.) obtained is PhD in 1998, from the University of Lisboa. Since then, he has served as Associate Professor at Instituto Universitário Egas Moniz (IUEM), teaching at graduate and postgraduate level in statistics, mathematics, physics and chemistry. He is currently also President of the Pedagogical Council of IUEM. To date, he is co-author of more than 75 articles published in peer-reviewed indexed journals (Web of Science/Scopus). His current research focuses on information and statistical data analysis as applied in biomedical, clinical and field multidisciplinary studies. He is also interested in numeracy, digital transformation and the use of pedagogical innovative approaches in Healthcare Higher Education.

José João Mendes

José João Mendes (Prof. Dr.) has served as President of the Egas Moniz – Cooperativa de Ensino Superior, CRL, since 2017 and was elected President of the Centro de Investigação Interdisciplinar Egas Moniz research center. Regarding his education and research background, he has completed a DDS at Egas Moniz University in Portugal in 1995, postgraduate studies in Implantology at the Universität Bern (Swtzerland. 1997), an MBA in Health Unit Management from Universidade Católica Portuguesa (2002) and a PhD in Biomedical Sciences from ICBAS School of Medicine and Biomedicine Sciences (2010). He is Section Editor of the European Journal of Dentistry and Associate Editor of Frontiers in Oral Medicine. To date, he has authored more than 80 articles and served as supervisor/co-supervisor of 52 master's and 10 PhD students. Furthermore, he was designated Assistant Professor of Conservative Dentistry (in the MSc in Dentistry of the ISCSEM/IUEM) in 1996, Assistant Professor of Physiology (MSc in Dentistry of the ISCSEM/IUEM) in 1999, and Head of the Integrated Dental Clinic Curricular Unit (MSc in Dentistry of the ISCSEM/IUEM) in 2008. Since 2010, he has held the position of Clinical Director of the Egas Moniz Dental Clinic.

João Botelho

João Botelho (Prof. Dr.) completed his DDS in 2015 at Egas Moniz University in Portugal. Dr. Botelho obtained his PhD degree in Biomedical Sciences from the University of Porto, ICBAS School of Medicine and Biomedicine Sciences. He was a visiting researcher in the laboratory of Prof. Jacques Nör at Michigan University, USA. Since 2017, Dr Botelho has been a consultant for Research and Education at Egas Moniz – Cooperativa de Ensino Superior, CRL. Since 2021, Dr. Botelho has been Associate Editor of BMC Systematic Reviews and PLOS Global Public Health and Review Editor for Frontiers in Dental Medicine. Since 2021, he has served as a Collaborator Member of Global Burden of Disease. Professor Botelho's research focuses mainly on the mechanisms of the association between oral health and systemic health, particularly periodontal diseases, inflammatory processes and the burden to systemic health from oral sources.

Vanessa Machado

Vanessa Machado (Prof. Dr.) completed her DDS in 2015 at Egas Moniz University in Portugal. Dr. Machado obtained her PhD degree in Biomedical Sciences from the University of Porto, ICBAS School of Medicine and Biomedicine Sciences. Since 2017, Dr Machado has been a consultant for Research and Education at Egas Moniz – Cooperativa de Ensino Superior, CRL. Since 2021, Dr. Machado has served as Associate Editor of BMC Oral Health and Frontiers in Dental Medicine. Since 2021, she has served as a Collaborator Member of Global Burden of Disease. Her research focuses mainly on the mechanisms of the association between periodontal conditions and female infertility, inflammatory processes and the burden to systemic health from oral sources.

Preface to "E-learning and Digital Training in Healthcare Education: Current Trends and New Challenges"

This book is dedicated to the current trends and new challenges that have emerged from the new e-learning environment, focusing on its potential to revolutionize Healthcare Education and exploring how it may help to better prepare future healthcare professionals for their daily practice. "E-learning and Digital Training in Healthcare Education: Current Trends and New Challenges" contains several research articles focused on new insights into the use of interactive and intuitive e-learning tools and innovative teaching methodologies that engage healthcare students in the new web-based environment training. It also includes several case studies of 'pathfinder' e-learning initiatives and surveys related to the penetration and acceptance of digital training in Healthcare Education.

Luís Proença, José João Mendes, João Botelho, and Vanessa Machado
Editors

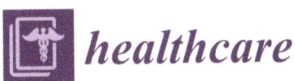

Article

Analysis of User Satisfaction with Online Education Platforms in China during the COVID-19 Pandemic

Tinggui Chen [1,*], Lijuan Peng [1], Xiaohua Yin [1], Jingtao Rong [1], Jianjun Yang [2] and Guodong Cong [3]

1. School of Statistics and Mathematics, Zhejiang Gongshang University, Hangzhou 310018, China; Cherrylijuanpeng@163.com (L.P.); yinxh0213@163.com (X.Y.); rjt323@126.com (J.R.)
2. Department of Computer Science and Information Systems, University of North Georgia, Oakwood, GA 30566, USA; Jianjun.Yang@ung.edu
3. School of Tourism and Urban-Rural Planning, Zhejiang Gongshang University, Hangzhou 310018, China; cgd@mail.zjgsu.edu.cn
* Correspondence: ctgsimon@mail.zjgsu.edu.cn

Received: 9 June 2020; Accepted: 2 July 2020; Published: 7 July 2020

Abstract: The outbreak of Corona Virus Disease 2019 (COVID-19) in various countries at the end of last year has transferred traditional face-to-face teaching to online education platforms, which directly affects the quality of education. Taking user satisfaction on online education platforms in China as the research object, this paper uses a questionnaire survey and web crawler to collect experience data of online and offline users, constructs a customer satisfaction index system by analyzing emotion and the existing literature for quantitative analysis, and builds aback propagation (BP) neural network model to forecast user satisfaction. The conclusion shows that users' personal factors have no direct influence on user satisfaction, while platform availability has the greatest influence on user satisfaction. Finally, suggestions on improving the online education platform are given to escalate the level of online education during the COVID-19 pandemic, so as to promote the reform of information-based education.

Keywords: public health emergencies; online education platform; user satisfaction prediction; emotion mining

1. Introduction

The global spread of COVID-19 resulted in the suspension of classes for more than 850 million students worldwide, disrupting the original teaching plans of schools in these countries and regions. Soon later, many countries started to offer online teaching to students by Zoom, Skype, FaceTime, etc. in order to promote online education and restore the normal teaching order, and on 6 February 2020, the Ministry of Education of the People's Republic of China announced to vigorously support information-based education and teaching, and enhance the platform's service capacity to support online teaching. In response to the outbreak of the epidemic, the online classroom has become a necessary way to maintain normal teaching order. Ding Ding, Fanya, and other office meeting software tools in China deliver services such as an online classroom and online teaching. However, these online education platforms have problems such as system jams and the inability to replay live broadcasts. It is necessary to study whether these network education platforms can meet the needs of teachers and students, whether the network teaching can complete the teaching tasks with high quality, whether the network education can become an effective means of special period education, and put forward suggestions to promote the development of network education according to the research results.

At present, scholars in various counties have carried out studies on online education platform evaluation, including using an analytic hierarchy process (AHP) and the partial least square method to establish the satisfaction evaluation system of online education platforms. For example, Wilbur [1] conducted a structured self-assessment and peer review using an instrument systematically devised according to Moore's principles of transactional distance to evaluate the online component of a blended-learning degree program for pharmacists, and he found that a number of course elements for modification could enhance the structure, dialog, and autonomy of the student learning experience. Ryan et al. [2] reported the results of a pre-post-test questionnaire designed to evaluate the impact of the professional development intervention, and the analysis showed high scoring means with many items in the questionnaire statistically significant ($p < 0.05$, CI = 95%). Chiao et al. [3] constructed a virtual reality tour-guiding platform and 391 students from a technological university in Taiwan participated in the study. The results indicated their learning effectiveness and technology acceptance within the education system. However, these traditional methods have some shortcomings in the evaluation process, such as complex calculation and unreasonable weight determination. In addition, the main forms of online education in the past were watching public classes of famous universities and tutorial videos of institutions. However, during the epidemic period, online education is mainly in the form of class-based teaching by teachers of their own school, which is an extension of the original offline education. Previous studies on the satisfaction of online education platforms did not take the new factors brought by the epidemic into account, such as ease of use and quality of interaction.

Based on this, combined with the background of public health emergencies, this paper evaluates the online education platform in China from the perspective of students. First of all, the emotional analysis of online user comments was conducted to find out the factors affecting the satisfaction of online education platforms. Then, the satisfaction evaluation system was established on its basis. The index coefficient was determined by using the structural equation, and the back propagation (BP) neural network model was further used to predict the satisfaction of online education platforms.

The structure of this paper is organized as follows: Section 2 is a literature review. Section 3 collects and processes users' online and offline data. Section 4 conducts emotional analysis of online comments. Section 5 carries out an empirical analysis of user satisfaction. Section 6 is the summary of the paper and the prospect of future work.

2. Literature Review

2.1. Online Education Platform

Many experts and scholars including Anderson [4] and Sultan [5] etc. from various counties have conducted research on online education with the vigorous development of the online education industry. Some typical studies are as follows: Chan et al. [6] described a novel technique combining Internet- and cloud-based methods to digitally augment the classic study group used by final-year residents studying for the Royal College of Physicians and Surgeons of Canada examination. Gofine and Clark [7] piloted the integration of Slack into their research team of one faculty member, one research coordinator, and approximately 20 research assistants. Statistics describing the app's usage were calculated twelve months after its implementation and their results indicating heavy usage by both research professionals and assistants were presented. Thor et al. [8] investigated the impact of the online format on the discussion quality and the survey results showed that students preferred using Voice Thread for presenting, learning from other presentations, and discussing presentation content by performing this process in the classroom. Botelho et al. [9] assessed the usefulness, ease of use, ease of learning and satisfaction of a cloud-based clinical progression practice record when compared to a traditional paper practice record. The results suggested that a digital clinical book, using free cloud-based collaboration tools, was more useful, easier to use and learn from and more satisfactory than a traditional paper recording system. Chapman et al. [10] proposed four important dimensions of coverage, participation, quality and student achievement, and constructed a massive open online course (MOOC) quality assessment framework, helping MOOC organizations make a series of measures for monitoring and improving. Hrastinski [11] put forward a theory in his research: if we wanted to enhance online learning, we needed to enhance online learner participation. Miri and Gizell [12] showed in their research the need for rethinking the way conventional online ethics courses are developed and delivered; encouraging students to build confidence in learning from distance, engaging them in online active and interactive experiences. Anderson et al. [13] pointed out that healthcare professionals could share their expertise through online education and incorporate this teaching into their annual learning. Kamali and Kianmehr [14] pointed out that the public's interest in online education was growing, while educational institutions' interest in online education was going down. They held the view that in order to change the negative effect of online education, it was necessary to provide students with a suitable network environment, and discussed online education from the perspective of students. Alcorn et al. [15] evaluated satisfaction of online education from the number of class participants, the participation rate of homework, the completion rate and the improvement of grades. Asarbakhsh and Sars [16] believed that the broken-down system, failed video connection or unusable use affected user satisfaction. From the perspective of users and designs, David and Glore [17] pointed out visual content was quite important to improve participation and interaction of users. Based on the technology acceptance model and taking 172 online learning users as the objects, Roca et al. [18] analyzed online learning satisfaction. The results showed that the user's online learning satisfaction was mainly determined by the user's perception of the usefulness and quality of the course, the quality of the platform and the website service and the degree of expected achievement. Lin and Wang [19] believed that students' satisfaction would be influenced by the difference of technology, the characteristics of teachers, students and courses. Panchenko [20] held the view that the MOOC teaching mode could develop teachers' careers, improve teaching skills, and enable teachers to consider and examine their teaching activities from more perspectives. Kravvaris and Kermanidis [21] testified that social networks contributed to MOOC development. The literatures [22,23] found that learners' autonomy played an important role in learning through the empirical study of MOOC. Through exploratory factor analysis (EFA) and confirmatory factor analysis (CFA), Parra-González and Segura-Robles [24] concluded that "game" was regarded as a motivating factor in the educational process, which could promote students to participate in the learning process more actively.

According to the above research results, many scholars study online education and establish many evaluation models. However, in the process of carrying out online education during this epidemic, many new problems arise in the new form of online education. This requires that new factors affecting user satisfaction be taken into account in the study. Based on this, this paper collects online user comment data to obtain the new factors affecting user satisfaction and establishes an evaluation system that can better reflect the satisfaction of online education platforms during the epidemic.

2.2. Customer Satisfaction

Customer satisfaction is the state of pleasure or disappointment formed by the comparison of the perceived effect of a product or service with the expected value. Previous scholars and experts have conducted many studies on customer satisfaction and established models, which can be divided into macro- and micro-models. Macro model: since the 1990s, many countries have carried out a national customer satisfaction index measurement work, regarding customer satisfaction index as a macroeconomic indicator to measure the customer satisfaction degree of a product or service. For instance, in 1989, Fornell [25] put forward the customer satisfaction index (CSI) by considering customer expectation, post-purchase perception and purchase value. Under the guidance of professor Fornell, based on the annual customer survey data of more than 100 enterprises over 32 industries, a Swedish Customer Satisfaction Barometer (SCSB) was constructed by using the Fornell model and calculation method. Under the guidance of Anderson and Fornell [26], America published the American Customer Satisfaction Index (ACSI) on the basis of the SCSB. The ACSI added perceived quality to measure the reliability of a product or service, as well as customer satisfaction. In 1992, Germany constructed the Deutche Kundenbarometer (DK) model, which consisted of 31 industries [27]. The European Union constructed the European Customer Satisfaction Index (ECSI) by adopting a comparative advantage over a wide variety of countries. This model omitted customer complaints but added company image, dividing perceived quality into perceived hardware quality and perceived software quality [28]. Micro model: the measurement model of customer satisfaction in micro fields is abundant. For instance, Tversky [29] put forward a variation model in 1969. Oliver [30] established a general model for measuring subjective inconsistencies in 1980. Sasser et al [31] proposed customer model with service level. Parasuram et al. [32] created the SERVQUAL scale to evaluate service quality. They divided the factors that determine service quality into five categories: reliability, responsiveness, assurance, empathy and tangibility.

From the above research outcomes, many scholars and institutions of various counties study the satisfaction evaluation system and establish many models. However, previous studies did not consider the impact of public health emergencies. On the basis of full reference to previous studies, this paper, in the context of the COVID-19 pandemic, optimizes the indicators used in previous studies and establishes a satisfaction evaluation model by considering the impact of public health emergencies.

3. Data Collection and Processing

In this paper, data are obtained through a questionnaire survey and web crawler. The online data obtained by web crawler technology are trustable and objective without restriction. Therefore, this paper uses the data obtained by web crawler to make a macro analysis of the user experience on the current online network teaching platform, and finally summarizes the main factors affecting the user experience satisfaction. Although the traditional questionnaire has many limitations, the obtained data are more targeted, diverse and abundant, which can test the ranking of impact factors summarized by the crawler data. Therefore, this paper combines the two methods to comprehensively acquire online and offline experience data of users.

3.1. Collecting Comments on Online Teaching Platforms

3.1.1. Platform Selection

At present, there are a large number of online teaching platforms in China, such as MOOC, and Tencent Class. We are unable to assess all platforms. Thus, it is necessary to select representative platforms to evaluate. In this study, data samples of online education platforms were selected on ASO100 (a big data service platform for analyzing the App Store, Qimai, Beijing, China), and the ranking of the education category (updated on 17 April 2020) was screened based on the download volume, comments and popularity of the platform as the representative measurement criteria of the platform. The platform ranking results are presented in Table 1.

Table 1. Rank of teaching platform.

Teaching Platform	Platform List	Classification Ranking	Keyword Coverage	Total Scores
Ding Ding	1	1(General list)	18.799	1,730,000
Tencent Meeting	2	2(General list)	8526	382,000
Tencent Class	1	1(Education)	10.276	167,000
Chaoxing Learning	7	7(Education)	2043	437,000
Chinese MOOC	13	13(Education)	7031	818,000

As illustrated in Table 1, in this study, Ding Ding (Alibaba, Hangzhou, China), Tencent Meeting (Tencent, Shenzhen, China), Tencent Class (Tencent, Shenzhen, China), Chaoxing Learning (Chaoxing, Beijing, China) and MOOC (Chaoxing, Beijing, China) were selected as the representative platforms for online teaching. These platforms have both synchronous and asynchronous learning capabilities, with no difference in system quality.

3.1.2. Collecting Comment Data

In China, schools began to implement online teaching on 17 February 2020; therefore, this study collected comments on those teaching platforms from 17 February 2020 to 17 March 2020.

3.2. Questionnaire Data Collection and Processing

3.2.1. Questionnaire Design

From the comments on ASO100, it is difficult to determine all the factors that affect an online teaching platform. To obtain a more targeted evaluation of user experience, this study adopted a questionnaire survey, whose targets were primary school, middle school, high school, university, and postgraduate students. By sorting and analyzing relevant literature, we designed the questionnaire with three parts, as demonstrated in Table 2.

Table 2. Questionnaire.

Classification of Investigation	Content of Investigation
User's behavior on network teaching platform	Usage intention, device, learning effect, learning content
User experience	Degree of satisfaction, interactivity, platform availability, perceived value and so on
Basic information	Age, gender, education background

In the second part, user experience satisfaction questions used a Likert scale. The scoring system was 1–5, where 5 represented strong agreement and 1 represented strong disagreement. The higher the score was, the more strongly the respondents agreed with the statement.

3.2.2. Questionnaire Validity Test

During the epidemic period, the questionnaire tool named Wenjuanxing was used to collect information. After investigation, a total of 800 questionnaires were received, with 712 remaining after the removal of invalid questionnaires. After data collection, 712 questionnaires were coded and entered into SPSS statistical software (SPSS Statistics 25.0 HF001 IF007, IBM, Armonk, NY, USA) to perform descriptive analysis, and reliability and validity analysis.

Reliability Test

The reliability test, which measures data reliability, is used to test the stability and consistency of questionnaire data. In this study, Cronbach's α was used to test the internal consistency of the questionnaire data, whose coefficient was between 0 and 1. In general, a coefficient greater than 0.7 indicates that the questionnaire can passes the internal consistency test. In contrast, a coefficient less than 0.7 indicates that some questions must be discarded. The reliability test results are presented in Table 3. In this questionnaire, six Cronbach's α coefficients were all greater than 0.7, indicating that the internal reliability of each first-level indicator of the questionnaire was high.

Table 3. Questionnaire data reliability information.

Index	Cronbach's α Coefficient	Number of Questions
Degree of satisfaction	0.712	3
Intention of continuous use	0.771	2
Quality of interaction	0.781	3
Quality of service	0.751	4
Platform availability	0.786	4
Personal factors of users	0.727	5

Validity Test

Validity Test

The validity test can be divided into content validity and structure validity. The questions in this questionnaire scale used relevant literature for reference to ensure high content validity. The structure validity passed the KMO (Kaiser–Meyer–Olkin) test and the Bartlett test. Generally, when KMO is greater than 0.5, and the significance level of the Bartlett test meets the significance requirement of a two-tailed test, it is considered that the questionnaire passes the validity test. The results of the validity test are presented in Table 4. It can be seen that the test values of the KMO and Bartlett test of the six first-level indicators in the questionnaire all met the requirements, indicating that they passed the validity test.

Table 4. Data validity test.

Index	KMO	Bartlett Test of Sphericity
Degree of satisfaction	0.599	0.000
Intention of continuous use	0.500	0.000
Quality of interaction	0.500	0.000
Quality of service	0.500	0.000
Platform availability	0.765	0.000
Personal factors of users	0.500	0.000

3.2.3. Data Analysis

Referring to Bawa's method of data analysis which includes descriptive statistics, analysis of variance (ANOVA) and T-tests [33], this paper analyzes the questionnaire data as follows: In this questionnaire survey, 26.6% of respondents were male while 73.4% of respondents were female. The majority of the participants were middle and high school students, junior college students, undergraduate students, and graduate students. Primary school students may produce invalid questionnaires due to their difficulties in text comprehension. According to the survey on the terminal types of online teaching platforms used by participants, mobile phones accounted for 84.62%, followed by laptop computers and tablet computers. The key questions in the questionnaire were analyzed to understand the data characteristics, as illustrated in Figure 1.

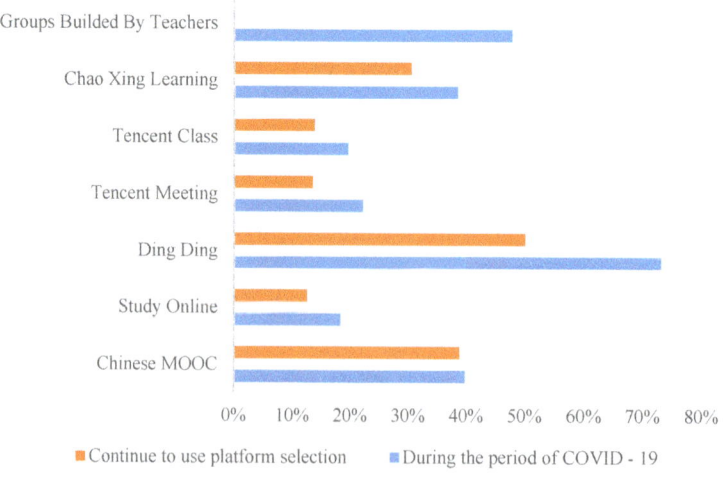

Figure 1. Choice of online teaching platform.

As can be seen from Figure 1, during the epidemic period, teachers mainly taught online using Ding Ding and self-established social groups (such as QQ group and WeChat group). As work management software, Ding Ding added on online teaching function in a timely manner in view of the epidemic. The results demonstrate that more than 50% of users continued using Ding Ding as an online learning platform after the epidemic ended.

As can be seen from Figure 2, most of the online teaching platforms can provide five learning modes and eight online interactive modes, which can effectively meet the existing teaching needs and provide feedback at any time. The two main teaching methods are online live broadcasting and existing courses on the platform. The MOOC platform contains rich teaching resources and has thus been favored and used as an online education platform for a long time.

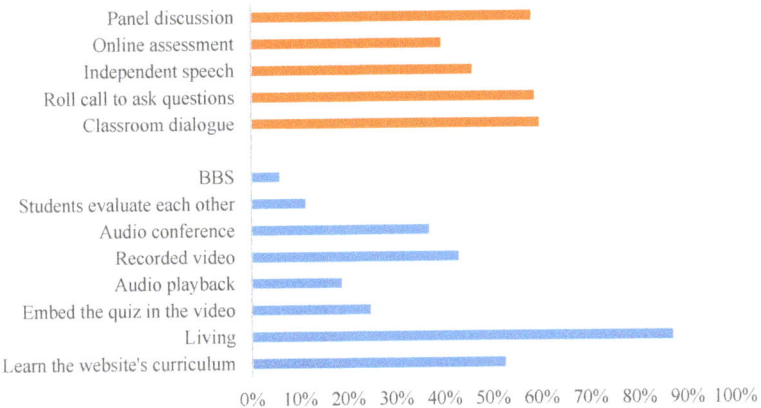

Figure 2. Online teaching and interaction.

As can be seen from Figure 3, there are 11 types of common problems regarding online teaching and courses that can be attributed to the problems mentioned in online comments, such as "network congestion", "live interactive stuck" and "unable to log in personal information". Therefore, to improve these issues, the five online teaching platforms can begin by addressing their live broadcast functions, system quality, and capacity enhancement.

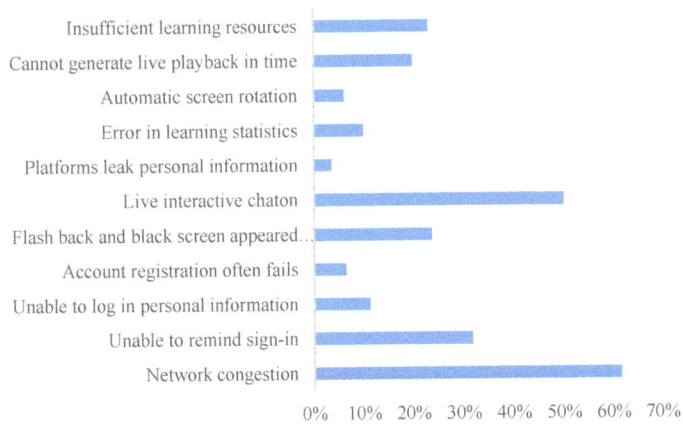

Figure 3. The use of online teaching platform.

4. User Emotion Analysis

The relationship between tutoring work and student emotions is of great significance to the cognitive re-evaluation of students. All comments were divided into different topics through data processing, and the key content in the comments was observed. In this study, the ROST (Regional Operations Support Team) [34] software was used to divide the emotional tendencies into three critical sets: positive, neutral and negative. Because the emotion dictionary of ROST is limited, the NLPIR-Parser(Natural Language Processing and Information Retrieval) [35] was used to score the emotion, which can be divided into the total score, positive score and negative score, to identify the platforms with better user experience. Using word frequency analysis, the advantages and disadvantages of platforms were extracted based on good or poor user experience.

4.1. Emotional Comment Analysis Based on ROST CM5.8.0

4.1.1. Comments Analysis

It was shown that those students who carried out activities related to their emotions and the improvement of coexistence in tutoring had a greater cognitive reevaluation. Therefore, this paper makes an emotional analysis of user comments [36]. Based on the analysis results of ROST, this study integrated the positive, neutral and negative comments of the five platforms, as illustrated in Table 5.

Table 5. ROST CM (Regional Operations Support Team Content Mining) Emotional comments analysis.

Teaching Platform	Ding Ding	Tencent Meeting	Tencent Class	Chaoxing Learning	Chinese MOOC
Positive comments	6161	1703	1623	1289	471
Neutral comments	1915	43	558	28	30
Negative comments	3809	2531	1185	3628	2051

Analysis of the positive, neutral, and negative comments indicated that Ding Ding and Tencent Class had more positive comments than negative comments, while Tencent Meetings, Chaoxing Learning, and Chinese MOOC demonstrated the opposite trend. In particular, Chaoxing Learning, and Chinese MOOC had more negative comments than positive comments.

4.1.2. Analysis of Visualization for Semantic Network

A semantic network expresses the structure of human knowledge through the network. It is composed of nodes and arcs among the nodes. Nodes stand for concepts (e.g., events, things), while arcs represent the relationship between them. Mathematically, a semantic network is a directed graph, corresponding to a logical representation. In this study, the semantic network relationship diagrams of the five platforms were obtained through ROST analysis. A partial image of the MOOC semantic network relationship is presented in Figure 4.

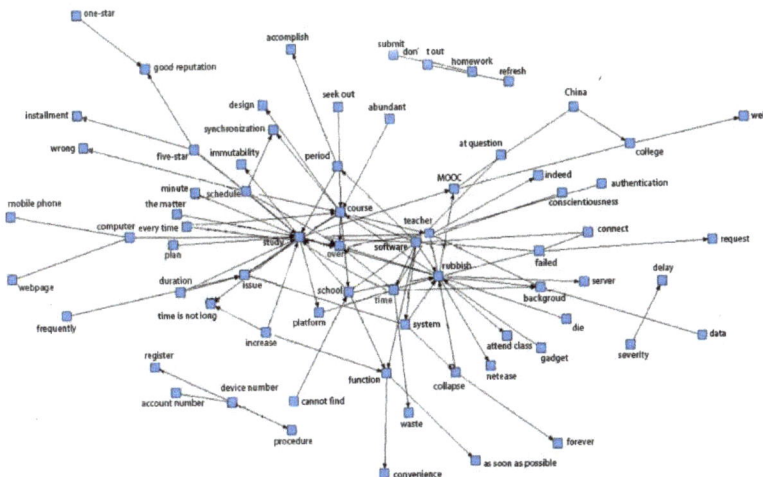

Figure 4. MOOC semantic network relationship.

(1) According to the semantic network relationship graph of Ding Ding, we use "study" as a node, and keywords that are close to this node are "epidemic" and "convenience". This is because during the epidemic, Ding Ding expanded the educational function on its platform, enabling colleges to use it as an online teaching platform. Taking "software" as a node, a closer keyword is "live broad cast", which also reflects that the teaching method of Ding Ding is mainly a live broadcast rather than students watching videos on their own. This method also increases the interactivity of online teaching, better mobilizes the learning atmosphere, and improves the quality of teaching. At the same time, due to the network congestion and negative user experience, most users gave a one-star rating to Ding Ding. This was explained by a Ding Ding official in time, leading to the popularity of the topic of "five-star payment by installment" on Weibo. It was due to the timely response that more users gave a five-star rating.

(2) According to the semantic network relationship graph of Tencent Meeting, we see that "five-star" and "meeting" are important nodes for Tencent Meeting evaluation. Taking "five-star" as a node, close keywords are "good reputation" and "epidemic", indicating that during the epidemic, users felt positively about the platform. Taking "meeting" as a node, the keywords are "convenience" and "screen", indicating that the Tencent Meeting platform was more convenient to use, and the quality and manner of screen presentation will affect the user experience.

(3) According to the semantic network relationship graph of Tencent Class, "teacher", "software" and "class" were important nodes, and close keywords were "epidemic", "attend class" and "many problems", indicating that users valued the attendance function of Tencent Class, however, there are also several problems.

(4) According to the semantic network relationship graph of Chaoxing Learning, "software", "rubbish", "study", and "course" were important nodes, and closer keywords were "submit", "server", "login", "collapse" which reflected the many problems that occurred in the Chaoxing Learning, such as server crashes, inability to log in, and inability to submit the learning duration, which all had a negative impact on the user experience.

(5) According to the semantic network relationship graph of MOOC, "learning", "rubbish", "course", and "software" were important nodes, and close keywords were "failed", "connect", "period", "server", and "progress". From these nodes, we can see that the MOOC platform often failed to connect, the learning time could not be submitted, and the server crashed. The independent nodes "account" and "homework" indicate that the platform was unable to register an account,

could not submit a job, and could not refresh. "Delay" and "severity" indicate that the delay in the MOOC platform was quite significant. "College" and "abundant" reflect that MOOC users were mainly college students, and the course types were abundant due to the characteristics of the MOOC platform. MOOC focuses on video teaching and conducts self-study courses, which are the primary reasons for its use.

Based on the analysis of the semantic network relationship graph obtained above, it can be seen that "epidemic", "student", "software", "teacher", "study", "five-star" and "every time" were important nodes that appeared together in the five platforms. The closer the nodes are to the words, the closer their relationship is. The presence of "every time" and "five-star" was caused by the timely response to problems in Ding Ding, thus indicating the large influence of the official Ding Ding group.

4.2. Emotion Analysis Based on NLPIR-Parser

NLPIR emotion analysis mainly uses two technologies. The first is the automatic recognition of emotion words and the automatic calculation of weights. The co-occurrence relationship and bootstrapping strategy is adopted to repeatedly produce new emotion words and weights. The second technology is a deep neural network for emotion discrimination. Based on a deep neural network, the extended calculation of emotion words is performed, which is integrated into the final result.

By analyzing the comment data of the online teaching platforms, the emotion scores of the five teaching platform reviews were obtained, including the total emotion score, positive score, and negative score, as displayed in Table 6.

Table 6. NLPIR-Parser emotional scores

Teaching Platform	Ding Ding	Tencent Meeting	Tencent Class	Chaoxing Learning	Chinese MOOC
Total emotional score	10,454.5	870	933.5	−2190.5	−642
Positive score	56.319	7374	10,898.5	9022	1148
Negative score	45,864.5	−6504	−9965	−11,212.5	−1790

From the above emotion scores, it can be seen that the total emotion scores of Ding Ding, Tencent Meeting, and Tencent Class were all positive, while the total emotion scores of Chaoxing Learning and MOOC were negative, indicating that Ding Ding, Tencent Meeting and Tencent Class provided good user experience. In addition, the shortcomings of Chaoxing Learning and MOOC were more evident, as these platforms were not satisfactory for users. Because the negative score of Chaoxing Learning was much lower than the positive score, it is important to analyze the problems in the Chaoxing Learning platform to propose corresponding improvement measures.

4.3. Semantic Association Expansion

NLPIR adopts POS-CBOW (Problem Oriented System, Continuous Bag of Words), integrating the distribution characteristics of speech and words, using the word2vectormodel to train educational corpora, and automatically extracting semantic association relations.

This paper expands the relevant semantics of high-frequency words on Ding Ding, Tencent Meeting, Tencent Class, Chaoxing Learning and MOOC. In addition, it captures new words and keywords with higher weight, and summarizes the factors that affect user experience. The part of the semantic graph related to Ding Ding is presented in Figure 5.

According to the relevant semantic expansion of the five platforms, the following words and phrases had the highest weight and the most frequent occurrence: "flash back", "convenient and swift", "customer service", "projection screen", "peep screen", "horizontal screen", "pop-up windows", "staff service", "prevention and control", "interactive panel", "dark mode", "abnormal network", "mobile office", "Ding mail", "call the camera", "bundled software", "shared screen", "client end", "verification code", "vertical screen" and "network anomaly", "recording", "web version", "screen recording", "no privacy", "blocking sight", "rotating the screen", "black screen", "background playback", "failed to load", "scan code", "system halted", "submit a job", "close microphone", "network fluctuations", "gesture check-in", "personal information", "submit homework", "main interface experience", "incompatibility", "lost connection", "self-rotating screen" and "mobile end".

NewWord	Part-Of-Speech	Weight	Frequency	KeyWord	Part-Of-Speech	Weight	Frequency
what	n_new	467.47	1968	teacher	n	497.77	3009
online classes	n_new	374.05	631	what	n_new	467.47	1968
online course	n_new	325.53	806	students	n	418.12	2447
bad review	n_new	325.05	859	learning	v	410.84	3263
the five-star high praise	n_new	323.43	1321	online classes	n_new	374.05	631
thanks DingDing	n_new	286.36	562	no	v	363.4	1755
video conference	n_new	125.3	136	software	n	361.18	6121
Submit a job	n_new	109.29	105	Ding	v	343.04	23,700
developers	n_new	107.18	154	can	v	338.44	2104
ghost livestock	n_new	100.55	143	one	aq	330.74	2359
flash back	n_new	94.27	109	online course	n_new	325.53	806
teasing	n_new	70.83	67	bad review	n_new	325.05	859
payment by installment	n_new	67.96	225	the five-star high	n_new	323.43	1321
customer service	n_new	67.55	60	have a class	vi	302.3	1753
frigging awesome	n_new	66.84	81	thanks DingDing	n_new	286.36	562
assign homework	n_new	62.18	63	homework	n	269.23	1563
uninstall	n_new	60.03	63	five-star	b	266.67	3500
social animals	n_new	58.71	53	living	v	265.28	1187
bear children	n_new	57.49	62	function	n	264.91	1350
ask for forgiveness video	n_new	53.33	95	now	t	247.96	804
special period	n_new	52.93	99	work	vn	209.04	779
anti-addiction system	n_new	52.62	41	video	n	203	1017
lump sum	n_new	49.41	67	hope	v	199.25	1072
DouYin	n_new	48.18	49	school	n	198.46	795

Figure 5. Comparison between new word and key word.

By classifying the new words and phrases mentioned above, we summarize the influencing factors that affect user experience, namely platform suitability, platform service type, platform privacy, platform teaching type, platform functionality, platform design environment, and network technology environment. By summarizing the factors influencing user experience for online teaching platforms during the epidemic, we determine the following Table 7.

Table 7. Influencing factors.

Factor	Description
Platform Suitability	"computer", "web", "tablet", "mobile terminal", "incompatibility"
Platform privacy	"peep screen", "prevention", "call the camera", "personal information"
Platform service type	"online customer service", "staff service"
Platform teaching type	"recorded broadcast", "live streaming"
Platform design environment	"blocking sight", "simple", "convenient and swift", "dark mode", "sharing the screen", "main interface experience", "interactive panel"
Platform functionality	"projection screen", "horizontal screen", "verification code", "close microphone", "vertical screen", "rotating screen", "scan a code", "submit homework", "self-rotating screen"
Network technology environment	"pop-up windows", "network anomaly", "bundled software", "server exception", "blank screen", "load fail", "system halted", "network fluctuation", "lost connection"

By classifying the new words mentioned above, we summarize the influencing factors that affect user experience, namely, platform suitability, platform service type, platform privacy, platform teaching type, platform functionality, platform design environment, and network technology environment. By summarizing the factors influencing user experience for online teaching platforms during the epidemic, we can determine the following:

(1) The design environment of the platform should be more concise and easy to operate, and additional modes should be designed for different users at different times. For example, a "dark mode" at night can have better protective effect on the eyesight of students.

(2) At present, the types of electronic devices continue to rise. To expand the use of the platform, it is necessary to increase the development of each port of the tablet. In addition, to make students more comfortable during an online class, the platform should be able to adjust the horizontal and vertical screen any time.

(3) To improve the utilization and popularity of online teaching education platforms, customer services are essential. In the use of the platform, online customer service should always be available to address problems to prevent the wasting of learning time.

(4) During the epidemic, not only college students and graduate students, but also primary and secondary school students, must study online. However, the concentration abilities of the latter groups are relatively limited, therefore, teachers cannot blindly teach by rote and lecturing, but must use a variety of different methods, such as "you ask me to answer", "face to face", "students record learning videos", and "real-time lecture". The platform should enhance the type of functions and improve the quality of interactive devices while setting software functions.

(5) A stable network technology environment is the most important basis for improving teaching quality. If "network congestion" or "flash back" often occur in the use of the platform, the user experience as well as the usage rate will decrease accordingly.

5. Empirical Research on User Satisfaction

5.1. Building a User Experience Satisfaction Index System

Based on the factors influencing user experience obtained by emotion, the advantages and disadvantages of online education noted by the users in the questionnaire (as illustrated in Figures 1–3), and a large number of documents, this study aims to establish an effective but non-redundant index system. It combines Webqual 4.0 (availability, information quality, interaction quality) and the D&M (DeLone and McLean) system success model (information quality, system quality, service quality) to refine the influencing indicators. The indicators at each level correspond to the questions in the questionnaire. Among them, information quality and system quality are expressed together with subjective multiple choice questions, while others are expressed on Likert scales, as illustrated in Table 8.

Table 8. Evaluation indicators affecting user satisfaction

The Primary Variable	The Secondary Variables	Indicators
User's willingness to continue using	Recommend to others	Loy1—During the COVID-19 pandemic, target the online education platform you are satisfied with, you would like to recommend it to others
	Increase the frequency of use	Loy2—During the COVID-19 pandemic, the online teaching platform you are using will be used more in the future
User satisfaction	Learning needs	Sat2—During the COVID-19 pandemic, you think the existing functions of the online teaching platform can meet your learning needs
	Use feeling	Sat3—During the COVID-19 pandemic, you are very satisfied with the online teaching platform
	Attractive	Sat1—Compared with offline learning, you think online teaching during the COVID-19 pandemic is more attractive
Platform availability	Learnability	Pq2—During the COVID-19 pandemic, the steps of the online teaching platform you are using are easy to learn
	Easy to browse	Pq3—During the COVID-19 pandemic, the navigation system of online network teaching platform you use is clear, without confusion, and the page is easy to browse
	Interface design	Pq1—During the COVID-19 pandemic, the interface design of the online network teaching platform you are using is very reasonable
	Learning record	Pq4—During the COVID-19 pandemic, the online teaching platform you use can accurately record your learning time, learning content and learning information

Table 8. Cont.

The Primary Variable	The Secondary Variables	Indicators
The quality of interaction	Learner participation	Int1—During the COVID-19 pandemic, while learning online, you will actively answer the teacher's questions and participate in the classroom learning
	Practice feedback	Int2—During the COVID-19 pandemic, you will complete the online study assignment assigned by the teacher on time
Information quality	Accuracy	A1—During the COVID-19 pandemic, which of the following difficulties and problems have you encountered while studying online?
	Integrity	A2—During the COVID-19 pandemic, according to your common online teaching platform, what are the main ways to learn online?
	Timeliness	A3—During the COVID-19 pandemic, in the course of online teaching, what online interactions did you mainly participate in?
	Completeness	
System quality	High concurrent access	A5—During the COVID-19 pandemic, which terminal can the online teaching platform you are using support for online learning?
	Security	
	Stability	
	Responsiveness	
The quality of service	Course management	Cq2—During the COVID-19 pandemic, the online teaching platform you use can recommend relevant courses according to what you watch
	Artificial service	Cq1—During the COVID-19 pandemic, when the online teaching platform fails, the customer service will help you to solve the problem in time
User personal factors	Education level	Per1—What kind of student are you?
	Use frequency	Per2—How often did you use an online teaching platform before COVID-19?
	Satisfaction tendency	Per3—When you use the online teaching platform for the first time, you will hold a completely negative attitude towards the platform because of some dissatisfaction with the use of the platform (such as registration trouble, slow login, etc.)
	Platform choice	A6—What platforms will you use as learning aids during and after the COVID-19 pandemic?

5.2. Structural Equation Model

Structural equation modeling (SEM) is a common method to solve complex multivariable problems in social sciences. For example, in research fields such as social science, it is sometimes necessary to explore the relationship between more than one dependent variable and the influence path between hidden variables that cannot be directly measured. SEM can estimate abstract hidden variables through observable variables [37].

According to the above user satisfaction indicators, this paper uses the structural equation model to build the indicator system model and obtains the influence path coefficient of the latent variables on user satisfaction to draw the conclusion that the effects on user experience satisfaction weights are different. By using path analysis for the structural equation to determine the correlation between the indicators, and by decreasing the number of indicators to avoid redundant indicator construction, suggestions for improving the main influencing factors are proposed.

The IS (information systems) success model proposed by DeLone and McLean [38] measured user satisfaction on a website in terms of the service quality. McKnight and Chervany [39] constructed the factors influencing customer belief and supplier intention from the perspective of psychology and sociology, and each structure was further decomposed into two to four measures. Lao et al. [40] used text mining technology to establish a curriculum quality evaluation model that included five first-level indicators: curriculum content, instructional design, interface design, media technology, and curriculum management to provide a base standard for learners to evaluate the quality of the curriculum. Huang et al. [41] constructed an overall evaluation index system based on online education using four primary indices: system structure, educational resources, interactive mode, and market environment.

Based on the above analysis, this paper examines the factors influencing user satisfaction with the continuous usage of the intention of online teaching platforms by examining the four aspects of interaction quality, service quality, availability, and personal factors, and proposes the following hypotheses:

Hypothesis 1. *The interactive quality of the online teaching platform has a significantly positive influence on user satisfaction.*

Hypothesis 2. *The service quality of the online teaching platform has a significantly positive influence on user satisfaction.*

Hypothesis 3. *The availability of the online teaching platform has a significantly positive influence on user satisfaction.*

Hypothesis 4. *The personal factor of the online teaching platform has a significantly negative influence on user satisfaction.*

Hypothesis 5. *The user satisfaction with the online teaching platform has a significantly positive influence on the user's willingness to continue using the platform.*

5.2.1. Model Estimation and Significance Test of Parameters

A structural equation model can effectively deal with the relationship of latent variables in the theoretical model of user satisfaction of an online network teaching platform. In this study, AMOS (Analysis of Moment Structures, IBM, Armonk, NY, USA) software was used to empirically study the structural equation model. On the premise that the reliability and validity analysis of the sample data met the requirements, parameter estimation of the model was performed based on the influencing factors of user satisfaction established previously. The estimated results of the model are presented in Figure 6.

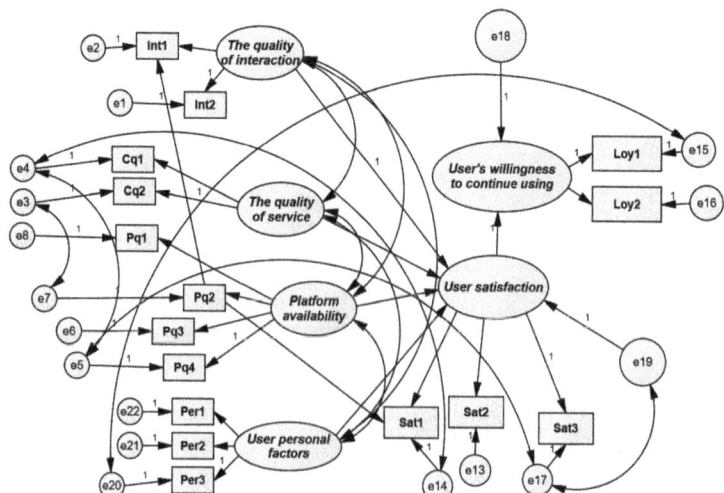

Figure 6. Parameter estimation of the model.

The parameter analysis results of the initial model are listed in Table 9. After estimating the initial model, the significance test of the path coefficient and load coefficient was required. The "C.R." (critical ratio) value was obtained by the disparity between the estimated parameter and standard parameter. When the absolute value of "C.R." was greater than 1.96 and the corresponding probability p value was less than 0.05, it can be stated that there was a significant difference between the path coefficient and the estimated parameter value of 0 at 95% confidence. Therefore, it is assumed that the influence of the path coefficient was significant. It can be seen that the path coefficient of "user personal factors" on user satisfaction was unable to pass the significance test.

Table 9. Parameter analysis results.

Influence Elements	Path Coefficient	Influence Elements	Estimate	S.E.	C.R.	p
User satisfaction	<—	The quality of interaction	1.000		1.989	***
User satisfaction	<—	The quality of service	0.389	0.187	2.078	***
User satisfaction	<—	Platform availability	−0.236	0.224	2.032	***
User satisfaction	<—	User personal factors	0.760	0.382	0.417	0.047
User's willingness to continue using	<—	User satisfaction	1.000			
The quality of interaction	<->	The quality of service	0.273	0.049	5.557	***
The quality of service	<->	Platform availability	0.262	0.042	6.225	***
The quality of interaction	<->	Platform availability	0.217	0.035	6.276	***
Platform availability	<->	User personal factors	0.002	0.016	0.102	0.918
The quality of service	<->	User personal factors	−0.083	0.033	−2.528	0.011
The quality of interaction	<->	User personal factors	−0.066	0.025	−2.639	0.008

Note that *** reflects the significance level when $p < 0.001$. C.R is the abbreviation of critical ratio. S.E is the abbreviation of Standard Error. <-> reflects the influencing factors are correlated. <— reflects a causal relationship between the influencing factors.

5.2.2. Modified Structural Equation Model

After the structural equation model was completed, it was used to test the fitness degree of the sample data and perform model path analysis by calculating the fitness effect parameters. In AMOS, there are three evaluation indices for the fitness degree of a model: the absolute fitness index, value-added fitness index, and simple fitness index. Common fitness indices include χ^2 (degree of freedom ratio) and GFI (goodness-of-fit index), AGFI (adjusted goodness-of-fit index), NFI (Normed fit index), RMSEA (Root Mean Square Error of Approximation), and CFI (comparative fit index). In this study, several common fitness indices were selected from the three fitness indices, and the calculation results are presented in Table 10.

Table 10. Fitness degree of model.

Indicators		Judgment Standard	Revised Model Results
Absolute fitness index	χ^2	the smaller the better	127.452
	χ^2/df	1–3	2.360
	GFI	>0.9 better fit >0.8 can accept	0.938
	RMR	<0.08	0.054
	RMSEA	<0.08	0.066
Value-added fitness index	NFI	>0.9 better fit >0.8 can accept	0.914
	TLI	>0.9	0.925
	CFI	>0.9	0.948
Simple fitness index	PCFI	>0.5	0.633
	PNFI	>0.5	0.656

Note that χ^2/df is the abbreviation of degree of freedom ratio; GFI: goodness-of-fit index; RMR: Root Mean Residual; RMSEA: Root Mean Square Error of Approximation, NFI: Normed fit index; TLI: Nonstandard fitting index; CFI: comparative fit index; PCFI: Simple adjustment comparison fit index; PNFI: parsimonious normed fit index.

It can be seen that after deleting the path of "user personal factors," all fitness indices were improved after the model was modified. According to the calculation results of all fitness indices, all reached the fitness standard of the model. The modified model is presented in Figure 7.

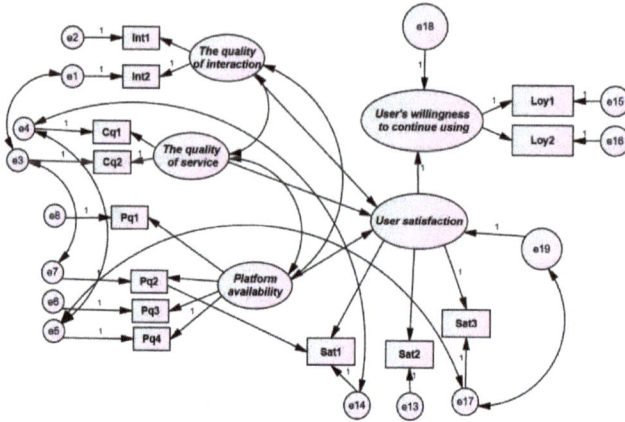

Figure 7. Modified results.

5.2.3. Results Analysis

By modifying and testing the structural equation model and studying the sequence proposed by the research hypothesis, the path coefficients of the influencing factors are summarized in Table 11.

Table 11. Path coefficients of the affecting factors.

Influence Elements	Path Coefficient	Influence Elements	Affect the Path
User satisfaction	<—	The quality of interaction	0.238
User satisfaction	<—	The quality of service	0.329
User satisfaction	<—	Platform availability	0.703
Pq2	<—	Platform availability	0.41
User's willingness to continue using	<—	User satisfaction	1.000
Int2	<—	The quality of interaction	0.35
Int1	<—	The quality of interaction	0.10
Cq2	<—	The quality of service	0.5
Cq1	<—	The quality of service	0.4
Pq4	<—	Platform availability	0.34
Pq3	<—	Platform availability	0.33
Pq1	<—	Platform availability	0.63
Sat3	<—	User satisfaction	0.13
Sat2	<—	User satisfaction	0.64
Sat1	<—	User satisfaction	0.55
Loy1	<—	User's willingness to continue using	0.55
Loy2	<—	User's willingness to continue using	0.78
The quality of interaction	<->	The quality of service	0.273
The quality of service	<->	Platform availability	0.262
The quality of interaction	<->	Platform availability	0.217

Note that <-> reflects the influencing factors are correlated. <— reflects a causal relationship between the influencing factors.

From the above analysis, we draw the conclusion that among the four major factors, personal factors had no direct influence on user satisfaction, indicating that users had a fair attitude and were not emotionally biased. Instead, platform availability had the largest influence on user satisfaction. In terms of availability, the function design and reasonable operation of the online teaching platform were the most important problems for users. In terms of interaction quality, the feedback for the homework assigned by teachers was the main factor affecting the sense of interaction experience. The influence of service quality on user satisfaction was mainly caused by matters such as timely response to problems, diverse course types, and learning extension. Users mainly hoped that the platform could meet their learning needs and provide necessary functions for learning; however, they did not have high expectations for the interface design of the platform. The correlation between the overall interaction quality, service quality, and availability was not high, indicating that the influence on user satisfaction was not high and that the construction of the structural equation was reasonable.

5.3. Predicted Satisfaction Model Based on the BP Neural Network

According to the above structural equation model results, the influence index of user satisfaction mainly involved platform availability, interaction quality, and service quality; personal factors had no direct effect on satisfaction. Therefore, this paper only regards the first three key indicators as input nodes and the degree of satisfaction as the output node by using the BP neural network model to forecast the degree of satisfaction.

5.3.1. Overview of the BP Neural Network Algorithm

A BP neural network [42], a type of artificial neural network, is a multi-layer network with one-way propagation, which is widely used in many fields such as public opinion [43–45], personalized recommendations [46], health monitoring [47], social network [48], feature subset selection [49,50] and emergency logistics [51,52]. A typical neural network consists of three layers: an input layer, hidden layer, and output layer. Each layer is composed of multiple neurons that are connected to each other by the weight coefficient; however, each neuron in the same layer is independent. The structure of a BP neural network is presented in Figure 8.

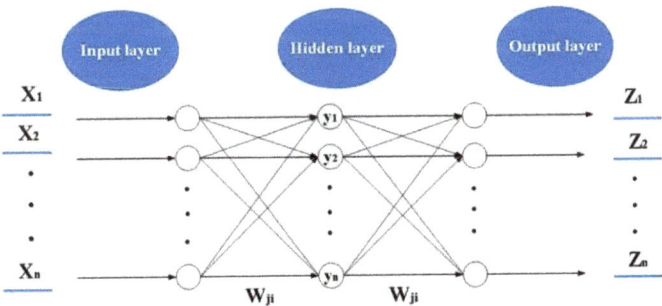

Figure 8. BP neural network structure.

In the Figure 8, $X_1, X_2 \cdots X_n$ is the input layer neuron, $y_1, y_2 \cdots y_n$ is the activation function, W_{ji} is the weight connecting the input layer, hidden layer and output layer, $W_1, W_2 \cdots W_n$ is the output layer neuron. The working principle of a BP neural network includes forward-propagation and back-propagation processes. Forward-propagation mainly refers to the input of training samples from the input layer, and the result of the output layer can be obtained through the connection of the weight coefficient between neurons and the activation function. If the prediction results of the output layer are not satisfactory, the back-propagation process is activated. The error signals of each unit are returned layer by layer along the original neuron connection pathway, and the weight coefficients of the neurons between layers are adjusted by calculating the error value. This training is repeated several times according to the training function until the network output error reaches a predetermined accuracy or the training times reach the set maximum iteration times. The algorithm steps are as follows:

Step 1: Data normalization;
Step 2: Data classification, extraction of normal training data, and data testing;
Step 3: Establishment of the neural network, including setting the number of nodes in each layer, activation function, etc.;
Step 4: Specifying parameters for training;
Step 5: Using training results, inputting test data after completing the training;
Step 6: Data anti-normalization;
Step 7: Error analysis, drawing, etc.

5.3.2. Data Processing of the Predicted Model

Because each key index of the input layer corresponds to two or three questions in the questionnaire, each index actually corresponds to two or three data points. To obtain the index data of the input layer, the average value of the actual measured data in the questionnaire is used as the actual score data of this index in this paper. The actual scoring principle is as follows:

$$X = \frac{\sum_{i=1}^{n} s_i}{n} \tag{1}$$

where n represents the number of questions corresponding to the key indicator and s_i represents the score of the ith question corresponding to the key indicator. With this formula, the data of each node in the input layer of the BP neural network can be obtained.

In addition, the satisfaction results obtained from the questionnaire survey are hierarchical data, while the data in the BP neural network are normalized. As the result, the satisfaction data predicted by the output layer may not be classified. Therefore, this study used the existing literature [53] to classify the satisfaction level. The specific division is shown in Table 12.

Table 12. Division of satisfaction level.

Satisfaction Level	Descriptive	Divide the Scale
1	Very dissatisfied	$x \leq 1.5$
2	Dissatisfied	$1.5 \leq x \leq 2.5$
3	General	$2.5 \leq x \leq 3.5$
4	Satisfied	$3.5 \leq x \leq 4.5$
5	Very satisfied	$x \geq 4.5$

5.3.3. Implementation and Evaluation of Model

In this study, after several simulation experiments to compare the prediction effects, tansig was selected as the spread function of the input layer and hidden layer, purelin was selected as the spread function of the output layer, traingdx (self-adjusting learning efficiency method) was selected as the training function of the BP neural network (whose number of nodes in the hidden layer was set to six), and the maximum number of iterations epochs was 20,000.

The key indicator data were divided into a training group and test group, and the predicted results were obtained through training the set parameters, as illustrated in Figure 9.

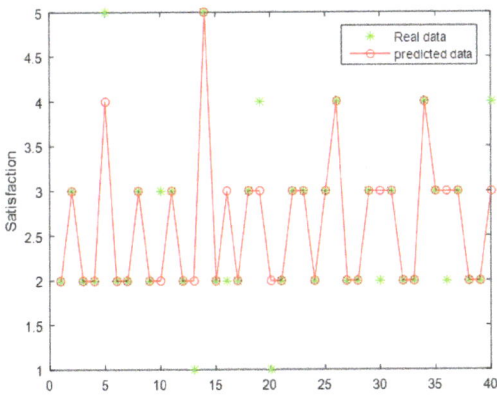

Figure 9. Predicted results.

As seen from Figure 9, the satisfaction level is mainly distributed in level 2 and level 3, indicating that the majority of users were dissatisfied with the existing online teaching platforms. Therefore, user satisfaction must be improved, and this study can be of great practical significance. In addition, the prediction results were generally accurate, but the prediction accuracy was only 77.5%, and the prediction effect was moderate, which may be due to the lack of training data in this study. If the proposed system is widely used in online education platform satisfaction prediction, the sample size can be increased, and the prediction accuracy may increase.

In addition, error analysis was performed on the prediction results of the BP neural network, and the results are presented in Figure 10.

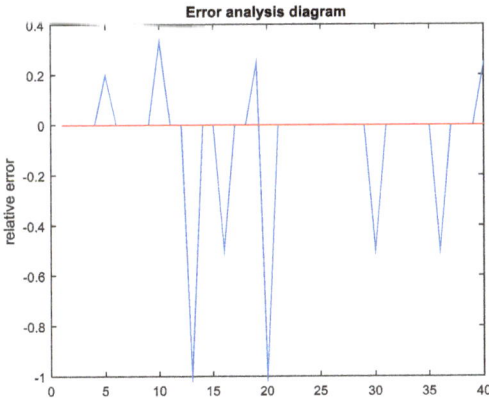

Figure 10. Error analysis diagram.

As can be seen from Figure 10, the MSE only fluctuated in the range (−0.5, 0.4) with a small error value, indicating that the satisfaction prediction model established in this paper is effective. Other error index data are provided in Table 13.

Table 13. Error indicator data.

Error Indicator	MSE	MAPE	RMSE	MSPE	SSE
Result	0.225	0.08	2.1213	0.55864	9

MAPE: Mean Absolute Percentage Error; RMSE: Root Mean Square Error; MSPE: Pure mean square error; SSE: The sum of squares due to error.

6. Discussion

In this section, we will discuss four issues. First of all, in order to summarize the outstanding contributions of this paper based on the previous literature, we compared the conclusions of relevant literatures and discuss the relationship between the existing literatures and this paper. Secondly, in order to highlight the unique factors that affect the user satisfaction of online education platforms during the COVID-19 pandemic, we discussed the differences between online education during the COVID-19 pandemic and general online education, which is also the outstanding contribution of this paper. Once more, in order to solve the problem of capital investment in platform availability, we discussed several financing methods from the perspective of online education platform enterprises, and put forward feasible financing suggestions. Finally, in order to show that the conclusion of this paper can be applied to other countries in the world, we discussed the internationalization of conclusions.

6.1. Relationship with the Existing Literature

It is a priority to discuss the connections with other research on the topic. Previous studies, such as literature [16] and literature [18], focused on the satisfaction of users' normal use of online education platforms when there was no public health disaster such as COVID-19. The influencing factors mainly include system fluency, visual content, curriculum usefulness, etc. The influencing factors considered in this paper are more combined with the problems in the online education teaching process during the COVID-19 pandemic, and the influencing factors such as platform availability, interaction quality, information quality, system quality, service quality and user personal factors are put forward. After structural equation analysis, it is found that platform availability is the most important factor, while user personal factors have little effect on satisfaction.

We will discuss it based on the relevant models mentioned in the above literatures. There are two basic antecedents of customer satisfaction in the SCSB model: expected quality and perceived value. User satisfaction is determined by the difference between perceived value and expected quality. Customer complaint and customer loyalty are outcome variables of customer satisfaction. The ACSI model is based on the SCSB model. The main innovation of the ACSI model is its ability to increase the quality of perception. The ECSI model inherits the basic structure and some core concepts of ACSI model, such as user expectation, perceived quality, perceived value, user satisfaction and user loyalty. Compared with the ACSI model, the ECSI model firstly removes the potential variable of user complaint in the ACSI model. Secondly, the ECSI model adds another potential variable, enterprise image, and divides the perceived quality into the quality evaluation of hardware and software.

The model used in this paper is constructed after referring to the above model, and combines emotional analysis and structural equation analysis. In the emotional analysis, we found that the factors that affect the satisfaction of online education platforms were platform availability, interaction quality, information quality, system quality, service quality and user personal factors. Combined with the relevant literatures, the platform availability, interaction quality, service quality and user personal factors are selected. Furthermore, after the structural equation analysis, the user's personal factors are eliminated. Thus, in the model of this paper, the platform availability, interaction quality and service quality are the three major factors that determine user satisfaction. User satisfaction then affects the user's willingness to continuously use the platform.

All in all, compared with the traditional SCSB, ACSI and ECSI models, the model constructed in this paper can better reflect the characteristics of an online education platform during the COVID-19 pandemic and, thus, it can better reflect the satisfaction of an online education platform.

6.2. Characteristics of Online Educationduring the COVID-19 Pandemic

In the past, teachers and students individualized and chose online education in a small range. At present, it has become a necessary choice for everyone. The seemingly helpless choice provides an opportunity for people to re-examine online education. Therefore, based on the COVID-19 situation, this paper studies the user satisfaction of online education platforms, which is different from the focus of user satisfaction under ordinary circumstances. When using an online education platform without COVID-19, more attention should be paid to the characteristics of the platform and the diversity of learning materials. According to the conclusion of this paper, the availability of the platform during the COVID-19 situation is the main factor affecting user satisfaction, which also reflects that users focus more on mobile terminal equipment, platform load, technology proficiency and other aspects. This study not only summarizes the weaknesses and constraints exposed by the online education platform during the COVID-19 pandemic, but also makes a significant contribution to the upgrading and optimization of online education, improving people's cognition of online education, and increasing the acceptance and satisfaction of online education.

Due to the significant social impact of COVID-19, learners will have emotional problems at different levels due to the influence of home isolation and other factors, thus affecting the effectiveness of online learning. Therefore, educators are more concerned about the emotional changes of students in this unique period and put the physical and mental health of students first. Therefore, this study conducts relevant emotional analysis on online user comments. Additionally, the emotional factors caused by external factors were added to the study of user satisfaction. This is also different from other studies.

In the past, the teachers who provided courses on the online education platform system were specially trained by enterprises and only taught for a certain type of course. However, this COVID-19 outbreak is sudden. Teachers who use the online education platform are transformed into ordinary offline teachers. The preparation time of ordinary teachers is not enough. In addition, a considerable number of teachers lack sufficient knowledge of information technology, so the concept of online teaching is relatively weak. In the face of sudden online teaching, problems emerge, such as how to arrange classes, how to carry out online teaching according to the plan, which online teaching platform to choose, and how to monitor the effect and quality of online teaching, which will lead to the decrease in user satisfaction. Therefore, in this study, the impact of COVID-19 on user satisfaction is not only in the context of COVID-19, but it is also concluded that the usability of the platform is the main factor affecting users' satisfaction with the online education platform in a unique period.

6.3. Education Financing Methods

Based on the research of online education satisfaction during the COVID-19 pandemic, we found that the platform availability is the most essential factor that affects the user satisfaction; therefore, we suggest that the enterprise that develops the online education platform puts more money into the technology research and development of platform availability in order to provide users with more satisfaction of online teaching services. To solve this problem, online education platform enterprises can consider several financing ways to raise funds. Online education platforms can be divided into two categories according to whether they charge fees or not. Therefore, this paper discusses the financing of online education platforms from two aspects. For online education platforms that charge tuition fees, there exist literatures that examine education financing problem. For example, Barr [54] set out the core lessons of financing higher education derived from economic theory and compares them with lessons of experiences of various countries. Jacobs and Wijnbergen [55] showed that public equity financing of education coupled with the provision of income insurance was the optimal way to finance education when private markets failed due to adverse selection. For online education platforms that do not charge fees, enterprises can consider the following ways of financing: (1) Enterprises can give priority to internal financing and rely on internal accumulation for financing, which includes three forms: capital, replacement investment converted by depreciation funds and new investment converted by retained earnings. Compared with external financing, internal financing can reduce information asymmetry and related incentive problems. (2) The enterprise may consider the way of introducing investment and seeking partner investment. During the COVID-19 pandemic, almost all college teaching activities have been transferred to online teaching. Enterprises can provide more detailed online teaching services to some well-known colleges to improve their online teaching quality. Hence, enterprises can find college partners to attract investment from colleges and universities. A practical example of this is as follows: Baidu Lecture Transfer reached a cooperation agreement with Georgia Institute of Technology, one of the three major American universities of science and Technology. Both sides will carry out in-depth cooperation in course introduction, technical research and joint exploration of an online education mode. (3) Enterprises can consider debt financing and obtain sufficient funds to research and develop technologies to improve the availability of online education platforms by issuing bonds or borrowing money for investments.

6.4. Internationalization of Conclusions

The analysis in this paper is based on the user data of Chinese online education platforms during the COVID-19 situation. In order to show that the conclusion of this paper is international, this part discusses whether the research results of this paper can be extended to other countries.

First of all, this paper finds that platform availability is the most important factor affecting the satisfaction of the online education platform, while the user personal factors have no significant impact on the satisfaction. In view of the similar online teaching methods adopted by countries all over the world, most of them adopt the forms of video conferences or live broadcasts. Therefore, the above conclusions can be extended to all countries in the world.

Secondly, this paper obtains the satisfaction evaluation system and satisfaction prediction model of an online education platform during the COVID-19 pandemic. Because this form of online education is still used in other countries, the evaluation system and prediction model obtained in this paper can be applied to the countries that have not yet recovered offline teaching. As long as relevant data are available, the BP neural network prediction model can be used.

7. Conclusions

This study collected user experience data on online education platforms in China during the COVID-19pandemic. Through emotion data analysis of online user reviews, we concluded that Ding Ding and Tencent Class provided high quality service, while Chaoxing Learning and MOOC encountered several problems, such as the inability to submit the learning time, lags, and a significant video delay. We extracted the factors influencing satisfaction and established a scientific and effective satisfaction index system using the existing literature. In addition, the data obtained from an offline questionnaire were examined and analyzed, and a structural equation model was built for quantitative analysis of the relationship between various indicators. It was found that users' personal factors had no direct impact on their satisfaction, while platform availability had the greatest impact on user satisfaction. In addition, a BP neural network model was used to predict user satisfaction with online education platforms, and the prediction accuracy reached 77.5%. The model is thus highly effective.

Based on the above analysis and research, this paper proposes the following suggestions, which are expected to improve user satisfaction with online education platforms during public health emergencies:

(1) Platform technology problems cannot be ignored. Although an online education platform provides available teaching methods, there are still many problems in the platform technology. The design environment of the platform should be more concise and easy to operate, and the development of a dark mode is recommended. In terms of platform adaptability, there is the

problem that mobile devices cannot switch between horizontal and vertical orientations. In terms of platform privacy, user authorization is required to control the user's camera and microphone. Currently, there is a lack of platform customer service, and it is thus impossible to obtain timely feedback for problems with the platform. In terms of the platform function, the head portrait cannot be modified, the video progress bar cannot be synchronized, and other problems must be improved. In terms of the network technology environment, some platforms frequently encounter problems such as internet lags and network congestion. Technical problems in these platforms are the main factors affecting user experience that lead to students' dissatisfaction and significantly reduce the efficiency and quality of teaching. Therefore, improving the platform technology is the primary problem to be solved. As for the above technical problems of the online education platform, the enterprises that belong to the platform should improve these problems, increase the investment in the online education platform and develop the function of the online system. Companies can obtain education financing through online crowd funding, initial coin offerings and other means, and use these financing methods to improve the quality and availability of online systems. As a result, these online education systems used in China can be extended to the world, increasing the use of the platform.

(2) The two-way interaction of teaching must be improved. Using a questionnaire of offline users, we analyzed eight first-level indicators selected by the structural equation, and determined that the main factors influencing user satisfaction with the online teaching platforms were system quality, interaction quality, service quality, and platform availability. Interaction environment refers to the effective communication environment in the process of knowledge acquisition. An increase in interaction can improve students' learning enthusiasm and concentration. In a traditional classroom, there are various teaching interaction modes, such as reversed classroom, random questions, and group reports. However, in a network environment, the platform has few settings for teaching interaction, and teachers' input teaching is the main teaching mode. Therefore, the platform must actively develop various interactive formats, such as "you ask me to answer", "face to face", "students record learning videos" and "real-time lecture" to promote efficient learning and further improve the quality of education.

8. Future Works

However, this paper still has the following limitations, which require further research:

(1) This paper only studies the satisfaction of online learning platforms from the perspective of students. In fact, the opinions of teachers and parents are also impactful. Therefore, future studies can comprehensively analyze the satisfaction of online education platforms from the perspective of multiple subjects.
(2) In this paper, the structural equation is used to predict the user satisfaction of the online learning platform, and the validity of the model is proved through analysis and verification. However, the questionnaire design and algorithm prediction need to be further improved.

Author Contributions: T.C. described the proposed framework and wrote the whole manuscript; L.P. implemented the simulation experiments; X.Y. and J.R. collected data; J.Y. and G.C. revised the manuscript; All authors have read and agreed to the published version of the manuscript.

Funding: This research is supported by the National Social Science Foundation of China (Grant No. 19ZDA122), Contemporary Business and Trade Research Center and Center for Collaborative Innovation Studies of Modern Business of Zhejiang Gongshang University of China (Grant No. 14SMXY05YB), Key project of Higher education research of Zhejiang Gongshang University in 2020 ("the construction path and influence promotion Mechanism of curriculum thought and politics driven by big data", Grant No. Xgz005) as well as Research and Innovation Fund for Postgraduates of Zhejiang Gongshang University of China in 2020 (Grant No. 19020040032).

Conflicts of Interest: The authors declare that they have no competing interests.

References

1. Wilbur, K. Evaluating the online platform of a blended-learning pharmacist continuing education degree program. *Med. Educ. Online* **2016**, *21*, 31832. [CrossRef] [PubMed]
2. Ryan, C.; Young, L.; McAllister, M. The impact of an online learning platform about nursing education on enrolled nurse preceptor teaching capabilities: A pre-post-test evaluation. *Contemp. Nurse* **2017**, *53*, 335–347. [CrossRef] [PubMed]
3. Chiao, H.M.; Chen, Y.L.; Huang, W.H. Examining the usability of an online virtual tour-guiding platform for cultural tourism education. *J. Hosp. Leis. Sport Tour. Educ.* **2018**, *32*, 29–38. [CrossRef]
4. Andersen, P. What is Web 2.0? Ideas, technologies and implications for education. *JISC Technol. Stand. Watch* **2007**, *1*, 1–64.
5. Sultan, N. Cloud computing for education: A new dawn? *Int. J. Inf. Manag.* **2010**, *30*, 109–116. [CrossRef]
6. Chan, T.; Sennik, S.; Zaki, A.; Trotter, B. Studying with the cloud: The use of online Web-based resources to augment a traditional study group format. *Can. J. Emerg. Med.* **2015**, *17*, 192–195. [CrossRef]
7. Gofine, M.; Clark, S. Integration of Slack, a cloud-based team collaboration application, into research coordination: A research letter. *J. Innov. Health Inf.* **2017**, *24*, 252. [CrossRef]
8. Thor, D.; Xiao, N.; Zheng, M.; Ma, R.; Yu, X.X. An interactive online approach to small-group student presentations and discussions. *Adv. Physiol. Educ.* **2017**, *41*, 498–504. [CrossRef]
9. Botelho, J.; Machado, V.; Proenca, L.; Rua, J.; Delgado, A.; Joao, M.J. Cloud-based collaboration and productivity tools to enhance self-perception and self-evaluation in senior dental students: A pilot study. *Eur. J. Dent. Educ.* **2019**, *23*, e53–e58. [CrossRef]
10. Chapman, S.A.; Goodman, S.; Jawitz, J. A strategy for monitoring and evaluating massive open online courses. *Eval. Programplan.* **2016**, *57*, 55–63. [CrossRef]
11. Hrastinski, S. A Theory of Online Learning as Online Participation. *Comput. Educ.* **2009**, *52*, 78–82. [CrossRef]
12. Miri, B.; Gizell, G. Novice Researchers' Views About Online Ethics Education and the Instructional Design Components that May Foster Ethical Practice. *Sci. Eng. Ethics* **2020**, *26*, 1403–1421.
13. Anderson, E.S.; Lennox, A.; Petersen, S.A. New opportunities for nurses in medical education: Facilitating valuable community learning experiences. *Nurse Educ. Pract.* **2004**, *4*, 135–142. [CrossRef]
14. Kamali, A.; Kianmehr, L. The Paradox of Online Education: Images, Perceptions, and Interests. *US China Educ. Rev.* **2015**, *15*, 591–601. [CrossRef]
15. Alcorn, B.; Christensen, G.; Emanuel, E.J. The Real Value of Online education. *Atlantic* **2014**, *317*, 58–59.
16. Asarbakhsh, M.; Sars, J. E-learning: The essential usability perspective. *Clin. Teach.* **2013**, *10*, 47–50. [CrossRef]
17. David, A.; Glore, P. The Impact of Design and Aesthetics on Usability, Credibility, and Learning in Online Courses. In Proceedings of the E-Learn 2010—World Conference on E-Learning in Corporate, Government, Healthcare, and Higher Education, Orlando, FL, USA, 18–22 August 2010; Association for the Advancement of Computing in Education: Orlando, FL, USA, 2010; p. 42.
18. Roca, J.C.; Chiu, C.M.; Marthnez, F.J. Understanding e-learning continuance intention: An extension of the Technology Acceptance Model. *Int. J. Hum. Comput. Stud.* **2013**, *64*, 683–696. [CrossRef]
19. Lin, W.S.; Wang, C.H. Antecedence to continued intentions of adopting e-learning system in blended learning instruction: A contingency framework based on models of information system success and task-technology fit. *Comput. Educ.* **2012**, *58*, 88–99. (in Chinese). [CrossRef]
20. Panchenko, L.F. Massive open online course as an alternative way of advanced training for higher educational establishment professors. *Educ. Pedagogical Sci.* **2013**, *156*, 1–17.
21. Kravvaris, D.; Kermanidis, K.L. How MOOCs Link with Social Media. *J. Knowl. Econ.* **2014**, *7*, 461–487. [CrossRef]
22. Mackness, J.; Mak, S.; Williams, R. The ideals and reality of participating in a MOOC. In Proceedings of the 7th International Conference on Networked Learning 2010, Aalborg, Denmark, 3–4 May 2020; University of Lancaster: Lancaster, UK; pp. 266–275.
23. Kop, R.; Carroll, F. Cloud Computing and Creativity: Learning on a Massive Open Online Course. *Eur. J. Open Distance E Learn.* **2011**, *14*, 111–131.
24. Parra-González, M.E.; Segura-Robles, A. Translation and evaluation criteria of bigamy experience (GAMEX). *Bordon J. Educ.* **2019**, *71*, 87–99.

25. Fornell, C. A national customer satisfaction barometer: The Swedish experience. *J. Mark.* **1992**, *56*, 6–21. [CrossRef]
26. Anderson, W.; Fornell, C. Foundations of the American Customer Satisfaction Index. *Total Qual. Manag.* **2000**, *11*, 869–882. [CrossRef]
27. Meyer, A. *Das Deutsche Kundenbarometer*; Ludwig-Maximilians-Universitat Munchen: Munich, Germany, 1994.
28. Eklof, J.A. *European Customer Satisfaction Index Pan-European Telecommunication Sector Report Based on the Pilot Studies 1999*; European Organization for Quality and European Foundation for Quality Management: Stockholm, Sweden, 2000; pp. 34–35.
29. Tversky, T. Intransitivity of Preferences. *Psychol. Rev.* **1969**, *76*, 31–48. [CrossRef]
30. Oliver, R.L. A cognitive model of the antecedents and consequences of satisfaction decisions. *J. Mark. Res.* **1980**, *17*, 460–469. [CrossRef]
31. Sasser, W.E.; Olsen, R.P.; Wyckoff, D.D. The Management of Service Operations. *Meas. Bus. Excell.* **2001**, *5*, 177–179. [CrossRef]
32. Parasuraman, A.; Berry, L.L.; Zeithaml, V.A. More on improving service quality measurement. *J. Retail.* **1993**, *69*, 140–147. [CrossRef]
33. Kuyini, A.B.; Yeboah, K.A.; Das, A.K.; Alhassan, A.M.; Mangope, B. Ghanaian teachers: Competencies perceived as important for inclusive education. *Int. J. Incl. Educ.* **2016**, *20*, 1–15. [CrossRef]
34. Liu, M.Q. *Presentation and Implementation of Geography Classroom Teaching Objectives—Based on Rost Software and Case Analysis*; Shanghai Normal University: Shanghai, China, 2019. (in Chinese)
35. Zhang, H.P.; Shang, J.Y. NLPIR-Parser: Big data semantic intelligent analysis platform. *Corpus Linguistics* **2019**, *1*, 87–104. (in Chinese).
36. Aguaded-Ramírez, E.M.; López, J.E.; Cuberos, R.C. Tutorial Action and Emotional Development of Students as Elements of Improved Development and Preventing Problems Related with Coexistence and Social Aspects. *Eur. J. Investig. Health Psychol. Educ.* **2020**, *10*, 615–627.
37. Evermann, J.; Tat, M. Assessing the predictive performance of structural equation model estimation. *J. Bus. Res.* **2016**, *69*, 4565–4582. [CrossRef]
38. Delone, W.H.; Mclean, E.R. The Delone and Mclean model of information systems success: A ten-year update. *J. Manag. Inf. Syst.* **2003**, *19*, 9–30.
39. McKnight, D.H.; Chervany, N.L. Conceptualizing trust: A typology and e-commerce customer relationships model. In Proceedings of the 34th Hawaii International Conference on System Sciences, Maui, HI, USA, 6 January 2010; pp. 23–31.
40. Lao, K.; Li, S.Z.; Li, Y.H. Research on MOOC evaluation model. *Fudan Educ. Forum* **2017**, *15*, 65–71. (In Chinese).
41. Huang, W.; Liu, X.; Shi, P. Research on the evaluation of online education model under the background of "Internet +". *J. Intell.* **2016**, *35*, 124–129. (In Chinese).
42. Moutinho, L.; Davies, F.; Curry, B. The impact of gender on car buyer satisfaction and loyalty: A neural network analysis. *J. Retail. Consum. Serv.* **1996**, *3*, 135–144. [CrossRef]
43. Chen, T.; Wang, Y.; Yang, J.; Cong, G. Modeling Public Opinion Reversal Process with the Considerations of External Intervention Information and Individual Internal Characteristics. *Healthcare* **2020**, *8*, 160. [CrossRef]
44. Chen, T.; Li, Q.; Fu, P.; Yang, J.; Xu, C.; Cong, G.; Li, G. Public Opinion Polarization by Individual Revenue from the Social Preference Theory. *Int. J. Environ. Res. Public Health* **2020**, *17*, 946. [CrossRef]
45. Chen, T.; Li, Q.; Yang, J. Modeling of the Public Opinion Polarization Process with the Considerations Individual Heterogeneity and Dynamic Conformity. *Mathematics* **2019**, *7*, 917. [CrossRef]
46. Xu, C. A novel recommendation method based on social network using matrix factorization technique. *Inf. Process. Manag.* **2018**, *54*, 463–474. [CrossRef]
47. Maria-Giovanna, M.; Albert, B.; Luís, R.F.; Amado-Mendes, P.; Paulo, L.B. An overview on structural health monitoring: From the current state-of-the-art to new bio-inspired sensing paradigms. *Int. J. Bio. Inspir. Comput.* **2019**, *14*, 1–26.
48. Chen, T.; Shi, J.; Yang, J.; Li, G. Enhancing network cluster synchronization capability based on artificial immune algorithm. *Hum. Centric Comput. Inf. Sci.* **2019**, *9*, 3. [CrossRef]
49. Israel, E.A.; Richard, M.C.; James, F.S.; Hongji, Y. Integration of Kestrel-based search algorithm with artificial neural network for feature subset selection. *Int. J. Bio. Inspir. Comput.* **2019**, *13*, 222–233.

50. Xue, J.; Jiang, Y.; Zhang, Y.; Hua, J.; Li, W.; Zhang, Z.; Wang, L.; Qian, P.; Muzic, R.F., Jr.; Sun, Z. Intelligent diagnosis of cardiac valve calcification in ESRD patients with peritoneal dialysis based on improved Takagi-Sugeno-Kang fuzzy system. *Int. J. Bio. Inspir. Comput.* **2019**, *13*, 277–286. [CrossRef]
51. Chen, T.; Wu, S.; Yang, J.; Cong, G.; Li, G. Modeling of Emergency Supply Scheduling Problem Based on Reliability and Its Solution Algorithm under Variable Road Network after Sudden-Onset Disasters. *Complexity* **2020**, *2020*, 7501891. [CrossRef]
52. Chen, T.; Wu, S.; Yang, J.; Cong, G. Risk Propagation Model and Its Simulation of Emergency Logistics Network Based on Material Reliability. *Int. J. Environ. Res. Public Health* **2019**, *16*, 4677. [CrossRef]
53. Zhu, C.W. *Research on User Satisfaction Evaluation of Taxi-Hailing Software Based on SEM*; Liaoning Technical University of Engineering: Fuxin, China, 2017. (in Chinese)
54. Barr, N. Higher Education Funding. *Oxford Rev. Econ. Policy* **2004**, *20*, 264–283. [CrossRef]
55. Jacobs, B.; van Wijnbergen, S.J.G. Capital-Market Failure, Adverse Selection, and Equity Financing of Higher Education. *Public Finance Anal.* **2007**, *63*, 1–32. [CrossRef]

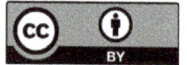

© 2020 by the authors. Licensee MDPI, Basel, Switzerland. This article is an open access article distributed under the terms and conditions of the Creative Commons Attribution (CC BY) license (http://creativecommons.org/licenses/by/4.0/).

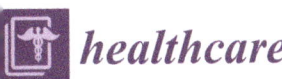

Article

Online Problem-Based Learning in Clinical Dental Education: Students' Self-Perception and Motivation

Mariana Morgado [1], José João Mendes [1,2] and Luís Proença [2,3,*]

1. Clinical Research Unit (CRU), Centro de Investigação Interdisciplinar Egas Moniz (CiiEM), Egas Moniz—Cooperativa de Ensino Superior CRL, Campus Universitário, Quinta da Granja, 2829-511 Caparica, Portugal; mmorgado@egasmoniz.edu.pt (M.M.); jmendes@egasmoniz.edu.pt (J.J.M.)
2. Evidence-Based Hub, CiiEM, Egas Moniz—Cooperativa de Ensino Superior CRL, Campus Universitário, Quinta da Granja, 2829-511 Caparica, Portugal
3. Quantitative Methods for Health Research (MQIS), CiiEM, Egas Moniz—Cooperativa de Ensino Superior CRL, 2829-511 Almada, Portugal
* Correspondence: lproenca@egasmoniz.edu.pt

Abstract: The physical closure of higher education institutions due to coronavirus disease 2019 (COVID-19) shed a brighter light on the need to analyze, explore, and implement strategies that allow the development of clinical skills in a distance learning situation. This cross-sectional study aims to assess dental students' self-perception, motivation, organization, acquired clinical skills, and knowledge using the online problem-based learning method, through the application of a 41-item questionnaire to 118 senior students. Answers were subjected to descriptive and inferential statistics analysis. Further, a principal component analysis was performed, in order to examine the factor structure of the questionnaire. Results show that online problem-based learning can be considered a relevant learning tool when utilized within the specific context of clinical dental education, displaying benefits over the traditional learning strategy. Overall, dental students prefer a hybrid system over the conventional one, in a distance learning context, and assume self-responsibility for their own learning, while knowledge thoroughness is perceived as inferior. This online active learning method is successful in improving information and clinical ability (visual/spatial and auditory) advancement in the scope of dental education, with similar results to presential settings. Further studies are required to assess clinical skill development through active learning methods, in a distance learning context.

Keywords: problem-based learning; dental education; e-learning; innovation in teaching; clinical teaching

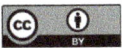

1. Introduction

Education is rooted in a social context, in particular its innovation. In the post-war era of the 1960s and 1970s, in line with the new values of cognitive psychology, passive learning and the reward concepts of behaviorism have been replaced by active, student-centered learning, with growing prominence given to individuality, equality, and personal development rather than authority and deductive learning. Problem-based learning (PBL) was part of this context of change [1,2].

Medical education has long been a stronghold of conventional methods. Nonetheless, in the aforementioned period, there were many changes in this specific field that led to the inevitable reform and innovation in the teaching of prospective medical practitioners, which included social critique, the rise and fall of clinical medicine, as well as the volume and changeability of medical knowledge [3,4].

Problem-based learning originated in 1966, at McMaster University, Canada [5], and groundbreaking work was later carried out at Newcastle University (Australia), Michigan State University (United States), and Maastricht University (The Netherlands) [6]. The first PBL-based medical curriculum was introduced in 1969 at McMaster University, while only in 1990 did the first PBL-based dental curriculum arise at the Faculty of Odontology in Malmö, Sweden [7].

While there are parallels between medical and dental education, there is a need to emphasize that the qualifications students need to learn are not exactly the same. Clinical skills in medical education, for example, are generally defined as clinical thinking and problem-solving, both of which are connected to doing and accurate physical assessment and performing a correct diagnosis [8]. While these clinical skills are also important for dental students to acquire, there is a need to further develop visual/spatial, auditory, and kinesthetic skills [9], which sums up to the point that dental education is quite different from medical education, mainly in the pre-clinical and clinical years [10].

Advances in technology have led to changes, not only inevitable but exponential [11], at all levels of education, but namely in higher education [12]. Emerging technologies, by allowing ubiquitous connections between individuals, content and digital/intelligent objects, in addition to enhancing learning [13], have created new teaching–learning dynamics, where students have different needs depending on the specific area of training, for example, the health area [14,15].

In the context of medical and medical–dental education, this paradigm shift has been explored through the implementation of active learning methods [16], such as self-guided study [17]; problem-based learning (PBL) [18]; mixed learning strategies, such as blended learning (BL) [19]; using asynchronous digital tools (e-Learning); and "inverted" or flipped classrooms [20], using didactic material previously available online, as well as simulation instruments [21] and gamification [22].

With the advent of the coronavirus disease 2019 (COVID-19) pandemic that we currently live in, and the physical closure of higher education institutions (HEIs), it is necessary to analyze, explore, and implement strategies that allow the development of clinical skills, even in face of a distance learning situation [23–25].

This study was aimed to assess dental students' self-perception on learning, motivation, organization, tool acquisition, clinical skills, and knowledge using the PBL method, through online/digital channels in a distance learning context, as well as the identification of limitations and difficulties in this context.

2. Materials and Methods

2.1. Course Description

The participants of this cross-sectional study, students of the Dentistry Integrated Master Course at Instituto Universitário Egas Moniz (IUEM), a higher education institution located in the southern Lisbon Metropolitan Area (Portugal), were enrolled during the fifth and final, year of their course. The study took place during the 2019/2020 term, from March to September 2020. In Portugal, by March 2020, a national lockdown was imposed due to the COVID-19 pandemic. As a result, from that date, higher education schools had to close and started teaching exclusively online, through digital platforms. This exclusively online teaching lasted for 10 weeks. Thus, the final year of the Dentistry Integrated Master Course at IUEM, during the 2019/2020 term, spanned over 33 weeks and was divided in three periods, according to the type of teaching that was implemented: six fully clinical (presential) weeks, 10 fully online synchronous weeks, and 17 hybrid (presential/online) weeks, as depicted in Figure 1.

During clinical practice weeks, students underwent six hours of live-patient encounters (LPE) *per* day at the University Dental Clinic. On online PBL weeks, students had six synchronous hours of real clinical case presentation and discussion *per* day. On mixed weeks, half of the students had clinical practice, while the other half had online lectures. Every week, the student groups switched, as indicated in the schedule (Figure 1).

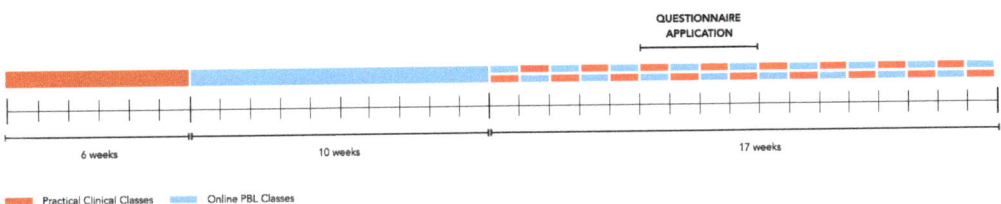

Figure 1. Dentistry Integrated Master Course final year schedule (33 weeks). Every space represents a week. Red boxes represent practical (presential) clinical classes. Blue boxes represent online problem-based learning (PBL) classes.

2.2. Study Design

The study was conducted through the application of an online questionnaire, via Google Forms. All of the 211 senior dental students of the Dentistry Integrated Master Course at IUEM were enrolled to participate, from which 118 (55.9%) answered the questionnaire. The exclusion criteria for participating in the study were as follows: refusal to provide informed consent and being enrolled in other university study programs. None of the students that answered the questionnaire were excluded.

A 41-item online questionnaire was constructed after a detailed literature review by using web-based search engines like PubMed and Google Scholar. The keywords "problem-based learning", "conventional lectures", "medical education", "dental education", "clinical education", and "student's perception" were used to search the literature. The final group of 41 close-ended questions were assembled from a 66-item database, collected from previously conducted surveys [26–31]. Exclusion criteria for the questions included lack of relevance to the scope of the study and duplicates, as shown in Figure 2. The content validity and clarity of the questionnaire was ensured by a review done by experts in medical education. Answers were coded following a five-point Likert rating scale (1 = "strongly disagree", 2 = "disagree", 3 = "neither agree nor agree", 4 = "agree", 5 = "strongly agree").

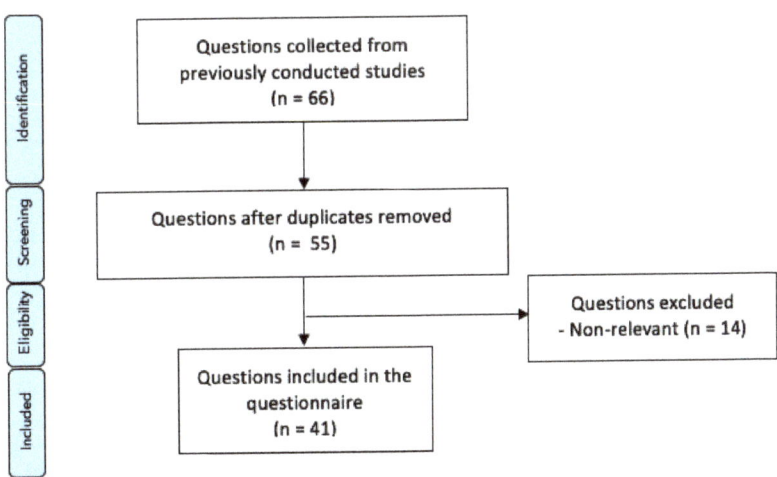

Figure 2. Preferred Reporting Items for Systematic Reviews and Meta-Analyses (PRISMA) flow chart. Presentation of the procedure of question selection with number of questions at each stage.

The description of the 41 items/questions included in the online questionnaire are presented in Table 1.

Table 1. Items included in the online questionnaire.

ID	Item
Q01	PBL is interesting.
Q02	PBL provides an interactive clinical learning environment.
Q03	PBL facilitates the use of learning resources for clinical learning.
Q04	PBL helps the achievement of curriculum outcomes.
Q05	PBL helps understand basic concepts.
Q06	PBL helps clinical exam preparation.
Q07	PBL helps to have a better understanding about the subject.
Q08	With PBL, students assume responsibility for their own learning.
Q09	PBL is a reliable tool that can facilitate visual/spatial learning in a clinical context.
Q10	PBL is a reliable tool that can facilitate auditory learning in a clinical context.
Q11	PBL is a reliable tool that can facilitate kinesthetic learning in a clinical context.
Q12	PBL helps convert from a passive to active lifelong learner in a clinical context.
Q13	PBL increases the learning motivation in a clinical context.
Q14	PBL helps to create clinical interest in the lectured lessons.
Q15	PBL enhances the ability to find information using the internet/library.
Q16	PBL enhances ability for public speaking in the clinical context.
Q17	PBL increases the ability to manage time effectively in the clinical context.
Q18	PBL improves decision-making skills in the clinical context.
Q19	PBL enhances clinical problem-solving ability in the clinical context.
Q20	PBL helps develop linguistic skills and self-confidence in the clinical context.
Q21	PBL enhances clinical reasoning ability in the clinical context.
Q22	A PBL hybrid system, composed by joining PBL and the conventional learning methods, is better than an exclusively conventional learning method.
Q23	When compared to the exclusively conventional learning method, the knowledge achieved with PBL is more thorough.
Q24	When compared to the exclusively conventional learning method, the focus of PBL on real medical/dental cases, makes it more relevant and interesting.
Q25	When compared to the exclusively conventional learning method, the subject objectives are better understood with PBL.
Q26	When compared to the exclusively conventional learning method, PBL is more time-consuming.
Q27	PBL is effective without having any conventional lectures on the subject.
Q28	With PBL, learners become active processors of information.
Q29	PBL helps identify knowledge weak areas for further improvement.
Q30	PBL enables the learners to establish a concrete action plan to achieve their learning goals.
Q31	PBL enhances the practical and clinical application of the ideas.
Q32	PBL helps develop clinical thinking, logical thinking, and abstract concepts.
Q33	PBL fulfills an effective integration between different subjects of basic medical sciences (horizontal integration).
Q34	PBL fulfills an effective integration between basic medical sciences with clinical sciences (vertical integration).
Q35	PBL is a reliable tool for developing scientific reading and writing skills.
Q36	PBL facilitates the development of interpersonal skills.
Q37	PBL facilitates the development of intrapersonal skills.
Q38	With PBL, knowledge activates prior knowledge around a problem, rather than specific subjects.
Q39	PBL allows learners to activate prior knowledge and learn to elaborate and organize their knowledge.
Q40	PBL enhances the retention of knowledge by practice, feedback, and evaluation.
Q41	PBL increases the extent of more related knowledge.

2.3. Ethical Considerations

The questionnaire was sent directly, via e-mail, to each one of the participants, from a third party not involved in the present study. The anonymous, voluntary, self-completion questionnaire was preceded by informed consent, which had to be provided in order to participate. The present work is part of an ongoing research project regarding the implementation and evaluation of learning methodologies for clinical dental teaching, approved by the Scientific Council of IUEM.

2.4. Statistical Analysis

Data analysis was performed using IBM SPSS Statistics software version 26.0 for Windows (IBM Corp., Armonk, NY, United States). Descriptive and inferential statistics methodologies were applied. Furthermore, a principal component analysis (PCA) was performed to examine the factor structure of the questionnaire.

All of the items were distributed, according to the rotated component matrix, via Varimax, with Kaiser normalization methods. The obtained Kaiser–Meyer–Olkin (KMO) validity test value was 0.902, falling into the range between 0.8 and 1.0, that deems a sample adequate for factor analysis. The extraction and retention of factors were based on visual examination of the scree plot, and eigenvalues >1.0 were retained. Factor loadings approximately equal to or higher than 0.50 dictated the assignment to a certain component. For questions with similar scores, a decision was made upon the contextualization of the question within each component, thus making its assignment to each one of two components possible.

3. Results

The mean age of the respondents was 28.7 (±7.6) years, and the majority (65.3%) were females (Table 2). Although 11% were not native Portuguese speakers, those participants had full understanding of the language, since the great majority (96%) self-reported an advanced (C1: 20%) or proficient (C2: 76%) level of Portuguese language reading skills.

Table 2. Sociodemographic characteristics of the participants in the study (n = 118).

		n	(%)
Gender	Female	77	65.3
	Male	41	34.7
Nationality	Portuguese	68	57.6
	Brazilian	37	31.4
	Other	13	11.0
		Mean	SD
Age	Years	28.7	7.6

The results of the answers to the 41-item questionnaire, based on a five-point Likert scale, are presented in Table 3. In general, a relatively high score was obtained for most of the questions (median, equal to, or higher than 4.0). The highest values were recorded for questions Q08 (student knowledge responsibility), with a median of 5.0, followed by Q22 (comparison of the PBL hybrid system with the conventional method), with a median of 4.5. The lowest score was obtained for questions Q11 (kinesthetic learning in a clinical context), Q23 (comparison of knowledge thoroughness gain), Q26 (time consumption comparison), and Q27 (effectiveness comparison), with a median of 3.0.

When comparing the answers as a function of gender, no statistically significant differences were found ($p > 0.05$, Mann–Whitney test).

Table 3. Questionnaire answers (n = 118). For each question, the correspondent median, interquartile range (IQR), minimum, and maximum values are presented.

ID	Item	Median (IQR)	Range (Min–Max)
Q01	PBL interest	4.0 (0)	1–5
Q02	Interactive clinical learning environment	4.0 (0)	1–5
Q03	Use of learning resources for clinical learning	4.0 (0)	1–5
Q04	Achievement of curriculum outcomes	4.0 (1)	1–5
Q05	Understanding of basic concepts	4.0 (0)	1–5
Q06	Clinical exam preparation	4.0 (1)	1–5
Q07	Subject understanding	4.0 (0)	1–5
Q08	Student knowledge responsibility	5.0 (1)	1–5
Q09	Visual/spatial learning in a clinical context	4.0 (1)	1–5
Q10	Auditory learning in a clinical context	4.0 (1)	1–5
Q11	Kinesthetic learning in a clinical context	3.0 (2)	1–5
Q12	Conversion to active lifelong learner in a clinical context	4.0 (2)	1–5
Q13	Learning motivation in a clinical context	4.0 (1)	1–5
Q14	Clinical interest in the lectured lessons	4.0 (1)	1–5
Q15	Ability to find information using the internet/library	4.0 (1)	1–5
Q16	Ability for public speaking	4.0 (2)	1–5
Q17	Time-management skills	4.0 (1)	1–5
Q18	Decision-making skills	4.0 (1)	1–5
Q19	Clinical problem-solving ability	4.0 (1)	1–5
Q20	Development of linguistic skills and self-confidence in a clinical context	4.0 (1)	1–5
Q21	Clinical reasoning ability, in a clinical context	4.0 (1)	1–5
Q22	Comparison of the PBL hybrid system with the conventional method	4.5 (1)	1–5
Q23	Comparison of knowledge thoroughness gain	3.0 (2)	1–5
Q24	Comparison of relevance and interest	4.0 (2)	1–5
Q25	Comparison of understanding of objectives	4.0 (1)	1–5
Q26	Time consumption comparison	3.0 (2)	1–5
Q27	Effectiveness comparison	3.0 (2)	1–5
Q28	Active processing of information	4.0 (1)	1–5
Q29	Identification of weakness areas	4.0 (1)	1–5
Q30	Establishment of a concrete action plan for the achievement of learning goals	4.0 (1)	1–5
Q31	Practical and clinical application of ideas	4.0 (1)	1–5
Q32	Development of clinical thinking, logical thinking, and abstract concepts	4.0 (0)	1–5
Q33	Horizontal integration effectiveness	4.0 (1)	1–5
Q34	Vertical integration effectiveness	4.0 (0)	1–5
Q35	Development of scientific reading and writing skills	4.0 (1)	1–5
Q36	Development of interpersonal skills	4.0 (1)	1–5
Q37	Development of intrapersonal skills	4.0 (1)	1–5
Q38	Prior knowledge activation around a problem	4.0 (0)	1–5
Q39	Knowledge organization	4.0 (1)	1–5
Q40	Knowledge retention by practice, feedback, and evaluation	4.0 (0)	1–5
Q41	Extension of related knowledge	4.0 (1)	1–5

The PCA results are presented in Table 4. Eight components were identified, according to the established criteria. As presented, in Component 1, Q13 (learning motivation, in a clinical context), Q14 (clinical interest in the lectured lessons), Q24 (comparison of relevance and interest), Q19 (clinical problem-solving ability), Q25 (comparison of understanding of objectives), Q27 (effectiveness comparison), Q23 (comparison of knowledge thoroughness gain), Q30 (establishment of a concrete action plan for the achievement of learning goals), and Q29 (identification of weakness areas) were categorized. In Component 2, Q01 (PBL interest), Q03 (use of learning resources for clinical learning), Q06 (clinical exam preparation), Q04 (achievement of curriculum outcomes), Q05 (understanding of basic concepts), Q02 (interactive clinical learning environment), Q07 (subject understanding), Q41 (extension of related knowledge), and Q40 (knowledge retention by practice, feedback, and evaluation) were categorized. In Component 3, Q16 (ability for public speaking), Q20 (development of linguistic skills and self-confidence in a clinical context), Q15 (ability to find information using the internet/library), Q17 (time-management skills), Q18 (decision-making skills), Q21 (clinical reasoning ability in a clinical context), and Q35 (development of scientific reading and writing skills) were categorized. In Component 4, Q33 (horizontal integration effectiveness), Q34 (vertical integration effectiveness), Q31 (practical and clinical application of ideas), Q32 (development of clinical thinking, logical thinking, and abstract concepts), Q39 (knowledge organization), Q38 (prior knowledge activation around a problem), and Q22 (comparison between the PBL hybrid system and the conventional method). In Component 5, Q09 (visual/spatial learning in a clinical context), Q12 (conversion to active lifelong learner in a clinical context), Q11 (kinesthetic learning in a clinical context), and Q10 (auditory learning in a clinical context) were categorized. In Component 6, Q36 (development of interpersonal skills) and Q37 (development of intrapersonal skills) were categorized. In Component 7, Q08 (student knowledge responsibility) and Q28 (active processing of information) were categorized. In Component 8, a single question was categorized: Q26 (time consumption).

Table 4. Items overall distribution among components, after principal component analysis (PCA), according to the rotated component matrix, via Varimax with the Kaiser normalization method (cumulative variance (%) = 73.644, Kaiser–Meyer–Olkin (KMO) value = 0.902).

Component	Item	Factor Loadings	Eigenvalue	Variance (%)	Communality
Component 1	Learning motivation in a clinical context (Q13)	0.773	19.251	46.955	0.824
	Clinical interest in the lectured lessons (Q14)	0.762			0.781
	Comparison of relevance and interest (Q24)	0.654			0.671
	Clinical problem-solving ability (Q19)	0.625			0.842
	Comparison of understanding of objectives (Q25)	0.623			0.707
	Effectiveness comparison (Q27)	0.601			0.568
	Comparison of knowledge thoroughness gain (Q23)	0.560			0.700
	Establishment of a concrete action plan for the achievement of learning goals (Q30) *	0.498			0.664
	Identification of weakness areas (Q29)	0.463			0.625
Component 2	PBL interest (Q01)	0.700	2.299	5.607	0.727
	Use of learning resources for clinical learning (Q03)	0.697			0.732
	Clinical exam preparation (Q06)	0.693			0.771
	Achievement of curriculum outcomes (Q04)	0.671			0.763
	Understanding of basic concepts (Q05)	0.671			0.691
	Interactive clinical learning environment (Q02)	0.666			0.733
	Subject understanding (Q07)	0.646			0.683
	Extension of related knowledge (Q41)	0.525			0.765
	Knowledge retention by practice, feedback, and evaluation (Q40)	0.486			0.733
	Prior knowledge activation around a problem (Q38) *[1]	0.406			0.664
Component 3	Ability for public speaking (Q16)	0.860	1.981	4.833	0.800
	Development of linguistic skills and self-confidence in a clinical context (Q20)	0.807			0.828
	Ability to find information using the internet/library (Q15)	0.650			0.592
	Time-management skills (Q17)	0.632			0.685
	Decision-making skills (Q18)	0.611			0.696
	Clinical reasoning ability in a clinical context (Q21)	0.516			0.800
	Development of scientific reading and writing skills (Q35)	0.470			0.707
	Establishment of a concrete action plan for the achievement of learning goals (Q30) *[1]	0.454			0.664

Table 4. Cont.

Component	Item	Factor Loadings	Eigenvalue	Variance (%)	Communality
Component 4	Horizontal integration effectiveness (Q33)	0.769	1.632	3.980	0.854
	Vertical integration effectiveness (Q34)	0.671			0.729
	Practical and clinical application of ideas (Q31)	0.605			0.769
	Development of clinical thinking, logical thinking, and abstract concepts (Q32)	0.549			0.741
	Knowledge organization (Q39)	0.513			0.835
	Prior knowledge activation around a problem (Q38) *	0.418			0.664
	Comparison between the PBL hybrid system with the conventional method (Q22)	0.418			0.555
Component 5	Visual/spatial learning in a clinical context (Q09)	0.711	1.598	3.899	0.748
	Conversion to active lifelong learner in a clinical context (Q12)	0.754			0.743
	Kinesthetic learning in a clinical context (Q11)	0.753			0.808
	Auditory learning in a clinical context (Q10)	0.504			0.713
Component 6	Development of interpersonal skills (Q36)	0.643	1.316	3.210	0.865
	Development of intrapersonal skills (Q37)	0.587			0.839
Component 7	Student knowledge responsibility (Q08)	0.841	1.104	2.692	0.795
	Active processing of information (Q28)	0.522			0.750
Component 8	Time consumption (Q26)	0.932	1.012	2.468	0.891

* Question assigned to the corresponding component; *1 question not assigned to the corresponding component.

In ascending order, the percent of Component 1 for total variance was approximately 49.96%, Component 2 was approximately 5.61%, Component 4 was 3.98%, Component 5 was approximately 3.90%, Component 6 was 3.21%, Component 7 was approximately 2.69%, Component 8 was approximately 2.47%, and Component 3 was approximately 1.99%. The cumulative variance of total factors was approximately 73.64%.

4. Discussion

Amid the lockdown imposed due to the COVID-19 pandemic, the physical closure of higher education institutions (HEIs) has shed a brighter light on the need of pedagogical innovation. Given the specificity of medical and dental education, this crisis is necessary to analyze, explore, and implement strategies that allow the development of clinical skills, even in face of a distance learning situation.

The present study was aimed at assessing dental students' self-perception on learning, motivation, organization, tool acquisition, clinical skills, and knowledge using an active learning method, such as PBL, through online/digital channels in a distance learning context, as well as the identification of the limitations and difficulties in this context.

Given the primacy of the present investigation, all of the results were compared to presential PBL method studies.

When comparing the answers as a function of the gender, no statistically significant differences were found ($p > 0.05$, Mann–Whitney test), contrary to previous evidence [27].

Concerning the items categorized to Component 1, 63.6% of the students agreed that the PBL method increased learning motivation in a clinical context (Q13), which supports previously conducted studies that reported 65.2%, but is inferior to those reported before of 95.6% [28] and 88.0% [30]. As for Q14, 71.2% agreed that the PBL method helps to create clinical interest, which supports previous evidence, but nonetheless is inferior to 95.6% reported [28]. Of the responding students, 71.2% agreed that the PBL method enhances clinical problem-solving abilities (Q19), which is in line with previously conducted study values of 66.7% [27] and 73.2% [31]. All of the remaining items from this component did not support previous evidence. As to comparing the knowledge thoroughness gained by the PBL method versus the conventional method (Q23), only 36.4% of the present study students agreed, which is inferior to the percentage of 53.3% previously reported [27]. The same tendency is verified in Q24 (comparison of relevance and interest), with 67.8% versus 83.4% previously [27]. When comparing to the subjects' understanding of objectives to the conventional method (Q25), 58.5% of the students of the present study agreed that the PBL method is better, facing 43.4% reported before [27]. As to the PBL method's effectiveness without a conventional lecture (Q27), 46.6% agreed, while only 20.0% was reported in a previous study [27]. Also, in Q29, while assessing if the PBL method helped identify areas of weakness for further improvement, our results found that 72.0% agreed, while only 50.0% was reported in a previous study [27].

The majority of the items categorized in Component 2 support previous evidence, namely PBL interest (Q01: 89.0% vs. 70.0% [27]), interactive clinical learning environment (Q02: 81.4% vs. 79.5% [31]), use of learning resources for clinical learning (Q03: 76.3% vs. 82.1% [31]), achievement of curriculum outcomes (Q04: 63.6% vs. 65.2% [31]), and extension of related knowledge (Q41: 83.1% vs. 83.0% [31]). As for Q40, 81.4% of the students agreed that the PBL method enhances knowledge retention by practice, feedback, and evaluation, which is consonant to what has been reported—85.7% [31]—but contrary to other results of 60.0% [30]. In what concerns Q07 (subject understanding), the results of the present study find that 76.3% agreed that the PBL method allows a better understanding about the subject, which is inferior to previous results of 97.2% [28]. This question was also mentioned in other previous studies, and even though strict data comparison is not possible. Due to the ordinary nature of the Likert scale, results (3.87 ± 0.79) are inferior to those presented of 4.42 ± 1.13 [26] and higher than 3.23 ± 0.57 [29]. Regarding Q05 (understanding basic concepts), our results (3.97 ± 0.78) are inferior to those previously reported of 4.24 ± 0.88 [26].

Most of the items categorized in Component 3 did not support previous evidence, with results inferior to those reported, namely ability to find information using the internet/library (Q15: 61.0% vs. 90.0% [27]), ability for public speaking (Q16: 52.5% vs. 93.3% [27] and 77.6% [26]), time-management skills (Q17: 55.9% vs. 90.1% [27] and 90.6% [26]), clinical reasonability in a clinical context (Q21: 76.3% vs. 90.6% [26]), and development of scientific reading and writing skills (Q35: 68.6% vs. 80.3% [31]). The exceptions for this tendency can be observed in Q18 (decision-making skills), where 66.1% of the students agreed that the PBL method helped in developing linguistic skills and self-confidence, in accordance with 60.0% [27] and 73.2% [31] previously, as well as in Q20 (development of linguistic skills and self-confidence in a clinical context), where the results obtained by the present study (58.5%) are superior to those reported earlier (48.5% [31]).

The majority of the items categorized in Component 4 support previous evidence, namely the practical and clinical application of ideas (Q31: 64.4% vs. 73.2% [31]); development of clinical thinking, logical thinking, and abstract concepts (Q32: 81.4% vs. 83.0% [31]); and prior knowledge activation around a problem (Q38: 76.3% vs. 73.3% [27] and 83.0% [31]). Regarding horizontal integration effectiveness (Q33: 86.4%), vertical integration effectiveness (Q34: 78.0%), and knowledge organization (Q39: 84.7%), our results were higher than those reported of 75.0% [31], 60.7% [31], and 73.3% [27], respectively. In regards to Q22, 81.4% of the students of the present study agree that a PBL hybrid system is better than an exclusively conventional method, which is a significantly higher percentage than the reported value of 46.4% [27].

Regarding the items categorized in component 5, 66.9% of the students agreed that the PBL method can facilitate auditory learning in a clinical context (Q10), and only 39.0% agreed on the facilitation of kinesthetic learning, which supports previous evidence of 79.5% [31] and 44.7% [31], respectively. The results obtained in Q9, visual/spatial learning in a clinical context (71.2%), support those reported (76.5%) from a previous study [26], while being superior to other results of 55.4% [31]. In relation to Q12, 70.3% of the students of the present study agree that the PBL helps the conversion from a passive to active lifelong learner in a clinical context, which is a significantly higher percentage than the 50.0% reported previously [27].

All of the items categorized in Component 6 did not support previous evidence, showing inferior results in Q36, development of interpersonal skills (53.4%), and Q37, development of intrapersonal skills (61.0%), to those reported in previous studies of 88.4% [31] and 87.5% [31], respectively.

Meanwhile, all of the items categorized in Component 7 support previous evidence, showing significantly higher results in Q8, student knowledge responsibility (90.7%), and Q28, active processing of information (83.1%), than those reported in previous studies of 70.0% [27] and 63.0% [27].

The only item categorized in Component 8 was not comparable, since the previous conducted study [32] compared all items as one, instead of an isolated analysis.

These findings deserve further reflection, hence the fact that even if there are other goals that can be accomplished with PBL, clinical reasoning (Q21), self-directed learning (Q08), and most of the factors referred to in Component 4 represent essential medical skills, while students' motivation (Q13) expands their internal learning drive, thus encouraging extraction and comprehension of data from learning platforms (Q03). All of these variables have been tested in the present study, and have shown positive results in online PBL settings. Regarding the four domains of VARK (visual, auditory, reading/writing, and kinesthetic), which represent essential skills for the dental field, our results demonstrate that PBL, even in a distance learning context, can facilitate visual/spatial, auditory, and reading/writing domains, while not easing the development of the kinesthetic domain due to the lack of tools that allow at-home, hands-on practice. Concerning the comparison to conventional methods in this particular setting, students self-perceived benefiting in regards to knowledge thoroughness (Q23) and subjects' understanding of objectives (Q25), while considering online PBL to be more relevant and interesting (Q24). This summed up to a majority belief that the hybrid method is better than the conventional one (Q22), with significantly superior results in this setting (81.4%), than in a previous one (46.4%) [27].

Several limitations must be taken into account when interpreting the findings. The most important is that the present study has a low response rate and is limited as to the sample size, which may not fully allow generalization for the whole population of dental students.

5. Conclusions

This study's results demonstrate that online PBL can be considered a relevant learning tool to be utilized within the specific context of clinical dental education, displaying benefits over traditional learning strategies.

Overall, dental students prefer a PBL hybrid system over the conventional one, in a distance learning context, and assume self-responsibility for their own learning. On the other hand, knowledge thoroughness is perceived as inferior to that gained through the conventional method.

The online PBL method is not a reliable tool to facilitate kinesthetic learning in a dental clinical setting, as compared to other methods.

Nonetheless, the online PBL strategy can be viewed as a successful instrument to improve information and clinical ability (visual/spatial and auditory) advancement in the scope of dental education, with similar results to those obtained in a presential setting.

Further studies are needed to assess clinical skills and knowledge development through active learning methods, such as PBL, in a distance learning context, as well as to design and implement effective complementary kinesthetic distance learning tools, namely through haptic technology, and also with a greater focus on the development of communication and personal skills, such as video-based online approaches, that have been showing promising results.

Author Contributions: Conceptualization, M.M., J.J.M. and L.P.; methodology, M.M., J.J.M. and L.P.; software, L.P.; formal analysis, L.P.; investigation, M.M. and J.J.M.; resources, J.J.M.; data curation, J.J.M. and L.P.; writing—M.M. and L.P.; writing—review and editing, M.M., J.J.M. and L.P.; supervision, J.J.M. and L.P. All authors have read and agreed to the published version of the manuscript.

Funding: This research received no external funding.

Institutional Review Board Statement: Not applicable.

Informed Consent Statement: Informed consent was obtained from all subjects involved in the study.

Data Availability Statement: The data used to support the findings of this study are available from the corresponding author (L.P.) upon request.

Conflicts of Interest: The authors declare no conflict of interest.

References

1. Hillen, H.; Scherpbier, A.; Wijnen, W. History of problem-based learning in medical education. In *Lessons from Problem-Based Learning*; Oxford University Press (OUP): Oxford, UK, 2010; pp. 5–12.
2. Norman, G.R.; Schmidt, H.G. The psychological basis of problem-based learning: A review of the evidence. *Acad. Med.* **1992**, *67*, 557–565. [CrossRef] [PubMed]
3. Foucault, M.; Sheridan, A. *The Birth of the Clinic: An Archaeology of Medical Perception [Naissance de la Clinique.]*; Presses Universitaires de France: Paris, France, 1963.
4. McKeown, T. *The Role of Medicine: Dream, Mirage, or Nemesis?* Princeton University Press: Princeton, NJ, USA, 2014.
5. Neufeld, V.R.; Barrows, H.S. The "McMaster Philosophy": An approach to medical education. *Acad. Med.* **1974**, *49*, 1040–1050. [CrossRef]
6. Boudier, H.A.J.S.; Smits, J.F.M. Problem-based learning: The Maastricht experience. *Trends Pharmacol. Sci.* **2002**, *23*, 164. [CrossRef]
7. Rohlin, M.; Petersson, K.; Svensäter, G. The Malmö model: A problem-based learning curriculum in undergraduate dental education. *Eur. J. Dent. Educ.* **1998**, *2*, 103–114. [CrossRef]
8. Holmboe, E.S. Faculty and the Observation of Trainees' Clinical Skills: Problems and Opportunities. *Acad. Med.* **2004**, *79*, 16–22. [CrossRef]
9. Suksudaj, N.; Townsend, G.C.; Kaidonis, J.; Lekkas, D.; Winning, T.A. Acquiring psychomotor skills in operative dentistry: Do innate ability and motivation matter? *Eur. J. Dent. Educ.* **2012**, *16*, e187–e194. [CrossRef]
10. Rich, S.K.; Keim, R.G.; Shuler, C.F. Problem-Based Learning Versus a Traditional Educational Methodology: A Comparison of Preclinical and Clinical Periodontics Performance. *J. Dent. Educ.* **2005**, *69*, 649–662. [CrossRef]
11. Kurzweil, R. The Law of Accelerating Returns. In *Alan Turing: Life and Legacy of a Great Thinker*; Springer: New York, NY, USA, 2004; pp. 381–416.
12. Renes, S.L.; Strange, A.T. Using Technology to Enhance Higher Education. *Altern. High. Educ.* **2010**, *36*, 203–213. [CrossRef]
13. Schmid, R.F.; Bernard, R.M.; Borokhovski, E.; Tamim, R.M.; Abrami, P.C.; Surkes, M.A.; Wade, C.A.; Woods, J. The effects of technology use in postsecondary education: A meta-analysis of classroom applications. *Comput. Educ.* **2014**, *72*, 271–291. [CrossRef]
14. Anderson, T.; Dron, J. Three generations of distance education pedagogy. *Int. Rev. Res. Open Distrib. Learn* **2011**, *12*, 80–97. [CrossRef]
15. Chhetri, S.K. E-learning in neurology education: Principles, opportunities and challenges in combating neurophobia. *J. Clin. Neurosci.* **2017**, *44*, 80–83. [CrossRef] [PubMed]
16. Restrepo, D.; Hunt, D.; Miloslavsky, E. Transforming traditional shadowing: Engaging millennial learners through the active apprenticeship. *Clin. Teach.* **2020**, *17*, 31–35. [CrossRef] [PubMed]
17. Mehta, N.B.; Hull, A.L.; Young, J.B.; Stoller, J.K. Just Imagine: New paradigms for medical education. *Acad. Med.* **2013**, *88*, 1418–1423. [CrossRef]
18. Blumberg, P.; Pontiggia, L. Benchmarking the Degree of Implementation of Learner-Centered Approaches. *Altern. High. Educ.* **2010**, *36*, 189–202. [CrossRef]
19. Thistlethwaite, J.E.; Davies, D.; Ekeocha, S.; Kidd, J.M.; MacDougall, C.; Matthews, P.; Purkis, J.; Clay, D. The effectiveness of case-based learning in health professional education. A BEME systematic review: BEME Guide No. 23. *Med. Teach.* **2012**, *34*, e421–e444. [CrossRef] [PubMed]
20. Ramnanan, C.J.; Pound, L.D. Advances in medical education and practice: Student perceptions of the flipped classroom. *Adv. Med. Educ. Pract.* **2017**, *8*, 63–73. [CrossRef] [PubMed]
21. Jones, F.; Passos-Neto, C.E.; Braghiroli, O.F.M. Simulation in medical education: Brief history and methodology. *Princ. Pract. Clin. Res. J.* **2015**, *1*, 56–63. [CrossRef]
22. Hung, A.C.Y. A critique and defense of gamification. *J. Interact. Online Learn.* **2017**, *15*, 57–72.
23. Ahmed, H.; Allaf, M.; Elghazaly, H. COVID-19 and medical education. *Lancet Infect. Dis.* **2020**, *20*, 777–778. [CrossRef]
24. Alkhowailed, M.S.; Rasheed, Z.; Shariq, A.; Elzainy, A.; El Sadik, A.; Alkhamiss, A.; Alsolai, A.M.; Alduraibi, S.K.; Alduraibi, A.; Alamro, A.; et al. Digitalization plan in medical education during COVID-19 lockdown. *Inform. Med. Unlocked* **2020**, *20*, 100432. [CrossRef]
25. Bennardo, F.; Buffone, C.; Fortunato, L.; Giudice, A. COVID-19 is a challenge for dental education—A commentary. *Eur. J. Dent. Educ.* **2020**, *24*, 822–824. [CrossRef] [PubMed]
26. Ma, X.; Luo, Y.; Wang, J.; Zhang, L.; Liang, Y.; Wu, Y.; Yu, H.; Cao, M. Comparison of student perception and performance between case-based learning and lecture-based learning in a clinical laboratory immunology course. *LaboratoriumsMedizin* **2016**, *40*, 283–289. [CrossRef]

27. Banabilh, S.M.; Alkhuwaiter, S.S.; Aljuailan, R.I. Problem-based learning: Dental student's perception of their education environments at Qassim University. *J. Int. Soc. Prev. Community Dent.* **2016**, *6*, 575–583. [CrossRef] [PubMed]
28. Preeti, D.; Ashish, A.; Shriram, G. Problem Based Learning (PBL)—An Effective Approach to Improve Learning Outcomes in Medical Teaching. *J. Clin. Diagn. Res.* **2013**, *7*, 2896–2897. [CrossRef]
29. Kim, Y.J. Observational Application Comparing Problem-Based Learning with the Conventional Teaching Method for Clinical Acupuncture Education. *Evid.-Based Complement. Altern. Med.* **2019**, *2019*, 1–6. [CrossRef] [PubMed]
30. Khoshnevisasl, P.; Sadeghzadeh, M.; Mazloomzadeh, S.; Feshareki, R.H.; Ahmadiafshar, A. Comparison of Problem-based Learning with Lecture-based Learning. *Iran. Red Crescent Med. J.* **2014**, *16*, e5186. [CrossRef] [PubMed]
31. Asad, M.R.; Tadvi, N.; Amir, K.M.; Afzal, K.; Irfan, A.; Hussain, S.A. Medical Student's Feedback towards Problem Based Learning and Interactive Lectures as a Teaching and Learning Method in an Outcome-Based Curriculum. *Int. J. Med. Res. Health Sci.* **2019**, *8*, 78–84.
32. Usmani, A.; Sultan, S.T.; Ali, S.; Fatima, N.; Babar, S. Comparison of students and facilitators' perception of implementing problem based learning. *J. Pak. Med. Assoc.* **2011**, *61*, 332–335.

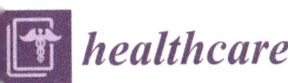

Article

Workshop on Blood Loss Quantification in Obstetrics: Improving Medical Student Learning through Clinical Simulation

Javier Ruiz-Labarta [1,2,3,4], Ana Martínez Martín [1], Pilar Pintado Recarte [1,2,3,4], Blanca González Garzón [1,2,3,4], Juan Manuel Pina Moreno [1,2,3,4], Mercedes Sánchez Rodríguez [1,2,3,4], África Vallejo Gea [1], Luis Sordo [1,3], Melchor Álvarez-Mon [5,6,7], Miguel A. Ortega [5,6,*], Coral Bravo Arribas [1,2,3,4,*] and Juan A. De León-Luis [1,2,3,4]

1. Department of Public and Maternal and Child Health, School of Medicine, Complutense University of Madrid, 28040 Madrid, Spain; franciscojavier.ruiz@salud.madrid.org (J.R.-L.); anmart22@ucm.es (A.M.M.); ppintado@salud.madrid.org (P.P.R.); bgonzalezg@salud.madrid.org (B.G.G.); juanmanuel.pina@salud.madrid.org (J.M.P.M.); mariamercedes.sanchez.rodriguez@salud.madrid.org (M.S.R.); africava@ucm.es (Á.V.G.); lsordo@ucm.es (L.S.); jaleon@ucm.es (J.A.D.L.-L.)
2. Department of Obstetrics and Gynecology, University Hospital Gregorio Marañón, 28009 Madrid, Spain
3. Health Research Institute Gregorio Marañón, Consortium for Biomedical Research in Epidemiology and Public Health (CIBERESP), 28009 Madrid, Spain
4. Maternal and Infant Research Investigation Unit, Alonso Family Foundation (UDIMIFFA), 28009 Madrid, Spain
5. Department of Medicine and Medical Specialties, Faculty of Medicine and Health Sciences, University of Alcalá, 28801 Madrid, Spain; mademons@gmail.com
6. Ramón y Cajal Institute of Healthcare Research (IRYCIS), 28034 Madrid, Spain
7. Immune System Diseases-Rheumatology and Oncology Service, University Hospital Príncipe de Asturias, CIBEREHD, 28805 Alcalá de Henares, Spain
* Correspondence: miguel.angel.ortega92@gmail.com (M.A.O.); cbravoarribas@gmail.com (C.B.A.); Tel.: +34-91-885-45-40 (M.A.O.); Fax: +34-91-885-48-85 (M.A.O.)

Abstract: Purpose: To assess whether a clinical simulation-based obstetric blood loss quantification workshop for medical undergraduate trainees improves theoretical–practical knowledge, along with self-assurance and self-confidence. Methods: This was a quasi-experimental pre-post learning study conducted at the Gynaecology and Obstetrics Unit of the Hospital Gregorio Marañón, Madrid, Spain. Participants were volunteer students in their fourth year of a 6-year degree course in Medicine. The study period was divided into the stages: pre-workshop, intra-workshop, 2 weeks post-workshop and 6 months post-workshop. In the pre-workshop stage, students completed a brief online course in preparation for the workshop. The effectiveness of the workshop was assessed through multiple choice tests and self-administered questionnaires. Data were compared between time-points using statistical tests for paired samples. Results: Of the 142 students invited (age 21.94 ± 3.12 years), 138 accepted the offer of the workshop (97.2%), and 85.4% had no experience in managing blood loss. Between the stages pre- and 2 weeks post-workshop, significant improvements were observed in theoretical–practical knowledge ($\mu = 1.109$), self-assurance and self-confidence. At the 6 months post-workshop stage, theoretical–practical knowledge diminished compared with 2 weeks post-workshop, returning to pre-workshop levels, while self-assurance and confidence failed to vary significantly in the longer term. Conclusions: The obstetric workshop improved theoretical–practical knowledge and the self-assurance and confidence of the medical students. Results 2 weeks post-workshop were maintained up until 6 months after the training intervention. The clinical simulation-based workshop was perceived by the students as useful and necessary.

Keywords: clinical simulation; blood loss quantification; obstetric haemorrhage; knowledge; self-assurance; self-confidence; usefulness; feedback

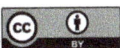

1. Introduction

In the past decade, clinical simulation as a learning method for medical undergraduates has advanced tremendously at universities and teaching hospitals across the world. Clinical simulation is the fictitious performance of a complex clinical procedure with sufficient realism to facilitate the acquisition of theoretical–practical skills, including communication and coordination with medical staff, through immersion, practice and feedback, while avoiding risks inherent to real healthcare situations. Among others, its benefits are learning curve shortening, improved patient confidence and competitive results [1].

Since 2017, the Gynaecology and Obstetrics Unit of the Hospital Universitario Gregorio Marañón (HUGM), Madrid, Spain, has been holding a series of clinical simulation workshops for undergraduates of medicine from the Universidad Complutense de Madrid (UCM), aimed at improving their understanding of maternal–neonatal health. These workshops are popular and seem subjectively to improve the theoretical–practical skills and self-assurance and confidence of participants. However, to date, no effort has been made to assess their effectiveness in an objective manner.

This study sought to assess the results of the workshop on "Quantification of blood loss in Obstetrics" conducted in 2020–2021 with the participation of students in their fourth year of a 6-year degree course in Medicine. The hospital teaching staff selected this workshop on the grounds of the importance of adequately managing obstetric haemorrhage [2,3]. There is no consensus in the literature when it comes to defining postpartum haemorrhage; however, one of the most accepted definitions is the one that defines it as a blood loss that exceeds 500 mL after a vaginal delivery, or 1000 mL if it is a caesarean section9. Postpartum haemorrhage appears in 1–5% of deliveries in our setting.

This complication of childbirth is the leading cause of maternal mortality, both in emergent and industrialized countries [4,5]. The workshop strives to teach students the necessary tools to learn how to diagnose an obstetric haemorrhage through the gravimetric quantification of blood loss in different settings (postpartum or during a caesarean birth).

The HUGM is a tertiary hospital that serves patients with special risk of the appearance of obstetric haemorrhage (induced labour, caesarean birth, twin birth or older maternal age). Our department is currently working towards instructing all healthcare workers on how to quantify blood loss by weighing fluids and sterile gauze during every delivery, in an attempt to reduce maternal morbidity and mortality. We also have an established multidisciplinary protocol for severe obstetric haemorrhage to help with the prevention, diagnosis and treatment of patients with this complication of childbirth [6,7].

Visual estimation of obstetric-related blood loss alone is poorly sensitive and specific, as it tends to underestimate real blood loss [3]. Thus, a more objective and accurate method of estimating excessive bleeding is needed [8]. Gravimetric quantification consists of weighing fluid losses collected in a calibrated under-buttocks drape or suction canister and adding this volume to that measured by weighing blood-soaked items or gauzes. This is the preferred method, recommended by guidelines issued by many national and international institutions, such as the American College of Obstetricians and Gynaecologists [9,10]. In effect, many studies have shown that this tool improves the skills and confidence of healthcare professionals [11,12].

The present study was designed to assess if the "Quantification of blood loss in Obstetrics workshop" (hereafter "the workshop") offered to medical students is useful in terms of improving theoretical–practical knowledge, along with the self-assurance and self-confidence of students when managing blood loss postpartum or during a caesarean delivery.

2. Materials and Methods

The study design was quasi-experimental pre–post, with longitudinal follow up from just before to several months after participating in the workshop implemented at the Gynaecology and Obstetrics Dept. of the HUGM, during the academic year 2020–2021. The recruited participants were 4th-year medical students enrolled in the subject of Obstetrics and Gynaecology, who were offered the workshop as part of their practical training in the subject, and who were able to attend voluntarily. The author MM. was in charge of controlling the lists of participants and verifying the correct completion of the tests and questionnaires that they had to fill out through a virtual platform. Later, they were downloaded in order to analyse the answers.

The workshop was divided into four consecutive stages which were described previously to the students (Figure 1). The stages were: (1) pre-workshop, (2) workshop, (3) up to 2 weeks after the workshop (short term), and (4) 6 months after the workshop (long term):

1. Stage 1: This was executed "on-line" via a virtual platform (www.aleesca.es/moodle, accessed on 18 August 2021). Here, the students had access to descriptions of the workshop along with the theory (presentations and videos) related to blood loss quantification in obstetrics. The tasks to be completed were:

    A. Multiple choice test (MCT), in which 20 questions should be answered in 30 min to assess theoretical–practical knowledge pertaining to the subject. For each correct answer, 0.5 points were added (no points were subtracted for incorrect answers).

    B. Two self-administered questionnaires to assess the self-assurance and self-confidence of the students when facing a similar clinical situation. Replies were scored according to a semiquantitative Likert scale [13] (Appendix A).

2. Stage 2: This was the actual clinical simulation workshop completed. Over a period of 1.5 hours, the students, in groups of 8–10, were given a brief lecture on how to quantify blood loss postpartum or during a caesarean section. The students then put their understanding of the topic into practice in different clinical scenarios with the help of a mannequin and artificial blood. Students were encouraged to ask questions during the task. A clinical scenario of a patient who had experienced postpartum haemorrhage after a normal vaginal delivery was depicted. To do this, a mannequin in the shape of a female pelvis was used, with a plastic blood collection bag located under the pelvis and textile material (compresses, gauze pads and underpads) soaked in blood. The student had to perform a gravimetric quantification of the blood lost by the patient during the immediate postpartum period. Subsequently, the students were able to design other simulated clinical scenarios (caesarean section, instrumental delivery) with the same material, to continue practicing gravimetric quantification in other situations.

3. Stages 3 and 4: These stages were completed on-line and included tasks such as:

    C. A similar MCT to that of stage 1, but with questions designed to compare the student's understanding of the topic and practical skills before and at two time points after the workshop.

    D. Three self-administered questionnaires designed to assess their self-assurance, self-confidence and perception of usefulness of the workshop, and to gain feedback (Appendix A).

Assistance and completion of each workshop stage were noted, so that students missing some of the tasks could be withdrawn from the study. Other exclusion criteria were: students completing the MCT in under 3 min or over 30 min, and those needing more than one attempt at the test.

The variables analysed were (Table 1): sex, age, prior experience, theoretical–practical knowledge, self-assurance, self-confidence, perception of workshop usefulness and feedback.

Replies to the MCT and questionnaires were collected online and transferred to an Excel sheet for their analysis. Statistical tests were performed using the software package SPSS Version 21.0 (IBM Corp., Armonk, NY, USA). Quantitative variables were expressed as the mean ± standard deviation, and categorical variables as their number and percentage. To assess the changes produced in theoretical–practical knowledge (assessed through MCT) between the different stages, we used the Student t-test for paired samples with significance set at $p < 0.05$. These statistical tests were also used to assess changes in self-assurance and self-confidence between the different study stages (assessed through self-administered questionnaires). The Kolmogorov–Smirnov test was used to check the normality of the data.

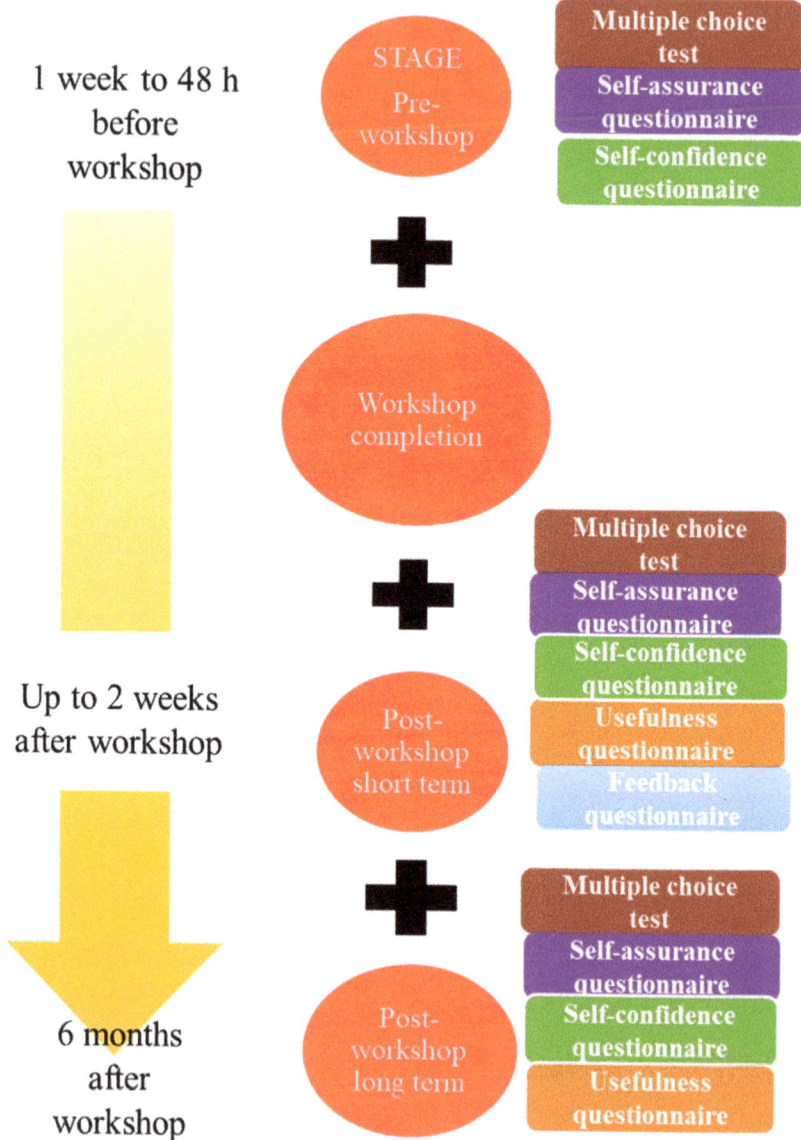

Figure 1. Stages and content of the blood loss quantification workshop.

Table 1. List of study variables along with their assessment method and qualifying measures.

Variable	Assessment Method	Qualifier
Sex	Student characteristic	Qualitative nominal
Age	Student characteristic	Quantitative discrete
Previous passive or active experience with clinical situations involving more than 1 L of blood loss	Student characteristic	Quantitative discrete 0 occasions; ≥1 occasion
Theoretical–practical knowledge	Multiple choice test	Quantitative discrete Score of 0–10 in 0.5-point steps
Self-assurance	Self-administered questionnaire	Quantitative discrete Likert scale (0–10) Poor (0–2), medium (3–4), good (5–6), very good (7–8) and excellent (9–10)
Self-confidence	Self-administered questionnaire	Quantitative discrete Likert scale (0–10) Not at all confident (0–2), scarcely confident (3–4), somewhat confident (5–6), confident (7–8) and very confident (9–10)
Perceived utility	Self-administered questionnaire	Quantitative discrete Likert scale (0–10) Not at all useful (0–2), not really useful (3–4), indifferent (5–6), useful (7–8) and definitely useful (9–10)
Feedback	Self-administered questionnaire	Three questions with different non-exclusive answers (students could mark as many options as they wished) Three questions with open answers

3. Results

Of the 147 students enrolled in the subject, 142 (97.2%) took part in the workshop. After applying the exclusion criteria, the rate of participation was high (>95%), both at the pre-workshop and workshop stages, and thereafter dropped slightly in the long-term post-workshop stage (78.2%) (Figures 2 and 3).

The mean age of the students was 21.94 ± 3.12 years. Scores obtained in the MCT were high, both in the pre- (mean = 7.47 out of 10) and post-workshop stages (8.52 and 7.47 at 2 weeks and 6 months, respectively). Between the stages pre-workshop and 2 weeks post-workshop, a significant improvement was observed in theoretical–practical knowledge ($p < 0.05$). At 6 months post-workshop, pre-workshop scores in response to the on-line course were maintained (Tables 2 and 3).

Table 2. MCT results and improvements during the study course.

	Results of Multiple Choice Test						
	Pre-WS (N = 142)	Post-WS 2 Weeks (N = 137)	Short-Term Improvement (μ post—μ pre) (N = 137)	p	Post-WS 6 Months (N =111)	Long-Term Improvement (μ 6 mo—μ 2 wk) (N =111)	p
Score (/10)	7.47 ± 1.66	8.52 ± 1.06	1.01 ± 1.60 (8.52–7.47)	<0.05	7.47 ± 1.51	−1.15 ±1.24 (7.47–8.52)	<0.05

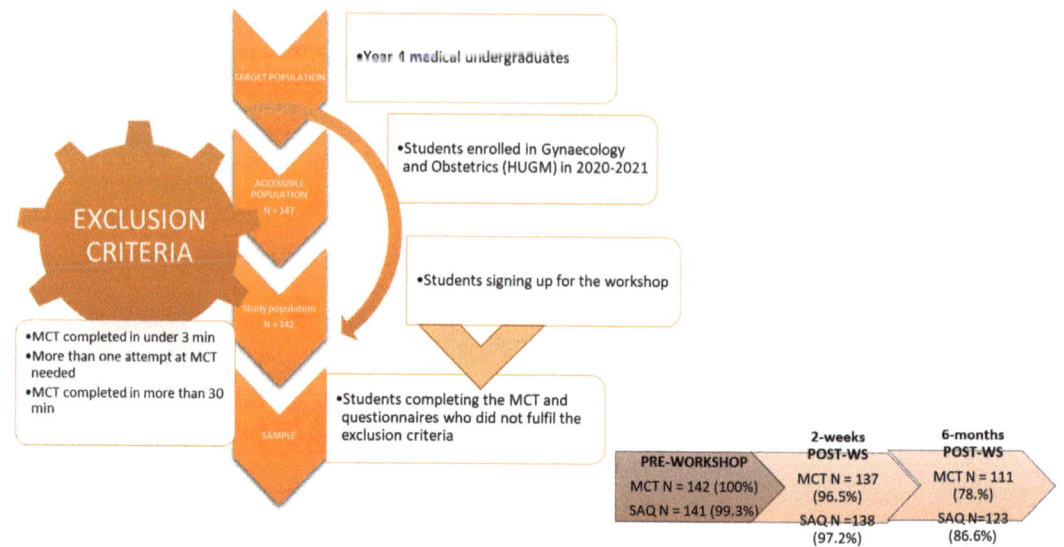

MCT: multiple choice test; SAQ: self-administered questionnaire; WS: workshop

Figure 2. Participant recruitment.

Table 3. Results of the self-assurance questionnaire and improvements during the study course. WS = workshop; wk = weeks; mo = months; BLQ = blood loss quantification.

	Self-Assurance Questionnaire						
	Pre-WS (N = 141)	Post-WS 2 Weeks (N = 138)	Short-Term Improvement (μ post—μ pre) (N = 138)	p	Post-WS 6 Months (N = 123)	Long-Term Improvement (μ 6 mo—μ 2 wk) (N = 121)	p
1. Theoretical BLQ knowledge	4.69 ± 2.21	7.37 ± 1.34	2.68 (7.37–4.69)	<0.05	7.47 ± 1.38	0.02 ± 1.36 (7.47–7.37)	0.88
2. Practical BLQ knowledge	4.71 ± 2.27	7.72 ± 1.13	2.98 (7.72–4.71)	<0.05	7.58 ± 1.31	−0.18 ± 1.16 (7.58–7.72)	0.09
3. Practical management skills	2.79 ± 2.26	6.87 ± 1.44	4.10 (6.87–2.79)	<0.05	6.68 ± 1.53	−0.27 (6.68–6.87)	<0.05

Results for self-reported confidence were similar. A significant improvement in scores was observed between pre-workshop and 2 weeks post-workshop ($p < 0.05$). Between the short- and long-term post-workshop stages, results remained practically stable, with a slight non-significant decrease observed at 6 months (Table 4).

When asked about the workshop's utility, in both the short and long term after the workshop, close to 90% of the participants considered it useful, this type of intervention being perceived as an essential part of medical training (Table 5, Figure 4).

Table 4. Results of the self-confidence questionnaire and improvements during the study course. WS = workshop; wk = weeks; mo = months; BLQ = blood loss quantification; PP = postpartum.

	Self-Confidence Questionnaire						
	Pre-WS (N = 141)	Post-WS 2 Weeks (N = 138)	Short-Term Improvement (μ post—μ pre) (N = 138)	p	Post-WS 6 Months (N =123)	Long-Term Improvement (μ 6 mo—μ 2 wk) (N = 121)	p
4. Experience with BLQ	3.65 ± 2.3	6.58 ± 1.43	3.02 (6.59–3.57)	<0.05	6.45 ± 1.66	−0.29 (6.43–6.71)	<0.05
5. Controlling blood loss	2.82 ± 2.13	6.09 ± 1.58	3.29 (6.09–2.80)	<0.05	6.00 ± 1.79	−0.26 (5.98–6.24)	0.093
6. Controlling initial situation	2.94 ± 2.07	6.05 ± 1.68	3.18 (6.06–2.88)	<0.05	5.86 ± 1.84	−0.31 (5.84–6.15)	0.065
7. Visual BLQ	3.70 ± 2.20	6.40 ± 1.62	2.79 (6.39–3.60)	<0.05	6.46 ± 1.65	−0.11 (6.43–6.55)	0.457
8. Gravimetric BLQ	4.60 ± 2.51	7.91 ± 1.30	3.35 (7.92–4.57)	<0.05	7.24 ± 1.61	−0.76 (7.24–8.00)	<0.05
9. Differentiating between mild and severe blood loss	4.52 ± 2.22	7.30 ± 1.37	2.79 (6.39–3.60)	<0.05	7.11 ± 1.59	−0.23 (7.10–7.32)	0.10
10. Coordinating with other staff	4.84 ± 2.35	7.37 ± 1.43	2.58 (7.38–4.80)	<0.05	7.32 ± 1.57	−0.14 (7.30–7.44)	0.31
11. Preventing severe blood loss	3.28 ± 2.16	6.36 ± 1.77	3.11 (6.36–3.24)	<0.05	6.52 ± 1.60	0.11 (6.49–6.38)	0.52
12. Assisting a physician during blood loss	4.62 ± 2.44	7.20 ± 1.61	2.66 (7.22–4.56)	<0.05	6.99 ± 1.64	−0.36 (6.98–7.34)	<0.05
13. Managing blood loss under supervision of obstetrician	4.94 ± 2.46	7.25 ± 1.62	2.39 (7.26–4.88)	<0.05	7.10 ± 1.79	−0.28 (7.08–7.36)	0.10
14. Managing blood loss under supervision of a medical intern	4.55 ± 2.33	6.90 ± 1.66	2.42 (6.91–4.49)	<0.05	6.92 ± 1.80	−0.10 (6.89–6.99)	0.55
15. Managing blood loss without supervision	1.65 ± 1.90	4.93 ± 1.96	3.38 (4.94–1.57)	<0.05	4.59 ± 2.20	−0.48 (4.56–5.04)	<0.05

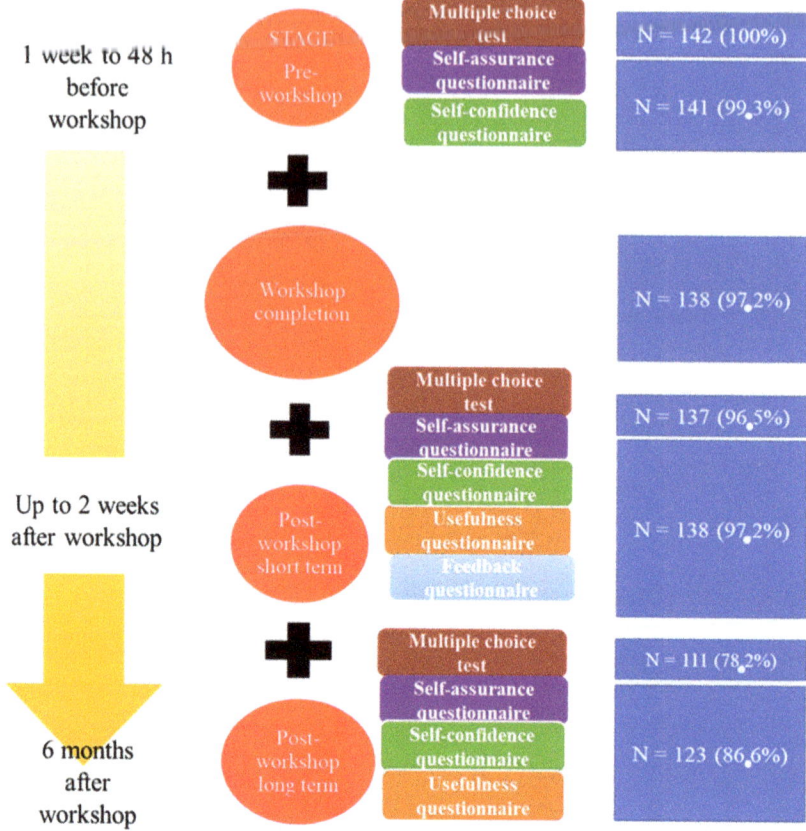

Figure 3. Workshop stages, tasks and participation.

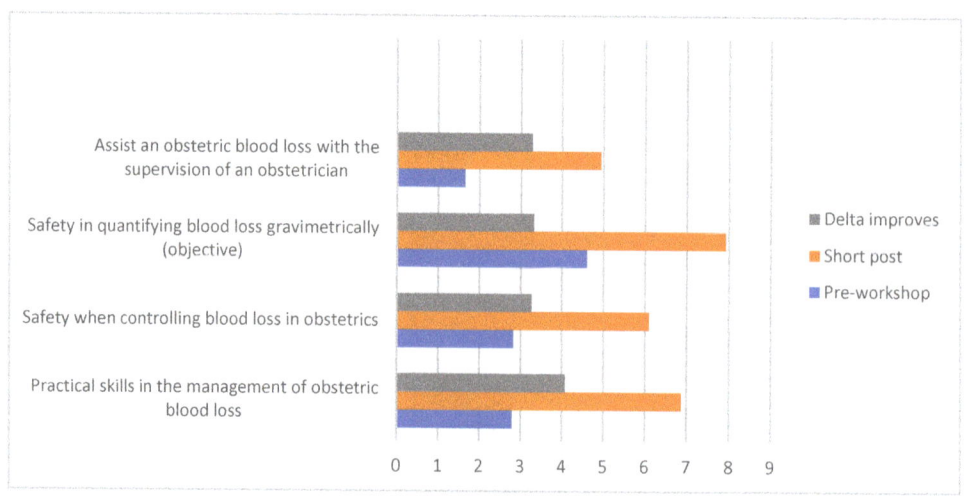

Figure 4. Aptitudes returning the greater improvement delta for pre-workshop vs. 2 weeks post-workshop.

Table 5. Results of the perceived usefulness questionnaire and improvements during the study course. WS = workshop; wk= week; mo = month; BLQ = blood loss quantification.

	Perceived Usefulness Questionnaire			
	Post-WS 2 Weeks (N = 138)	Post-WS 6 Months (N = 123)	Long-Term Improvement (μ 6 mo—μ 2 wk) (N = 121)	p
16. WS usefulness	9.14 ± 1.02	8.98 ± 1.19	−0.16 ± 1.19 (8.98–9.14)	0.13
17. Improved BLQ theoretical knowledge	8.97 ± 1.20	8.99 ± 1.11	0.06 ± 1.31 (8.98–8.93)	0.63
18. Improved BLQ practical knowledge	9.04 ± 1.06	8.68 ± 1.39	−0.34 ± 1.41 (8.67–9.02)	<0.05
19. Reduced stress when faced with blood loss	8.38 ± 1.30	8.07 ± 1.56	−0.34 ± 1.45 (8.06–8.39)	<0.05
20. WS needed in theoretical terms	8.96 ± 1.38	8.81 ± 1.57	−0.14 ± 1.82 (8.80–8.94)	0.40
21. WS needed in practical terms	9.31 ± 1.04	9.23 ± 1.11	−0.12 ± 1.08 (9.22–9.34)	0.24
22. WS should be obligatory	9.02 ± 1.39	8.85 ± 1.41	−0.16 ± 1.36 (8.84–8.99)	0.21

4. Discussion

Initially, 142 medical students signed up for the simulation-based workshop on blood loss quantification in Obstetrics. Participation was high in most study stages (>95%), although this proportion decreased to 78.2% in the long-term stage after the workshop. Theoretical and practical knowledge assessed in the MCT improved significantly from the pre- to short-term post-workshop stages, although this improvement did not persist over time. The self-assurance and confidence of the students also showed significant improvement from before to 2 weeks after the workshop, and these two improvements continued in the long term. The questionnaire designed to assess how useful the workshop was perceived by the students was clear in indicating that they found it useful and necessary for their training.

Despite the high workload involving three MCTs and nine questionnaires to be completed over 6 months, the participation rate in all consecutive stages of this study was high. This high participation highlights how receptive our medical students were to simulation-based training extending for a period of 6 months. The teaching unit of the HUGM hosts a large number of students every year. Furthermore, the division of the workshop into several stages offers continuity in the follow up of students, and the *"on-line"* platform (www.aleesca.es/moodle, accessed on 18 August 2021) offers rapid easy access to the teaching material. Other studies that have assessed a simulation-based approach to blood loss quantification in Obstetrics include one conducted in 44 medicine undergraduates [14], and another one in a setting of midwifery with 65 participants [15]. These studies, nevertheless, had different objectives and procedures than our investigation.

According to the MCT results regarding the acquisition of theoretical–practical knowledge, we should mention that starting from a high mean pre-workshop score of 7.47, this score went up significantly in the short term by one point, and thereafter returned to baseline values at 6 months post-workshop. While this increase may seem unsurprising, we should not forget that the students maintained a high grade (7–9 out of 10) throughout the process, even in the long term, when they had not recently revised the theory of blood loss quantification. Certainly, the study proves the necessity to organize similar repeated training, since the results obtained before the workshop and after 6 months are almost identical (7.47 ± 1.66 vs. 7.47 ± 1.24). This highlights the importance of periodic training to update the management of many obstetric emergencies.

According to the results of other studies [14], student understanding of this topic did not significantly improve after clinical simulation. However, in a study with participants who were midwives, an improvement in understanding along with improved efficiency was observed compared with a group of midwives not completing the clinical simulation course [12].

For most of the questionnaire items related to the self-assurance and confidence of our participants, scores increased by a mean of more than 2.5 points. This has also been observed by others who observed the improved confidence of midwives assisting a simulation-based course on postpartum blood loss management, although the method used to assess confidence was not specified [15]. In our study, not only were participant replies collected adequately in terms of time and manner, but we also performed a comparative analysis and obtained statistical significance.

Among the limitations of this study is the drop out of some participants at 6 months post-workshop. This loss of students to follow up was likely due to a loss of motivation over time, or the lack of interest of a minority of students whose performance was below the average. In an analysis of the 25 students lost to follow up, it was observed that their mean MCT score at 2 weeks post-workshop was 7.8, while the mean for the whole group was 8.5.

Another limitation was the lack of a control group of students who did not complete the workshop. As the workshop was offered to all students in their fourth year of Medicine, a participation bias of the most applied students was assumed. We, nevertheless, consider the excellent participation rate of 97.2% a main strength of this study.

As only medical students were enrolled, we could not assess the role of this simulation-based workshop in improving the routine management of real patients with obstetric haemorrhage. This could be resolved if this workshop was offered to resident doctors, obstetricians or midwives. This issue was addressed in a rural hospital in Tanzania, and the authors concluded that clinical simulation can lead to a 38% reduction in the number of patients experiencing postpartum haemorrhage [16].

Among the study strengths, as far as we are aware, no published study has had the same objectives and methods as ours. We should also mention the larger sample size than described in most published reports [14,15], and highlight the excellent response shown by the students throughout the whole study period.

Finally, our students perceived the simulation-based workshop as useful and necessary. To our knowledge, these characteristics have not been assessed previously in similar studies in the field of obstetrics. We feel that exploring factors such as these is essential to determine the impact of this type of intervention on student behaviour and learning.

5. Conclusions

This simulation-based blood loss quantification workshop designed for medical students in their fourth year resulted in significant improvements in the theoretical–practical learning curve in the short term. Further improvements noted were the increased self-assurance and self-confidence of the students when facing this clinical situation. The workshop was also perceived as useful and necessary for their academic training. Based on these findings, we would recommend the use of more clinical reconstruction teaching interventions in faculties of medicine, as they seem much appreciated by students.

Author Contributions: Conceptualization, J.R.-L., C.B.A., J.A.D.L.-L.; methodology, J.R.-L., C.B.A., J.A.D.L.-L.; investigation, A.M.M., P.P.R., B.G.G., J.M.P.M., M.S.R., Á.V.G., L.S., M.Á.-M., M.A.O., C.B.A., J.A.D.L.-L.; resources, M.Á.-M., C.B.A., J.A.D.L.-L.; writing—original draft preparation, J.R.-L., A.M.M., P.P.R., B.G.G., J.M.P.M., M.S.R., Á.V.G., L.S., M.Á.-M., M.A.O., C.B.A., J.A.D.L.-L.; writing—review and editing, J.R.-L., A.M.M., P.P.R., B.G.G., J.M.P.M., M.S.R., Á.V.G., L.S., M.Á.-M., M.A.O., C.B.A., J.A.D.L.-L.; supervision, M.Á.-M., C.B.A., J.A.D.L.-L.; project administration, M.A.O.; funding acquisition, M.Á.-M. All authors have read and agreed to the published version of the manuscript.

Funding: This study (FIS-PI18/00912, PI21/01244) was supported by the Instituto de Salud Carlos III (Plan Estatal de I + D+I 2013–2016) and cofinanced by the European Development Regional Fund "A way to achieve Europe" (ERDF) and B2017/BMD-3804 MITIC-CM, B2020/MITICAD-CM funded as part of the Union response to the pandemic of COVID-19 and Halekulani S.L.

Institutional Review Board Statement: Not applicable.

Informed Consent Statement: Not applicable.

Data Availability Statement: The data used to support the findings of the present study are available from the corresponding author upon request.

Acknowledgments: Juan Laso Perez; Ignacio Cueto Hernandez; Nieves Cuesta Campins; Barbara Maricalva; Esther Garcia Ruiz; Maria del Carmen Muñoz Serrano; Carmen Viñuela Beneitez; Raquel Pérez Lucas; Elisa Sáez Cereceda; Francisco José Amor Valera; Carlos Alonso Mayo; Ignacio Romero Martínez; María López Altuna; Marina Inmaculada Díaz Perdigón; Mireia Bernal Claverol; Irene Aracil Moreno; María Ruiz Minaya; Camilo Galvis Isaza; Rocío Aracil Rodríguez; Laura Pérez Burrel; Ainoa Sáez Prat; Andrea Fraile López; Beatriz Gutiérrez Del Río; María Fernández Muñoz; Marta Feltrer Hidalgo; Zuriñe Raquel Reyes Angulo.

Conflicts of Interest: The authors declare no conflict of interest.

Appendix A. Self-Confidence, Self-Assurance, Usefulness and Feedback Questionnaires

	Self-assurance					
	Question			Reply		
1.	How would you describe your theoretical knowledge of blood loss quantification?	Poor (0–2)	Medium (3–4)	Good (5–6)	Very good (7–8)	Excellent (9–10)
2.	How would you describe your practical knowledge of blood loss quantification?	Poor (0–2)	Medium (3–4)	Good (5–6)	Very good (7–8)	Excellent (9–10)
3.	How would you describe your practical skills in managing obstetric blood loss?	Poor (0–2)	Medium (3–4)	Good (5–6)	Very good (7–8)	Excellent (9–10)
	Self-confidence					
	Question			Reply		
1.	How confident are you at dealing with obstetric blood loss?	Not at all (0–2)	Scarcely (3–4)	Somewhat (5–6)	Confident (7–8)	Very (9–10)
2.	How confident are you at controlling blood loss?	Not at all (0–2)	Scarcely (3–4)	Somewhat (5–6)	Confident (7–8)	Very (9–10)
3.	How confident are you at controlling the initial situation?	Not at all (0–2)	Scarcely (3–4)	Somewhat (5–6)	Confident (7–8)	Very (9–10)
4.	How confident are you at quantifying blood loss visually (subjective)?	Not at all (0–2)	Scarcely (3–4)	Somewhat (5–6)	Confident (7–8)	Very (9–10)
5.	How confident are you at quantifying blood loss gravimetrically (objective)?	Not at all (0–2)	Scarcely (3–4)	Somewhat (5–6)	Confident (7–8)	Very (9–10)
6.	How confident are you at differentiating between mild and severe blood loss?	Not at all (0–2)	Scarcely (3–4)	Somewhat (5–6)	Confident (7–8)	Very (9–10)
7.	How confident are you at coordinating with the medical staff present?	Not at all (0–2)	Scarcely (3–4)	Somewhat (5–6)	Confident (7–8)	Very (9–10)
8.	How confident are you at preventing severe blood loss?	Not at all (0–2)	Scarcely (3–4)	Somewhat (5–6)	Confident (7–8)	Very (9–10)
9.	How confident would you feel assisting a clinician during a blood loss episode?	Not at all (0–2)	Scarcely (3–4)	Somewhat (5–6)	Confident (7–8)	Very (9–10)

	Question			Reply		
		Self-confidence				
10.	How confident would you feel assisting an obstetrician during a blood loss episode?	Not at all (0–2)	Scarcely (3–4)	Somewhat (5–6)	Confident (7–8)	Very (9–10)
11.	How confident would you feel under the supervision of a resident doctor?	Not at all (0–2)	Scarcely (3–4)	Somewhat (5–6)	Confident (7–8)	Very (9–10)
12.	How confident would you feel assisting a blood loss episode without supervision?	Not at all (0–2)	Scarcely (3–4)	Somewhat (5–6)	Confident (7–8)	Very (9–10)

	Statement			Agreement level		
		Perceived usefulness				
1.	I found the workshop useful	No, not at all (0–2)	No, not really (3–4)	Indifferent (5–6)	Yes (7–8)	Yes, definitely (9–10)
2.	My theoretical knowledge of obstetric blood loss has improved	No, not at all (0–2)	No, not really (3–4)	Indifferent (5–6)	Yes (7–8)	Yes, definitely (9–10)
3.	My practical knowledge of obstetric blood loss has improved	No, not at all (0–2)	No, not really (3–4)	Indifferent (5–6)	Yes (7–8)	Yes, definitely (9–10)
4.	This workshop will reduce my stress levels when dealing with a blood loss episode in the future.	No, not at all (0–2)	No, not really (3–4)	Indifferent (5–6)	Yes (7–8)	Yes, definitely (9–10)
5.	This workshop is necessary to gain theoretical knowledge	No, not at all (0–2)	No, not really (3–4)	Indifferent (5–6)	Yes (7–8)	Yes, definitely (9–10)
6.	This workshop is necessary to gain practical knowledge	No, not at all (0–2)	No, not really (3–4)	Indifferent (5–6)	Yes (7–8)	Yes, definitely (9–10)
7.	This workshop should be obligatory for all medical undergraduates	No, not at all (0–2)	No, not really (3–4)	Indifferent (5–6)	Yes (7–8)	Yes, definitely (9–10)

	Question		Reply (mark one or several)		
		Feedback			
1.	How did you feel about assisting the workshop?	Curious	Unsure	Anxious	None of these
2.	How did you feel when conducting the simulation?	Sure of yourself	Confused	Stressed/tense	None of these
3.	How do you feel about the feedback session?	It was useful	It helped me connect with my peers and share our ideas	It was an opportunity to confront each other	None of these

References

1. Vázquez-Mata, G.; Guillamet-Lloveras, A. El entrenamiento basado en la simulación como innovación imprescindible en la formación médica. *Educ. Méd.* **2009**, *12*, 149–155. [CrossRef]
2. Hemorrhage, P. Practice bulletin no. 183: Postpartum hemorrhage: Postpartum hemorrhage. *Obstet. Gynecol.* **2017**, *130*, e168–e181.
3. Bose, P.; Regan, F.; Paterson-Brown, S. Improving the accuracy of estimated blood loss at obstetric haemorrhage using clinical reconstructions. *BJOG* **2006**, *113*, 919–924. [CrossRef] [PubMed]
4. Say, L.; Chou, D.; Gemmill, A.; Tunçalp, Ö.; Moller, A.-B.; Daniels, J.; Gülmezoglu, A.M.; Temmerman, M.; Alkema, L. Global causes of maternal death: A WHO systematic analysis. *Lancet Glob. Health* **2014**, *2*, e323–e333. [CrossRef]

5. Larroca, S.G.-T.; Amor Valera, F.; Herrera, E.A.; Hernandez, I.C.; Lopez, Y.C.; De Leon-Luis, J. Human Development Index of the maternal country of origin and its relationship with maternal near miss: A systematic review of the literature. *BMC Pregnancy Childbirth* **2020**, *20*, 224.
6. Ruiz Labarta, F.J.; Pintado Recarte, M.P.; Joigneau Prieto, L.; Bravo Arribas, C.; Bujan, J.; Ortega, M.A.; De León-Luis, J.A. Factors associated with failure of Bakri balloon tamponade for the management of postpartum haemorrhage. Case series study and systematic review. *Healthcare* **2021**, *9*, 295. [CrossRef]
7. Ruiz Labarta, F.J.; Pintado Recarte, M.P.; Alvarez Luque, A.; Joigneau Prieto, L.; Perez Martín, L.; Gonzalez Leyte, M.; Abizanada Palacio, F.; Ramirez Morillas, F.; Perez Corral, A.; Quintana Ortiz, L.; et al. Outcomes of pelvic arterial embolization in the management of postpartum haemorrhage: A case series study and systematic review. *Eur. J. Obstet. Gynecol. Reprod. Biol.* **2016**, *206*, 12–21. [CrossRef]
8. American College of Obstetricians and Gynecologists. *Quantitative Blood Loss in Obstetric Hemorrhage: Acog Committee Opinion, Number 794*; ACOG: Washington, DC, USA, 2019. [CrossRef]
9. American College of Obstetricians and Gynecologists. ACOG Practice Bulletin: Clinical Management Guidelines for Obstetrician-Gynecologists Number 76, October 2006: Postpartum hemorrhage. *Obstet. Gynecol.* **2006**, *108*, 1039–1047.
10. Street, N.W. Quantification of blood loss: AWHONN practice brief number 1. *J. Obstet. Gynecol. Neonatal. Nurs.* **2015**, *44*, 158–160. [CrossRef] [PubMed]
11. Al-Kadri, H.M.; Dahlawi, H.; Al Airan, M.; Elsherif, E.; Tawfeeq, N.; Mokhele, Y.; Brown, D.; Tamim, H.M. Effect of education and clinical assessment on the accuracy of post partum blood loss estimation. *BMC Pregnancy Childbirth* **2014**, *14*, 110. [CrossRef] [PubMed]
12. Kato, C.; Kataoka, Y. Simulation training program for midwives to manage postpartum hemorrhage: A randomized controlled trial. *Nurse Educ. Today* **2017**, *51*, 88–95. [CrossRef] [PubMed]
13. Matas, A. Diseño del formato de escalas tipo Likert: Un estado de la cuestión. *Rev. Electrón. Investig. Educ.* **2018**, *20*, 38–47. [CrossRef]
14. Mclelland, G.; Tremayne, A.; Carr, B.; Hall, H.; Plummer, V.; Kumar, A.; Corlass, A.; East, C.; Buttigieg, H.; Fernando, S.; et al. Learning together to manage simulated postpartum haemorrhage: Undergraduate midwifery and medical students' satisfaction with simulation and impact upon self-efficacy. *Women Birth.* **2019**, *32*, S6–S7. [CrossRef]
15. Mohamed, A.E.E.; Mostafa, E.H. Effect of simulation based training on maternity nurses' performance and self-confidence regarding primary postpartum hemorrhage management. *Am. J. Nurs. Res.* **2018**, *6*, 388–397. [CrossRef]
16. Nelissen, E.; Ersdal, H.; Mduma, E.; Evjen-Olsen, B.; Twisk, J.; Broerse, J.; van Roosmalen, J.; Stekelenburg, J. Clinical performance and patient outcome after simulation-based training in prevention and management of postpartum haemorrhage: An educational intervention study in a low-resource setting. *BMC Pregnancy Childbirth* **2017**, *17*. [CrossRef] [PubMed]

A Preliminary Italian Cross-Sectional Study on the Level of Digital Psychiatry Training, Knowledge, Beliefs and Experiences among Medical Students, Psychiatry Trainees and Professionals

Laura Orsolini [1], Silvia Bellagamba [1], Virginia Marchetti [2], Giulia Menculini [3], Silvia Tempia Valenta [1], Virginio Salvi [1] and Umberto Volpe [1,*]

1 Unit of Clinical Psychiatry, Department of Neurosciences/DIMSC, Polytechnic University of Marche, 60126 Ancona, Italy; l.orsolini@staff.univpm.it (L.O.); silvibella95@gmail.com (S.B.); silvia.tempia@gmail.com (S.T.V.); v.salvi@staff.univpm.it (V.S.)
2 School of Medicine and Surgery, Polytechnic University of Marche, 60126 Ancona, Italy; virginiamarchettivm@gmail.com
3 Department of Psychiatry, University of Perugia, 06100 Perugia, Italy; giuliamenculini@gmail.com
* Correspondence: u.volpe@staff.univpm.it

Abstract: The COVID-19 pandemic led to the implementation of digital psychiatry (DP), resulting in the need for a new skilled healthcare workforce. The purpose of this study was to investigate the level of training, knowledge, beliefs, and experiences of young mental health professionals and medical students in DP. An ad hoc cross-sectional survey was administered and descriptive analyses, Student's t and ANOVA tests were conducted, together with an exploratory factor analysis, bivariate correlations and linear regression. Most of the sample (N = 239) declared that DP was never discussed within their academic training (89.1%), mainly revealing an overall lack of knowledge on the issue. Nevertheless, subjects mostly declared that DP represents a valuable therapeutic tool in mental health (80%) and that their training should include this topic (54.4%). Moreover, most subjects declared that digital interventions are less effective than face-to-face ones (73.2%), despite the emerging evidence that being trained in DP is significantly associated with the belief that digital and in-person interventions are comparable in their effectiveness ($p \leq 0.05$). Strong positive correlations were found between the knowledge score (KS) and perceived significance index (PSI) (r = 0.148, $p < 0.001$), and KS and Digital Psychiatry Opinion (DPO) index (r = 0.193, $p < 0.001$). PSI scores statistically significantly predicted KS total scores (F(1, 237) = 5.283, R^2 = 0.022, p = 0.022). KS scores statistically significantly predicted DPO total scores (F(1, 237) = 9.136, R^2 = 0.037, p = 0.003). During the current pandemic, DP represented an ideal response to the forced physical distancing by ensuring the advantage of greater access to care. However, this kind of intervention is still uncommon, and mental health professionals still prove to be skeptical. The lack of formal training on DP during the academic years could be a limiting factor.

Keywords: digital psychiatry; education; psychiatry training; telepsychiatry; trainees

1. Introduction

The term telemedicine (TM) refers to a way of providing healthcare services through the use of innovative technologies, particularly Information and Communication Technologies (ICTs), in those circumstances in which the health professional and the patient are not in the same place. The term TM, literally meaning "healing at a distance", was coined in 1970, referring to care programs addressed to geographically isolated patients [1]. The origins of this technology date back to the early 20th century, and in the subsequent decades rapidly evolved from the spread of the Erickson's Bakelite telephones, the advent of the Internet and ICTs until the development of online video-communication services (e.g., Zoom

Cloud Meeting, Google LLC Meet). This innovation has implemented increasingly effective remote health care, which nowadays represent a valid and cost-effective alternative to the traditional in-patient interventions in various specialty areas of medicine [2–4]. In recent years, before the COVID-19 pandemic, the annual number of TM visits has increased enormously, with an estimated compound annual growth rate of 52% from 2005 to 2014 and 261% from 2015 to 2017 [5]. The current health emergency is rapidly transforming the medical care system, driving the use of TM to a further exponential increase, the full extent of which is still being measured with the present knowledge [6]. Early estimates conducted by McKinsey & Company suggested that telehealth increased 38-fold during the timeframe winter 2020 and winter 2021, with a usage peak during April 2020 and subsequent stabilization in the subsequent months [6].

Telepsychiatry (TP) refers to the usage of ICTs in mental health care and treatment. It represents one of the earliest adaptations of TM in the field of medicine [7]. Nowadays, TP is the second most applicable type of TM globally (following teleradiology) [8,9]. If compared to TP, the concept of telemental health (TMH) has a more recent origin and a broader meaning, encompassing all technology-mediated modes of communication and referring to the use of ICTs for diagnostic, therapeutic, preventive, educational, and administrative purposes. The services supplied by TMH are provided not only by psychiatrists but also by a broader range of professionals. Further, TMH includes both synchronous (that take place simultaneously in different locations—such as videoconferencing or via telephone) and asynchronous modalities (that occur at different places and times—such as messaging or smartphone apps) [10]. Videoconferencing represents the most frequently applied modality, approaching the traditional setting of the doctor-patient interview [11]. The latest denomination of TMH is e-mental health (EMH), which similarly relates to the provision of care services through electronic media. EMH refers to a user-centered model of care, increasingly personalized to the user's needs [12]. Another contemporary terminology is digital psychiatry (DP), defining a highly tailored and confidential care relationship through the use of an intuitive interface, and Digital Health Interventions (DHI) which include all health interventions virtually delivered [13].

The COVID-19 pandemic disproportionately impacted mental health services worldwide [14–17]. The pandemic-related outbreak and relative restrictive measures determined, on the one hand, the abrupt discontinuation in the traditional mental health care; on the other hand, the rapid modification of services to guarantee both the continuity of treatment in usual patients and the access of new ones [18–20]. Among these adaptations, the implementation of TMH and TP services has allowed the substitution of traditional in-person interventions in respect of the norms of physical distancing [21]. However, not all countries and mental health services, including Italy, were adequately prepared for this "digital revolution" since TP-related topics are rarely included in academic formation. Therefore, the primary objective of the present work aims to preliminarily explore the level of training, knowledge, beliefs, and experiences in the field of DP and related topics (i.e., TM, TP, TMH, EMH, DP, DHIs) at different stages of training in a cohort of Italian medical students, psychiatry trainees, and early career psychiatrists (ECPs). Secondly, explore if any determinants (i.e., the level of training, the level of clinical practice experience) may influence the level of knowledge of DP and related topics. Finally, explore if any determinants (i.e., the level of training, the level of clinical experience, the level of knowledge in DP and related topics) may influence the beliefs and/or opinions of Italian medical students, psychiatry trainees, and early career psychiatrists (ECPs) in the field of DP and related topics (i.e., TM, TP, TMH, EMH, DP, DHIs).

2. Materials and Methods

An ad hoc cross-sectional online survey was designed using Google LLC Forms and disseminated, in both digital and paper form, from 28 September 2020 to 7 April 2021. The link to participate was shared using social platforms, such as Facebook, WhatsApp, and Instagram. The survey was also administered in paper form to all medical students who attended the SOD Unit of Clinical Psychiatry at the Azienda Ospedaliero-Universitaria "Ospedali Riuniti", in Ancona, Italy.

All recruited participants met the following inclusion criteria: (a) being an Italian medical student, a medical doctor waiting to start a psychiatry training program, a psychiatry trainee, or an ECP (i.e., a young psychiatrist within five years of their psychiatry training program or less than 40 years old); (b) being able and willing to provide consent to participate in the study and authorization to analyze data for research purposes; (c) filling out all sections and questions of the survey.

The survey consisted of four main sections. The first focused on sociodemographic data and included ten questions (seven multiple-choice and three open-ended questions). This first section was designed to collect general data on participants (i.e., sex, age, civil status, socio-economic status, current year of university study, current year of psychiatry training, how many years post-psychiatry training program were passed, country of origin, country of university studies, and so forth).

The second section consisted of 20 questions (14 multiple-choice and six 5-point Likert rating scale questions) designed to collect information regarding academic training (if any) in the field of DP and related topics (i.e., TM, TP, TMH, EMH, DP, DHIs). The six 5-point Likert rating scale items (items 9–14 of the second section) were developed to assess the level of participant's perceived significance derived by the implementation of DP and related topics (i.e., TM, TP, TMH, EMH, DP, DHIs) during the Faculty of Medicine and during the Psychiatry Training Program, that it was named 'Perceived Significance Index' (PSI). The PSI is the sum of items 9–14 of the second section and ranges 5–25. The internal consistency was determined from Cronbach's alpha calculation, considering that a Cronbach's alpha of 0.70 or higher was adequate if the objective of the scale is for use in research [22].

The third section included 19 multiple-choice questions designed to explore participants' level of knowledge on the topic. This section was used to build an index named Knowledge Score (KS), indicating the overall level of knowledge of the participants based on the sum of their correct answers. The KS represents a continuous variable that was developed to compare the level of knowledge in the field of DP and related topics according the level of training (i.e., the four subgroups constituted by medical students, medical doctors waiting to start a psychiatry training program, psychiatry trainees and ECPs), and according to the level of clinical experiences in the field of DP and related topics (i.e., TM, TP, TMH, EMH, DP, DHIs), as measured by the exploratory items contained in the second section specifically investigating which topics of DP and at which levels of training have been taught.

The fourth section consisted of 34 questions (5-point Likert rating scale) designed to investigate participants' opinions on DP and related topics (i.e., TM, TP, TMH, EMH, DP, DHIs). The total score derived by the sum of all items of the fourth section was named Digital Psychiatry Opinion index (DPO). The Kaiser-Mayer-Olkin (KMO) measure of sampling adequacy suggested that the sample was favourable (KMO = 0.936) and the Bartlett's test of Sphericity was highly significant (χ^2 = 6723.041, df = 561, $p < 0.001$). Thereafter, an exploratory factor analysis (EFA) was performed with the principal components extraction method and the Kaiser-Varimax rotation method. The number of factors was determined by the size of eigenvalues (>1) and the variance explained by each factor, as well as the coherence and interpretability of the factors. Items allocated to a specific factor were based on a loading of more than 0.50 on the corresponding factor, and items were excluded when the difference of factor loadings was less than 0.49. Lastly, the internal consistency was determined from Cronbach's alpha calculation, considering that a Cronbach's alpha of 0.70 or higher was adequate [22].

Statistical analysis, including EFA, was conducted using Statistical Package for Social Sciences (SPSS) software for macOS (version 26.0, IBM Corp., Armonk, NY, USA, 2019). Categorical variables were summarized as frequencies and percentages (N; %), while continuous variables (age, PSI, KS, DPO and related factors) were reported as mean and standard deviation (S.D.). The normality of continuous variables was analyzed by using the Kolmogorov-Smirnov and Shapiro-Wilk normality tests. Student's *t*-test or analysis of variance (ANOVA), when appropriate, were used to compare the KS according to: (1) the level of training (i.e., the four subgroups constituted by medical students, a medical doctor waiting to start a psychiatry training program, psychiatry trainees and early career psychiatrists; (2) the level of theoretical and/or practical training experiences (i.e., whether and which DP and related topics were taught from a theoretical and/or practical point of view). Mann-Whitney U or Kruskal-Wallis test, when appropriate, were used to compare the PSI, DPO and related factors according to: (1) the level of training (i.e., the four subgroups constituted by medical students, a medical doctor waiting to start a psychiatry training program, psychiatry trainees and early career psychiatrists; (2) the level of theoretical and practical training experiences (i.e., whether and which DP and related topics were taught from a theoretical and/or practical point of view). Bivariate Pearson's correlations were used to investigate potential relationships between DPO and KS, DPO and PSI, and KS and PSI scores. Linear regression analysis was performed to investigate the associations between DPO and KS, DPO and PSI, and KS and PSI scores. The level of significance was set at $\alpha \leq 0.05$, and all hypotheses were two-tailed.

3. Results

3.1. Sociodemographic Results

Key sociodemographic characteristics are summarized in Table 1. The final sample included 239 subjects, of which the majority were female. The mean age was 26.6 ($\pm$SD = 3.9) years, ranging from 19 to 41 years. Regarding marital and economic status, the majority were single/unmarried and belonging to the middle class. Regarding current college/work status, slightly over a half were medical students, and the remaining were newly qualified doctors, psychiatry trainees, and ECPs, approximately one-third each one. Among medical students, the majority attended the fifth or sixth year. Within the sample of psychiatry trainees, most reported attending the first year of their psychiatry training program. The majority of the sample stated that they were studying/working in Italy.

3.2. Training in Digital Psychiatry

Most of the sample stated that the topics of TM, EH, EMH, and DP had not been taught within their medical school training, and, whereas these topics were discussed in the academic setting, the time dedicated to them was little, i.e., less than 20% of the total training time (N = 222; 92.9%). Nevertheless, more than half of the sample declared that implementing a course/module about TM (N = 133; 55.6%) or EH (N = 148; 62%) within the medical school would be important. Similarly, almost all the sample stated that no training in DP was provided within the psychiatry training program or they were unaware of it (N = 230; 96.2%). However, the majority declared that implementing a course/module on TP (N = 174; 72.8%), DP (N = 182; 76.2%), or EMH (N = 185; 77.4%) within the psychiatry training program would be important. Furthermore, 33 subjects reported to have applied their DP-related knowledge in their clinical practice (13.8%), and 11 declared to have used it moderately (i.e., about 1–2 times/month) even before the onset of the COVID-19 pandemic (4.6%). Finally, 15 subjects reported that they had never applied DP before the COVID-19 pandemic (6.3%), and 11 declared that the pandemic slightly intensified the use of DP (4.6%). The PSI score showed an excellent internal consistency (Cronbach's α of 0.92). The mean average of PSI was 23.1 (SD = 4.7), without any significant sex-based differences ($p = 0.496$) (Table 2). Interestingly, psychiatry trainees showed significantly lower PSI scores compared to ECPs ($p = 0.007$) and newly qualified M.D. waiting for a psychiatry training program ($p = 0.011$); while medical students showed significantly lower PSI scores compared to ECPs ($p = 0.047$) (Table 3).

Table 1. Socio-demographic data of the sample.

Socio-Demographic Data of the Sample			
Variable	Answer	N	%
Sex	Male	92	38.5
	Female	147	61.5
Marital status	Single/unmarried	202	84.5
	Married/cohabiting	37	15.5
Economic status (optional item)	Low	15	6.3
	Average	175	73.2
	High	41	17.2
	Not known	8	3.3
Current position	Medical students	140	58.6
	First year	1	0.7
	Second year	1	0.7
	Third year	5	3.6
	Fourth year	10	7.1
	Fifth year	25	17.9
	Sixth year	98	70
	Newly qualified doctors	34	14.2
	Psychiatry residents	39	16.3
	First year	22	56.4
	Second year	7	18
	Third year	8	20.5
	Fourth year	2	5.1
	ECPs	26	10.9
	<1 year	8	30.8
	1–2 years	4	15.4
	2–3 years	2	7.6
	4–5 years	4	15.4
	3–4 years	8	30.8
Medical school country	Italy	236	98.7
	Foreign	3	1.3
Psychiatry residency country	Italy	63	96.9
	Foreign	2	3.1

N: frequency; %: percentage; ECP: Early Career Psychiatrist.

Table 2. Perceived Significance Index according to socio-demographic and training variables.

	Mean	SD	p-Value *,**
Male	22.8	4.8	* 0.496
Female	23.2	4.7	
Single/unmarried	22.9	4.7	* 0.150
Married/cohabiting	24	5	
Low income	22.9	4.8	** 0.680
Medium income	23.2	4.7	
High income	22.8	5.2	
Medical Students	22.8	4.8	** 0.015
Newly qualified M.D.	24.6	3.6	
Psychiatry residents	21.7	4.4	
ECP	24.7	5.3	

Table 2. Cont.

	Mean	SD	p-Value *,**
Medical Students			
First Year	n.m.	n.m.	
Second Year	n.m.	n.m.	
Third Year	21.6	5.4	** 0.558
Fourth Year	24.6	3.4	
Fifth Year	21.6	5.1	
Sixth Year	22.9	4.8	
Psychiatry residents			
First Year	22	4.1	
Second Year	20.6	5.7	** 0.968
Third Year	21.6	4.5	
Fourth Year	23	7.1	
ECP			
<1 year	23.5	5.8	
1–2 years	22	6.7	
2–3 years	22	7	** 0.575
3–4 years	26.2	5	
4–5 years	26.5	4.2	
Taught TM in Medicine Faculty			
Yes	22.6	4.4	* 0.446
No	23.1	4.8	
Taught EH in Medicine Faculty			
Yes	20.4	4.5	* **0.025**
No	23.2	4.7	
Taught EMH in Psychiatry Training Programme			
Yes	20.4	4.7	* 0.308
No	23.2	4.7	
Taught DP in Psychiatry Training Programme			
Yes	21.8	5.7	** 0.882
No	23.2	4.7	
Type of DP Training			
Only theoretical	18	0	
Only Practical	n.m.	n.m.	** 0.151
Theoretical and Practical	23.2	3.6	
Clinical Practice in DP			
Qualified, Yes	24.3	4.7	
Qualified, No	23	4.7	** 0.235
Not Qualified, No	22.8	4.8	
How much COVID-19 pandemic favoured the implementation of DP in my clinical practice?			
None change	23.8	4	
Slight change	21.7	6.7	** 0.324
Moderate change	26.3	3.7	
Substantial change	25.6	4	

M: mean; SD: standard deviation; ECP: Early Career Psychiatrists; n.m.: not measurable. * Mann Whitney's U-test; ** Kruskal-Wallis test. Bold number indicates significant p-value.

Table 3. Pairwise comparisons PSI according to the level of training.

Sample 1–Sample 2	Statistics of Test	Standard Error	Statistics of Standard Test	p-Value
Psychiatry Trainee vs. Medical Student	18.017	12.472	1.445	0.149
Psychiatry Trainee vs. Newly qualified medical doctor	41.127	16.162	2.545	**0.011**
Psychiatry Trainee vs. ECP	−47.192	17.440	−2.706	**0.007**
Medical Student vs. Newly qualified medical doctor	−23.110	13.170	−1.755	0.079
Medical Student vs. ECP	−29.175	14.710	−1.983	**0.047**
Newly qualified medical doctor vs. ECP	−6.066	17.946	−0.338	0.735

ECP: early career psychiatrist. Each line runs a statistical test according to the null hypothesis that the distribution between sample 1 and sample 2 are identical. The asymptotic significance (2-way) are represented in the table with a significance level set at 0.05. Bold number indicates significant p-value.

3.3. Level of Knowledge on Digital Psychiatry

More than half of the sample (N = 134; 56.1%) gave an incorrect definition of EH; conversely, most of the sample correctly defined TP (N = 176; 73.6%) and TM (N = 137; 57.3%). Regarding the main targets of TM, the majority of the sample indicated most of the correct answers. Concerning the sub-specialties included in the DP, over half of the sample correctly identified TP, EMH, and TM, while only the minority of the sample indicated phone-, chat-, and email-based psychiatric counseling, smartphone apps, social media. Regarding DHIs, only 24.3% (N = 58) of the participants correctly replied that they require neither physical nor temporal co-presence of clinician and patient. There were conflicting responses regarding which platforms/tools could be included in DHIs.

Obsessive-compulsive disorder (OCD), post-traumatic stress disorder (PTSD), and phobias were correctly identified by the majority of the sample (N = 175; 73.2%) as mental health conditions that may be treated by using digital interventions. The majority of the sample (N = 136; 56.9%) correctly identified PTSD and attention deficit hyperactivity disorder (ADHD) as conditions for which TP is recommended. The majority of the sample (N = 164; 68.6%) also indicated paranoia and the paranoid state as contraindicated conditions in TP, in line with the International Psychoanalytic Association (IPA) guidelines. Conversely, only 22.2% of the sample (N = 53) indicated severe trauma as contraindicated conditions in TP.

Almost all the sample could not determine the historical origin of TP, while most of the sample recognized the country in which TP was born and identified videoconferencing as the most commonly used mode of communication in TP; only one-fifth of the participants were able to indicate Zoom as the platform recommended by the European Association for Psychotherapy (EAP) guidelines.

According to most participants, the patient should be able to access the Internet and use the electronic device independently (N = 210; 87.9%) and has to be skilled in electronic device characteristics and the management of their sensitive data (privacy and confidentiality) (N = 204; 85.4%). Most of the sample believe that the mental health professional should investigate the patient's attitude towards online treatment (N = 177; 74.1%) and obtain informed consent (written form) before providing a TP consultation (N = 172; 72%). In contrast, over half of the sample erroneously declared that the clinician should attend a training course/obtain a certification to use DP (N = 141; 59%).

The mean average KS was 9.9 (SD = 2.7), with statistically significantly higher scores in women ($p = 0.023$), psychiatry trainees and ECPs (in both cases, $p < 0.001$) (Table 4). As expected, statistically higher KS were reported among those who gave a correct definition of DP ($p = 0.01$), TP ($p = 0.02$), and DHIs ($p < 0.001$). Time dedicated to the topic during the training did not influence KS, even though a trend was observed ($p = 0.07$). Higher KS scores were observed in those who had applied their knowledge in digitally-delivered mental health interventions, acquired during their university and post-lauream studies, into their clinical practice ($p < 0.001$), had applied digital interventions moderately even before the COVID-19 pandemic ($p = 0.04$), had moderately or substantially increased the frequency in their use of DP during the pandemic ($p = 0.03$) (Table 4).

Table 4. Knowledge Score according to socio-demographic and training variables.

	Mean KS	SD	Statistical Test *,**	p-Value
Male	9.5	2.5	* t(237) = −2.281	0.023
Female	10.3	2.8		
Single/unmarried	9.7	2.7	** F(1) = 12.403	0.001
Married/cohabiting	11.4	2.7		
Low income	9.9	2		
Medium income	9.9	2.8	** F(3) = 0.377	0.77
High income	10.3	2.5		
Medical Students	9.1	2.4		
Newly qualified M.D.	10.4	2.9	** F(3) = 15.046	<0.001
Psychiatry residents	11.2	2.2		
ECP	12.1	2.8		
Medical Students				
First Year	10.2	n.m.		
Second Year	9.3	n.m.		
Third Year	7.8	2.6	** F(5) = 0.492	0.782
Fourth Year	9.1	2.7		
Fifth Year	8.7	2		
Sixth Year	9.2	2.6		
Psychiatry residents				
First Year	11.1	2.4		
Second Year	10.4	2.1	** F(3) = 0.176	0.912
Third Year	11.3	3.6		
Fourth Year	10.8	2.2		
ECP				
<1 year	10.8	3.2		
1–2 years	12.7	1.8		
2–3 years	9.5	5	** F(4) = 1.407	0.265
4–5 years	11	0.5		
3–4 years	13.5	3.3		
Taught TM in Medicine Faculty				
Yes	9.7	2.3	* t(237) = −0.570	0.569
No	10	2.8		
Taught EH in Medicine Faculty				
Yes	9.3	3.5	* t(237) = −0.848	0.397
No	10	2.7		
Taught EMH in Psychiatry Training Programme				
Yes	8.9	2.7	* t(213) = −1.177	0.24
No	10.1	2.7		
Taught DP in Psychiatry Training Programme				
Yes	8	2.8	* t(216) = −1.786	0.075
No	10.2	2.7		
Type of DP Training				
Only theoretical	2.6	4.2	** F(2) = 0.977	0.429
Only Practical	11.7	n.m.		
Theoretical and Practical	11.7	4.7		

Table 4. *Cont.*

	Mean KS	SD	Statistical Test *,**	*p*-Value
Clinical Practice in DP				
Qualified, Yes	11.2	3	** F(2) = 8.827	**<0.001**
Qualified, No	10.5	2.9		
Not Qualified, No	9.3	2.4		
How much COVID-19 pandemic favoured the implementation of DP in my clinical practice?				
None change	9.5	3.7	** F(3) = 3.327	**0.033**
Slight change	10.6	1.8		
Moderate change	13.2	1.5		
Substantial change	12.2	2.8		

M: mean; SD: standard deviation; ECP: Early Career Psychiatrists; n.m.: not measurable. * Student's *t*-test; ** ANOVA. Bold number indicates significant *p*-value.

3.4. The Digital Psychiatry Opinion

The majority of the sample declared that TM might improve healthcare in various conditions. Responses were uneven regarding DP's potential to provide interventions comparable to those in-person and ensure adequate privacy. More than half of the sample agreed (N = 134; 56.1%) that DP did not affect the building of a good therapeutic alliance with the patient. However, most of the sample stated that, before providing DP interventions, the clinician should accurately assess the risks versus benefits of the digital tool (N = 200; 83.7%). They also declared that DP should mainly be used for follow-up visits of already known and stable patients (N = 192; 80.4%) and that it should not be recommended during a first assessment visit (N = 179; 74.9%).

Overall, most participants declared that DP cannot wholly replace traditional in-person interventions (N = 170; 71.2%). Moreover, more than half of the sample believe that DP synchronous interventions are more effective than the asynchronous ones (N = 151; 63.1%), and a substantial part of the sample declared that DP should be provided just in synchronous mode (N = 100; 41.9%). Only 28.4% of the sample (N = 68) correctly declared that digital interventions are effective as in-person interventions, being significantly reported among those participants who declared to have received training in DP ($p = 0.01$).

EFA and scree plot indicated that 30 items out of the initial 34 items of the fourth section, loaded onto five factors with eigenvalues greater than one should be retained, accounting for 67.6% of the total variance (Figure S1). Factor 1 (named 'Mental Health Services Improvement of Digital Interventions', F1) consisted of 10 items (range 10–50) explaining 45.6% of the total variance. Factor 2 (named, 'Preliminary needed technical requirements and indications for delivering digital mental health interventions', F2) consisted of six items (range 6–30) and accounted for 9.3% of the total variance. Factor 3 (named, 'Basic needed training requirements for delivering digitally-mediated mental health interventions', F3) consisted of six items (range 6–30) accounting for 5.6% of the total variance. Factor 4 (named, 'Opinions regarding the comparable efficacy between in-person versus digitally-delivered mental health interventions', F4) consisted of four items (range 4–20) and explained 3.8% of the total variance. Factor 5 (named, 'Usability of digitally-delivered mental health interventions in special/critical situations', F5) consisted of four items (range 4–20) and accounted for 3.3% of the total variance. Pearson's correlations analyses showed that there were significant positive correlations among these five factors. Analysis of the internal consistency showed an excellent internal reliability in the DPO index (Cronbach's α of 0.961), and excellent reliability in the following retained factors (Cronbach's α of 0.945 for F1, Cronbach's α of 0.903 for F3, Cronbach's α of 0.910 for F5. While a good internal consistency was shown for F2 (Cronbach's α of 0.887) and acceptable for F4 (Cronbach's α of 0.786).

The mean average of DPO was 111.40 (SD = 19.2), without any significant sex-based differences ($p = 0.414$), neither for the level of training ($p = 0.373$), the type of training provided during medical school and/or psychiatry training programs ($p = 0.118$), clinical practice experience before the COVID-19 pandemic ($p = 0.376$) and after COVID-19 pandemic ($p = 0.658$). The mean average of F1 was 38.4 (SD = 8.1), without any significant differences for sex ($p = 0.392$), for level of training ($p = 0.261$), for the presence/absence of TM ($p = 0.699$), EH ($p = 0.378$), EMH ($p = 0.937$), DP training ($p = 0.533$). No significant differences were found depending on the type of training acquired in DP (theoretical/practical) ($p = 0.410$) or the level of clinical practice in DP ($p = 0.647$).

The mean average of F2 was 23.7 (SD = 4.5), without any significant differences for sex ($p = 0.199$), for level of training ($p = 0.831$), for the presence/absence of TM ($p = 0.537$), EH ($p = 0.373$), EMH ($p = 0.263$), DP training ($p = 0.155$). No significant differences were found depending on the type of training acquired in DP (theoretical/practical) ($p = 0.424$) or the level of clinical practice in DP ($p = 0.239$).

The mean average of F3 was 22.6 (SD = 4.5), without any significant differences for sex ($p = 0.730$), for level of training ($p = 0.768$), for the presence/absence of TM ($p = 0.378$), EH ($p = 0.131$), except for EMH ($p = 0.019$) and DP training ($p = 0.010$). No significant differences were found depending on the type of training acquired in DP (theoretical/practical) ($p = 0.109$) or the level of clinical practice in DP ($p = 0.601$).

The mean average of F4 was 10.5 (SD = 3.2), without any significant differences for sex ($p = 0.571$), for level of training ($p = 0.336$), for the presence/absence of TM ($p = 0.935$), EH ($p = 0.354$) and DP training ($p = 0.230$), except for EMH ($p = 0.027$). No significant differences were found depending on the type of training acquired in DP (theoretical/practical) ($p = 0.118$) or the level of clinical practice in DP ($p = 0.185$).

The mean average of F5 was 16.3 (SD = 3.3), without any significant differences for sex ($p = 0.534$), for level of training ($p = 0.259$), for the presence/absence of TM ($p = 0.592$), EMH ($p = 0.109$) training, except for EH ($p = 0.015$) and DP training ($p = 0.046$). F5 scores were significantly higher in psychiatry trainees belonging to the first year of their psychiatry training program, compared to senior psychiatry trainees ($p = 0.007$) and in those who declared to have already used DP before the COVID-19 pandemic ($p = 0.011$). No significant differences were found depending on the type of training acquired in DP (theoretical/practical) ($p = 0.666$) or the level of clinical practice in DP ($p = 0.370$).

3.5. Associations between KS, PSI and DPO

Bivariate correlations analyses demonstrated strong positive significant correlations between KS and PSI ($r = 0.148$, $p < 0.001$), KS and DPO ($r = 0.193$, $p < 0.001$) and KS and each factor of DPO (Figure 1). Linear regression analysis demonstrated that PSI scores statistically significantly predicted KS total scores ($F(1, 237) = 5.283$, $R^2 = 0.022$, $p = 0.022$) (Figure 2). Linear regression analysis demonstrated that KS scores statistically significantly predicted DPO total scores ($F(1, 237) = 9.136$, $R^2 = 0.037$, $p = 0.003$) (Figure 3).

	KS	F1	F2	F3	F4	F5	DPO	PSI
F1	0,191	--	0,523	0,613	0,514	0,726	0,897	0,33
F2	0,168	0,523	--	0,645	0,183	0,651	0,747	0,135
F3	0,187	0,613	0,645	--	0,443	0,721	0,841	0,264
F4	-0,021	0,514	0,183	0,443	--	0,449	0,607	0,308
F5	0,19	0,726	0,651	0,721	0,449	--	0,873	0,268
DPO	0,193	0,897	0,747	0,841	0,607	0,873	--	0,33
PSI	0,148	0,33	0,135	0,264	0,308	0,268	0,33	--

Figure 1. Pearson's Correlations' Heatmap. KS: Knowledge Score; DPO: Digital Psychiatry Opinion; PSI: Perceived Significance Index; F1: factor 1; F2: factor 2; F3: factor 3; F4: factor 4; F5: factor 5. Higher correlations are marked with darker shades, while lower correlations are marked with lighter shade.

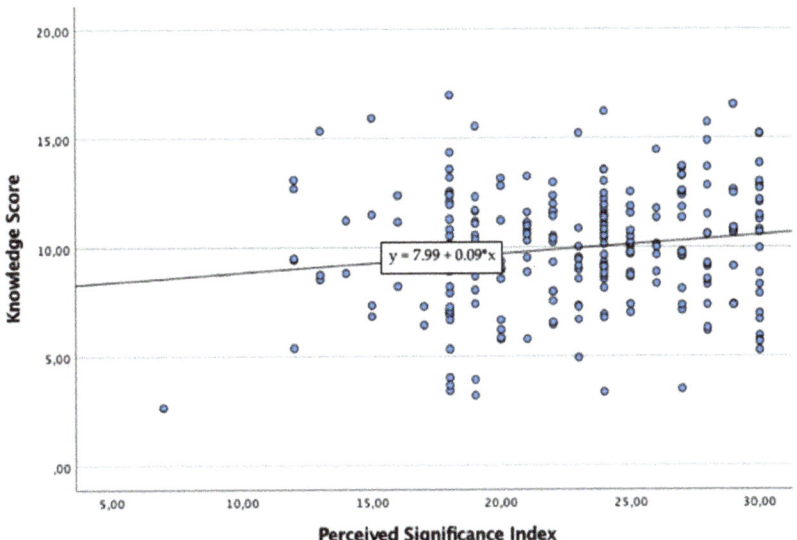

Figure 2. Linear Regression Model between Knowledge Score (dependent variable) and Perceived Significance Index (independent variable/predictor).

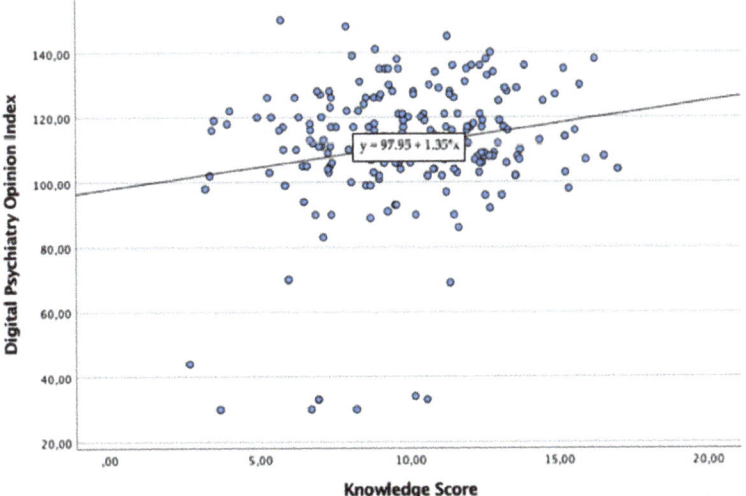

Figure 3. Linear Regression Model between Digital Psychiatry Opinion Index (dependent variable) and the Knowledge Score (independent variable/predictor).

4. Discussion

At the time of writing, this study represents the first Italian one to investigate the level of training and attitudes of medical students and young mental health professionals in the field of DP. Despite their long history, DP-related disciplines appear to be poorly addressed within the Italian academic formation, leading to a lack of knowledge on the topic. Although some participants possess general notions regarding TM and TP, specialty and detailed knowledge are often lacking. In addition, only a limited number of subjects demonstrated awareness about the recent introduction of digital tools in clinical practice. Nevertheless, most participants expressed interest in having these topics addressed during their training, particularly ECPs and newly qualified medical doctors waiting to start a psychiatry training program. The reason would be mainly explained by the same starting working condition of both categories who are going to start working on the frontline and may feel the need to possess more technical skills also in the field of DP, due to the current COVID-19 pandemic. Moreover, early career (and inexperienced) health professionals are those more prone to consider DP and related disciplines significantly important to be implemented in medicine courses and/or psychiatry training programmes, being those who showed higher PSI scores, compared to more senior (mental) health professionals. PSI significantly predicts KS, probably due to the fact that a positive and propositive attitude towards DP and related disciplines can predispose mental health professionals to deepen this topic, also independently by a formal academic DP training. In particular, our findings demonstrated that to be female and trained in DP-related topics is significantly associated with higher KS. Significantly higher KS scores were also found among ECPs and psychiatry trainees and this could reflect the initial hypothesis that at a later stage of psychiatry training each participant could have received a formal (practical and/or theoretical) DP training. Interestingly, the most significantly higher KS scores were found among those who declared to have received a practical (formally and/or informally) clinical experience in delivering digital mental health interventions. Furthermore, KS significantly predicts DPO, by underlining how knowing and to be informed about DP can significantly influence participant's DP opinion and attitude and, hence, their application of DP interventions in their routinely clinical practice. In fact, those participants who declared to be trained in DP and EMH showed significantly positive opinions regarding which professional and training skills are needed to provide digital mental health interventions (factor 3), think that in-person versus remote digital mental health interventions are comparable in terms of efficacy (factor 4) and that digital mental health interventions may represent a useful tool in those critical/emergency situation, such as the current COVID-19 pandemic (factor 5). Indeed, the current COVID-19 pandemic may have influenced our findings as the study was carried out during the second Italian COVID-19 pandemic wave, as demonstrated by the highest opinions towards the usability of digital mental health interventions during crisis/emergency situations provided by psychiatry trainees at their early stage.

Overall, the present findings of the inadequate DP training in Italy are in line with data collected in other European countries, such as France [23], and in non-European countries, such as India [24], Sri Lanka [25] and Asia-Pacific Regions [26]. Similarly, the overall interest in implementing the field of DP is consistent with past findings in samples of medical students and psychiatry trainees [24–31]. Conversely, different data emerge from U.S. studies conducted in the last decade. According to these, one-fifth of respondents had received formal training in TP already during medical school [27] and almost half of them during psychiatry training programs [32].

Most participants shared the same beliefs regarding both advantages and limitations of DP. The large majority declared that the application of ICTs could facilitate treatment access and continuity in case of reduced mobility, geographic isolation, or health emergencies. Moreover, most participants believe that digitalization could result in cost-saving, bringing a concrete benefit to the National Health Service, and a better rationalization of social and health care processes. These findings are in accordance with those emerging from previous studies [15,29,33,34].

At the same time, in line with earlier findings [35,36], data showed a general hesitation and lack of confidence regarding digital interventions. In particular, the perplexities concerned the effectiveness of digital interventions compared to in-person ones, despite the evidence proving that the two modes are equally effective in terms of outcomes, treatment adherence, and symptomatology improvement [37]. Only a tiny percentage of the sample declared that digital interventions are as effective as in-person ones, following data emerging from existing literature [30,38,39].

In this regard, the present work showed that being trained in DP is significantly associated with the belief that DP is equally effective to in-person care. Indeed, the knowledge acquired through adequate (mainly practical) training on DP can favorably influence the perception of its usefulness and validity in clinical practice [40]. It therefore seems undeniable that the lack of education and clinical practice in this field, leading to a negative influence on clinicians' opinions, is a critical limiting factor in the process of psychiatry digitization [36,41].

Moreover, data revealed a general concern about achieving a good therapeutic alliance through digital tools. These results are consistent with existing literature [11,30,34,35,39], and in contrast with the evidence that patients treated via videoconferencing tend to consider the therapeutic alliance valid [42]. Other perplexities were related to data and privacy protection and the appropriateness of using DP during the first psychiatric visit rather than just in follow-up visits in already stable patients. Likewise, those concerns are in line with previous research [34,35,40].

These preliminary findings should also be considered in light of the limitations that this first study presents. First, the choice of a mixed-mode data collection (both hand-to-hand and digital form). In fact, the digital form did not allow to verify the actual occupational/work belonging and, hence, to ensure the respect of inclusion criteria. In addition, the digital modality does not prevent filling out the questionnaire more than once. Second, the study's cross-sectional nature allowed us to have the current snapshot of the Italian situation but did not provide an observation over time (i.e., comparison between before and after academic training). Third, the period of data collection during the COVID-19 pandemic may have determined an overestimation of the KS and level of interest/attitude towards DP (i.e., the recent rapid spread of DP could have impacted KS). Fourth, the small sample size may have undermined the sample's representativeness, which may vary in its characteristics on a regional basis. Finally, the sample of medical students and psychiatry trainees was widely more represented than ECPs. This may explain the low values of KS and the poor training on the issue. Similarly, among psychiatry trainees, most of the sample was represented by those attending the first year, i.e., at the very beginning of their training.

Therefore, our findings may interestingly address more specific changes in DP training, as they underline how it is significant to implement education and clinical practice in DP and related disciplines since the course of medicine and then during psychiatry training programmes. Another important point regards the presence of a mentorship program within psychiatry training programmes which could significantly improve the PSI as well as DPO among early career (mental) health professionals, as it has been demonstrated that own a positive attitude towards the importance to implement DP and related disciplines in university and post-university courses may significantly improve the level of knowledge and, then, the overall opinion in digital mental health interventions and, hence, incentivize their use in the routinary clinical practice. The current COVID-19 pandemic taught that digitalization is an essential part of the (mental) health services and infrastructures which should be greatly implemented as it may ensure the continuity to access and care in (mental) health services that could be abruptly discontinued due to the crisis/emergency situation and represent a protective factor towards the recrudescence of mental health conditions. Further studies with a greater sample size and more homogeneous geographic representation are needed to confirm what emerged from this research. Moreover, further longitudinal studies should appropriately stratify the results, considering the different academic and occupational categories and the variations in participants' KS and attitudes over time.

5. Conclusions

In conclusion, the present study demonstrated the lack of formal training in DP within medical school and psychiatry training programmes, despite the recent digitalization of several health care services and medical specialties. The lack of theoretical and practical education during the academic years may represent a limiting factor to the spread of DP, resulting in a vast digitalization gap in today's clinical practice. These findings reported that those who had received academic training had a more favorable opinion about digital mental health interventions and were more inclined to use them in their clinical practice. Overall, developing a toolkit of core competencies in the field of DP and including it within the formal training should be encouraged. Starting from a good education, we may see impressive increases in the digitization of psychiatry in the coming years.

Supplementary Materials: The following supporting information can be downloaded at: https://www.mdpi.com/article/10.3390/healthcare10020390/s1, Figure S1: Scree Plot.

Author Contributions: Conceptualization, L.O. and U.V.; methodology, L.O. and V.M.; formal analysis, L.O.; investigation, V.M., L.O. and G.M.; data curation, L.O., S.T.V. and S.B.; writing—original draft preparation, L.O.; writing—review and editing, L.O. and S.B.; visualization, V.S.; supervision, U.V. All authors have read and agreed to the published version of the manuscript.

Funding: This research received no external funding.

Institutional Review Board Statement: The study was conducted according to the guidelines of the Declaration of Helsinki, and approved by the Institutional Review Board of the Department of Clinical and Experimental Medicine of the Polytechnic University of Marche (protocol code ACPS-D-21-00347, 28 September 2021).

Informed Consent Statement: Informed consent was obtained from all subjects involved in the study.

Data Availability Statement: Data supporting reported results are available, upon request to corresponding author.

Acknowledgments: We would like to acknowledge all medical students and colleagues who voluntarily agree to participate in the study.

Conflicts of Interest: The authors declare no conflict of interest.

References

1. Strehle, E.M.; Shabde, N. One hundred years of telemedicine: Does this new technology have a place in paediatrics? *Arch. Dis. Child.* **2006**, *91*, 956–959. [CrossRef] [PubMed]
2. Lupton, D.; Maslen, S. Telemedicine and the senses: A review. *Sociol. Health Illn.* **2017**, *39*, 1557–1571. [CrossRef] [PubMed]
3. Kaplan, B. Revisiting health information technology ethical, legal, and social issues and evaluation: Telehealth/telemedicine and COVID-19. *Int. J. Med. Inform.* **2020**, *143*, 104239. [CrossRef] [PubMed]
4. O'brien, M.; McNicholas, F. The use of telepsychiatry during COVID-19 and beyond. *Ir. J. Psychol. Med.* **2020**, *37*, 250–255. [CrossRef] [PubMed]
5. Barnett, M.L.; Ray, K.N.; Souza, J.; Mehrotra, A. Trends in telemedicine use in a large commercially insured population, 2005–2017. *JAMA* **2018**, *320*, 2147–2149. [CrossRef] [PubMed]
6. Ortega, G.; Rodriguez, J.A.; Maurer, L.R.; Witt, E.E.; Perez, N.; Reich, A.; Bates, D.W. Telemedicine, COVID-19, and disparities: Policy implications. *Health Policy Technol.* **2020**, *9*, 368–371. [CrossRef]
7. Chakrabarti, S. Usefulness of telepsychiatry: A critical evaluation of videoconferencing-based approaches. *World J. Psychiatry* **2015**, *5*, 286–304. [CrossRef]
8. Chen, J.A.; Chung, W.-J.; Young, S.K.; Tuttle, M.C.; Collins, M.B.; Darghouth, S.L.; Longley, R.; Levy, R.; Razafsha, M.; Kerner, J.C.; et al. COVID-19 and telepsychiatry: Early outpatient experiences and implications for the future. *Gen. Hosp. Psychiatry* **2020**, *66*, 89–95. [CrossRef]
9. Spivak, S.; Spivak, A.; Cullen, B.; Meuchel, J.; Johnston, D.; Chernow, R.; Green, C.; Mojtabai, R. Telepsychiatry use in U.S. mental health facilities, 2010–2017. *Psychiatr. Serv.* **2020**, *71*, 121–127. [CrossRef]
10. Barrera-Valencia, C.; Benito-Devia, A.V.; Vélez-Álvarez, C.; Figueroa-Barrera, M.; Franco-Idárraga, S.M. Costo-efectividad de telepsiquiatría sincrónica frente a asincrónica para personas con depresión privadas de la libertad. *Rev. Colomb. Psiquiatr.* **2017**, *46*, 65–73. [CrossRef]
11. Caroppo, E.; Lanzotti, P.; Janiri, L. *Interventi a Distanza in Salute Mentale*; Alpes Italia: Roma, Italy, 2020.
12. Catwell, L.; Sheikh, A. Evaluating eHealth interventions: The need for continuous systemic evaluation. *PLoS Med.* **2009**, *6*, e1000126. [CrossRef] [PubMed]
13. Dave, S.; Abraham, S.; Ramkisson, R.; Matheiken, S.; Pillai, A.S.; Reza, H.; Bamrah, J.S.; Tracy, D.K. Digital psychiatry and COVID-19: The big bang effect for the NHS? *BJPsych Bull.* **2021**, *45*, 259–263. [CrossRef] [PubMed]
14. Adiukwu, F.; de Filippis, R.; Orsolini, L.; Bytyçi, D.G.; Shoib, S.; Ransing, R.; Slaih, M.; Jaguga, F.; Handuleh, J.I.M.; Ojeahere, M.I.; et al. Scaling up global mental health services during the COVID-19 pandemic and beyond. *Psychiatr. Serv.* **2022**, *73*, 231–234. [CrossRef] [PubMed]

15. Ayatollahi, H.; Sarabi, F.Z.P.; Langarizadeh, M. Clinicians' knowledge and perception of telemedicine technology. *Perspect. Health Inf. Manag.* **2015**, *12*, 1c. [PubMed]
16. Pereira-Sanchez, V.; Adiukwu, F.; El Hayek, S.; Bytyçi, D.G.; Gonzalez-Diaz, J.M.; Kundadak, G.K.; Larnaout, A.; Nofal, M.; Orsolini, L.; Ramalho, R.; et al. COVID-19 effect on mental health: Patients and workforce. *Lancet Psychiatry* **2020**, *7*, e29–e30. [CrossRef]
17. Kuzman, M.R.; Vahip, S.; Fiorillo, A.; Beezhold, J.; da Costa, M.P.; Skugarevsky, O.; Dom, G.; Pajevic, I.; Peles, A.M.; Mohr, P.; et al. Mental health services during the first wave of the COVID-19 pandemic in Europe: Results from the EPA ambassadors survey and implications for clinical practice. *Eur. Psychiatry J. Assoc. Eur. Psychiatr.* **2021**, *64*, e41. [CrossRef]
18. Vindegaard, N.; Benros, M.E. COVID-19 pandemic and mental health consequences: Systematic review of the current evidence. *Brain Behav. Immun.* **2020**, *89*, 531–542. [CrossRef]
19. Gorwood, P.; Fiorillo, A. One year after the COVID-19: What have we learnt, what shall we do next? *Eur. Psychiatry J. Assoc. Eur. Psychiatr.* **2021**, *64*, e15. [CrossRef]
20. Fiorillo, A.; Sampogna, G.; Giallonardo, V.; Del Vecchio, V.; Luciano, M.; Albert, U.; Carmassi, C.; Carrà, G.; Cirulli, F.; Dell'osso, B.; et al. Effects of the lockdown on the mental health of the general population during the COVID-19 pandemic in Italy: Results from the COMET collaborative network. *Eur. Psychiatry J. Assoc. Eur. Psychiatr.* **2020**, *63*, e87. [CrossRef]
21. Ramalho, R.; Adiukwu, F.; Bytyçi, D.G.; El Hayek, S.; Gonzalez-Diaz, J.M.; Larnaout, A.; Grandinetti, P.; Nofal, M.; Pereira-Sanchez, V.; Da Costa, M.P.; et al. Telepsychiatry during the COVID-19 pandemic: Development of a protocol for telemental health care. *Front. Psychiatry* **2020**, *11*, 552450. [CrossRef]
22. Tavakol, M.; Dennick, R. Making sense of Cronbach's alpha. *Int. J. Med. Educ.* **2011**, *2*, 53–55. [CrossRef]
23. Yaghobian, S.; Ohannessian, R.; Mathieu-Fritz, A.; Moulin, T. National survey of telemedicine education and training in medical schools in France. *J. Telemed. Telecare* **2020**, *26*, 303–308. [CrossRef] [PubMed]
24. Zayapragassarazan, Z. Awareness, knowledge, attitude and skills of telemedicine among health professional faculty working in teaching hospitals. *J. Clin. Diagn. Res.* **2016**, *10*, JC01–JC04. [CrossRef] [PubMed]
25. Edirippulige, S.; Marasinghe, R.B.; Smith, A.C.; Fujisawa, Y.; Herath, W.B.; Jiffry, M.T.M.; Wootton, R. Medical students' knowledge and perceptions of e-health: Results of a study in Sri Lanka. *Stud. Health Technol. Inform.* **2007**, *129*, 1406–1409.
26. Orsolini, L.; Jatchavala, C.; Noor, I.M.; Ransing, R.; Satake, Y.; Shoib, S.; Shah, B.; Ullah, I.; Volpe, U. Training and education in digital psychiatry: A perspective from Asia-Pacific region. *Asia Pac. Psychiatry* **2021**, *13*, e12501. [CrossRef] [PubMed]
27. Glover, J.A.; Williams, E.; Hazlett, L.J.; Campbell, N. Connecting to the future: Telepsychiatry in postgraduate medical education. *Telemed. J. e-Health J. Am. Telemed. Assoc.* **2013**, *19*, 474–479. [CrossRef]
28. Sunderji, N.; Crawford, A.; Jovanović, M. Telepsychiatry in graduate medical education: A narrative review. *Acad. Psychiatry* **2014**, *39*, 55–62. [CrossRef]
29. Crawford, A.; Sunderji, N.; López, J.; Soklaridis, S. Defining competencies for the practice of telepsychiatry through an assessment of resident learning needs. *BMC Med. Educ.* **2016**, *16*, 28. [CrossRef]
30. Cruz, C.; Orchard, K.; Shoemaker, E.Z.; Hilty, D.M. A survey of residents/fellows, program directors, and faculty about telepsychiatry: Clinical experience, interest, and views/concerns. *J. Technol. Behav. Sci.* **2021**, *6*, 327–337. [CrossRef]
31. Orchard, K.; Cruz, C.; Shoemaker, E.Z.; Hilty, D.M. A survey comparing adult and child psychiatry trainees, faculty, and program directors' perspectives about telepsychiatry: Implications for clinical care and training. *J. Technol. Behav. Sci.* **2021**, *6*, 338–347. [CrossRef]
32. Hoffman, P.; Kane, J.M. Telepsychiatry education and curriculum development in residency training. *Acad. Psychiatry* **2015**, *39*, 108–109. [CrossRef] [PubMed]
33. Cloutier, P.; Cappelli, M.; Glennie, J.E.; Keresztes, C. Mental health services for children and youth: A survey of physicians' knowledge, attitudes and use of telehealth services. *J. Telemed. Telecare* **2008**, *14*, 98–101. [CrossRef] [PubMed]
34. Das, N. Telepsychiatry during COVID-19—A brief survey on attitudes of psychiatrists in India. *Asian J. Psychiatry* **2020**, *53*, 102387. [CrossRef] [PubMed]
35. Wagnild, G.; Leenknecht, C.; Zauher, J. Psychiatrists' satisfaction with telepsychiatry. *Telemed. J. e-Health Off. J. Am. Telemed. Assoc.* **2006**, *12*, 546–551. [CrossRef]
36. Feijt, M.; De Kort, Y.; Bongers, I.; Bierbooms, J.; Westerink, J.; Ijsselsteijn, W. Mental health care goes online: Practitioners' experiences of providing mental health care during the COVID-19 pandemic. *Cyberpsychol. Behav. Soc. Netw.* **2020**, *23*, 860–864. [CrossRef]
37. Hilty, D.M.; Ferrer, D.C.; Parish, M.B.; Johnston, B.; Callahan, E.J.; Yellowlees, P.M. The effectiveness of telemental health: A 2013 review. *Telemed. J. e-Health Off. J. Am. Telemed. Assoc.* **2013**, *19*, 444–454. [CrossRef]
38. Baer, L.; Elford, R.D.; Cukor, P. Telepsychiatry at forty: What have we learned? *Harv. Rev. Psychiatry* **1997**, *5*, 7–17. [CrossRef]
39. Brooks, E.; Turvey, C.; Augusterfer, E.F. Provider barriers to telemental health: Obstacles overcome, obstacles remaining. *Telemed. J. e-Health Off. J. Am. Telemed. Assoc.* **2013**, *19*, 433–437. [CrossRef]
40. Gibson, K.; O'Donnell, S.; Coulson, H.; Kakepetum-Schultz, T. Mental health professionals' perspectives of telemental health with remote and rural first nations communities. *J. Telemed. Telecare* **2011**, *17*, 263–267. [CrossRef]

41. Jameson, J.P.; Farmer, M.S.; Head, K.J.; Fortney, J.; Teal, C.R. VA community mental health service providers' utilization of and attitudes toward telemental health care: The gatekeeper's perspective. *J. Rural Health Off. J. Am. Rural Health Assoc. Natl. Rural Health Care Assoc.* **2011**, *27*, 425–432. [CrossRef]
42. Simpson, S.; Richardson, L.; Pietrabissa, G.; Castelnuovo, G.; Reid, C. Videotherapy and therapeutic alliance in the age of COVID-19. *Clin. Psychol. Psychother.* **2021**, *28*, 409–421. [CrossRef] [PubMed]

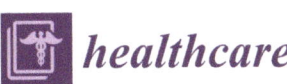

Article

Students' and Examiners' Experiences of Their First Virtual Pharmacy Objective Structured Clinical Examination (OSCE) in Australia during the COVID-19 Pandemic

Vivienne Mak [1,*], Sunanthiny Krishnan [2] and Sara Chuang [1]

[1] Faculty of Pharmacy and Pharmaceutical Sciences, Monash University, Parkville, VIC 3052, Australia; sara.chuang@monash.edu
[2] School of Pharmacy, Monash University Malaysia, Bandar Sunway, Subang Jaya 47500, Malaysia; Sunanthiny.S.Krishnan@monash.edu
* Correspondence: vivienne.mak@monash.edu

Abstract: Objective Structured Clinical Examinations (OSCEs) are routinely used in healthcare education programs. Traditionally, students undertake OSCEs as face-to-face interactions to assess competency in soft skills. Due to physical distancing restrictions during COVID-19, alternative methods were required. This study utilized a mixed-method design (online survey and interviews) to evaluate second-year pharmacy students' and examiners' experiences of their first virtual OSCEs in Australia. A total of 196 students completed their first virtual OSCE in June 2020 of which 190 students completed the online survey. However, out of the 190 students, only 88% ($n = 167$) consented to the use of the data from their online survey. A further 10 students and 12 examiners were interviewed. Fifty-five students (33%) who participated in the online survey strongly agreed or agreed that they preferred the virtual experience to face-to-face OSCEs while 44% ($n = 73$) neither agreed nor disagreed. Only 20% ($n = 33$) felt more anxious with the virtual OSCEs. Additionally, thematic analysis found non-verbal communication as a barrier during the OSCE. Positive aspects about virtual OSCEs included flexibility, decreased levels of anxiety and relevance with emerging telehealth practice. The need for remote online delivery of assessments saw innovative ways of undertaking OSCEs and an opportunity to mimic telehealth. While students and examiners embraced the virtual OSCE process, face-to-face OSCEs were still considered important and irreplaceable. Future opportunities for OSCEs to be delivered both face-to-face and virtually should be considered.

Keywords: e-learning; healthcare education; telehealth; OSCE; pharmacy; communication

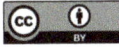

1. Introduction

Objective Structured Clinical Examinations (OSCEs) have been used routinely in healthcare education programs. Traditionally, students undertake OSCEs as face-to-face interactions to assess competency in soft skills including problem solving, empathy and communication. Students move through a circuit of purposely designed stations to assess them in a standardized simulated environment. At each station, students complete a clinical task within a predetermined time in the presence of a simulated patient. These simulated patients adhere to a strict script to ensure that each student is assessed in a standardized manner. In the pharmacy course, an OSCE is used to evaluate students simulating a patient–pharmacist encounter in a community or hospital pharmacy setting. There may also be instances where the student will simulate a pharmacist encounter with another healthcare professional. These OSCEs assess content knowledge as well as problem solving, communication skills and empathy. OSCEs are considered the gold standard in assessing skills development in clinical students due to their objectivity and reliability [1].

Due to physical distancing restrictions during the COVID-19 pandemic, alternative methods of conducting OSCEs were required as face-to-face OSCEs were no longer possible at many institutions. Fortunately, due to the advances in technology and the rising demand for telehealth solutions, conversion of OSCEs to virtual or online formats occurred quickly. Utilizing telecommunication platforms such as Zoom, traditional face-to-face OSCE scenarios were adapted for online delivery. This was proven to be done successfully in other health professions such as in a medical faculty [2]. There are many considerations before conducting a virtual OSCE, including ensuring that both examiners and students have the appropriate resources, including a functional device compatible with Zoom, a video camera, audio capabilities, and a good and stable internet connection. This reduces any potential for technological challenges that may occur during the OSCE. As this was the first time pharmacy students and examiners were undertaking their OSCEs in a virtual format, it was important to provide clear instructions and training on how the virtual OSCEs would be conducted [3].

While this swift adaptation to virtual OSCEs afforded reasonable continuity of the assessment, there were considerable challenges with this mode of examination that course coordinators had to navigate in order to achieve the learning outcomes of these performance-based competency assessments. In particular, it is difficult to capture the full range of non-verbal communication skills on synchronous video conferencing media, due to audio-visual limitations such as screen size, position of the student on screen as well as potential poor video quality [4,5].

Poor internet connectivity further impedes the smooth process of "live interactive" assessments. Low bandwidth connections, especially among students living in rural areas with limited internet access, could be particularly challenging and stressful during time-sensitive assessments such as OSCEs. There have been previous reports that poor internet access could be a potential for concern around equity in assessments [6,7]. In a survey conducted among 307 agricultural graduates from different universities in India, a lack of internet connectivity was reported as the major hindrance to online learning, more acutely affecting those from remote areas [7]. Technology and connection issues are of concern regardless of location. In reporting the outcome of a virtual teaching OSCE (vTOSCE) with pharmacy students at Ferris State University, the authors noted that both students as well as faculty members experienced connectivity issues during the vTOSCE [8]. Similarly, another study reported that many students experienced internet connectivity issues during their first remote OSCE in the United States, thus further highlighting the global nature of the problem [9].

Furthermore, academic integrity is also a serious cause for concern with virtual OSCEs as non-invigilated remote assessments are subject to cheating and collusion among students [6,10]. Many studies have shown that students in unproctored online assessments perform better compared to those in proctored environments [11–13]. Notably, students who undertake the OSCE at a later examination schedule may have an advantage due to the potential for students who have completed their examination prior to share exam information with others who have not [14]. Updike et al. (2021) reported an incident of a possible breach of OSCE integrity in a high-stakes assessment where students could potentially have taken screenshots or photos of electronically shared OSCE case materials [15]. The authors have suggested various approaches, including creating different case scenarios and reducing administration time during examinations to limit discussions among students and to protect the integrity of the virtual OSCEs [15].

Given these challenges, the conversion from conventional face-to-face to virtual OSCEs requires varying degrees of modifications to the assessment format, as the former is not entirely replicable virtually. Several papers described the functional processes of adaptation and the changes necessitated by the online delivery. Some of these amendments include fewer OSCE stations, conversion of interactive stations to passive stations, written stations examinable via the institution's Learning Management System (LMS), changes to testing procedures using proctoring software (e.g., ExamSoft), video recording of the examination as well as recruiting internal faculty members as simulated patients instead [1,15,16]. There have been many innovative OSCE conversions during the pandemic, including one in the

United States where students were "advised to recruit an adult within their residence to be their patient" [17] (p. 247) as part of a physical examination on a simulated patient. Evidently, many modifications were essentially driven by the logistical complexity of implementing "live interactive" online assessments and their feasibility during the pandemic.

At the Faculty of Pharmacy and Pharmaceutical Sciences, Monash University, second-year pharmacy students completed an OSCE in June 2020. This OSCE consisted of two stations situated within the community pharmacy setting. The examination was designed to assess students' skills in problem solving, oral communication and empathy as a pharmacist, using role play with a simulated patient suffering from asthma or eczema. As with other faculties during the pandemic, the options were to either delay the OSCE until lockdown restrictions were lifted or to continue the assessment virtually. Given that there was a closure on international borders, shutdown of non-essential services and movement restrictions in Melbourne, Australia [18], we decided to convert the OSCE to an online format and utilized the Zoom video conferencing platform as the medium for the assessment. Students were then able to be assessed synchronously by examiners who also played the role of the patients.

Whilst students had previously experienced OSCEs via face-to-face delivery in the first year of their pharmacy degree, this was their first exposure to the online format. To prepare faculty and students for the online format of the OSCE, training was conducted online. Students practised and were formatively assessed on their role plays in weekly workshops conducted over Zoom with a pharmacist facilitator. They were also provided an OSCE overview video that showcased the process and what to expect in a virtual OSCE. Faculty completed an online training module that consisted of the virtual OSCE process, how to assess online and the case content.

There have been many international reports describing the experiences of undertaking a virtual OSCE during the pandemic; however, this is an Australian study that adds to the literature on pharmacy students' and examiners' experiences of their first virtual OSCE utilizing a mixed-method study design. The aim of our study was to evaluate pharmacy students' and OSCE examiners' experiences of their first virtual OSCE.

The research questions for this study were as follows:

1. What were the pharmacy students' experience of undertaking a virtual OSCE?
2. What were the examiners' experience of the virtual OSCEs?
3. Were there differences in experiences between the virtual OSCEs and face-to-face OSCEs?

2. Materials and Methods

2.1. Virtual OSCE Process

The virtual OSCE process involved five steps, as summarized in Table 1 [3]. A day prior to the OSCE, the examination times were published to the students. The published times were given only a day prior to the OSCE to minimize any opportunities for collusion. We also had a Zoom license that allowed for administrators to host concurrent meetings and be dialled into multiple Zoom Meetings at the same time.

Table 1. Zoom OSCE process for each student [3].

Step	Description
1	Students dial into the "Zoom OSCE Lobby" Meeting link at their allocated time
2	Technology (audio/visual) and identification checks are conducted
3	Students are sent to their "Zoom OSCE Room" for their examination
4	OSCE interaction with the examiner occurs in the Zoom OSCE Room
5	Students leave the Zoom OSCE Room at the conclusion of their OSCE

On the day of the OSCE, the students dialled into the Zoom Meeting using the link provided to them at their published time. The Zoom Meeting was referred to as the "Zoom

OSCE Lobby". Once they dialled into the Zoom Meeting, they immediately appeared in a Zoom "waiting room". Students waited until the administrators admitted them into the Zoom OSCE Lobby. If there were delays, the administrators communicated with those in the waiting room using the Zoom chat function.

Once admitted into the Zoom OSCE Lobby, an administrator would check their identifications and also test that their internet connection was stable, as well as their audio and visual capabilities were sufficient for the examination. This was to determine if there was obvious lag in the student's internet connection or if there was any problem with their audio and video. In the event that there were issues, a member of staff assisted the student virtually to overcome the technical difficulties. The students were then given a quick briefing of the processes for the day.

When the identification process and technical set up was completed, the students were then sent to their Zoom OSCE Room. This was a new Zoom Meeting link where the examiner was located. An administrator provided this Zoom Meeting link to the student via a private chat. This administrator was dialled into the Zoom OSCE Lobby and also the Zoom OSCE Room. This meant that once the student clicked the Zoom OSCE Room link, the administrator was able to observe the student transporting themselves virtually to their exam room.

Once the student arrived in the Zoom OSCE Room, they automatically appeared in another Zoom waiting room. The students were briefed to wait patiently until the examiner admitted them into the exam room. This often occurred either immediately or up to 5 min post arrival. Once admitted into the Zoom OSCE Room, the examiner would ask for their full name and student ID number to confirm that they had the correct student. The examiner then provided a quick introduction to the exam and informed the student once the timer began. In this OSCE, the timer was set for seven minutes and the examiner was also simulating the patient. Marking was conducted on Qualtrics and a link was provided to the examiners prior to the commencement of the assessment. At the end of the seven minutes, the examiner would end the interaction and the students were asked to leave the Zoom OSCE Room. The examiner then completed their marking and repeated the process by admitting the next student from the Zoom waiting room.

2.2. Study Design

This study employed a mixed-method design. An online survey via Qualtrics and semi-structured interviews were conducted.

At Monash University, after each OSCE, students complete a post-OSCE reflection online survey where they reflect and rate their own performance. As part of this usual online survey, additional questions were included to explore their experiences of their first virtual OSCE for this study. These questions were developed by the course instructors and evaluated for face validity. These questions included statements ranked using the 5-point Likert scale, as well as opportunities for open-ended comments to elaborate on their answers pertaining to the virtual OSCE:

1. (a) I prefer virtual OSCEs compared to face-to-face OSCEs
   (b) Please elaborate on the reasons for your answer
2. (a) I felt more anxious during the virtual OSCE compared to face-to-face OSCE
   (b) Please elaborate on the reasons for your answer
3. (a) The virtual OSCE felt more challenging compared to a face-to-face OSCE
   (b) Please elaborate on the reasons for your answer

   Complete the following:
4. The best thing about the virtual OSCE is . . .
5. If I could improve something about the virtual OSCE, I would . . .
6. Please provide final comments (if any) about the virtual OSCE

As part of this online survey, students were invited to consent to a follow-up semi-structured interview to further explore their experiences. All examiners received an invitation to participate in a semi-structured interview to discuss the benefits and disadvantages of virtual OSCEs, as well as how they conducted the virtual OSCE as an examiner.

2.3. Data Collection and Analysis

The OSCE was conducted in June 2020. The online survey was administered to 196 second-year pharmacy students immediately after completion of their first virtual OSCE. All students completed the survey as part of the routine quality improvement process for the course but were required to consent to the use of their data for this study. The quantitative online survey data were analyzed descriptively.

Students who completed the online survey were also invited to participate in a further interview. A total of 25 students indicated that they were interested in being interviewed. All 18 OSCE examiners who examined in the OSCE were invited to participate in an interview.

All interviews were conducted via Zoom Meetings and transcribed verbatim using a speech to text transcription service called Otter.ai. All open-ended comments in the online survey and interviews were included in the qualitative data analysis. Qualitative data were thematically analyzed, where open-ended comments from the online survey and interview transcripts were read repeatedly for initial familiarization and coded. The codes were then grouped into themes and discussed with the project team until consensus was reached.

3. Results

A total of 190 students (96.9%) completed the online survey; however, only 87.9% (n = 167) of those who completed the online survey consented to the use of their survey data.

Ten of the 25 students who indicated their interest to be interviewed were contacted and interviews arranged. A total of 12 examiners agreed to be interviewed.

3.1. Quantitative Data

The survey results showed that 33% of students strongly agreed or agreed that they preferred the virtual OSCE experience to face-to-face OSCE while 44% showed no preference to either methods. Only 20% felt more anxious compared to the face-to-face OSCE while 12% agreed that the virtual OSCE felt more challenging (Table 2).

Table 2. Online survey results (n = 167).

Item	Strongly Disagree/Disagree n (%)	Neither Agree/Disagree n (%)	Strongly Agree/Agree n (%)
I prefer virtual OSCEs compared to face-to-face OSCEs	38 (23%)	74 (44%)	55 (33%)
I feel more anxious during the virtual OSCE compared to face-to-face OSCE	79 (47%)	55 (33%)	33 (20%)
The virtual OSCE felt more challenging compared to face-to-face OSCE	63 (38%)	84 (50%)	20 (12%)

3.2. Qualitative Themes

There were five themes that arose from the open-ended survey comments from students and the interviews with both students and examiners. Positive aspects about virtual OSCEs included flexibility, decreased levels of anxiety and the relevance with emerging practice such as telehealth. Many students also indicated that they practiced with their peers online in preparation for the virtual OSCEs. Non-verbal communication was seen to be challenging virtually.

3.2.1. Theme 1: Flexibility, Convenience and Comfort

One of the main themes in this study was the increased flexibility and convenience of the virtual OSCEs. There were several students and examiners who expressed that the opportunity to undertake the examinations at home was seen as a benefit (Table 3, Subtheme 1.1).

Table 3. Subthemes from Theme 1 and representative quotes.

Subthemes	Participant Group	Representative Quotes
1.1. Benefit of virtual OSCE at home	Students	"More flexible, less stress when at home"—Online Survey "Well, for me, I travel, you know, if I had to come to university I would have to travel around an hour or so. So that you know if when you take that out of the picture I get that extra time to maybe prepare. And so that was, I really appreciated that from my perspective. I've been able to save up a lot of time because I don't have to go to university."—Interview Student 8 "Virtual OSCE is pretty good because it saves a lot of time like on traffic. That's one of the best parts."—Interview Student 3 "Convenient, just have to show up at the allocated time without worrying about public transport etc."—Online Survey
	Examiners	"Flexibility I suppose, flexibility in terms of the fact that again, I was able to examine from the home, students were able to sit from their place of choosing, I was able to put in my background a nice pharmacy environment, which may be looked a bit more realistic than just being in a counselling suite. I think that was all a positive experience to come out of it."—Interview Examiner 3
1.2 Comfort	Students	"I would say seamless online learning, it's being able to conduct the OSCE in the comfort of your own home. I think you get to have that full sleep in. For me it's to get to uni. It's quite far. It's about an hour and 40 or so minutes. So by the time I get there on public transport, and they give you can get quite fatigued and then having to be so I guess surrounded by friends can be a good thing ... So I think doing it at home, you see people briefly get to be at home, get to sleep well and then go into your OSCE. I think it's more comfortable in that sense."—Interview Student 7
1.3 Convenience	Students	"How easy it is to access our notes and other resources."—Online Survey
	Examiners	"Certainly, more convenience and I guess a better use of my time in that setting. I found it very easy to be having them on the screen there. And like I've got two screens here. So I think having two screens is a good advantage as opposed to just one. So having like the rubric open on one screen, and student on the other screen, I thought worked really well. And it was quite easy for me to do both simultaneously."—Interview Examiner 2 "But I did set up two computers and made sure that I actually connected through different internet connections, so that if one went down, you know ... "—Interview Examiner 4 "I think that flexibility and the, I guess also the ability to really have what you need on your screens, and I know some people have three screens. And so that perhaps as an examiner, you may appear to sort of be able to look at a few things without distracting as much because I guess if you're looking at your notes, or trying to confirm something, in person, that's really obvious ... "—Interview Examiner 7
1.4 Reliance on Technology	Students	"I felt like with the technical, I understand like, it's completely unavoidable in some cases as well. But it just threw me off a little bit. Because then I'm like, Am I missing my OSCE? Is the examiner waiting for me? But aside from that, it was just the whole ... I was pretty comfortable during the OSCE."—Interview Student 4 "Convenient but then the internet connection was not always stable."—Online Survey

Table 3. Cont.

Subthemes	Participant Group	Representative Quotes
1.5 Flexibility	Examiners	"I like the fact that, because it was conducted virtually, I have a bit of control over the timing. If the students came in, you know, a little bit later they were flustered, I could say you know calm down and then I can start the seven minutes. I always stuck to the 7 min allowance but it was good to have a little bit of flexibility even to say to the student before I can you just give me a minute to catch up on my marks with the previous students. So all in all, from my experience and I'm doing this, honestly, it was seamless."—Interview Examiner 1
1.6 Future practice	Students	"And I definitely think we should have a combination of face to face and telehealth like communication, because like if someone's working, you know in the city and they have to talk to someone who's in a rural area. This is the best way of communication and like we're gonna have to deal with technology, it's like already prominent now."—Interview Student 4 "Zoom OSCEs are more convenient and perhaps more comfortable for me, but I think the face to face OSCEs can better prepare us for future practice."—Online Survey

A student further described that they felt less fatigued due to not needing to travel to university and that they felt that it was a better use of their time. The ability to undertake the OSCEs in the comfort of their own home was also seen to be a preference in a number of students (Table 3, Subtheme 1.2).

Examiners on the other hand also found it convenient conducting virtual OSCEs as they were able to have the examination materials they require on their screens/monitors. This is unlike a face-to-face examination where they had to either memorize the materials or assess the student after the interaction. Additionally, they were able to have the comfort of setting up a backup plan at home in case of technical difficulties. As with examiners and their convenience in materials, students also expressed the convenience in their ability to access their notes and resources from home (Table 3, Subtheme 1.3).

Nevertheless, even though students were in the comfort of their own home, technical difficulties and challenges were still possible. One student identified that the inability to see the physical examiner meant that they were questioning if their technology was working before the examination while in the Zoom waiting room. Another student indicated that even in the convenience of their home, the internet connection could still be an issue (Table 3, Subtheme 1.4).

As OSCEs are time-sensitive assessments, where each station needs to commence at a specific time, the examiners felt that there was flexibility in when the student commences the interaction. Examiners had to admit the students from the Zoom waiting room and thus had control of the assessment times to some extent (Table 3, Subtheme 1.5).

Students were not only thinking about flexibility and convenience for their own personal examinations. A couple of students were also expressing flexibility and convenience for their future practice (Table 3, Subtheme 1.6).

3.2.2. Theme 2: Decreased Anxiety and Nerves

A number of students expressed that doing the OSCE virtually made them feel secure as they felt that they were in a safe environment. Interestingly, they expressed that not being able to speak to their peers or be around other nervous students helped them stay calm and mentally prepared for the assessment (Table 4, Subtheme 2.1).

Table 4. Subthemes from Theme 2 and representative quotes.

Subthemes	Participant Group	Representative Quotes
2.1 Sense of security	Students	"I think it was good how, because I was at home, I was like, in a safe environment. Like there was no one else around me that stressed me out like it was just me. So I feel like it was less stressful than like being in a room with lots of people nervous waiting for it. Just like I feel like you just like sit and look at everyone's faces and you're like, oh, like they're worried too. Like, should I be as worried as them kind of thing."—Interview Student 1 "I guess the best stuff is that I don't have to talk with my peers before and after. Talking to them before, most of them are really nervous. And I'm kind of person to not put myself in a nervous state. But if people keep talking too much around me, I get nervous as well. And the best thing is after is that because after my test I don't want to talk about it anymore. I just want to get rid of it. And if that's OSCE during in school, I have to talk with my peers, Oh how did you go … yeah"—Interview Student 3 "I did feel anxious for the virtual OSCE however it was to a lesser extent compared to the face to face. I think the environment of the real life OSCE makes me more anxious whereas with the virtual one it was more calm and collected. The virtual OSCE allowed me to mentally prepare myself without being surrounded by others"—Online Survey "Quick and easy process. Low stress environment because there weren't other stressed students around."—Online Survey
2.2 Reduced nerves	Examiners	"Well, the students mostly do struggle with communication … If anything, maybe some of the students were more confident on screen than they would have a person, well at least seems that way. And some get very nervous in person … . So that's certainly a difference."—Interview Examiner 4 "But then I think of all the times when the poor things are so, so nervous. And what I feel more like is that I'm seeing them suffer, whereas, I don't know whether they were more relaxed (virtually) or it's just that, you know, you don't see things like their hands actually shaking when it's on video … but I suppose you don't get the full feel of how they are feeling because you can't see the whole body and you know, whether they're absolutely shaking literally in their boots or not."—Interview Examiner 8 "I personally find it quite a positive experience … I thought it was a positive experience for me. It was more comfortable. Like, doing the timing itself on the phone … When you're actually there physically in the OSCE is quite confronting, and quite like everything needs to happen so quickly. Whereas, when you're there, on your own, and you've got the dual screens and you've got the capacity to do things. It becomes a lot easier."—Interview Examiner 10
	Students	"But being at home, I think did help my nerves."—Interview Student 8 "I felt not as stressed as I would in normal face to face physical environment. Um, I had my phone with the timer on my desk as well. And I think that helped, like calm my nerves because I was like, I'm travelling like well for time as compared to the physical like environment where you don't have a counter like, time. Usually the thing is the timing is the source of stress. But because I had like, I was able to look at it this time it was less stressful."—Interview Student 2 "So I think for some people, and like for me, in some ways that was a bit more better because I had time to relax in my own room. And, you know, have my own prep before, before going into the room, and also in some way that was a bit informal, which that was another aspect of it, but it was great like to see that whole lead up being avoided … So like before, I have an assessment, or maybe I like play my music and like I'll nibble on something. And so I just like get myself in the zone"—Interview Student 4 "Doing the OSCE in a familiar environment encouraged me to feel more relaxed and at ease"—Online Survey

Examiners also noticed that students appeared less nervous during the virtual OSCEs compared to face-to-face OSCEs. Both students and examiners felt that having set up their surroundings to be familiar to them, including setting up their own timer for the OSCE and having their own ways of preparing themselves, helped them with their nerves; they were less stressful (Table 4, Subtheme 2.2).

3.2.3. Theme 3: Skill Development and Future Training for Telehealth

Many students saw this first opportunity to undertake virtual OSCEs as good training for their future as pharmacists and with the evolving roles with the use of technology and digital health (Table 5, Subtheme 3.1).

Table 5. Subthemes from Theme 3 and representative quotes.

Subthemes	Participant Group	Representative Quotes
3.1 Pharmacists in training	Students	"This is also one of the great ways to learn as a pharmacist in training"—Online Survey "Although it was a different experience, I am glad that we were given a chance to do a virtual OSCE as in practice, there may be cases where we have to counsel online so it really was beneficial in preparing us for what to expect in the future"—Online Survey "It feels appropriate to the challenges of today—having to complete telehealth consultations"—Online Survey "We are in a, I guess, electronic technology age where we do depend on our phones, our laptops, the internet pretty much everything. And what I do see from the virtual OSCE is I do see pharmacists in the future, using technology, such as this to talk to patients who are unable to come into the pharmacy. So, maybe in a community, or maybe even in a hospital if let's say, like there is with coronavirus, they want to limit the amount of people with each other. This covers how you know health professionals can get in contact with patients."—Interview Student 6 "I like that this is preparation for telehealth in my future career."—Online Survey "I think that virtual OSCEs will really help in terms of the growing telehealth which is emerging especially in times like this with the Coronavirus and will allow me to practice communicating with patients especially if you are not talking to them directly."—Online Survey
3.2 Telehealth	Students	"... since like now telehealth is such a big thing. I feel like there's benefits face to face and by Zoom because if there are cases such like the Coronavirus, telehealth is so important. So we would have to learn how to communicate with other people online and still be able to give patient centred care, I guess, to the best of our abilities but just through a different medium. And I feel like having this opportunity to actually do that, has been really beneficial"—Interview Student 9 "Doing the OSCE virtually was a great opportunity for me to learn more about Telehealth and it taught me how to be flexible. For example what to do if the patient can't hear us, how to explain certain medications without having the patient physically in front."—Online Survey "Telehealth is becoming far more common in modern day pharmacy and an OSCE that involves it would be very useful for developing online communication skills."—Online Survey "In recent years telehealth has been coming especially due to the COVID-19 situation and the future I think may be a staple of pharmacy practice. In my own country, it is actually used pretty often. So for example, pharmacy technicians will be stationed at the pharmacy or pharmacists can be called in from a different location. So this will allow for more flexible workings and it's a lot easier on the pharmacy side as well."—Interview Student 5
	Examiners	"To prepare students for telehealth and it would be interesting actually to compare how the students, you know conduct themselves, and you know whether they meet the same criteria in the virtual versus non virtual world."—Interview Examiner 1

Table 5. Cont.

Subthemes	Participant Group	Representative Quotes
3.3 Hybrid OSCE for skill development	Examiners	"If telehealth becomes like, you know, the normal for pharmacists, then that's brilliant, because like, I think it's a really great way to train them . . . I think, you know, for what we, you know, for the unprecedented sort of time that we have. The assessments were quite good. But I wouldn't sort of think that they would be sufficient for the future training of other students. I think the face to face assessments are still superior. That's just from just because some of them clearly are having sort of trouble talking to people in person already. And then online, that is a bit harder. So, because they are obviously quite young and have less life experience and things like that. So I think my experience overall with the virtual OSCEs, 100%, like I'm very happy, but in terms of helping out the students, I think, then it might not be as sufficient sort of way of training them and assessing them in the course overall."—Interview Examiner 5 "I think it's something we could certainly build into the course and it's a good one for like telehealth and all that kind of stuff. But I think it does take away from the fact that you do see a real person in front of you. So I still think face to face contact is essential to improve students' empathy, and improve those kinds of skills."—Interview Examiner 2
	Students	"So I think it's a great concept. And I think it's so relevant, but I'd like a mix of face to face."—Interview Student 4 "A mix it would be more preferable. So maybe alternating time because sometimes there is two OSCEs we have a period of time. So one physical one virtual, so to experience two parts of what could be possible in the future. So something more holistic in nature."—Interview Student 5

They saw the pandemic to have allowed for this opportunity to keep up with practice considering that uptake to telehealth was accelerated during COVID-19. In addition, it was considered to be a flexible way of working in the future. Examiners' views were also consistent with how students viewed the future of telehealth and felt that this was a great way to train students (Table 5, Subtheme 3.2).

Nevertheless, examiners were concerned about the training of pharmacy students solely on the use of virtual OSCEs. They felt that a mix of both virtual and face-to-face OSCEs would be most beneficial. Similarly, students expressed that they would ideally like to have a combination of face-to-face and virtual OSCEs (Table 5, Subtheme 3.3).

3.2.4. Theme 4: Non-Verbal Communication a Barrier

Although there were many positives with the virtual OSCEs, both examiners and students identified non-verbal communication as the main barrier during the OSCE. Students expressed challenges in displaying good non-verbal skills while examiners found difficulty evaluating these skills virtually (Table 6, Subtheme 4.1). Empathy was highlighted as a skill that was difficult to assess virtually from an examiner's perspective. Students also expressed difficulty in picking up empathy cues from simulated patients (Table 6, Subtheme 4.2).

3.2.5. Theme 5: Practice in Preparation for Virtual OSCE

Many students also said that they practised online before the virtual OSCEs to be more familiar with the technology and also to mimic the style of assessments they were going to undertake (Table 7).

Table 6. Subthemes from Theme 4 and representative quotes.

Subthemes	Participant Group	Representative Quotes
4.1 Difficulty displaying good non-verbal skills	Students	"When you're doing online, like video, interviewing and things like that, it's always harder to gauge people's non-verbal cues. I think in person you can kind of sense when someone's about to start talking, or how someone's responding to what you're saying. But when it's online, I find it much more difficult . . . . I would pick traditional OSCEs for the human interaction. Because I think it's, you're better able to, I guess, show yourself and your energy and your personality and I guess non-verbal cues and things like that in person."—Interview Student 7 "You aren't able to really see the bottom half, the hands, you're only able to see the face, most of the time so without that, non-verbal communication has been cut off. But still I feel that even though just seeing the face, you are still able to get the information, or able to understand what you have said . . . But, obviously it's not perfect."—Interview Student 5 "I don't mind doing either as the process is still similar. However non-verbal communication may not be delivered as readily through the computer screen."—Online Survey
	Examiners	"The face to face had a massive advantage in terms of being able to have that interpersonal you know, non-verbal communication skills showing off and that was quite difficult to do in the virtual OSCE. As obviously, but it's, you know, to be expected. So it was a bit harder to . . . Yeah, just have that interpersonal skills coming out from the students, so it (was) harder to sort of connect with them as well. And when you're playing the patient or you know, yeah, I thought that was the biggest, most noticeable effect of that."—Interview Examiner 5 "But the only thing I noticed was students were probably more reliant on resources around, because I'm sure the visual OSCE gave them more opportunities to have everything around them and so they were very concerned because you could see their eyes moving. In person you know they'd be very fixated on speaking to you, whereas in the virtual ones not everyone, but sometimes there would be looking elsewhere, and not so much, paying attention to the patient that was in front of them."—Interview Examiner 9
4.2 Empathy	Students	"It was harder to understand the patient, and show empathy over a computer screen"—Online Survey "I guess compared to being a real patient, on screen does make a patient's emotion less easier for me to observe. Their statement are quite straightforward though . . . . normally if we were sitting face to each other face to face, it's easier to observe like the, like eye contact, like through the like tiny movement. Yeah."—Interview Student 3 "It's different to when you're in person. And I guess it doesn't tone down how empathetic you are and I guess it just, it can't . . . some people may come up as different if it's in a camera or if it's face to face."—Interview Student 6
	Examiners	"The potential for lack of engagement that you might get, and that's of empathy and non-verbal communication, those sort of aspects that you probably do pick up better in person"—Interview Examiner 4 "The fact that I did notice that some of the poorer English language students were obviously reading off a script, which if you think about that from a real life perspective . . . Although they did look quite formulaic, and I had one student who she seriously sounded like a robot, I thought the way in which there was little emotion that she showed throughout the OSCE interview . . . The fact that she was so robotic, and maybe that's that would have been the same from a face to face OSCE but it was clearly noticeable in the OSCE last week that was run via zoom. That formulaic nature and just showing very little emotion to any response that I gave, which was quite, just quite, quite concerning and disappointing, but again, I don't know whether that same student would have performed the same way if it was a face to face OSCE."—Interview Examiner 3 "Trying to pick up on some of the students' non-verbal language is maybe not quite as easy. I probably took a very, almost digital approach in that. You know, it's hard with cameras because cameras can be at different points. And so you're looking at the person, but, you know, they're looking at their screen rather than the camera so they don't always look like they're making eye contact with you."—Interview Examiner 8 "I was more conscious that I needed to engage the student, which is kind of strange because I think for me, I find it quite strange because in person that happens naturally anyway because you're in front of a physical person whereas this is behind the screen. And so I think perhaps I was more aware to, to be friendly and sort of use gestures and normally you can see body language really easily in front of the person but in this case you have a screen so I was making sure that, you know, if I was sneezing (for the case) or whatever it was and it was quite, quite obvious as well."—Interview Examiner 9

Table 7. Theme 5 and representative quotes.

Participant Group	Representative Quotes
Students	"Yes, so me and a few of my peers, we decided to jump on to Zoom and then pretend that we were in the Zoom OSCEs. Not necessarily through the meeting format, but all the breakout room formats, but more so just some general meeting. And so we, one person would pretend to be the patient and then the other person would be unfamiliar with what the patient was presenting with. And then we just play it out within the seven minutes. And we take turns doing that . . . . we decided that because the OSCE was going to be done over zoom, we would jump over to zoom meetings and then try it out and put up our backgrounds and yeah, test everything out, test the waters before we started."—Interview Student 7 "Did practice on Zoom with my friend. And that helped a lot."—Interview Student 3 "I prepared for it a bit differently compared to the face to face OSCE that I prepared for last year . . . as you progress through university, your strategies do change over time. But in this case, what I did was, I did have zoom calls with my colleagues, and we practice the OSCE with each other. And I think that really helped me understand my tone of voice, how, how loud I should be speaking for the other person to be able to understand through the screen. I also wrote a script, which was sort of going which would help me organise my thoughts and the things that I'll see."—Interview Student 8 "We went on a zoom call, not unlike this one. And we timed ourselves using our phones. And we came up with scenarios . . . So yes, I'm just trying to like reenact the environment of an OSCE"—Interview Student 2

4. Discussion

This study found that it was still feasible to conduct OSCEs virtually and both examiners and students felt that this alternative assessment method had many positive aspects compared to face-to-face OSCEs. Nevertheless, there was still a preference for traditional methods and a desire for a hybrid version with both virtual and face-to-face OSCEs in the future. A major benefit of virtual OSCEs felt by students was a decrease in anxiety and nerves for the assessment. Students who were interviewed all indicated less anxiety during virtual OSCEs, which was consistent with the survey results, where only 20% of the students agreed that they felt more anxious during the virtual OSCEs compared to face-to-face OSCEs. Studies in other countries also found that students were less anxious in online OSCEs [19,20], while traditional face-to-face OSCEs have always been intimidating and stressful [21]. The decreased stress levels expressed by the students in our study could potentially be due to a result of being in the comfort of their home surroundings and, in some cases, the absence of peer anxiety. However, it should be noted that a recent systematic review examining the relationship between OSCE-associated test anxiety and OSCE performance found that there was little influence on student performance [22]. Another study compared the performance of two cohorts of pharmacy students with one cohort in 2020 that undertook the OSCE virtually during the pandemic and the second cohort in 2019 with traditional methods [23]. The authors found that students who undertook their OSCE virtually performed as well as those who completed it in-person via traditional methods [23].

An emerging theme in our study was the increased flexibility of virtual OSCEs expressed by both students and examiners. The reduced travel time and the ability to complete the OSCE from almost any location appealed strongly to all participants. Given the situation during the pandemic whereby students were potentially located overseas due to the closure of international borders, this flexibility to conduct the examinations online was essential to prevent delays in students' course progressions. A study found that 60% of their academic staff members felt that working from home was more flexible than traditional methods during COVID-19 [24]. Flexibility to work from anywhere assisted faculty members especially if there was a need to manage family responsibilities [25]. This was particularly useful for faculty members with children that require home schooling during the pandemic. Virtual OSCEs also provided greater ease in logistical and spatial requirements, which is often a limiting factor to face-to-face OSCEs [26]. Nevertheless, our virtual OSCE was conducted with multiple Zoom Meetings hosted concurrently. This could be limited if other educators decide to replicate similar methods of conducting the virtual OSCEs as special scheduling privileges are required for administrators to host multiple concurrent Zoom Meetings and can cost more to institutions [27].

There was also recognition of virtual OSCE by our student participants as an avenue to develop skills in the direction of telehealth. Telehealth has been steadily redesigning the landscape of healthcare systems since the rapid advancements and utilization of telecommunication media over the past two decades, which was accelerated due to the COVID-19 pandemic [28]. Originally conceptualized to overcome barriers to healthcare access, particularly geographical distance and restricted mobility [28,29], the value of telemedicine has expanded to reduce waiting times, reduce the need for travel and time off work and greater overall convenience compared to face-to-face medical consultation [29,30]. More recently, telehealth models have emerged at the forefront at the outset of the COVID-19 pandemic, allowing delivery of healthcare services while containing the transmission of infection [30,31]. Pharmacists have also effectively embraced telehealth to provide ongoing monitoring and management to patients with chronic conditions during the pandemic [32,33]. The present dynamics of global healthcare has enabled students to appreciate telehealth as the next frontier in healthcare delivery. As one of the students stated in the interview, telehealth could also offer flexibility in working schedules for healthcare providers, thus enhancing their work–life balance. This reflection on the perceived benefits of telehealth beyond what it is credited for thus far underpins the larger potentials of digital health in the near future. Moving forward, it would be vital for faculties to consider incorporating education and training of telehealth skills into the pharmacy curriculum by means such as virtual OSCEs to future-proof pharmacy graduates. Future research could explore whether medical educators could utilise this form of virtual assessment for rural and remote students who are on placements.

While the majority of examiners also viewed the virtual OSCE as a great platform to upskill students in telehealth delivery, some were of the opinion that face-to-face interaction with patients is still essential for students to develop soft skills such as empathy. The importance of empathy in patient care is unquestionable. Research indicates that empathy has a significantly positive impact on patients' health outcomes [34,35]. Aside from increasing patient satisfaction and adherence, practitioner empathy also strengthens patient enablement [35]. However, with digitization of healthcare, there is a deep concern that interactions can become impersonal and expression of empathy is reduced [36].

As suggested by previous commentaries [4,5], it is challenging to capture non-verbal communication skills via video conferencing tools. In a study conducted at a tertiary hospital in Japan, comparing telemedicine consultation with face-to-face consultation among doctors and patients, the researchers reported that affective behaviour patterns, particularly empathy-utterances, were less evident in the telemedicine consultations [37]. Our study reinforces these views as both examiners and students mentioned difficulty in either expressing non-verbal communication, such as cues for empathy or giving eye contact, while examiners expressed the lack of ability to observe and assess students' non-verbal communication. Even though these challenges were mainly due to the limitations of the online platforms, such as the inability to observe the full body or difficulties with audio, making it more difficult to hear, students showed self-awareness of these challenges and a desire to improve.

It is positive that students were able to acknowledge that providing patient care via telehealth can be a challenge and that it requires a different set of skills than counselling a patient in person. This was evident with our students' motivation to practise virtually to mimic their actual assessments over Zoom. Additionally, faculty should consider targeted training focused on the development of virtual communication skills. Perhaps it is time for educators to consider integrating the construct of digital empathy in the pharmacy curriculum [36]. To this end, both students and examiners suggested that a combination of the traditional face-to-face and virtual OSCEs in the curriculum will be able to equip them holistically to render good patient and pharmaceutical care.

This study has its limitations. This study was only conducted within one pharmacy school in Melbourne, Australia. Although a high response rate was achieved, the findings might not be generalizable to other schools or countries, depending on the program and strategies in place to adapt during the pandemic. Nevertheless, this study adds to the qualitative findings from both students and examiners around their experiences of virtual OSCEs and provides insight into the potential usefulness of virtual OSCEs in future pharmacy programs.

5. Conclusions

The need for remote online delivery of assessments saw innovative ways of undertaking OSCEs. We found that the virtual OSCEs were an opportunity to mimic telehealth and current practice. While students and examiners embraced the virtual OSCE process, face-to-face OSCEs were still considered important and irreplaceable. This is most evident around aspects of the development of non-verbal communication skills, which was challenging to observe virtually. Future opportunities for OSCEs to be delivered both face-to-face and virtually should be considered.

Author Contributions: Conceptualization, V.M. and S.C.; methodology, V.M. and S.C.; data analysis, V.M. and S.C.; writing—original draft preparation, V.M., S.K. and S.C.; writing—review and editing, V.M., S.K. and S.C. All authors have read and agreed to the published version of the manuscript.

Funding: This research received no external funding.

Institutional Review Board Statement: The study was conducted according to the guidelines of the Declaration of Helsinki, and approved by the Monash University Human Ethics Low Risk Review (Project ID 24637).

Informed Consent Statement: Participants provide consent to the use of the data when completing the survey and when participating in the interviews. For this study, all data is de-identified.

Data Availability Statement: Original data are stored by the authors. Participants did not consent to have their raw data made publicly available.

Acknowledgments: The authors acknowledge the OSCE examiners and pharmacy students who have participated in the surveys and interviews.

Conflicts of Interest: The authors declare no conflict of interest.

References

1. Hsia, S.L.; Zhou, C.; Gruenberg, K.; Trinh, T.D.; Assemi, M. Implementation and evaluation of a virtual objective structured clinical examination for pharmacy students. *J. Am. Coll. Clin. Pharm.* **2021**, *4*, 837–848. [CrossRef]
2. Shaiba, L.A.; Alnamnakani, M.A.; Temsah, M.H.; Alamro, N.; Alsohime, F.; Alrabiaah, A.; Alanazi, S.N.; Alhasan, K.; Alherbish, A.; Mobaireek, K.F.; et al. Medical Faculty's and Students' Perceptions toward Pediatric Electronic OSCE during the COVID-19 Pandemic in Saudi Arabia. *Healthcare* **2021**, *9*, 950. [CrossRef] [PubMed]
3. Mak, V. Online objective structured clinical examination overview. *BMJ Simul. Technol. Enhanc. Learn.* **2021**, *7*, 461–462. [CrossRef]
4. Lucas, C.; Forrest, G. Virtual OSCEs—Challenges and Considerations for Pharmacy Education? Pulses. Currents in Pharmacy Teaching and Learning Scholarly Blog 2020. Available online: https://cptlpulses.com/2020/06/18/virtual-osces/ (accessed on 29 December 2021).
5. Skylar, J. 'Zoom Fatigue' Is Taxing the Brain. Here's Why That Happens. Available online: https://www.nationalgeographic.com/science/2020/04/coronavirus-zoom-fatigue-is-taxing-the-brain-here-is-why-that-happens/ (accessed on 29 December 2021).
6. Guangul, F.M.; Suhail, A.H.; Khalit, M.I.; Khidhir, B.A. Challenges of remote assessment in higher education in the context of COVID-19: A case study of Middle East College. *Educ. Assess. Eval. Account.* **2020**, *32*, 519–535. [CrossRef]
7. Muthuprasad, T.; Aiswarya, S.; Aditya, K.S.; Girish, K.J. Students' perception and preference for online education in India during COVID-19 pandemic. *Soc. Sci. Humanit. Open* **2021**, *3*, 100101. [CrossRef]
8. VanLangen, K.M.; Salvati, L.A. Virtual TOSCEs: This Wasn't the Plan! Pulses. Currents in Pharmacy Teaching and Learning Scholarly Blog 2020. Available online: https://cptlpulses.com/2020/04/09/virtual-tosces/ (accessed on 29 December 2021).

9. Savage, A.; Minshew, L.M.; Anksorus, H.N.; McLaughlin, J.E. Remote OSCE Experience: What First Year Pharmacy Students Liked, Learned, and Suggested for Future Implementations. *Pharmacy* **2021**, *9*, 62. [CrossRef]
10. Andreou, V.; Peters, S.; Eggermont, J.; Wens, J.; Schoenmakers, B. Remote versus on-site proctored exam: Comparing student results in a cross-sectional study. *BMC Med. Educ.* **2021**, *21*, 624. [CrossRef]
11. Brallier, S.A.; Schwanz, K.A.; Palm, L.J.; Irwin, L.N. Online Testing: Comparison of Online and Classroom Exams in an Upper-Level Psychology Course. *Am. J. Educ. Res.* **2015**, *3*, 255–258. [CrossRef]
12. Daffin, L.W.J.; Jones, A.A. Comparing student performance on proctored and non-proctored exams in online psychology courses. *Online Learn. J.* **2018**, *22*, 131–145. [CrossRef]
13. Dendir, S.; Maxwell, R.S. Cheating in online courses: Evidence from online proctoring. *Comput. Hum. Behav. Rep.* **2020**, *2*, 100033. [CrossRef]
14. Ghouri, A.; Boachie, C.; McDowall, S.; Parle, J.; Ditchfield, C.A.; McConnachie, A.; Walters, M.R.; Ghouri, N. Gaining an advantage by sitting an OSCE after your peers: A retrospective study. *Med. Teach.* **2018**, *40*, 1136–1142. [CrossRef] [PubMed]
15. Updike, W.H.; Cowart, K.; Woodyard, J.L.; Serag-Bolos, E.; Taylor, J.R.; Curtis, S.D. Protecting the Integrity of the Virtual Objective Structured Clinical Examination. *Am. J. Pharm. Educ.* **2021**, *85*, 8438. [CrossRef] [PubMed]
16. Deville, R.L.; Fellers, C.M.; Howard, M.L. Lessons learned pivoting to a virtual OSCE: Pharmacy faculty and student perspectives. *Curr. Pharm. Teach. Learn.* **2021**, *13*, 1498–1502. [CrossRef] [PubMed]
17. Morgan, K.; Adams, E.; Elsobky, T.; Darr, A.; Brackbill, M. Moving assessment online: Experiences within a school of pharmacy. *Online Learn.* **2021**, *25*, 245–252. [CrossRef]
18. Chuang, S.; Trevaskis, N.L.; Mak, V. The effects of the COVID-19 pandemic on pharmacy education, staff and students in an Australian setting. *Pharm. Educ.* **2021**, *20*, 87–90. [CrossRef]
19. Kakadia, R.; Chen, E.; Ohyama, H. Implementing an online OSCE during the COVID-19 pandemic. *J. Dent. Educ.* **2020**, *85*, 1006–1008. [CrossRef]
20. Elnaem, M.H.; Akkawi, M.E.; Nazar, N.; Ab Rahman, N.S.; Mohamed, M. Malaysian pharmacy students' perspectives on the virtual objective structured clinical examination during the coronavirus disease 2019 pandemic. *J. Educ. Eval. Health Prof.* **2021**, *18*, 6. [CrossRef]
21. Hanna, L.A.; Davidson, S.; Hall, M. A questionnaire study investigating undergraduate pharmacy students' opinions on assessment methods and an integrated five-year pharmacy degree. *Pharm. Educ.* **2017**, *17*, 115–124.
22. Martin, R.D.; Naziruddin, Z. Systematic review of student anxiety and performance during objective structured clinical examinations. *Curr. Pharm. Teach. Learn.* **2020**, *12*, 1491–1497. [CrossRef]
23. Scoular, S.; Huntsberry, A.; Patel, T.; Wettergreen, S.; Brunner, J.M. Transitioning Competency-Based Communication Assessments to the Online Platform: Examples and Student Outcomes. *Pharmacy* **2021**, *9*, 52. [CrossRef]
24. Almaghaslah, D.; Alsayari, A. The Effects of the 2019 Novel Coronavirus Disease (COVID-19) Outbreak on Academic Staff Members: A Case Study of a Pharmacy School in Saudi Arabia. *Risk Manag. Healthc. Policy* **2020**, *13*, 795–802. [CrossRef] [PubMed]
25. Irawanto, D.W.; Novianti, K.R.; Roz, K. Work from Home: Measuring Satisfaction between Work–Life Balance and Work Stress during the COVID-19 Pandemic in Indonesia. *Economies* **2021**, *9*, 96. [CrossRef]
26. Thomas, D.; Beshir, S.A.; Zachariah, S.; Sundararaj, K.G.; Hamdy, H. Distance assessment of counselling skills using virtual patients during the COVID-19 pandemic. *Pharm. Educ.* **2020**, *20*, 196–204. [CrossRef]
27. Scheduling Privilege. Available online: https://support.zoom.us/hc/en-us/articles/201362803 (accessed on 29 December 2021).
28. World Health Organization (WHO). Telemedicine: Opportunities and Developments in Member States: Report on the Second Global Survey on eHealth 2009. In *Global Observatory for eHealth Series*, 2nd ed.; WHO Press: Geneva, Switzerland, 2010.
29. Raven, M.; Butler, C.; Bywood, P. Video-based telehealth in Australian primary health care: Current use and future potential. *Aust. J. Prim. Health* **2013**, *19*, 283–286. [CrossRef]
30. Gajarawala, S.N.; Pelkowski, J.N. Telehealth Benefits and Barriers. *J. Nurse Pract.* **2021**, *17*, 218–221. [CrossRef]
31. Monaghesh, E.; Hajizadeh, A. The role of telehealth during COVID-19 outbreak: A systematic review based on current evidence. *BMC Public Health* **2020**, *20*, 1193. [CrossRef]
32. Bonner, L. Pharmacists embrace telehealth during COVID-19. *Pharm. Today* **2020**, *26*, 26–29. [CrossRef]
33. Elbeddini, A.; Yeats, A. Pharmacist intervention amid the coronavirus disease 2019 (COVID-19) pandemic: From direct patient care to telemedicine. *J. Pharm. Policy Pract.* **2020**, *13*, 23. [CrossRef]
34. Neumann, M.; Bensing, J.; Mercer, S.; Ernstmann, N.; Ommen, O.; Pfaff, H. Analyzing the "nature" and "specific effectiveness" of clinical empathy: A theoretical overview and contribution towards a theory-based research agenda. *Patient Educ. Couns.* **2009**, *74*, 339–346. [CrossRef]
35. Derksen, F.; Bensing, J.; Lagro-Janssen, A. Effectiveness of empathy in general practice: A systematic review. *Br. J. Gen. Pract.* **2013**, *63*, e76–e84. [CrossRef]
36. Terry, C.; Cain, J. The Emerging Issue of Digital Empathy. *Am. J. Pharm. Educ.* **2016**, *80*, 58. [CrossRef] [PubMed]
37. Liu, X.; Sawada, Y.; Takizawa, T.; Sato, H.; Sato, M.; Sakamoto, H.; Utsugi, T.; Sato, K.; Sumino, H.; Okamura, S.; et al. Doctor-patient communication: A comparison between telemedicine consultation and face-to-face consultation. *Intern. Med.* **2007**, *46*, 227–232. [CrossRef] [PubMed]

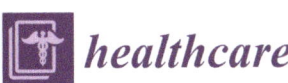

Article

A Video-Based Reflective Design to Prepare First Year Pharmacy Students for Their First Objective Structured Clinical Examination (OSCE)

Vivienne Mak *, Daniel Malone, Nilushi Karunaratne, Wendy Yao, Lauren Randell and Thao Vu

Pharmacy and Pharmaceutical Sciences Education, Faculty of Pharmacy and Pharmaceutical Sciences, Monash University, Parkville, VIC 3052, Australia; Dan.Malone@monash.edu (D.M.); nilushi.karunaratne@monash.edu (N.K.); wyao0001@student.monash.edu (W.Y.); lsran2@student.monash.edu (L.R.); Thao.Vu1@monash.edu (T.V.)
* Correspondence: Vivienne.Mak@monash.edu

Citation: Mak, V.; Malone, D.; Karunaratne, N.; Yao, W.; Randell, L.; Vu, T. A Video-Based Reflective Design to Prepare First Year Pharmacy Students for Their First Objective Structured Clinical Examination (OSCE). *Healthcare* **2022**, *10*, 280. https://doi.org/10.3390/healthcare10020280

Academic Editors: Luís Proença, Vanessa Machado, João Botelho and José João Mendes

Received: 24 December 2021
Accepted: 27 January 2022
Published: 31 January 2022

Publisher's Note: MDPI stays neutral with regard to jurisdictional claims in published maps and institutional affiliations.

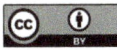

Copyright: © 2022 by the authors. Licensee MDPI, Basel, Switzerland. This article is an open access article distributed under the terms and conditions of the Creative Commons Attribution (CC BY) license (https://creativecommons.org/licenses/by/4.0/).

Abstract: We explored the use of a video-based reflective design in preparing first-year pharmacy students for their Objective Structured Clinical Examination (OSCE) in Victoria, Australia. This involved pre-workshop activities (a recording of themselves simulating the pharmacist responding to a simple primary care problem, written reflection, review of the OSCE video examples and pre-workshop survey); workshop activities (peer feedback on videos) and post-workshop activities (summative MCQ quiz and post-workshop survey). These activities took place three weeks before their OSCE. A mixed-method study design was employed with quantitative and qualitative analyses of the surveys and a focus group. A total of 137 students (77.4%) completed the pre- and post-workshop surveys, and ten students participated in the focus group. More student participants (54%) reported feeling prepared for the OSCE post-workshop than pre-workshop (13%). The majority (92%) agreed that filming, watching and reflecting on their video allowed them to learn and improve on their skills for the OSCE. The regression analysis found that video recording submissions and written reflections correlated positively with student OSCE performances, and the video-based reflective design learning experience was perceived to be beneficial in multiple ways. Thematic analysis of the focus group data revealed that students acquired metacognitive skills through the self-assessment of their video recordings, developed an awareness of their learning and were able to identify learning strategies to prepare for their first OSCE. Fostering students' feedback literacy could be considered in future educational designs.

Keywords: e-learning; healthcare education; OSCE; video; reflective practice; feedback

1. Introduction

Video-based reflective design incorporates the use of technology, in this instance, video recordings, as a medium for self-reflection and feedback. The observation of self-performance through video recordings allows for a review of how one's self is portrayed and to facilitate self-directed learning [1]. Multiple studies have outlined the benefits of improving self-evaluation and communication skills through the review of video recordings [2–6]. It is suggested that, when weaknesses are identified in one's own performance through self-evaluation, one is more likely to be motivated to consider steps to improve [7]. There is an increasing uptake in the utilisation of video recording and reviewing activities within teaching, nursing, medical and pharmacy courses globally. It is proposed that communication skills will improve in pharmacy students through the feedback and reflection of simulated role play recordings [8]. One study observed an increase in self-perception following a video review of a counselling activity conducted by first-year pharmacy students and supported the inclusion of an activity that reinforced self-evaluation [5]. The concept of metacognition, in which self-evaluation is an important component, continues to be explored as an important skill for pharmacy students to develop over time [9]. Metacognition has been defined in various ways but is generally considered to be the process of reflecting on and evaluating one's own learning [10]. The metacognitive process of self-regulation and reflection on knowledge and skills is important for health professional students for self-improvement [11].

In this current study, we implemented a video-based reflective design to prepare students for their first Objective Structured Clinical Examination (OSCE). OSCEs have been established as an effective means of evaluating pharmacy students' performances in a simulated environment [12,13]. OSCEs have been used as summative assessment tasks to assess problem-solving and communication at the Monash University Faculty of Pharmacy and Pharmaceutical Sciences since 2011 [14]. Preparing healthcare students in terms of developing their problem-solving and communication skills can be done in numerous ways. These include, but are not limited to, the use of online virtual tools, video exemplars, teaching or mock OSCEs, peer assessment and feedback [15–18]. On the other hand, preparing students for OSCEs using teaching or mock OSCEs and instructor feedback can be challenging due to resource constraints such as time barriers, additional staff workload and costs [19]. Generally, students with previous OSCE experiences, whether through an actual or mock OSCE, have experienced reduced anxiety and improved performances, although the implementation of mock OSCEs as described is limited by the associated costs [20].

Thus, self-directed learning and preparation for OSCEs by students themselves is important. The study strategies identified in the literature that students themselves use to prepare for OSCEs include practicing with other students, rehearsing routines, physical examination courses (practical classes), class notes/logs and skills labs [20,21]. Nevertheless, students found resources for gathering knowledge such as lectures or textbooks less helpful and spent less time studying as compared to multiple-choice question (MCQ) tests [20]. Many OSCE preparation techniques have been reviewed to help students achieve the optimal performance in OSCEs. These include various strategies reported that aim to improve metacognition in students as part of the OSCE preparation process. Teaching reflective skills and encouraging students to voluntarily practise and reflect on their clinical skills were shown to improve OSCE scores in medical students [22]. High achievements in pharmacy students have been linked to various metacognitive processes, including self-efficacy and self-evaluation [23]. A peer-led mock OSCE approach is a strategy identified to reduce the costliness of OSCE preparation whilst retaining the benefit of the mock OSCE experience [24,25]. However, peer-led mock OSCEs do not address any deficiency in students' self-reflective capacities [25–28] that pharmacists may carry throughout their careers [29]. Therefore, if metacognitive skills can be incorporated as part of the pharmacy curriculum, this may lead to the better preparation of students for high stakes assessment tasks such as OSCEs.

The purpose of this study was to explore the use of a structured video-based reflective design and its influence in preparing first-year pharmacy students for their first OSCE. To our knowledge, there is limited literature linking the impact of a structured video-based reflective design utilizing students' own video recordings, self-reflection of those video recordings and further reflection upon receiving peer feedback on those video recordings within Australian pharmacy programs on OSCE performances in pharmacy students.

The most common undergraduate pharmacy degree that is offered in Australia is the four-year Bachelor of Pharmacy (BPharm). At the Faculty of Pharmacy and Pharmaceutical Sciences, a new pharmacy program was developed that had its first cohort of year 1 students in 2017 [30]. One of the major distinguishing features of this new program is the whole degree flipped classroom delivery that includes self-directed learning, interactive lectures, weekly small group workshops and a skills coaching program that is focused on enhancing reflective practice and metacognitive skills. The new pharmacy program places an emphasis on skill development, including oral communication, empathy and problem-solving skills.

Students enter the pharmacy course without the experience of a skills-based performance exam such as the OSCEs. Therefore, providing guidance on how to undertake, and perform well in, their first-year OSCE is essential.

A structured video-based reflective design to prepare students for their first-year OSCE was introduced with a series of preparatory activities. These activities included providing students with tasks that are easy to complete in their own time, with the aim to equip them with OSCE preparation strategies that they can retain throughout their degree. This study provides insight into how health professional schools can prepare students for their first OSCE utilising a structured video-based reflective design.

The research questions for this study were:

(1) How did the video-based reflective design prepare students for first-year OSCEs as perceived by the students?
(2) What is the relationship between student engagement in the video-based reflective design activities and their OSCE performance?

2. Materials and Methods

2.1. Video-Based Reflective Design

We designed a video-based reflective design to prepare students for their first OSCE. This included pre-workshop tasks, workshop activities and a post-workshop task.

Pre-workshop: Students completed a summative assessment worth 2% of the course mark. There were two components to this summative assessment: (1) video recording submission and (2) written reflection submission. For the video recording, students had to film themselves performing a short *role play interaction* (5 min maximum) simulating a pharmacist responding to one simple primary care problem with a mock patient. The eight primary care topics included diarrhoea, threadworm, constipation, headache, tinea, hay fever, reflux and the common cold. Students were provided with one case topic and the corresponding script. Each student selected their own partner as the mock patient to complete the task. For the *written reflection*, students were asked to review their recordings and, based on their videos, respond to three structured points: reflect on their accomplishments, identify areas for improvement and identify strategies to improve. The 2% of the course mark was awarded as long as the student submitted both the video recording and written reflection (*summative pre-workshop video and reflection submission*). The content of the video recording and written reflection was not assessed. Although not compulsory, students were encouraged to self-evaluate the video using the *OSCE communication rubric* provided to them. Students then attended two face-to-face 50-min large class interactive lectures that included *watching a previous student's OSCE video as examples* and information on the OSCE process. Whilst watching the video examples, students were asked to formatively assess the performances in the videos using the OSCE communication rubric. Prior to attending the workshop, the students were invited to complete a 1-item survey asking how prepared they were for the OSCE (*pre-workshop survey*).

Workshop: Three days after the completion of the pre-workshop tasks, students attended a two-hour workshop (*workshop attendance*). At the commencement of the workshop, the workshop facilitator, who was also a practicing pharmacist, played two exemplar videos to the students, with one video more ideal than the other. Students were then asked to provide feedback on the exemplar videos using the same structure as their pre-workshop written reflections and with using the OSCE communication rubric. The workshop facilitator then provided the students with feedback on the quality of their feedback on the exemplar videos. Students were then divided into small groups of 5 to 6 students per group and were told to use the same feedback structure in the following workshop task. Each student then played their own recording to their peers, verbally shared their written reflections from the pre-workshop and received peer feedback on their video. Each student repeated this process until all the students played their own recordings.

Post-workshop: After completion of the workshop, students were invited to complete a 4-item survey evaluating how helpful the workshop was and how prepared they felt for the OSCEs (*post-workshop survey*). Students then had one week to complete a summative multiple-choice question (MCQ) quiz on the eight primary care topics. This was a content knowledge quiz with 20 MCQs with a 60-min time limit. Students could attempt this twice, with the final attempt counting towards their course mark and worth 8% (*summative post-workshop MCQ quiz mark*).

2.2. Study Design and Participants

This was a mixed-method study design where we triangulated both quantitative with qualitative analyses to answer our research questions. Participants in this study were first-year pharmacy students at Monash University Australia in 2017. A total of 177 students were invited to complete the pre- and post-workshop surveys. The same 177 students were invited to participate in the focus group. The study was approved by the Monash University Human Research Ethics Committee. As part of the standard quality improvement processes for the pharmacy degree and consistent with the Student Privacy Collection Statement, student performance data were collected and deidentified.

2.2.1. Pre- and Post-Workshop Survey

Students were invited to complete a 1-item perception survey about OSCE preparedness before the workshop commenced. Following the workshop, students were invited to complete a 4-item perception survey about the usefulness of the workshop activities. Specifically, these items were used to determine whether students self-recording and reflecting on their performance helped students learn and improve their skills for the OSCEs and, secondly, whether reviewing recordings of other students helped students learn and improve their skills for the OSCEs. Student perceptions on OSCE preparedness were also recorded at the completion of the workshop. Data were collected using a self-administered online survey based on the objectives of the research. This survey was conducted on the learning management system Moodle. Data were analysed using descriptive analysis (percentage agreement with each survey item).

Three regression analyses were performed to determine whether correlations existed between the students' OSCE performances and various video-based reflective design activities.

These analyses were completed with the three dependent variables:

(1) *OSCE communication mark*—graded using an OSCE communication rubric and assesses skills;
(2) *OSCE analytical checklist mark*—graded using a checklist that assesses clinical points;
(3) *Overall OSCE mark*—total mark combining both communication and analytical checklist marks.

For each analysis, the independent variables were *summative pre-workshop video and reflection submission, workshop attendance* and *summative post-workshop MCQ quiz mark* (as described in Section 2.1). Statistical significance was defined when $p < 0.05$. All statistical analyses were conducted using SPSS Version 23 (IBM Corporation, Armonk, NY, USA).

2.2.2. Focus Group

Ten students (seven female, three male) who had completed both the pre- and post-workshop surveys and their first-year OSCE volunteered to participate in an hour-long focus group facilitated by two researchers (T.V. and N.K.). These two researchers were not part of the students' direct teaching staff. As the students completed the same activity in their first year, their shared experience was conducive to facilitating an interactive reflection of their first-year OSCE preparation, which is essential for using the focus group data collection method [31]. To minimise bias due to potential pre-existing relationships among the student participants, a number of strategies were employed. Firstly, the students were briefed on the aims and the format of the focus group and were invited to participate in and cocreate a safe and nonjudgmental environment to share individual ideas about their experiences. Secondly, to ensure all students had the opportunity to share their personal perspectives, the students were asked to complete a list of individual brainstorming tasks before taking turns responding to open-ended questions prepared in advance by the researcher facilitators. Students were regularly prompted with "How?" and "Why?" questions to explain their own answers. Thirdly, students were frequently encouraged during the focus group to agree, disagree and elaborate on each other's ideas.

The focus group was audio-recorded with the student participants' consent. The audio recording was transcribed and deidentified. Focus group data as password-protected files were only accessible by the researchers. Two researchers (T.V. and N.K.) analysed the data together using thematic analysis [32] to answer the research question: How did the video-based reflective design prepare students for the OSCEs? The data was categorised according to the main components of the activity: (1) filming, watching and reflecting on their own role play video using a structured approach; (2) watching and evaluating example videos of student OSCE performances and (3) watching and evaluating example videos of student OSCE performances. Following this structure, a mutually agreed codebook was developed. Given the relatively small amount of qualitative data, the coding was conducted using a shared Google Doc, Google Sheet and extensive discussions between the two coders. The codes and the individually induced themes were thoroughly discussed, moderated and triangulated by the two coders to reach a consensus on the final themes [31,33]. The codes from the focus group data analysis are explained in Sections 3.1.1–3.1.3. Two emerging themes related to students acquiring metacognitive knowledge through self-reflection and feedback literacy are discussed in Section 4.

3. Results

A total of 137 students completed the pre- and post-workshop surveys (77.4%). Student performance and engagement data were collected from all 177 students. A total of ten students participated in the focus group.

3.1. How Did the Video-Based Reflective Design Prepare Students for the First Year OSCEs as Perceived by the Students?

This section presents the research findings in response to the first research question. The data from both the pre- and post-workshop survey results and focus group showed that the student participants felt more prepared for the first-year OSCE after the workshop and reportedly benefited from all the three components of the video-based design: the video recording, watching and reflecting on their own or their peers' role play videos (Table 1). When students were engaged in the activity and adopted a structured approach to reflect on their own video and their peers' videos, the learning experience was perceived to be beneficial in multiple ways that will be explained below. These research findings shed light on two interrelated emerging themes (discussed in Section 4) about the acquisition of metacognitive knowledge through self-reflection and feedback literacy that are essential to this activity.

Table 1. Pre- and post-workshop survey results (n = 137).

Survey	Item	Strongly Disagree/Disagree	Neutral	Strongly Agree/Agree
Pre-workshop	I currently feel prepared for the OSCEs	36%	51%	13%
Post-workshop	After the workshop, I feel prepared for the OSCEs	7%	39%	54%
	Watching student OSCE video examples helped me prepare for the OSCE	5%	9%	86%
	Filming, watching and reflecting on my role play video allowed me to learn and improve on my skills for the OSCE	4%	4%	92%
	Reviewing and providing feedback on my peers' role play videos allowed me to learn and improve on my skills for the OSCE	9%	4%	87%

Overall, a greater proportion of student participants (54%) who completed the survey reported feeling prepared for the OSCEs after the workshop compared to only 13% before the workshop.

To shed light on what specifically students found useful about these activities in helping them prepare for the OSCE, the focus group data showed that all the activities contributed to enhancing students' awareness of their own areas for improvement and their ability to reflect and provide feedback on an OSCE performance, which helped them feel more able to self-regulate their learning and practice of their skills.

3.1.1. Filming, Watching and Reflecting on Their Own Role Play Video Using a Structured Approach

In this activity, students filmed, watched and reflected on their own role play video with their own selected mock patient using the provided *OSCE communication rubric* and a structured approach. There was a strong consensus among the focus group students that this activity was *"very helpful"* (Student 5) for several reasons.

Most importantly, students reported that they became more **self-aware of the areas to improve in communication skills** and that they were able to **draw on their gained self-awareness to regulate their own practice for the OSCE**. For example, some students explained that they were able to observe their own performances objectively and become cognizant of specific behaviours that might affect their communication:

*"On the video **I saw I was fidgeting a lot; moving around in my chair**. So that was a good way to find out how to improve yourself."* (Student 7)

"I also thought videoing ourselves was really valuable ... I watched mine many times, I was like, That's another thing I can pick up, that's another thing I shouldn't be doing." (Student 2)

"I felt that was pretty good because you could actually see the mistakes you did throughout the actual video." (Student 5)

A student reportedly utilised this new knowledge of their own performance to inform their preparation for the OSCE:

" ... we were able to come to terms with where we were at the moment and we still had a few weeks until the OSCE to improve upon that for the OSCE." (Student 3)

In addition, the students also found filming their role play videos helpful because the activity **prompted them to practice and learn through practice**. For instance, one student said that, by working on the role play counselling video, they practised *"how to actually communicate to each other, how to set a structure as to how we go about collecting information and giving out information about medication"*. (Student 2). Another student contended that, by working with other students to film the video, they could *"pick up"* good strategies from their peers and *"incorporate"* those into their own counselling (Student 8).

Furthermore, by reflecting on their own video using the provided structured approach with the *OSCE communication rubric*, the student reported the **benefit of interacting with the rubric to be used in the exam** and became more aware of *"what we're looking for"* in terms of evaluating their own performance and *"what we should aim towards"* in terms of preparing for their future OSCE performances (Student 9). The gained awareness was then used to *"guide"* their own practices for the OSCE (Student 9).

3.1.2. Watching and Evaluating Example Videos of Student OSCE Performances

In this activity, students attended two interactive lectures where they were shown examples of past videos of student performances in the OSCEs and were instructed to use the OSCE communication rubric to evaluate the example performances. There was a strong agreement in the group that the knowledge gained from this activity *"demystified the whole OSCE process"* and provided them with a perspective of what worked and what could go wrong in an OSCE performance.

The students reflected that, because they had no prior experience with OSCEs, the opportunity to "*go through the exemplars ... what not to do and what to do*" was "*really invaluable*" (Student 4). Without this instruction, the students felt that they would have felt "*blank*" during in the actual exam (Student 6) and their performances could have been negatively affected because their first OSCE could be "*an overwhelming experience*" (Student 5).

The perspectives gained from various video examples were also reportedly helpful for students' self-reflection and sense of confidence. For example, one student commented:

> "*My favorite part was when they used to show us videos of a really bad OSCE and really good OSCE. They seem really obvious and people laugh at them, as if you would do an OSCE that bad, but **sometimes you can see something in yourself that you're doing in that video**, or it's a bit of confidence. At least I'm not doing that. They were really good, those videos.*" (Student 3)

Students suggested that the activity could be improved with the use of an audience engagement tool like Poll Everywhere to encourage more students to provide feedback and/or to ask for clarification. Another recommendation that some students shared was to make the example videos used in the lecture accessible afterwards for reviewing.

3.1.3. Reviewing and Providing Feedback on Peer's Role Play Videos

In this activity, students participated in a workshop where they worked in small groups and provided peer feedback on one another's videos that they had submitted in the previous activity. The most common view among the focus group participants was that, **when students were engaged** in sharing their own videos and providing structured feedback, they **benefited from gaining more awareness of what they could improve and what they could learn from their peers**. The students believed that this practice was helpful for both the **short-term OSCE preparation** and their **development of professionalism in the long run**. However, a few students found this activity not as helpful when they or their peers were hesitant to participate or when they perceived the provided feedback from peers was too general.

What the focus group students found most helpful about the peer feedback activity was **the various perspectives about how they could improve their performance**. For instance, one student reflected positively on the variety and objectivity of the feedback received from the students randomly allocated to their workshop group, which could be different from the feedback they usually received from their friends:

> "*... we were a group of six, so you **get more opinions** ... my friends focus more on the content, but ... they [other students in the workshop group] focus more on the other aspects of communication, like non-verbal, what you could do to improve your performance ... I personally felt it was good because I was given **different opinions from six different people that I don't really talk to** ... Their objective views were really nice because when I ask my friends about it [my OSCE video] they're like, Oh, that sounds great. When you ask someone else they're more like, You need to fix this, you need to fix that, and I was like, Okay, I shall do that next time round. So personally I liked it.*" (Student 9)

Similarly, another student acknowledged that the peer feedback helped them **understand their strengths and weaknesses better** so that they could prepare for their OSCE performance:

> "*... in my opinion, if you kept the video to yourself you wouldn't be able to understand what you did wrong. Whereas, my friend [student in the workshop group] told me what **I needed to work on as well as what I needed to fix up**. That then gave me **a good understanding of what I actually did well**.*" (Student 7)

Nevertheless, a minority of students held a different view that peer feedback group activity **might not be helpful when the feedback they received from their peers was not** specific enough. One student contended that *"showing that [the video] to someone else and having them say, Ah, you didn't really do a great job, is not helpful for me"* (Student 3). In this case, the workshop group appeared not to follow the structured approach using the OSCE communication rubric to provide feedback as instructed. Another hindrance to the usefulness of the workshop activity was that the students **declined to show their own videos** to the group or were **reluctant to provide peer feedback**. The same student who did not find peer feedback helpful admitted refusing to show their own video because they *"felt like they had a long way to go"* and *"having to show that to a peer, I just think it's embarrassing"* (Student 3). Another student observed that their group was *"reluctant to talk"* and *"reluctant to give feedback"* (Student 9). The obstacle to really benefiting from this activity seemed to relate to **the sense of safety** students have in terms of receiving and providing feedback in a group setting and, potentially, their **level of feedback literacy**.

Whilst exposing one's own potential weaknesses and receiving feedback can be *"daunting"* to students, the skill was believed to benefit the students' **long-term growth in professionalism**. One student reflected that it was important to develop this skill as part of their professionalism:

> *"Initially it's very daunting and to present [one's own video] in front of other people is even more daunting. I think from a professional standpoint, it's a skill that you have to develop because you're going to get feedback from people you do not want to get feedback from anyways."* (Student 5)

Moreover, some students acknowledged that providing peer feedback and observing others' performances was a useful learning experience in which they **transferred their feedback of other performances to what they could improve in their own performance**:

> *"I was able to see their OSCE videos as well, so I was able to see ... what they did in their video and I was like, Oh, okay, so I need to do that ... Or how to phrase some words when counseling patients, so that was nice."* (Student 9)

> *" ... by looking at other people's videos we could see, Okay, they did that, I want to do that. Or They didn't do that, I would have put that in my video."* (Student 10)

In summary, according to most of the student participants in both the survey and focus groups, the video-based reflective design was useful in preparing students for their first OSCE. When students were engaged in the activity and adopted the structured approach with the OSCE communication rubric to reflect on their own video and others' videos, the learning experience was perceived to be beneficial in multiple ways. Filming the video prompted students to practise what they had learnt during the course. Reflecting on their own performance and others' using the OSCE communication rubric helped enhance the awareness of their own and others' strengths and gaps in skills that informed their regulation of practising the skills to prepare for the OSCE. Providing peer feedback helped students learn from each other and potentially nurtured the necessary mindset and skill to receive feedback as part of their professionalism. From the focus group data, what appeared to be important influencing factors for the students to gain these benefits could be their sense of safety and ability in dealing with the discomfort of letting others see and evaluate their (perceived) *"imperfect"* performances, as well as their feedback literacy, particularly the ability to provide effective specific feedback to their peers.

3.2. What Is the Relationship between Student Engagement in the Video-Based Reflective Design Activities and Their OSCE Performance?

Multiple linear regression analyses found significant effects of the teaching activities on the *overall OSCE mark* ($F_{3,136} = 4.110$, $p < 0.05$), *OSCE communication mark* ($F_{3,136} = 4.024$, $p < 0.05$) and the *OSCE analytical checklist mark* ($F_{3,136} = 3.312$, $p < 0.05$). The *summative pre-workshop video and reflection submission* were the only significant predictors of the *overall OSCE mark* ($p = 0.001$), *OSCE communication mark* ($p = 0.001$) and *OSCE analytical checklist mark* ($p = 0.007$) (Table 2). This indicates that students that created a video and submitted a reflection performed better in the OSCEs, both from the perspective of communication and achieved scores on the OSCE analytical checklist, than students that did not.

Table 2. Multiple regression of OSCE teaching activities (independent variables) and OSCE performance (dependent variables).

Independent Variables	Overall OSCE Mark		OSCE Communication Mark		OSCE Analytical Checklist Mark	
	Std. B	p	Std. B	p	Std. B	p
Summative pre-workshop video and reflection submission	0.284	0.001	0.306	0.001	0.239	0.007
Workshop attendance	0.088	0.294	0.096	0.253	0.048	0.566
Summative post-workshop MCQ quiz mark	−0.011	0.894	−0.049	0.573	0.060	0.488

4. Discussion

This study offers several findings on the use of video-based reflective designs in preparing students for their first Objective Structured Clinical Examinations (OSCEs) in pharmacy education. It is an innovative structured video-based reflective design incorporating video recordings, self-assessment and exemplar videos with peer feedback, and this study linked the impact of this design on pharmacy students' first OSCE performance. This study found that more students perceived that they felt more prepared for their OSCE after the workshop compared to pre-workshop. It was found that the students' perceptions of their preparedness for the OSCEs drastically improved from 13 to 54% after participating in the workshop. Although 39% of student participants did not feel either way, most students (92%) agreed or strongly agreed that the process of filming, watching and reflecting on their role play videos allowed them to learn and improve on their skills for their OSCE. These findings are consistent with a previous study, albeit it was conducted on fourth-year pharmacy students, where video reviews of their simulated role plays were shown to be beneficial in facilitating awareness of their nonverbal communication [4]. This was further substantiated by the qualitative data in our study demonstrating that the video-based reflective design activities stimulated students' ability to identify their strengths and areas for improvement in their communication skills to consider the learning strategies for further improvement. They found the feedback received and given to their peers useful for their own learning and preparation for their OSCE. Importantly, our findings demonstrated better performances in the OSCEs by students who undertook the video-based reflective design activities, as evidenced by a regression analysis. A similar outcome was observed in a study with nursing students that found students were more satisfied with their learning and noticed a significant positive impact on summative grades for students who participated in the video-based self-assessment [3].

Our study provided empirical findings around the usefulness of the video-based reflective design as part of the wider programmatic approach in developing metacognitive skills amongst pharmacy students. Metacognition helps the individual be more aware of and control their thinking processes. Classically described metacognition frameworks involve two components of metacognition: knowledge of cognition (metacognitive knowledge) and regulation of cognition (metacognitive regulation). This study integrated metacognitive development into the undergraduate curriculum through a video-based reflective design to prepare first-year pharmacy students for their first OSCE.

The students acquired metacognitive knowledge through self-reflection, especially among their peers in a classroom setting, providing learners the opportunity to develop these soft skills through the self-identification of gaps to be filled. The learning strategies of peer assessment and self-reflection have been demonstrated to quicken the process of the development of metacognitive skills among learners [34,35]. This is because a peer assessment often leverages on social pressure associated with learners not wanting to lose face in front of their peers. Learners are motivated to focus on the processes of self-reflection and self-regulation to avoid the embarrassment of having their colleagues openly identify the probable gaps in their learning among their peers [31]. Students were further able to identify the strengths and weaknesses in relation to their OSCE preparations when working with peers. This provided students with more robust knowledge and more accurate self-assessments of their abilities. Furthermore, engaging students in discussions around their self-recorded videos allowed students to compare their own performances against their peers, as well as reflect on improving their own skills. Students were also able to practice providing and receiving constructive feedback, which is an important quality that is necessary for ongoing development [36].

The video-based reflective design learning activity also created opportunities for learners to regulate their acquired metacognitive knowledge. Students reviewed their performance of the task and understood how the performance would be assessed. The activity enabled students to use the OSCE communication rubric to guide them toward the goals from practice and provided guidance on how to achieve these goals. Through this reflective practice of evaluation, metacognitive knowledge is built and refined, which implicates a feedback loop where new and better knowledge is used for the regulation of cognition, for example, resulting in better planning in the future.

In this paper, we explored how a video-based reflective design prepared students for their first OSCE. We found further evidence on how incorporating feedback literacy in educational design as part of the video-based reflective design could benefit student learning. Feedback could be understood as *"a process through which learners make sense of information from various sources and use it to enhance their work or learning strategies"* [37] (p. 1315). Students' feedback literacy, which is fundamental to their learning and in their future work as a pharmacist, consists of four main dimensions: *"appreciating feedback; making judgments; managing affect; and taking action"* [37] (p. 1316). Our study showed that students' learning was enhanced through the process of providing and receiving feedback, and they appreciated this ability as part of their long-term development in professionalism. The two activities, peer feedback and analysing video exemplars, in our design, were recognised as activities that facilitated their development in feedback literacy. We also found that students' sense of safety and comfort in their peer group impacted their willingness to share their imperfect video recordings. Additionally, their perceived skill to provide actionable feedback influenced the quality and outcome of the learning experience. Previous literature has also described how a student is less likely to participate in providing peer feedback due to a lack of confidence in the task [38]. Therefore, we highly recommend including learning materials and activities to help students develop a positive mindset about receiving and giving feedback and the ability to "manage affect" feedback, as well as the skill to provide effective feedback at the outset of these activities [37] (p. 1316).

The results from the multiple regression analysis showed that there was no correlation between the *summative post-workshop MCQ quiz mark* and student performance in any aspects of the OSCE. It may have been expected to see a correlation between the *summative post-workshop MCQ quiz mark* and the *OSCE analytical checklist mark*, considering both were summative assessments based on students' content knowledge. However, the *MCQ quiz* tested the ability of students to remember and understand material related to the OSCEs, as opposed to the *OSCE analytical checklist*, which was designed to assess the ability of students to analyse information in, and apply knowledge to, a clinical case. It has been previously shown that pharmacy students perform differently on assessments that focus on recall compared with the application or analysis of information [39,40].

Despite there being no correlation between *workshop attendance* having an impact on the *overall OSCE mark*, the findings of the focus group discussion suggested otherwise. The majority of the focus group students expressed that the workshop activity provided multiple learning opportunities not only from watching other student videos but also from receiving and providing constructive feedback. This entire process allowed each student to critique their own performance and identify areas of improvement so as to assist in the preparation for their first OSCE. The results of the multiple regression analysis regarding attendance may be explained by the minority of focus group students who considered the workshop activity as unhelpful. Students found the workshop unhelpful when other students were unwilling to share their own videos or received nonspecific feedback with no indication of how to improve their performance. Thus, it is important for educators to create a safe environment during the learning activity so that students feel safe to share their self-recorded videos and feel confident in providing and receiving feedback.

A strength of this study was the focus on one approach, the video-based reflective design as part of a programmatic approach to developing the core skills and knowledge for the OSCE. However, it is important to acknowledge that skill development can be influenced by a number of factors, including engagement in other activities within the program, workplace experiences and prior exposure to patient care activities. Future research should evaluate the program's instructional design model as a whole in preparing students for the OSCE. A limitation of this research was that there was no guarantee that the peer feedback provided was constructive or helpful to students, as the quality of the feedback was not assessed. Nevertheless, there was an instructor present, but this instructor may not have provided oversight of every student. Additionally, the focus group consisted of 10 students in the cohort, and thus, the results may not be generalisable to the majority of students.

5. Conclusions

The video-based reflective design used in this study was found to be useful in the development of metacognitive skills, with video recordings and reflective tasks positively correlating with the OSCE performance outcomes. The video-based reflective practice helped enhance students' awareness of their learning and stimulated them to consider various learning strategies according to their own learning needs to prepare for their first OSCE. Educators may also consider students' feedback literacy in their educational design to further encourage student confidence in giving peer feedback so that a positive overall learning experience can be achieved.

Author Contributions: Conceptualization, V.M.; methodology, V.M., D.M., N.K. and T.V.; data analysis, V.M., D.M., N.K., L.R., W.Y. and T.V.; writing—original draft preparation, V.M., D.M., N.K., L.R., W.Y. and T.V. and writing—review and editing, V.M., D.M., N.K., L.R., W.Y. and T.V. All authors have read and agreed to the published version of the manuscript.

Funding: This research received no external funding. However, this project was part of a student's summer research project where the student received a weekly stipend ($240/week).

Institutional Review Board Statement: The study was conducted according to the guidelines of the Declaration of Helsinki and approved by the Monash University Human Ethics Low Risk Review (Project ID 16514).

Informed Consent Statement: Participant consent followed an opt out consent process due to the low-risk study. At the Monash University Faculty of Pharmacy and Pharmaceutical Sciences, the pharmacy program runs an education research registry. Each year, all the students are informed of education research projects and presented with the opportunity to opt out of having their student data used for education research. For this study, we removed any data from students who opted out of the education research registry. Students provide consent when participating in the focus group.

Data Availability Statement: The original data are stored by the authors. Participants did not consent to have their raw data made publicly available. However, data on this study may be available upon reasonable request in various forms.

Acknowledgments: The authors acknowledge the pharmacy instructors, teaching associates and pharmacy students who participated in the video-based reflective activity.

Conflicts of Interest: The authors declare no conflict of interest.

References

1. Hays, R.B. Self-evaluation of videotaped consultations. *Teach. Learn. Med.* **1990**, *2*, 232–236. [CrossRef]
2. Baecher, L.; Kung, S. C.; Jewkes, A.M.; Rosalla, C. The role of video for self-evaluation in early field experiences. *Teach. Teach. Educ.* **2013**, *36*, 189–197. [CrossRef]
3. Yoo, M.; Son, Y.; Kim, Y.; Park, J. Video-based self-assessment: Implementation and evaluation in an undergraduate nursing course. *Nurse Educ. Today* **2009**, *29*, 585–589. [CrossRef] [PubMed]
4. Hanya, M.; Yonei, H.; Kurono, S.; Kamei, H. Development of reflective thinking in pharmacy students to improve their communication with patients through a process of role-playing, video reviews, and transcript creation. *Curr. Pharm. Teach. Learn.* **2014**, *6*, 122–129. [CrossRef]
5. Mort, J.R.; Hansen, D.J. First-year Pharmacy Students' Self-Assessment of Communication Skills and the Impact of Video Review. *Am. J. Pharm. Educ.* **2010**, *74*, 78. [CrossRef] [PubMed]
6. Hanley, K.; Zabar, S.; Disney, L.; Kalet, A.; Gillespie, C. Students Who Develop Self-Assessment Skills In A Structured Videotape Review Improve Their Interviewing Skills With Standardized Patients. *J. Gen. Intern. Med. 33rd Annu. Meet. Soc. Gen. Intern. Med.* **2010**, *25*, 393–394. [CrossRef]
7. Duffy, F.D.; Holmboe, E.S. Self-assessment in Lifelong Learning and Improving Performance in Practice. *JAMA J. Am. Med. Assoc.* **2006**, *296*, 1137–1139. [CrossRef]
8. Kerr, A.; Kelleher, C.; Pawlikowska, T.; Strawbridge, J. How can pharmacists develop patient-pharmacist communication skills? A realist synthesis. *Patient Educ. Couns.* **2021**, *104*, 2467–2479. [CrossRef]
9. Nisly, S.A.; Sebaaly, J.; Fillius, A.G.; Haltom, W.R.; Dinkins, M.M. Changes in Pharmacy Students' Metacognition Through Self-Evaluation During Advanced Pharmacy Practice Experiences. *Am. J. Pharm. Educ.* **2020**, *84*, 7489. [CrossRef]
10. Tanner, K.D. Promoting Student Metacognition. *CBE—Life Sci. Educ.* **2017**, *11*, 113–120. [CrossRef]
11. Medina, M.S.; Castleberry, A.N.; Persky, A.M. Strategies for Improving Learner Metacognition in Health Professional Education. *Am. J. Pharm. Educ.* **2017**, *81*, 78. [CrossRef] [PubMed]
12. Austin, Z.; O'Byrne, C.; Pugsley, J.; Munoz, L.Q. Development and Validation Processes for an Objective Structured Clinical Examination (OSCE) for Entry-to-Practice Certification in Pharmacy: The Canadian Experience. *Am. J. Pharm. Educ.* **2003**, *67*, 642–649. [CrossRef]
13. Terry, R.; Hing, W.; Orr, R.; Milne, N. Do coursework summative assessments predict clinical performance? A systematic review. *BMC Med. Educ.* **2017**, *17*, 40. [CrossRef] [PubMed]
14. Hussainy, S.Y.; Crum, M.F.; White, P.J.; Larson, I.; Malone, D.T.; Manallack, D.; Nicolazzo, J.A.; McDowell, J.; Lim, A.S.; Kirkpatrick, C. Developing a Framework for Objective Structured Clinical Examinations Using the Nominal Group Technique. *Am. J. Pharm. Educ.* **2016**, *80*, 158. [CrossRef]
15. Lim, A.S.; Lee, S.W.H.; Karunaratne, N.; Caliph, S. Pharmacy Students' Perceptions and Performance on the Use of an Online Virtual Experience Tool for Practicing Objective Structured Clinical Examinations. *Am. J. Pharm. Educ.* **2020**, *84*, 7920. [CrossRef]
16. Hussainy, S.Y.; Styles, K.; Duncan, G. A Virtual Practice Environment to Develop Communication Skills in Pharmacy Students. *Am. J. Pharm. Educ.* **2012**, *76*, 202. [CrossRef]
17. Adrian, J.A.L.; Zeszotarski, P.; Ma, C. Developing Pharmacy Student Communication Skills through Role-Playing and Active Learning. *Am. J. Pharm. Educ.* **2015**, *79*, 44. [CrossRef]
18. Hess, R.; Hagemeier, N.E.; Blackwelder, R.; Rose, D.; Ansari, N.; Branham, T. Teaching Communication Skills to Medical and Pharmacy Students Through a Blended Learning Course. *Am. J. Pharm. Educ.* **2016**, *80*, 64. [CrossRef]
19. Sturpe, D.A. Objective Structured Clinical Examinations in Doctor of Pharmacy Programs in the United States. *Am. J. Pharm. Educ.* **2010**, *74*, 148. [CrossRef]
20. Müller, S.; Koch, I.; Settmacher, U.; Dahmen, U. How the introduction of OSCEs has affected the time students spend studying: Results of a nationwide study. *BMC Med. Educ.* **2019**, *19*, 1–7. [CrossRef]
21. Rudland, J.; Wilkinson, T.; Smith-Han, K.; Thompson-Fawcett, M. "You can do it late at night or in the morning. You can do it at home, I did it with my flatmate." The educational impact of an OSCE. *Med. Teach.* **2008**, *30*, 206–211. [CrossRef] [PubMed]
22. Tagawa, M.; Imanaka, H. Reflection and self-directed and group learning improve OSCE scores. *Clin. Teach.* **2010**, *7*, 266–270. [CrossRef] [PubMed]
23. Colthorpe, K.; Ogiji, J.; Ainscough, L.; Zimbardi, K.; Anderson, S. Effect of Metacognitive Prompts on Undergraduate Pharmacy Students' Self-regulated Learning Behavior. *Am. J. Pharm. Educ.* **2019**, *83*, 6646. [CrossRef] [PubMed]
24. Pegram, A.; Fordham-Clarke, C. Implementing peer learning to prepare students for OSCEs. *Br. J. Nurs.* **2015**, *24*, 1060–1065. [CrossRef]
25. Austin, Z.; Gregory, P.A.M. Evaluating the Accuracy of Pharmacy Students' Self-Assessment Skills. *Am. J. Pharm. Educ.* **2007**, *71*, 89. [CrossRef]
26. Davis, D.A.; Mazmanian, P.E.; Fordis, M.; Van Harrison, R.; Thorpe, K.; Perrier, L. Accuracy of Physician Self-assessment Compared with Observed Measures of Competence. *JAMA J. Am. Med. Assoc.* **2006**, *296*, 1094–1102. [CrossRef]
27. Pawluk, S.A.; Zolezzi, M.; Rainkie, D. Comparing student self-assessments of global communication with trained faculty and standardized patient assessments. *Curr. Pharm. Teach. Learn.* **2018**, *10*, 779–784. [CrossRef]
28. Eva, K.W.; Regehr, G. "I'll never play professional football" and other fallacies of self-assessment. *J. Contin. Educ. Health Prof.* **2008**, *28*, 14–19. [CrossRef]

29. Nash, R.; Chalmers, L.; Stupans, I.; Brown, N. Knowledge, use and perceived relevance of a profession's Competency Standards; implications for Pharmacy Education. *Int. J. Pharm. Pr.* **2016**, *24*, 390–402. [CrossRef]
30. Malone, D.; Galbraith, K.; White, P.J.; Exintaris, B.; Nicolazzo, J.A.; Brock, T.; Bruno-Tomé, A.; Short, J.L.; Larson, I. Development of a Vertically Integrated Pharmacy Degree. *Pharmaceuticals* **2021**, *9*, 156. [CrossRef]
31. Rosenthal, M. Qualitative research methods: Why, when, and how to conduct interviews and focus groups in pharmacy research. *Curr. Pharm. Teach. Learn.* **2016**, *8*, 509–516. [CrossRef]
32. Castleberry, A.; Nolen, A. Thematic analysis of qualitative research data: Is it as easy as it sounds? *Curr. Pharm. Teach. Learn.* **2018**, *10*, 807–815. [CrossRef] [PubMed]
33. Varpio, L.; Ajjawi, R.; Monrouxe, L.V.; O'Brien, B.C.; Rees, C.E. Shedding the cobra effect: Problematising thematic emergence, triangulation, saturation and member checking. *Med. Educ.* **2017**, *51*, 40–50. [CrossRef] [PubMed]
34. Oderda, G.M.; Zavod, R.M.; Carter, J.T.; Early, J.L.; Joyner, P.U.; Kirschenbaum, H.; Mack, E.J.; Traynor, A.P.; Plaza, C.M. An Environmental Scan on the Status of Critical Thinking and Problem Solving Skills in Colleges/Schools of Pharmacy: Report of the 2009–2010 Academic Affairs Standing Committee. *Am. J. Pharm. Educ.* **2010**, *74*, S6. [CrossRef] [PubMed]
35. Kasiar, J.B.; Lanfear, S.L. Using peer assessment to develop ability outcomes [abstract]. *Am. J. Pharm. Educ.* **2003**, *67*, 27S.
36. Altmiller, G.; Deal, B.; Ebersole, N.; Flexner, R.; Jordan, J.; Jowell, V.; Norris, T.; Risetter, M.J.; Schuler, M.; Szymanski, K.; et al. Constructive Feedback Teaching Strategy. *Nurs. Educ. Perspect.* **2018**, *39*, 291–296. [CrossRef]
37. Carless, D.; Boud, D. The development of student feedback literacy: Enabling uptake of feedback. *Assess. Evaluation High. Educ.* **2018**, *43*, 1315–1325. [CrossRef]
38. Mishra, S.D.; Rebitch, C.B.; Choi, I. Exploring student perceptions and attitude towards various aspects of peer feedback in a pharmacotherapy course. *Curr. Pharm. Teach. Learn.* **2020**, *12*, 701–708. [CrossRef]
39. Kim, M.-K.; Patel, R.A.; Uchizono, J.; Beck, L. Incorporation of Bloom's Taxonomy into Multiple-Choice Examination Questions for a Pharmacotherapeutics Course. *Am. J. Pharm. Educ.* **2012**, *76*, 114. [CrossRef]
40. Tiemeier, A.M.; Stacy, Z.A.; Burke, J.M. Using Multiple Choice Questions Written at Various Bloom's Taxonomy Levels to Evaluate Student Performance across a Therapeutics Sequence. *Innov. Pharm.* **2011**, *2*. [CrossRef]

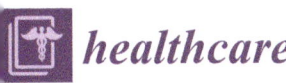

Article

Educational Videos as an Adjunct Learning Tool in Pre-Clinical Operative Dentistry—A Randomized Control Trial

Osama Khattak [1], Kiran Kumar Ganji [2,*], Azhar Iqbal [1], Meshal Alonazi [1], Hmoud Algarni [1] and Thani Alsharari [3]

[1] Department of Operative Dentistry & Endodontics, Jouf University, Sakaka 72345, Saudi Arabia; dr.osama.khattak@jodent.org (O.K.); dr.azhar.iqbal@jodent.org (A.I.); dr.meshal.alonazi@jodent.org (M.A.); dr.hmoud.algarni@jodent.org (H.A.)
[2] Department of Preventive Dentistry, Jouf University, Sakaka 72345, Saudi Arabia
[3] Restorative and Dental Materials Department, Faculty of Dentistry, Taif University, Taif 26571, Saudi Arabia; Thani.Alsharari@gmail.com
* Correspondence: dr.kiran.ganji@jodent.org

Citation: Khattak, O.; Ganji, K.K.; Iqbal, A.; Alonazi, M.; Algarni, H.; Alsharari, T. Educational Videos as an Adjunct Learning Tool in Pre-Clinical Operative Dentistry— A Randomized Control Trial. *Healthcare* **2022**, *10*, 178. https://doi.org/10.3390/healthcare10020178

Academic Editors: Luís Proença, José João Mendes, João Botelho and Vanessa Machado

Received: 12 December 2021
Accepted: 10 January 2022
Published: 18 January 2022

Publisher's Note: MDPI stays neutral with regard to jurisdictional claims in published maps and institutional affiliations.

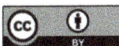

Copyright: © 2022 by the authors. Licensee MDPI, Basel, Switzerland. This article is an open access article distributed under the terms and conditions of the Creative Commons Attribution (CC BY) license (https://creativecommons.org/licenses/by/4.0/).

Abstract: Background: E-learning is an important adjunct used for teaching clinical skills in medicine dentistry. This study evaluated and compared the effectiveness of e-learning resources as an additional teaching aid to traditional teaching methods in male and female students and based on CGPA scores in a pre-clinical operative skill course. Methods: A randomized control trial was conducted in the College of Dentistry, Jouf University, to assess the impact of e-learning resources in learning clinical skills in a pre-clinical operative dentistry course. Fifty second-year dental students were randomly divided into two groups, with 25 students each. Group A (control group) was taught using traditional teaching methods, and Group B (intervention group) used e-learning resources along with traditional methods. Both groups were assessed using objective structured clinical examinations (OSCEs). Standardized forms prepared by faculty members were used to assess the students. The students also filled in a questionnaire afterwards to provide feedback regarding the e-learning resources. Results: The difference between both groups was statistically significant ($p < 0.05$). Female students performed better in three OSCE stations out of six. Furthermore, the students positively responded to the use of additional resources. Conclusion: The use of e-learning resources in pre-clinical operative dentistry courses can be a useful adjunct to traditional teaching methods and can result in better learning of dental pre-clinical operative skills.

Keywords: operative pre-clinical; competency-based education; e-learning

1. Introduction

There has been a paradigm shift in medical education in the last decade, with the incorporation of e-learning resources in teaching and learning [1,2]. E-learning entails teaching with the aid of electronic resources. Traditional teaching involves classroom teaching that includes monitoring. With the increasing use of computers and the Internet, e-learning has become common. The Bandura social learning theory emphasizes the dynamics of the learning process, particularly for self-confidence and learning from observation of one's own or others' failures and the success resulting from the acquisition of new abilities. Listening to podcasts, learning from viewing videos, and others are all part of the Bandura social learning concept [3]. Dental education is also undergoing a paradigm shift in learning where various dentistry fields are witnessing innovation in teaching and learning methods. Using e-learning resources has positively impacted students in terms of understanding the basic concepts of dentistry and their application in clinical scenarios [4]. However, students view e-learning as a helpful supplement to traditional teaching methods rather than a replacement for traditional teaching methods [5].

The outcome of systematic studies on selection techniques in medical education backed up the idea that past academic achievement is a predictor of success [6]. Even though overall cumulative grade point averages (CGPA) and CGPA in science are the strongest indicators of success in dentistry schools, these may not always represent a dental student's success in terms of clinical performance on regional tests [7].

As more importance is assigned to the impact of gender in academic achievement, research in this area is becoming more vital. As far as theoretical and practical examinations in dentistry are concerned, data show that female medical students perform better than their male classmates [8,9]. The study by Nuzhat et al. [10] in Saudi Arabia found gender-based differences in learning style preferences and the corresponding consequences on medical students' academic performance. This study emphasized that females have more diverse preferences than male students [10]. Furthermore, female Jordanian dental students surpass males in dentistry courses, according to the reports of Sawair [11].

Clinical competency is an individual's ability to work independently and without supervision in clinical practice. The ultimate objective of competency-based education is to enable dental students to be competent enough in the management of dental diseases. Therefore, the dental faculty must assess the same before students move from pre-clinical simulation to clinical courses. This process involves a series of progressive stages that begin with theory, then move toward pre-clinical simulation, and end at the clinical stage. Pre-clinical simulation courses provide a safe environment for students for learning clinical skills before moving on to the clinical stage [12]. Simulation labs provide an opportunity for the students to learn such skills. Operative dentistry is an extensive subject. It requires learning clinical skills, which begins from the second year of a Bachelor of Dental and Oral Surgery program (BDS). Operative dentistry skill is one of the basic skill courses in the undergraduate dental curriculum. It covers important topics, including knowledge about dental materials and their clinical application, various infection control measures for the dental unit, and the use of equipment related to operative dentistry. Students are expected to be competent in the skills mentioned above at the end of the course. It provides an opportunity to learn the basic skills of operative dentistry in pre-clinical simulation labs before proceeding to clinical courses. The objective structured clinical examination (OSCE) is an efficient method of assessing students' clinical competency and skills [13]. It is used routinely in dentistry for student assessment [14]. Studies have shown that students feel less confident about the skills they learn using traditional, didactic teaching methods, and this makes learning difficult [15]. An opportunity to start learning about teledentistry and virtual patient management is provided during the COVID 19 epidemic [16]. Blended learning, which involves traditional teaching along with electronic resources, has shown that it can transform traditional teaching experiences into technology-enhanced learning ones, which students today find beneficial [17]. Haptic technology, such as robotics, is also gaining traction, since it allows for two-way communication between the user and the environment, allowing for a more accurate simulation of the clinical setting for learning reasons. Current literature lacked information about use of e-learning tools as a additional teaching aid for the pre-clinical operative skills of dentistry.

This study aimed at:
1. Evaluating and comparing the effectiveness of e-learning resources as an additional teaching aid to traditional teaching methods in male and female students as well as based on the CGPA scores in a pre-clinical operative skill course.
2. Correlating the effectiveness of e-learning resources with CGPA scores of dental students.

2. Materials and Methods

This randomized control trial (Figure 1) was conducted at College of Dentistry, Jouf University, KSA, from 15 January to 28 February 2021. Ethical approval was obtained by the Local Committee of Bioethics, Jouf University. The study sample comprised all second-year dental students of the 2020–2021 Bachelor of Oral and Dental Surgery program who consented (n = 50) to the census technique. This is a method where all members of a population are analyzed. Students who did not volunteer were excluded. Recruitment was conducted by announcements through e-mail. Informed consent was obtained from students. They were randomly distributed into two groups: control and intervention. Randomization was undertaken using a computer-generated random number for the roll numbers as per their attendance list (Figure 1).

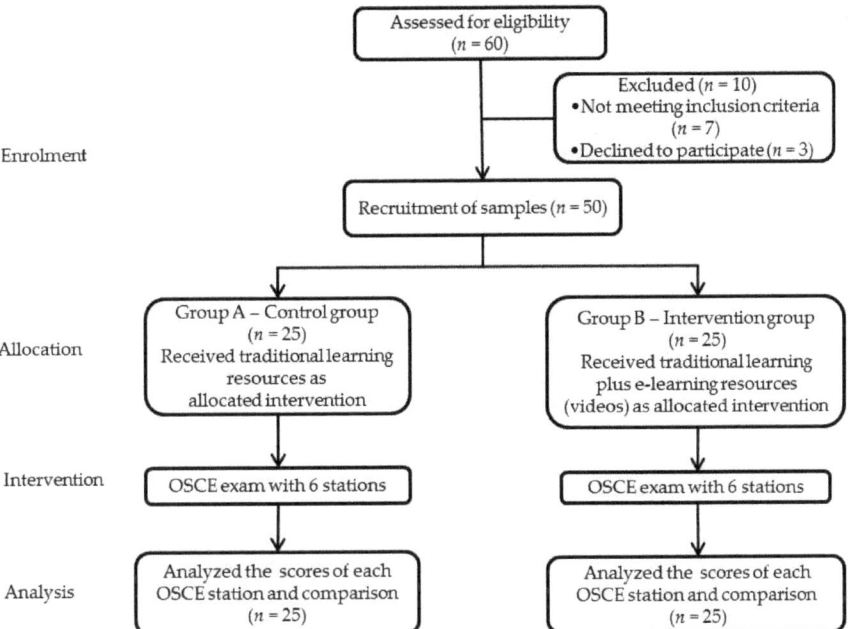

Figure 1. Consort chart for randomization, intervention and follow-up of study samples.

The skill lab was scheduled as per the calendar of the curriculum for teaching the operative dentistry skills using the traditional method. The traditional method included the demonstration of matrix band placement, dental dam application, application of retraction cord, mixing of glass ionomer restorative material, operator positioning for specific tooth and disinfection of dental unit using a simulation process. The intervention group (Group B) received an e-learning resource in the form of audiovisual aids such as videos in addition to traditional demonstration methods whereas the control group (Group A) were taught by the traditional demonstration method only. The e-learning resources comprised educational videos of the same skill procedures which were already taught employing traditional methods. These resources were selected by other faculty members of the department of operative dentistry who were not involved in the study process. The total duration of the videos was around 24 min. The videos were shared only with the intervention group (Group B) through the institutional e-learning app called Blackboard®, with statistics tracking enabled to confirm that students viewed this video for the minimum number of five views at their convenience. According to the statistics, a reminder email was issued to students who had not watched the videos. At the end of the videos, a quiz was administered to assess their understanding by using the adaptive release feature of Blackboard in which a student can take up the quiz if and only upon they had completed the minimum number of views. After 1 week, both the groups were assessed using OSCE (Figure 2), the standard method followed in College of Dentistry, Jouf University. For the examiners, the students of both groups were anonymized. To maintain a high level of objectivity, it was ensured that the examiners were not familiar with the students from previous academic courses. The students were assessed by two examiners to maintain inter-examiner reliability using checklists for each station. The average score of the two examiners was considered the score for that station. It was ensured that the examiners did not share the results. The average scores for each station were calculated, which did not contribute to the real grades of the students, as these OSCE exams were conducted during revision sessions before summative exams.

Number of Stations	Objective of the OSCE station	Components of OSCE station	Evaluation level	
			Satisfactory (2)	Unsatisfactory (0)
Station 1	Matrix band placement on the specified tooth	Wears gloves		
		Selects appropriate type of band and retainer for the specific tooth		
		Contours the band appropriately		
		Applies the band and retainer appropriately		
		Used the wedge to stabilize the band		
Station 2	Dental dam application on the specified tooth	Selects appropriate clamp		
		Ties Floss to secure the clamp		
		Punches the hole in right position		
		Secures the clamp and sheet to the tooth appropriately		
		Removes the clamp and sheet appropriately		
Station 3	Application of retraction cord	Selects appropriate size of the cord		
		Impregnates the cord in astringent solution		
		Places the cord in the gingival sulcus		
		Secures the cord within the sulcus		
		Removes the cord appropriately		
Station 4	Mixing of glass ionomer restorative material	Selects appropriate mixing glass slab or paper pad		
		Dispenses the appropriate ratio of power and liquid on the glass slab or paper pad		
		Incorporates the powder into the liquid quickly		
		Appropriate mixing time 45-60 seconds		
		Prepares glossy final mix		
Station 5	Operator positioning for working on specified tooth.	Properly positions himself/herself for working on the specified tooth (clock positioning)		
		Maintains proper height of the operator chair		
		Positions jaw appropriately to work on the specified tooth		
		Adjusts the light appropriately on the specified working area		
		Appropriate use to direct/indirect vision for the specified working area		
Station 6	Cleaning and disinfection of dental unit	Wears gloves / mask appropriately		
		Follows correct sequence of disinfecting dental chair		
		Uses multiple towels/cloths for cleaning the dental unit		
		Proper cleaning of bench surface		
		Discards used towels/cloth appropriately		

Figure 2. Sample description of objective structured clinical examination (OSCE) stations.

Thereafter, feedback was obtained using a Likert scale rating (1—strongly agree to 5—strongly disagree) from the students regarding the importance of e-learning resources.

The CGPA of all the students were categorized into three categories: low CGPA (<3), average CGPA (3–4), high CGPA (>4). The CGPA scores and gender information were used as dependent variables; OSCE scores were used as the outcome variable. The data were entered in Microsoft Excel and statistics were performed using Statistical Package for the Social Sciences (SPSS) IBM Corp. released 2017, version 25.0 Armonk, NY, USA. Results were presented as mean values with standard deviation. The test of significance for mean OSCE scores between the two groups and gender was assessed using Student's t-test. One way ANOVA was used to assess the test of significance for mean OSCE scores in 3 different CGPA groups. The mean OSCE scores of the two groups were compared using Student's t-test, and mean CGPA scores (low, average, and high) were compared using the ANOVA test. Pearson correlation test was used to correlate the OSCE scores with CGPA scores. The p-value of <0.05 was considered statistically significant, with 95% confidence intervals.

3. Results

Fifty second-year BDS students participated in the study: 33 male and 17 female students. Twenty-five students were allocated to each group, with 18 male and 7 female students in Group A and 15 male and 10 female students in Group B. This unequal distribution was due to randomization. The average score for all the students in both groups was 40.22, with a standard deviation of 4.46. The cumulative grade point average (CGPA) of the students in each group was considered. An independent-sample t-test was conducted to evaluate the homogeneity of the CGPA scores in both groups. There was no significant difference in the CGPA scores for Group A (M = 3.9, SD = 0.68) and Group B (M = 3.8, SD = 0.25), p = 0.24 (Table 1). These results suggest that both the groups were homogenous and identical concerning CGPA.

Table 1. Comparison of OSCE station scores with respect to Group A and Group B.

	Group	n	Mean	Std. Deviation	Std. Error Mean	F Value	p Value
Station#1	A	25	6.480	1.045	0.209	0.763	0.067 *
	B	25	7.000	0.912	0.182		
Station#2	A	25	6.200	0.500	0.100	3.903	0.000 *
	B	25	7.000	0.866	0.173		
Station#3	A	25	6.240	0.925	0.185	0.480	0.002 *
	B	25	7.040	0.840	0.168		
Station#4	A	25	6.480	0.822	0.164	0.071	0.025 *
	B	25	7.040	0.888	0.177		
Station#5	A	25	6.280	0.791	0.158	1.186	0.000 *
	B	25	7.280	0.936	0.187		
Station#6	A	25	6.320	0.627	0.125	2.790	0.002 *
	B	25	7.080	0.996	0.199		
CGPA	A	25	3.926	0.684	0.136	28.98	0.245
	B	25	3.834	0.255	0.051		

* Statistically significant (p < 0.05).

Table 1 shows the performance of students of each group at each of the six OSCE stations. All students passed, with the cut-off score set at 60%. Group B performed better at each station compared to Group A. For all six stations, the average score of the intervention group was higher than the control group. The female students performed significantly better at stations one, three, and five compared to the male students (Table 2), whereas there was no significant difference in the performance of male and female students at other stations. The three categories of students which were made based on CGPA (low, average and high) showed a significant difference in performance across all OSCE stations when one-way ANOVA was conducted (Table 3). This result also supports our hypothesis that students with better CGPA perform better in terms of skills.

Table 2. Comparison of OSCE station scores with respect to gender (male and female).

	Gender	n	Mean	Std. Deviation	Std. Error Mean	F Value	p Value
Station#1	Male	33	6.424	0.902	0.157	0.763	0.001 *
	Female	17	7.352	0.931	0.225		
Station#2	Male	33	6.484	0.833	0.145	3.903	0.163
	Female	17	6.823	0.727	0.176		
Station#3	Male	33	6.424	0.902	0.157	0.480	0.026 *
	Female	17	7.058	0.966	0.234		
Station#4	Male	33	6.666	0.924	0.160	0.071	0.308
	Female	17	6.941	0.826	0.200		
Station#5	Male	33	6.515	0.972	0.169	1.186	0.007 *
	Female	17	7.294	0.848	0.205		
Station#6	Male	33	6.697	1.045	0.181	2.790	0.974
	Female	17	6.705	0.587	0.142		

* Statistically significant ($p < 0.05$).

Table 3. Comparison of OSCE stations scores with respect to cumulative grade point averages (CGPA) groups (low, average and high).

OSCE	CGPA Score	n	Mean	Std. Deviation	Std. Error	95% Confidence Interval for Mean		p Value
						Lower Bound	Upper Bound	
Station#1	Low	5	5.400	0.547	0.244	4.719	6.080	0.000
	Average	11	6.272	0.646	0.194	5.838	6.707	
	High	34	7.088	0.933	0.160	6.762	7.413	
Station#2	Low	5	5.800	0.447	0.200	5.244	6.355	0.002
	Average	11	6.181	0.404	0.121	5.910	6.453	
	High	34	6.852	0.821	0.140	6.566	7.139	
Station#3	Low	5	5.200	0.447	0.200	4.644	5.755	0.000
	Average	11	6.181	0.603	0.181	5.776	6.586	
	High	34	7.000	0.852	0.146	6.702	7.297	
Station#4	Low	5	5.800	1.095	0.489	4.439	7.160	0.006
	Average	11	6.454	0.687	0.207	5.992	6.916	
	High	34	7.0000	0.816	0.140	6.715	7.284	
Station#5	Low	5	5.6000	0.547	0.244	4.919	6.280	0.000
	Average	11	6.272	0.646	0.194	5.838	6.707	
	High	34	7.117	0.945	0.162	6.787	7.447	
Station#6	Low	5	5.800	0.447	0.200	5.244	6.355	0.004
	Average	11	6.272	0.467	0.140	5.958	6.586	
	High	34	6.970	0.936	0.160	6.643	7.297	

A Pearson correlation coefficient was computed to assess the relationship between the CGPA score and individual station (Table 4). Overall, there was a positive correlation between them. An increase in stations scores were correlated with the increase in CGPA. There was a strong correlation ($r = 0.701$) with respect to station three, whereas moderate correlation was found with respect to stations one ($r = 0.563$), two ($r = 0.525$), four ($r = 0.509$), and five ($r = 0.620$) respectively. However, the correlation was weak with respect to station six ($r = 0.492$, $p < 0.00$). The response rate was 100% in the survey filled by the participating students who provided overall positive feedback regarding the use of additional aids.

Table 4. Correlation matrix between OSCE station scores and CGPA.

	Station#1	Station#2	Station#3	Station#4	Station#5	Station#6	CGPA
Station#1	1						
Station#2	0.647 **	1					
Station#3	0.722 **	0.493 **	1				
Station#4	0.542 **	0.401 **	0.466 **	1			
Station#5	0.655 **	0.700 **	0.532 **	0.490 **	1		
Station#6	0.605 **	0.778 **	0.573 **	0.362 **	0.534 **	1	
CGPA	0.563 **	0.525 **	0.701 **	0.509 **	0.620 **	0.492 **	1

** Statistically significant ($p < 0.01$).

4. Discussion

E-learning resources were helpful in enhancing dental students' understanding of fundamental concepts and their application to clinical scenarios [4]. We also believe that these will also help students engage in active learning with the faculty in the skill labs, enabling more discussion on the topic.

The results obtained from our study encourage us to believe that the students can perform better when they are taught using traditional methods along with additional e-learning resources. The students in Group B who were provided with the e-learning resources performed significantly better than the other group. The results of our study are similar to those of Qutieshat et al. [18] who found that the students who studied using the hybrid model (including traditional as well as e-learning methods) performed better. E-learning resources have been useful in enhancing dental students' understanding of fundamental concepts and their application to clinical scenarios [4]. We also believe that these will also help students engage in active learning with the faculty in the skill labs, enabling more discussion on the topic. They also found that the student's perception of the hybrid learning method was positive, similar to our study. The positive feedback received from our sample regarding the use of videos to teach skills is similar to a study by Jang et al. who found that students' overall perception regarding the use of videos was positive. They recommended the faculty use such resources [19]. The positive feedback emphasizes the importance of freely-available e-learning resources in teaching skills in operative dentistry. The students were able to access the videos whenever they wanted to. This helped them consolidate their knowledge through repetition. Unlike the case with traditional methods, they could watch the faculty demonstrate the skills more than once. Similar results have been yielded with the use of online videos in a pre-clinical prosthodontics course at a dental school in Germany [20]. Pre-clinical prosthodontics provides a set of skills very similar to pre-clinical operative dentistry courses, and hence their results provide external validity.

The students with better CGPA performed better than those with lower CGPA. This was expected because the students with better academic performance tend to be more academically groomed. Sound knowledge about the materials, equipment, and practical techniques forms the basis for good practical skills. They use multiple preparation techniques for their assessments and perform better. Previous studies have shown similar results in undergraduate medical education, with CGPA being a predictor of students' performance [21]. Our study showed that the female students performed better than the male students. This is similar to studies conducted in undergraduate dental education where female students' cumulative grades were significantly better than male students [11]. However, our results differ from a study on the effect of gender on performance in medicine in a medical college in Saudi Arabia [22], where the females performed only slightly better than their male counterparts. We believe that female students with better didactic knowledge perform better than males in dental skills, as shown in the results of our study. Our findings might potentially be utilized to garner more interest in studying gender-based differences in ability in practical courses taken by dentistry students. More exploratory studies are needed to relate gender to the performance of dental students.

We found a strong to moderate correlation between the CGPA and students' performance at each station. However, station six revealed a weak correlation. This station involved cleaning and disinfection of the workstation. The possible explanation is that this was the only component that was not taught in the lectures, and only a demonstration of the skill was provided. This is because the students had completed the knowledge and understanding part of this aspect in another course in the previous year. Knowledge about all other stations was provided in the lecture component of the skill course. This underlines the fact that only demonstrations or the use of videos are not sufficient to learn a skill. For competence, sound theoretical background, as well as clinical demonstration, is important. A major limitation of our study is the involvement of only one cohort of students. Our study does not correlate the impact of e-learning resources on the enhancement of clinical skills by prospective follow-up. More studies involving a larger group of students in different skill-related courses of dentistry are needed to conclude this assumption.

5. Conclusions

Students enrolled in in pre-clinical operative dentistry skills training performed significantly better when provided with additional e-learning tools than those who were not. Thus, resources that are easily accessible to students help them perform better in the assessments. We recommend that the additional e-learning resources should be part of the teaching methodology in the skill courses of dentistry colleges. This would help students become more competent in skill courses.

Author Contributions: Conceptualization, O.K. and K.K.G.; methodology, A.I., M.A., H.A. and T.A.; software, K.K.G.; validation, A.I., M.A. and H.A.; formal analysis, K.K.G.; investigation, A.I. and O.K.; resources, T.A.; data curation, M.A. and H.A.; writing—original draft preparation, O.K. and K.K.G.; writing—review and editing, M.A., H.A. and T.A.; visualization, A.I.; supervision, K.K.G.; project administration, O.K.; funding acquisition, K.K.G. All authors have read and agreed to the published version of the manuscript.

Funding: This work was funded by the Deanship of Scientific Research at Jouf University under grant No (DSR-2021-01-03177).

Institutional Review Board Statement: The study obtained ethical clearance from local committee of bioethics, Jouf University wide reference 1-5-42.

Informed Consent Statement: Informed consent was obtained from all subjects involved in the study.

Data Availability Statement: Data will be made available on request.

Conflicts of Interest: The authors declare no conflict of interest.

References

1. Ellaway, R.; Masters, K. AMEE Guide 32: E-Learning in medical education Part 1: Learning, teaching and assessment. *Med. Teach.* **2008**, *30*, 455–473. [CrossRef] [PubMed]
2. Ganji, K.K. Evaluation of reliability in structured viva voce as a formative assessment of dental students. *J. Dent. Educ.* **2017**, *81*, 590–596. [CrossRef] [PubMed]
3. Consorti, F. *Didattica Professionalizzante nei Corsi di Laurea in Medicina*; Edra: Milano, Italy, 2018.
4. Turkyilmaz, I.; Hariri, N.H.; Jahangiri, L. Student's perception of the impact of e-learning on dental education. *J. Contemp. Dent. Pract.* **2019**, *20*, 616–621. [CrossRef]
5. Asiry, M.; Hashim, H. Tooth size ratios in Saudi subjects with Class II, Division 1 malocclusion. *J. Int. Oral Health* **2012**, *4*, 29.

6. Al-Ansari, A.A.; El Tantawi, M.M. Predicting academic performance of dental students using perception of educational environment. *J. Dent. Educ.* **2015**, *79*, 337–344. [CrossRef] [PubMed]
7. Rudy, J.O.; Singleton, J.A.; Lewis, L.H.; Quick, R.N. Admissions criteria that influence dental hygiene students' performance on board examinations. *Am. Dent. Hyg. Assoc.* **2017**, *91*, 24–29.
8. Haq, I.; Higham, J.; Morris, R.; Dacre, J. Effect of ethnicity and gender on performance in undergraduate medical examinations. *Med. Educ.* **2005**, *39*, 1126–1128. [CrossRef] [PubMed]
9. McDonough, C.; Horgan, A.; Codd, M.; Casey, P. Gender differences in the results of the final medical examination at University College Dublin. *Med. Educ.-Oxf.* **2000**, *34*, 30–34. [CrossRef] [PubMed]
10. Nuzhat, A.; Salem, R.O.; Al Hamdan, N.; Ashour, N. Gender differences in learning styles and academic performance of medical students in Saudi Arabia. *Med. Teach.* **2013**, *35* (Suppl. S1), S78–S82. [CrossRef]
11. Sawair, F.A.; Baqain, Z.H.; Al-Omari, I.K.; Wahab, F.K.; Rajab, L.D. Effect of gender on performance of undergraduate dental students at the University of Jordan, Amman. *J. Dent. Educ.* **2009**, *73*, 1313–1319. [CrossRef]
12. Al-Elq, A.H. Simulation-based medical teaching and learning. *J. Family Community Med.* **2010**, *17*, 35. [CrossRef]
13. Plakiotis, C. Objective structured clinical examination (OSCE) in psychiatry education: A review of its role in competency-based assessment. *GeNeDis 2016* **2017**, *988*, 159–180.
14. Kemelova, G.; Tuleutaeva, S.; Aimbetova, D.; Garifullina, R. The objective structured clinical examination in dentistry: Strengths and weaknesses. *Stomatologiia* **2019**, *98*, 8–11. [CrossRef]
15. Shigli, K.; Jyotsna, S.; Rajesh, G.; Wadgave, U.; Sankeshwari, B.; Nayak, S.S.; Vyas, R. Challenges in learning pre-clinical prosthodontics: A survey of perceptions of dental undergraduates and teaching faculty at an Indian dental school. *J. Clin. Diagn. Res. JCDR* **2017**, *11*, ZC01.
16. Cervino, G.; Oteri, G. COVID-19 Pandemic and Telephone Triage before Attending Medical Office: Problem or Opportunity? *Medicina* **2020**, *56*, 250. [CrossRef]
17. Bock, A.; Modabber, A.; Kniha, K.; Lemos, M.; Rafai, N.; Hölzle, F. Blended learning modules for lectures on oral and maxillofacial surgery. *Br. J. Oral Maxillofac. Surg.* **2018**, *56*, 956–961. [CrossRef]
18. Qutieshat, A.S.; Abusamak, M.O.; Maragha, T.N. Impact of Blended Learning on Dental Students' Performance and Satisfaction in Clinical Education. *J. Dent. Educ.* **2020**, *84*, 135–142. [CrossRef]
19. Jang, H.W.; Kim, K.-J. Use of online clinical videos for clinical skills training for medical students: Benefits and challenges. *BMC Med. Educ.* **2014**, *14*, 56. [CrossRef]
20. Reissmann, D.R.; Sierwald, I.; Berger, F.; Heydecke, G. A model of blended learning in a pre-clinical course in prosthetic dentistry. *J. Dent. Educ.* **2015**, *79*, 157–165. [CrossRef]
21. Sladek, R.M.; Bond, M.J.; Frost, L.K.; Prior, K.N. Predicting success in medical school: A longitudinal study of common Australian student selection tools. *BMC Med. Educ.* **2016**, *16*, 187. [CrossRef]
22. Albalawi, M. Does gender difference have an effect in the academic achievements of undergraduate students' and later as interns? A single medical college experience, Taibah university, KSA. *Allied J. Med. Res.* **2019**, *3*, 20–25.

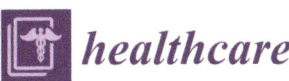

Article

An Abrupt Transition to Digital Teaching—Norwegian Medical Students and Their Experiences of Learning Output during the Initial Phase of the COVID-19 Lockdown

Henriette K. Helland [1], Thorkild Tylleskär [2], Monika Kvernenes [1] and Håkon Reikvam [3,4,*]

1. Faculty of Medicine, University of Bergen, 5020 Bergen, Norway; Henriette.K.Helland@student.uib.no (H.K.H.); Monika.Kvernenes@uib.no (M.K.)
2. Centre for International Health, University of Bergen, 5020 Bergen, Norway; Thorkild.Tylleskar@uib.no
3. Department of Clinical Science, University of Bergen, 5020 Bergen, Norway
4. Clinic for Medicine, Haukeland University Hospital, 5021 Bergen, Norway
* Correspondence: Hakon.Reikvam@uib.no; Tel.: +47-55-97-37-00

Abstract: Norwegian universities closed almost all on-campus activities on the 12 March 2020 following a lockdown decision of the Norwegian government in response to the COVID-19 pandemic. Online and digital teaching became the primary method of teaching. The goal of this study was to investigate how the transition to digital education impacted on medical students enrolled at the University of Bergen (UiB). Key points were motivation, experience of learning outcomes, and fear of missing out on important learning. Using an online questionnaire, students were asked to evaluate the quality of both lectures and taught clinical skills and to elaborate on their experience of learning output, examination, and digital teaching. Answers from 230 students were included in the study. Opinions on the quality and quantity of lectures offered and their experience of learning output varied based on gender, seniority and the amount of time spent on part time jobs. Students at UiB were generally unhappy with the quality of teaching, especially lessons on clinical skills, although both positive and negative experiences were reported. Securing a satisfying offer of clinical teaching will be important to ensure and increase the student experience of learning output in the time ahead.

Keywords: medical education; digital education; COVID-19 pandemic

Citation: Helland, H.K.; Tylleskär, T.; Kvernenes, M.; Reikvam, H. An Abrupt Transition to Digital Teaching—Norwegian Medical Students and Their Experiences of Learning Output during the Initial Phase of the COVID-19 Lockdown. *Healthcare* **2022**, *10*, 170. https://doi.org/10.3390/healthcare10010170

Academic Editors: Luís Proença, José João Mendes, João Botelho and Vanessa Machado

Received: 6 December 2021
Accepted: 14 January 2022
Published: 17 January 2022

Publisher's Note: MDPI stays neutral with regard to jurisdictional claims in published maps and institutional affiliations.

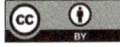

Copyright: © 2022 by the authors. Licensee MDPI, Basel, Switzerland. This article is an open access article distributed under the terms and conditions of the Creative Commons Attribution (CC BY) license (https://creativecommons.org/licenses/by/4.0/).

1. Introduction

Norway introduced a general lockdown on the 12 March 2020, in response to the global COVID-19 pandemic [1]. Despite the comprehensive restrictions, the universities were encouraged to keep up the pace in the educational programs. Emergency remote learning (ERL), a temporary shift from the traditional form of education into a remote one following a state of emergency, was implemented by the Norwegian universities to ensure the continuation of higher education [2]. This abrupt transition to emergency remote learning was a worldwide phenomenon. More than 1.9 billion students from 190 countries were forced to transfer their education from face-to-face to digital education to fight the ongoing pandemic, according to UNESCO [3]. In Norway, emergency digital education included the transition from a mainly physical learning environment to video recordings, live lectures on digital platforms and home exams [4]. Prohibition of physical attendance left students without an office, without the possibility of hands-on learning of clinical skills, without academic and social meeting places and with major changes in their daily study habits [4]. Transitioning to emergency digital education has been challenging in most countries. A study conducted on middle school students in Palestine reported that the quality of emergency remote learning has been low even compared to digital learning in normal circumstances. Course designs, assessment, and teaching strategies in schools and at universities are originally designed for face-to-face teaching. In addition, both educators and students are living under a high level of stress, anxiety, and uncertainty due to the state of emergency affecting all parts of society and normal life [5]. The challenges of emergency digital education have potentially been similar for medical students in Norway. The abrupt closing of Norwegian universities meant that medical schools had little or no time to restructure their education and prepare for digital education. In addition, medical training facilities in Norway were closed, and students were left without a place to practice clinical skills.

Face-to-face education is today a crucial part of medical education worldwide [6]. Acquiring practical skills is of utmost importance when learning how to practice medicine. However, according to the World Health Organization (WHO) digital education may be capable of supplying the estimated 4.3 million shortage in healthcare workers worldwide [7]. Student experience of digital education during the pandemic may provide useful information on how to develop and implement a potentially more digitalized medical education in the future.

We conducted a study to investigate how the period from the 12 March 2020 to the end of the spring semester (20 June 2020) affected the lives and the learning environment for medical students at the University of Bergen (UiB) in Bergen, Norway. The aims were to assess students' own experiences of learning output, motivation, and possible fear of missing out on important learning, due to the switch to digital education. In addition, we wanted the student's perspective on the positives and negatives of digital education, and their opinion on how this type of education could be improved in the future. This study is the first study to explore the student experience of the COVID-19 pandemic on medical students in Norway.

2. Subjects and Methods

2.1. Undergraduate Medical Program at UiB

The undergraduate medical program at UiB is a six-year long program divided into 12 terms, referred to as MED1, MED2 etc. It is organized as three columns that run parallel throughout the program (columns of profession, academics, and professionalism) and include elements of a spiral curriculum where key topics and subfields are revisited progressively. Teaching is offered using primarily lectures, Team-based learning [8], and clinical teaching. There is a final assessment after each term using multiple choice (MCQ) and short answer questions (SAQ). Objective structured clinical examinations are held after the 3rd and 6th year.

2.2. Setting and Application

Our study is a cross-sectional retrospective study, using a combination of qualitative and quantitative research methodology. We used a questionnaire to collect data for assessing the educational environment. The questionnaire was administered to all undergraduate medical students at UiB between the 12th of June 2020 and the 16th of August 2020 using the digital tool Skjemaker®, a local adaptation of MachForm (Appnitro software, Malang, East Java, Indonesia, Available online: www.machform.com (accessed on 5 January 2022)). Students were invited to participate in our study through a link sent to their student e-mail portal with a copy sent to their private e-mail address. Data was collected in relation to the 2020 spring semester when restrictions were most intense. The questionnaire was first shared a few days after the last exam of the semester to ensure that students would be able to answer questions about the final exam with the least amount of memory bias. Three reminders were sent out during the data-collecting period in effort to boost the response rate. In addition, a link to the study was published in relevant social media. The questionnaire was completed in approximately 15 min. The study was approved by the Norwegian Center for Research Data (NSD) and used voluntary consent. Participants were informed that they had the right to discontinue the study at any point without any consequences. Answers to the questionnaire are completely anonymous, and investigators has no way of identifying participating students.

2.3. Sample Size Determination

All medical students at UiB (958 in total) were invited to participate, which means there was no sampling. This was also done to ensure inclusion of the variations in teaching methods and adaptation to digital education between all six years of the program.

2.4. Questionnaire

A self-designed questionnaire was used in this study. Design and layout of the questionnaire was discussed several times between authors to maximize face validate. A small pre-test group of five students were used to standardize questions. The participants offered some amendments to the questionnaire which were considered and noted. The questionnaire was finalized after an in-depth discussion among the authors. The end-product consisted of 53 questions divided into five different categories, (Table 1), each addressing different aspects of digital education. 27 questions used a Likert type response scale, 10 were closed-ended questions, and 16 questions were open ended. Quantitative information was collected using either a 5-point Likert scale [9] or close-ended questions. Open-ended questions were used to collect qualitative data explaining the rationale behind answers to the other questions. The questionnaire was in Norwegian. Quotes, tables, and diagrams reported in the following are translated from Norwegian to English for the purpose of this article.

Table 1. The questionnaire was divided in five main categories. The table illustrates the different categories and includes an example of questions within each category.

Categories	Examples
General situation	How has your living situation been during the COVID-19 pandemic?
Teaching	On a scale of 1–5: How would you rate the quality of PowerPoint with sound?
Your own learning experience	My experience of learning output has been the same as during a normal semester
Exam	I am satisfied with my own achievement on my exam this semester
Digital education as a whole	What I enjoyed most about digital education was

2.5. Statistical Analysis

Quantitative data were analyzed using Stata (StataCorp, College Station, TX, USA). Comparison of ordinary data between groups was done using the Mann–Whitney U-test and the using Kruskal–Wallis test for analyzing more than two groups. Participants were categorized based on gender, years of study and whether they were providing care for children. Graded Likert scale questions are presented descriptively including mean values and a 95% confidence interval. Potential gender differences in student experience of digital education were investigated, as well as differences between years of studying medicine. Differences between students spending more, equal, or less hours at a part time job outside of studies was also investigated. Qualitative data were reviewed, sorted, and categorized thematically.

3. Results

3.1. Quantitative Response Data

A total of 230 students, a response rate of 24%, submitted answers to the questionnaire—169 women (73%) and 61 men (27%). The gender distribution among participants reflects the current gender distribution at the medicine program at UiB—75.7% women and 24.3% men [10]. Participation was somewhat uneven among students at different years of study. For instance, the response rate of students in their last semester (6th year, MED12) was 49% while the response rate of students in their second last semester (6th year, MED11) was only 13% (Table 2). 17 students cared for children during the lockdown, of which 13 were women and three were men. A total of 19% of students had spent more time, 41% less time and 40% equal amount of time in their paid part-time positions outside of study as before the lockdown. A total of 74 students were living with other students during the initial lockdown, and 102 students moved back in at their parents' house for some period.

Table 2. An overview of year progression for medical students at UiB. The table includes response rate for the specific year and distribution of each year in the study population.

Year	Semester [a]	Distribution in Study Population	Response Rate for Each Term
6th year	MED12	39 (17%)	49%
	MED11	9 (8%)	13%
5th year	MED10	11 (5%)	14%
	MED9	13 (6%)	18%
4th year	MED8	36 (16%)	44%
	MED7	17 (7%)	20%
3rd year	MED6	25 (11%)	15%
2nd year	MED4	24 (10%)	15%
1st year	MED2	46 (20%)	27%

[a] The medical students are in one group of 180 students during the first three years after which they split in two groups of 90 in each.

3.2. Quality of Digital Education Media

Different digital teaching methods, specifically pre-recorded PowerPoint slides with sound, pre-recorded video lectures, and live video lectures, were rated based on technical, academic, and pedagogical quality. Live video lectures had the highest mean score in pedagogical quality (3.69 (3.57–3.82)), while pre-recorded lectures scored the highest on both academic (4.02 (3.9–4.12)) and technical quality (3.94 (3.18–4.07)) (Figure 1). Female students were statistically significantly more satisfied with pedagogical quality of all digital education media than their male colleagues (Live video: $p = 0.002$. Video recording: $p = 0.05$. PowerPoint with sound: $p = 0.03$).

3.3. Teaching of Clinical Skills and Hands-on Education

The students were asked whether they agreed, disagreed or were indifferent to several statements regarding the quality of the clinical training. One statement read "In my experience, my benefit from clinical and practical education has been good compared to an ordinary, physical semester", on which 61.7% of students disagreed, 23.0% were indifferent and 14.8% agreed. Another statement "I believe that our clinical and practical education has been replaced in a satisfying manner", on which 59.1% of students disagreed, 22.6% were indifferent and 18.3% agreed (Figure 2). However, there was statistically significant differences between students in the different semesters. There was a statistically significant difference in both experience of benefit of clinical and practical lectures ($p = 0.003$), and in experience of satisfying replacement of clinical education ($p = 0.003$) between the different semesters (Figure 3).

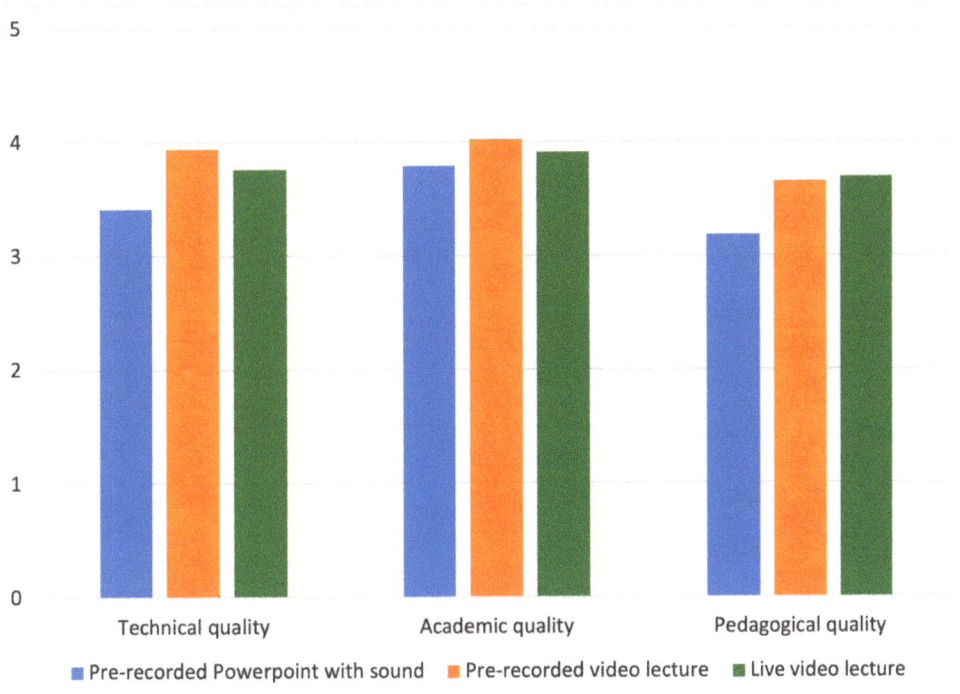

Figure 1. Student experience expressed on a Likert scale regarding technical, academic, and pedagogical quality on pre-recorded PowerPoint with sound, pre-recorded video lectures and live video lectures.

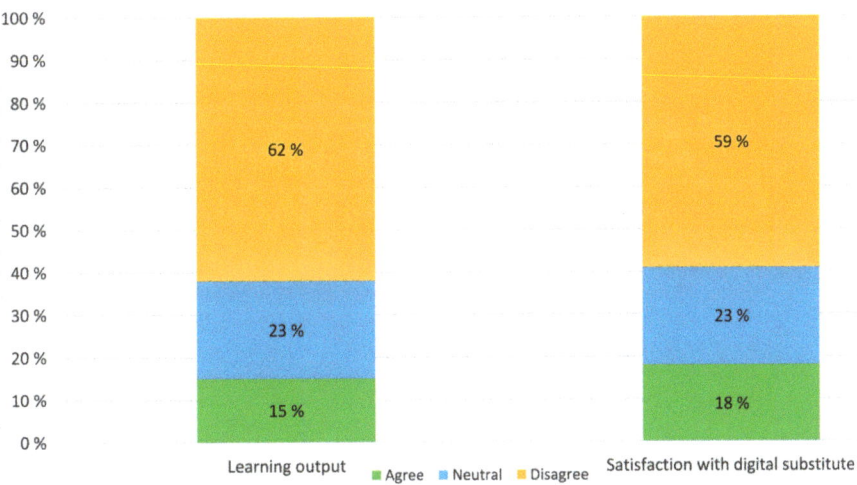

Figure 2. Distribution of agreement, disagreement, or neutral view on statements regarding clinical and practical education.

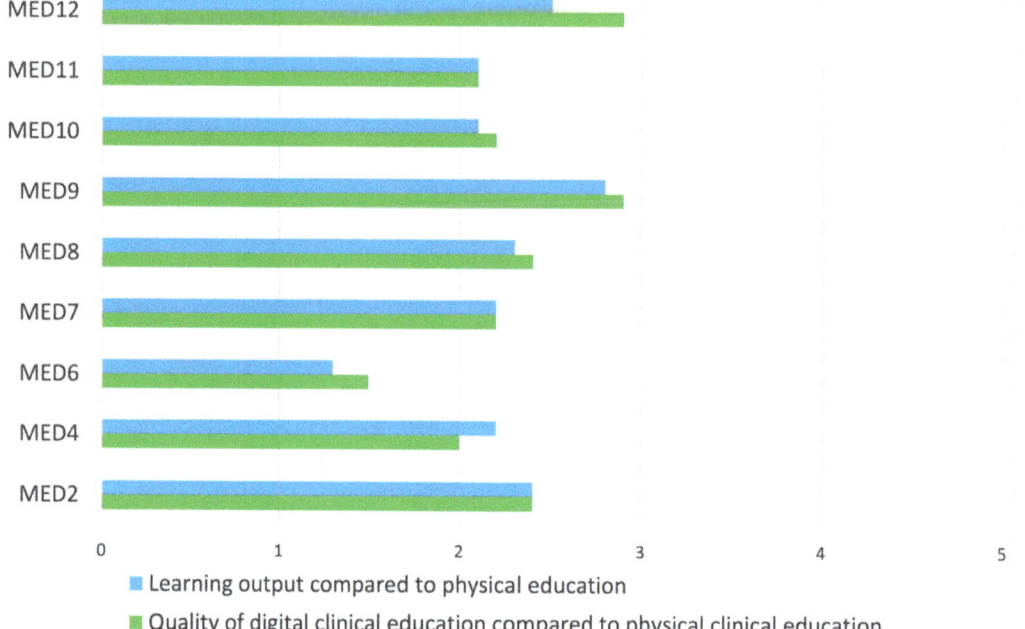

Figure 3. Likert scale mean value on student opinion regarding clinical and practical education depending on semester of study. Learning output: My learning output from digital clinical and practical teaching has been the same as with physical teaching.

3.4. Student Experience of Own Learning Output

Mean value of students' perceived learning output was 2.59 (Figure 4). Experienced learning output compared to an ordinary, physical semester correlated positively with satisfying information about changes in timetable and lectures ($p < 0.001$), student experience of their own motivation for learning ($p < 0.001$) and student experience of their own study efforts ($p < 0.001$). Motivated students, with enough and satisfying information given during the semester and with high own study efforts, experienced higher learning output than their counterparts. In addition, students who put in more hours in their part time job than during an ordinary semester had a lower learning outcome than students with fewer or the same hours ($p = 0.0025$) and had a more negative attitude towards digital education ($p < 0.001$).

Female students had a more positive attitude towards digital education than their male colleagues ($p = 0.04$), while at the same time being more anxious of having lost out on important learning because of digital education ($p = 0.05$). This fear of losing out on important learning also differed between the semesters ($p < 0.001$). Semesters MED7 and MED10 were generally more worried about potential gaps in their knowledge, while MED9 and MED12 where less anxious.

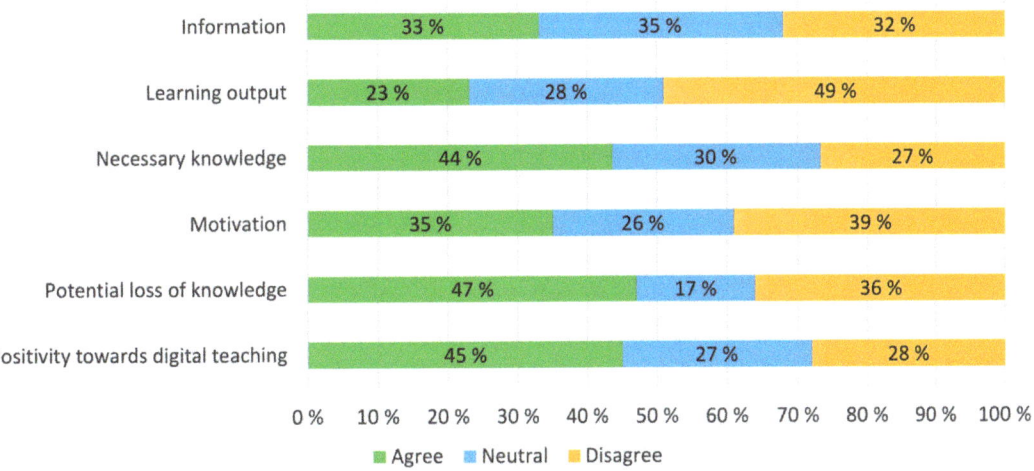

Figure 4. Student attitude to questions regarding their own learning experience this semester. Information: Necessary information about changes in education offer has been given; Learning output: My learning output during digital teaching has been equal to that of physical teaching; Knowledge acquired: I have acquired the necessary amount of knowledge during digital teaching; Motivation: I have been motivated for learning during digital teaching; Potential loss of knowledge: I am anxious that digital teaching has caused me to miss out on important knowledge; Positivity towards digital teaching: I have a positive attitude towards the possibility of digital teaching the next semester.

3.5. Student Feedback on How to Improve Digital Education

Several pros and cons were highlighted when students were asked about their experience with digital education. A majority emphasized the possibility of structuring their own study days as the biggest advantage, including choosing when to watch a lecture, being able to repeat when needed and being able to pause or rewind in case of ambiguity. Reduced possibility of socialization, lack of structure and canceled classes were, on the other hand, emphasized as factors that students disliked with digital education (Table 3).

Table 3. Five most common answers when students were asked about the pros and cons of digital education.

Pros	Cons
Increased opportunity to structure your own studies (67%)	Reduced possibility for socializing with fellow students (35%)
Increased time efficiency (15%)	Less day-to-day structure (17%)
Being able to decide time and place for study (9%)	Lessons deviating from the original timetable and/or being cancelled (14%)
Being more comfortable asking questions during lessons (8%)	Insufficient technical abilities in educators (11%)
Increased availability of lessons (2%)	A general feeling of distance to educator (10%)

Several proposals were made on how to improve digital education in the future. Improving teachers' technical skills, increased use of interactive teaching and improving the structure and flow of information on the learning management system (Canvas) (Available online: https://www.instructure.com/en-gb/canvas (accessed on 29 December 2021)), were some of the proposals made by several students (Table 4). In addition, students demanded that the faculty of medicine should ensure that all physical lectures receive some form of digital replacement, as opposed to just being cancelled. Digital education should correspond with the original timetable, and teachers should agree on one platform to present information to their students.

Table 4. Five most common answers when students were asked about how to improve digital education in the future.

	Proposals on How to Improve Digital Education	Number of Students
What should the teacher do to improve digital education?	Take advantage of opportunities for interactive teaching	44 (22.9%)
	Familiarize yourself with technical aids before the lesson	39 (20.3%)
	Ensure that students still get their 15-min breaks between lessons	24 (12.5%)
	Ensure that students may still ask questions, despite the lecture being a prerecorded video	19 (9.9%)
	Be sure to record and publish live video lectures	15 (7.8%)
What should the university/faculty do to improve digital education?	Ensure proper education in the use of digital media for educators	61 (35.5%)
	Try to prevent large deviations in scheduled education, and ensure that all teaching receive a digital substitute	46 (26.7%)
	Ensure that information reach the students by establishing a common system for information	23 (13.4%)
	Record and publish all live video lectures	23 (13.4%)
	Optimize video and sound quality	19 (11.0%)

4. Discussion

Medical students at UiB reported an experience of lower learning output because of emergency digital education the spring semester of 2020. This is despite that increased use of digital education is generally found to be a positive contribution to the learning environment at a university. Most of medical students in our study did report several positive factors regarding digital education. These included the increased opportunity to structure their own days, increased flexibility, and experience of increased time efficiency. Learning values, such as flexibility, usefulness and worthiness are found to have a positive effect on behavioral intention in context of digital learning. Behavioral intention is defined as the motivational factors that influence a given behavior [11]. Greater behavioral intention increases the likelihood of a desired behavior. In this context, increased behavior intention with increased learning values means that students that experience learning value are more likely to utilize digital education and learning platforms in a productive way [12]. Other studies have reported that an increased sense of time efficiency among medical students related to digital education have led to increased family time, better quality of sleep and increased opportunities for research [13,14]. Video lectures have shown the possibility of increasing learning output and speed of learning, especially when watching speed can be regulated and when students may repeat a lecture if they like [15].

Medical students in our study did also report a general satisfaction with the quality of theoretical teaching provided. Instructor characteristics are defined as qualities that makes a good instructor or teacher [16]. Qualities such as being able to fully utilize an eLearning platform and answering questions, are good instructor characteristics, and are found to increase behavioral intention in students in context of digital learning [12]. However, medical students in our study did request a higher degree of familiarization of technical aids from their teachers. They also requested the teachers to ensure the possibility to ask questions. Absence of good instructor characteristics may have reduced behavioral intention in medical students at UiB and contributed to the experience of a low learning output. A study by Bettinger et al. also show that to some extent, online learning might not compete with aspects of other learning, such as interactive knowledge building between teacher and student [17]. This finding is consistent with our study, with 22.9% of students reporting that teachers should take better advantage of the possibility of interactive learning in digital education.

Our study showed a correlation between lack of motivation and reduced learning output. Previous studies have shown that learning motivation is directing towards achievement and is therefore an essential part of perceived learning output and academic success [18–20]. Lack of motivation may have several possible explanations. Reduced motivation in students during the COVID-19 pandemic has been linked to for instance the individual student surroundings. Students possessing good internet access, a quiet and suitable place to study and with a high degree of digital social interaction have a higher degree of motivation during the pandemic [21]. A study by Khlaif et al. shows that poor internet connection and lack of technical support affect digital education in a major way [5]. Most of students in our study were living with other students during the initial lockdown, and 102 students moved back to their parents' house for some time. Lack of information from the university, moving back home to parents and constant changes in workload are likely linked to increased stress and consequently reduced motivation in for instance psychology students [22]. Living in dormitories with other students may also have caused a lack of a suitable study environment for students in our study. In addition, the unpredictability of emergency digital education and the pandemic in general may have caused an increased level of stress among students [5].

There was a major dissatisfaction with how clinical and practical teaching was replaced among medical students at UiB. Dissatisfaction with the practical teaching offered has been reported in several other studies, and several raise concern that the COVID-19 pandemic has resulted in a serious lack of clinical skills among medical students [14,23]. A study by AlQhani et al. showed that more than half of respondents thought that online learning was much or somewhat less effective in balancing practical and theoretical experience. Satisfaction was decreasing with increasing years of study and was especially low when practical aspects of teaching were at its highest [24]. A concern for the UiB students has been the forced cancellation of Objective Structured Clinical Examination (OSCE) for students in their final year of study. OSCE often serves as an additional motivation for students to practice clinical skills, and several studies fear that the cancellation of this exam will result in a generation of doctors unsure in their own clinical skills [25–28]. In this context, it should be mentioned that the graduating class in our study had generally low anxiety for having lost important skills and knowledge.

Our study showed a difference between male and female students. Female students were generally more satisfied with the pedagogical quality of teaching and had a more positive attitude towards more digital education in the future. At the same time, they were more anxious about potential important gaps in their knowledge. A study by Worly et al. has shown that female medical students have a higher risk of burnout and emotional exhaustion compared to male students [29]. In addition, female medical students have had a greater increase in stress levels and anxiety during the COVID-19 pandemic than their male colleagues [23]. A paradoxically more positive attitude towards digital education may be surfacing due to female students generally being more structured [30], and digital education demanding a higher degree of self-organization. However, earlier studies have not shown a difference in the usage of digital tools between male and female students [31].

A limitation to our study is that it did not assess students' performance. Their perceived learning output may not be the same as their actual learning output. However, subjective feedback is essential to map out student opinions and to investigate how to make digital education a better experience. It is essential to develop digital education further. Our study had a low response rate, with 24% of medical students at UiB. At the same time, our response rate and final number of participants is consistent with similar published studies. Gender distribution is consistent with gender distribution on the medical education of UiB.

5. Conclusions

Despite several studies showing the positive potential of digital education in the field of medicine, medical students at UiB generally reported an experience of reduced learning output during the COVID-19 pandemic. Our findings indicate that lack of motivation and lack of a sufficient offer in clinical education are the biggest contributing factors. Practical and clinical skills are essential to the field of medicine, and a lack of opportunity to rehearse and practice skills could potentially lead to a generation of insecure doctors with reduced experience in meeting and examining actual patients. However, if used correctly, digital education can be a most useful tool to increase flexibility and time efficiency among students and could even contribute to an increased learning output. With an increased focus on securing student motivation, learning values, and good instructor characteristics, as well as investigating and utilizing tools for clinical digital education, digital education may prove to be a most useful tool for educating medical students and other health workers in the future.

Author Contributions: Conceptualization, H.K.H., T.T., M.K. and H.R.; methodology, H.K.H., T.T., M.K. and H.R.; software, H.K.H. and H.R.; validation, H.K.H., T.T., M.K. and H.R.; formal analysis, H.K.H. and H.R.; investigation, H.K.H., T.T., M.K. and H.R.; resources, H.K.H., T.T., M.K. and H.R.; data curation, H.K.H. and H.R.; writing—original draft preparation, H.K.H., T.T., M.K. and H.R.; writing—review and editing, H.K.H., T.T., M.K. and H.R. visualization, H.K.H. and H.R.; supervision, T.T., M.K. and H.R.; project administration, H.R. All authors have read and agreed to the published version of the manuscript.

Funding: This research received no external funding.

Institutional Review Board Statement: The study was conducted according to the guidelines of the Declaration of Helsinki and approved by the Norwegian Center of Research Data (Reporting form 196323, approved 02.06.2020).

Informed Consent Statement: Informed consent was obtained from all subjects involved in the study.

Data Availability Statement: The data presented in this study are available on request from the corresponding author.

Acknowledgments: We are grateful for technical assistance from Dina-Kristin Topphol Midtflø at the Medical Faculty, University of Bergen.

Conflicts of Interest: The authors declare no conflict of interest.

References

1. Norwegian Department of Health. Norwegian Department of Health has Taken Comprehensive Measures to Prevent the Spread of COVID-19. 2020. Available online: https://www.helsedirektoratet.no/nyheter/helsedirektoratet-har-vedtatt-omfattende-tiltak-for-a-hindre-spredning-av-covid-19#stengingogforbudavulikearrangementerogtilbud (accessed on 16 November 2020).
2. Hodges, C.; Moore, S.; Lockee, B.; Trust, T.; Bond, A. The Difference between Emergency Remote Learning and Online Learning. 2020. Available online: https://er.educause.edu/articles/2020/3/the-difference-between-emergency-remote-teaching-and-online-learning (accessed on 20 November 2021).
3. UNESCO. #LearningNeverStops. 2021. Available online: https://en.unesco.org/covid19/educationresponse/globalcoalition (accessed on 5 January 2022).
4. University of Bergen. The University is to Close from the 12th of March 2020 at 6 p.m. 2020. Available online: https://www.uib.no/aktuelt/134112/universitetet-stenges-fra-12-mars-2020-kl-18 (accessed on 10 December 2021).
5. Khlaif, Z.N.; Salha, S.; Kouraichi, B. Emergency remote learning during COVID-19 crisis: Students' engagement. *Educ. Inf. Technol.* **2021**, *26*, 7033–7055. [CrossRef] [PubMed]
6. Adams, A.M. Pedagogical underpinnings of computer-based learning. *J. Adv. Nurs.* **2004**, *46*, 5–12. [CrossRef] [PubMed]
7. Shorbaji, N.A.; Atun, R.; Car, J.; Majeed, A.; Wheeler, E. eLearning for Undergraduate Health Professional Education: World Health Organization. 2015. Available online: https://www.who.int/hrh/documents/14126-eLearningReport.pdf (accessed on 12 December 2021).
8. Michaelsen, L.K.; Knight, A.B.; Fink, L.D. *Team-Based Learning: A Transformative Use of Small Groups in College Teaching*; Stylus Pub.: Sterling, VA, USA, 2004.

9. Jamieson, S. Likert Scale: Encyclopedia Brittanica. 2017. Available online: https://www.britannica.com/topic/Likert-Scale (accessed on 5 December 2021).
10. Skarsbø, A.M.; Johansen, H.M.; Dalheim, E.; Bakken, K. Equality at UiB: Action Plan for Gender Equality 2017–2020. 2017. Available online: https://www.uib.no/sites/w3.uib.no/files/attachments/us2017-037.pdf (accessed on 2 January 2022).
11. Shroff, R.H.; Deneen, C.C.; Ng, E.M.W. Analysis of the technology acceptance model in examining students' behavioural intention to use an e-portfolio system. *Australas. J. Educ. Technol.* **2011**, *27*, 600–618. [CrossRef]
12. Prasetyo, Y.T.; Roque, R.A.C.; Chuenyindee, T.; Young, M.N.; Diaz, J.F.T.; Persada, S.F.; Miraja, B.A.; Perwira Redi, A.A.N. Determining Factors Affecting the Acceptance of Medical Education eLearning Platforms during the COVID-19 Pandemic in the Philippines: UTAUT2 Approach. *Healthcare* **2021**, *9*, 780. [CrossRef]
13. Khalil, R.; Mansour, A.E.; Fadda, W.A.; Almisnid, K.; Aldamegh, M.; Al-Nafeesah, A.; Alkhalifah, A.; Al-Wutayd, O. The sudden transition to synchronized online learning during the COVID-19 pandemic in Saudi Arabia: A qualitative study exploring medical students' perspectives. *BMC Med. Educ.* **2020**, *20*, 285. [CrossRef] [PubMed]
14. Shahrvini, B.; Baxter, S.L.; Coffey, C.S.; MacDonald, B.V.; Lander, L. Pre-clinical remote undergraduate medical education during the COVID-19 pandemic: A survey study. *BMC Med. Educ.* **2021**, *21*, 13. [CrossRef]
15. Cardall, S.; Krupat, E.; Ulrich, M. Live Lecture Versus Video-Recorded Lecture: Are Students Voting With Their Feet? *Acad. Med.* **2008**, *83*, 1174–1178. [CrossRef]
16. Carrigan, S. Qualities of a Good Instructor. 2005. Available online: https://www.researchgate.net/publication/294408459_Qualities_of_a_good_instructor (accessed on 29 December 2021).
17. Bettinger, E.P.; Fox, L.; Loeb, S.; Taylor, E.S. Virtual Classrooms: How Online College Courses Affect Student Success. *Am. Econ. Rev.* **2017**, *107*, 2855–2875. [CrossRef]
18. Jun Xin, L.; Ahmad Hathim, A.A.; Jing Yi, N.; Reiko, A.; Noor Akmal Shareela, I. Digital learning in medical education: Comparing experiences of Malaysian and Japanese students. *BMC Med. Educ.* **2021**, *21*, 418. [CrossRef] [PubMed]
19. van der Burgt, S.M.E.; Kusurkar, R.A.; Wilschut, J.A.; Tjin A Tsoi, S.L.N.M.; Croiset, G.; Peerdeman, S.M. Motivational Profiles and Motivation for Lifelong Learning of Medical Specialists. *J. Contin. Educ. Health Prof.* **2018**, *38*, 171–178. [CrossRef]
20. Steinmayr, R.; Weidinger, A.F.; Schwinger, M.; Spinath, B. The Importance of Students' Motivation for Their Academic Achievement—Replicating and Extending Previous Findings. *Front. Psychol.* **2019**, *10*, 1730. [CrossRef] [PubMed]
21. Meeter, M.; Bele, T.; den Hartogh, C.; Bakker, T.; de Vries, R.E.; Plak, S. *College Students' Motivation and Study Results after COVID-19 Stay-at-Home Orders*; Vrije Universiteit Amsterdam: Amsterdam, The Netherlands, 2020.
22. Usher, E.L.; Golding, J.M.; Han, J.; Griffiths, C.S.; McGavran, M.B.; Brown, C.S.; Sheehan, E.A. Psychology Students' Motivation and Learning in Response to the Shift to Remote Instruction During COVID-19. *Scholarsh. Teach. Learn. Psychol.* **2021**, *33*. [CrossRef]
23. Harries, A.J.; Lee, C.; Jones, L.; Rodriguez, R.M.; Davis, J.A.; Boysen-Osborn, M.; Kashima, K.J.; Krane, N.K.; Rae, G.; Kman, N.; et al. Effects of the COVID-19 pandemic on medical students: A multicenter quantitative study. *BMC Med. Educ.* **2021**, *21*, 14. [CrossRef] [PubMed]
24. AlQhtani, A.; AlSwedan, N.; Almulhim, A.; Aladwan, R.; Alessa, Y.; AlQhtani, K.; Albogami, M.; Altwairqi, K.; Alotaibi, F.; AlHadlaq, A.; et al. Online versus classroom teaching for medical students during COVID-19: Measuring effectiveness and satisfaction. *BMC Med. Educ.* **2021**, *21*, 452. [CrossRef] [PubMed]
25. Sani, I.; Hamza, Y.; Chedid, Y.; Amalendran, J.; Hamza, N. Understanding the consequence of COVID-19 on undergraduate medical education: Medical students' perspective. *Ann. Med. Surg.* **2020**, *58*, 117–119. [CrossRef]
26. Raymond-Hayling, O. What lies in the year ahead for medical education? A medical student's perspective during the COVID-19 pandemic. *Med. Educ. Online* **2020**, *25*, 1781749. [CrossRef]
27. Zayyan, M. Objective structured clinical examination: The assessment of choice. *Oman Med. J.* **2011**, *26*, 219–222. [CrossRef] [PubMed]
28. Choi, B.; Jegatheeswaran, L.; Minocha, A.; Alhilani, M.; Nakhoul, M.; Mutengesa, E. The impact of the COVID-19 pandemic on final year medical students in the United Kingdom: A national survey. *BMC Med. Educ.* **2020**, *20*, 206. [CrossRef] [PubMed]
29. Worly, B.; Verbeck, N.; Walker, C.; Clinchot, D.M. Burnout, perceived stress, and empathic concern: Differences in female and male Millennial medical students. *Psychol. Health Med.* **2019**, *24*, 429–438. [CrossRef] [PubMed]
30. Nilsen, H.B.; Henningsen, I. Boy panic and girl pressure—Paradoxes and knowledge crisis. *Tidsskr. Kjønnsforskning* **2018**, *42*, 6–28. [CrossRef]
31. Turkyilmaz, I.; Hariri, N.; Jahangiri, L. Student´s perception on the impact of eLearning on dental education. *J. Contemporary Dent. Pract.* **2019**, *20*, 616–621. [CrossRef]

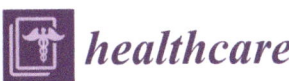

Article

Perception of E-Resources on the Learning Process among Students in the College of Health Sciences in King Saud University, Saudi Arabia, during the (COVID-19) Outbreak

Reham AlJasser [1,*], Lina Alolyet [2], Daniyah Alsuhaibani [2], Sarah Albalawi [2], Md. Dilshad Manzar [3] and Abdulrhman Albougami [3]

1. Department of Periodontics and Community Dentistry, Dental College, King Saud University, Riyadh 11545, Saudi Arabia
2. Department of General Dentistry, Dental College, King Saud University, Riyadh 11545, Saudi Arabia; Linaalolayet@hotmail.com (L.A.); Danzalsuhaibani@Gmail.com (D.A.); Albalawisarah@gmail.com (S.A.)
3. Department of Nursing, College of Applied Medical Sciences, Majmaah University, AlMajmaah 11952, Saudi Arabia; md.dilshadmanzar@gmail.com (M.D.M.); a.albougami@mu.edu.sa (A.A.)
* Correspondence: raljasser@ksu.edu.sa; Tel.: +966-534119922

Abstract: Aim: to assess the impact of e-learning through different e-resources among health sciences students. Methodology: A cross-sectional design was conducted among health science students (n = 211; 134 female and 77 male) at King Saud University, Saudi Arabia. The data was collected using a previously used structured questionnaire to assess the impact of e-resources on learning. Results: The four most frequently used e-resources were: Zoom (38%), YouTube (31%), Google applications (29%), and Blackboard (27%). More than one-third of the students (35%) reportedly used e-resources for three or more hours daily. The majority of the students (55.9%) recognized a gender-related and age-related difference among faculty members in terms of e-resources usage. The majority of the students (58.2%) believe that online resources recommended by faculty members were credible. The majority of students believed that their academic performance was primarily influenced by these features of the e-resources: organization/logic of the content (64.5%), the credibility of the video (64.5%), and up to date "look and feel" of the video (60.6%). The study identified the most frequently used e-resources, gender, and age-related differences in faculty members' use of e-resources, students' overwhelming reliance on faculty feedback regarding the credibility of e-resources, and three most important characteristics (organization, credibility, and updated status) of e-resources. Conclusion: e-learning resources had a significant impact on participating students' education as they were used very frequently during their health sciences' courses.

Keywords: e-resources; e-learning; credibility; academic performance; health sciences education

1. Introduction

Recently, the outbreak of the pandemic situation due to Coronavirus (COVID-19) had led to massive loss of human life worldwide. The result of this massive loss spurred economic and social disruption. Therefore, it was recommended to limit social gathering and apply social distancing with increased precaution protocols to control this virus's transmission. This recommendation was also applied globally at different levels of all educational systems as physical classes were stopped.

UNESCO estimates suggested that over 1.5 billion learners were affected during this period in the education system [1–3]. Therefore, alternatives have immediately been investigated and gathered to resume teaching and learning at different levels of education throughout the world.

Many educational institutes took the initiative to transfer traditional onsite learning to online education. This initiative was done in order to maintain the safety of their students and to fulfill their basic needs for education through distance learning.

Distance education, also known as distance learning, is defined as the education of students who may not always be physically present at a school [1,2]. Traditionally, this usually involved correspondence courses wherein the student corresponded with the school via mail, and today it usually involves online education.

Technological innovation has not only impacted social change in recent years but has been the prime driver of educational transformation [4–7]. There has been a growing interest in using Internet-based learning by universities over the past decade to supplement or replace traditional learning [8]. The development of new technologies marks the growth of the internet. E-learning is the use of internet-based resources in education. Internet-based learning for health professional education is increasing [9]. It offers advantages over traditional learning approaches, enables learning to be completed conveniently for the user, and improves accessibility, especially where facilities are geographically disparate [9,10]. It can also deliver a broad array of solutions that enhance knowledge and performance [8], increase accessibility to education, and improve self-efficacy [11] and clinical skills.

This results in improving practitioners' capabilities [12], cost-effectiveness, learner flexibility [7], satisfaction and promotion of student-to-student and student-to-instructor interactions [13]. Therefore, it is of utmost importance to integrate e-learning to acquire knowledge in the study of health sciences.

Some barriers can affect the development and implementation of online learning in education, such as poor technical skills, inadequate infrastructure, absence of institutional strategies and support, and negative attitudes of stakeholders [14–16]. On the other hand, the practical nature of health science education demands direct contact between students, instructors, and patients [17]. Therefore, traditional teaching methods in health sciences are essential.

The use of digital devices in the college of health sciences for teaching and learning purposes has been widely accepted in universities [18]. As a result of this development, it has become apparent in recent years that Internet-based learning or electronic learning (E-learning) has increased its attraction to students at large [19]. E-learning has recently been proposed as a primary complementary tool to improve medical and dental education [20], which has been defined as learning while "utilizing electronic technologies to access educational curriculum outside of a traditional classroom" [21,22]. These interactive teaching strategies have enhanced students' focus, amplified their attention, and maximized their long-term knowledge retention [20]. Therefore, most higher education institutions classify online learning as crucial for their educational strategy [23].

Electronic and virtual applications and sources can be compelling and entertaining in several educational fields. However, this can be very challenging in terms of application, especially in health science education which focuses on proper care, prevents the spread of diseases, and improves the lives of every patient to ensure the longevity of life or improvement in the life expectancy of individuals.

This field should provide students with technical skills, proper health care competencies, and various opportunities to obtain the knowledge needed for growth and development in the health sector [1]. It also aims to improve physical, mental, emotional, and social health by increasing their knowledge and influencing their attitudes by caring for their well-being [1,3].

King Saud University was one of the first universities in Saudi Arabia to transfer courses from traditional onsite to online education. Lectures were mainly given through live webinars to ensure proper interaction between the lecturer and the students. Assignments, quizzes, and exams were conducted through the BlackBoard website, which was previously activated during traditional education as a supportive tool for the educational process of the students. After the adoption of the online education system, the website became the backbone of the educational process.

With the ongoing spread of the coronavirus, online learning resources have become increasingly essential to ensure uninterrupted educational delivery to isolated students. This opportunity has expanded the learning offering beyond the limitations of the traditional methods. The literature revealed that learning technology has positively supported the health sciences curriculum [20]. Hence, it is crucial to evaluate its proper applicability in each specific education field and make a positive adjustment for maximum learning experience.

This study aims to assess the impact of e-learning through different e-resources among health sciences students attending King Saud University.

The objectives of the present study are as follows:

1. To understand the most prominent e-resources used among health sciences students attending King Saud University.
2. To assess the relationship between the age of faculty members related to given courses through e-resources and their use of these facilities.
3. To assess the relationship between the gender of faculty members related to given courses through e-resources and their use of these facilities.
4. To examine various e-resources and evaluate the effect of various sources of E-learning on health sciences students' ability to comprehend academic topics.

Therefore, the Null hypothesis is that there is no positive impact of e-learning through different e-resources among health sciences students attending King Saud University.

The Alternative Hypothesis is that there is a positive impact of e-learning through different e-resources among health sciences students attending King Saud University

2. Materials and Methods

2.1. Ethical Considerations

Institutional review board approval was obtained from King Saud University, Riyadh, Saudi Arabia (E-20-5052). Informed consent was required for the participants to proceed to answer the questionnaire. Therefore responses without the participants' consent were not recorded. The purpose and objectives of this study were explained, and the participants were informed that the information obtained was to be used for research purposes only, and the outcome would be presented in anonymous charts, figures, and tables.

2.2. Setting and Application

The survey was offered to undergraduate medical sciences students which included medical, dental, pharmacy, applied medical sciences, and nursing students from both female and male sections. An online survey was used, with all participants anonymously completing the survey at an opportune place and time for them.

A web-based survey with a link provided was distributed to participants through an e-mail and an invitation through social media platforms. Participants used a device and a browser of their choice and convenience. Investigators cannot identify participating students, and the survey was completely anonymous. Students were informed that they had the right to discontinue the study at any point in time without any consequences. The participation was sought to be voluntary, and the confidentiality of responses was maintained.

The proposed survey did not take more than five minutes to complete for the majority.

2.3. Sample Size Determination

The study focused on undergraduate students attending colleges of health sciences in King Saud University, Saudi Arabia. The sample size was determined by G Power software (Hinnerup, Denmark). The confidence level was set at 95%. The power level was set at 80% with a moderate effect size and a final sample size of 180 students. However, a larger sample was recruited to avoid the possibility of a low response rate that could affect the sample size. A final sample of 211 students was recruited using purposive sampling because the goal of this study focused on students in the college of health sciences [24].

2.4. Instrument to Be Used

A modified version was used after obtaining permission of the primary author of the survey for Student's Perception of the Impact of E-Learning on Dental Education [14].

The survey was comprised of 14 questions, including seven multiple-choice questions, two fill-in-the-blank questions, two open-ended questions, and three Likert scale questions. The purpose of the two open-ended questions was to allow students to share the applications they used during their dental education, their perceived impact on their academic achievement, and their opinion of online education.

The first part contains questions related to demographic information.

The second part contains questions related to students' use of E-learning resources (e-resources) and their perceptions of these resources.

The third part contained questions that asked students to mention the top three e-resources used for academic purposes. The questions explored several factors influencing the use of these e-resources which included the following: the time spent on these resources, the credibility of the e-resources recommended by faculty members, the influence of certain factors regarding e-resources on students' academic achievement, the effect of e-resources on students' ability to understand academic topics, students' observation of faculty members integration of e-resources in their courses and its relationship with the faculty members age, the relationship that the students observed between the faculty member's age and their dependence on social media for communication, the students' attendance preference, and finally the effects of e-resources on students' academic performance.

The modified version was sent to survey experts in the dental field to receive feedback and opinion about its clarity and easiness and recommendations for further adjustments. As a second step, a small sample of 20 students were chosen to pre-test the final version. This step showed that the questionnaire needed to become shorter and more straightforward. The participants also offered some amendments to the questionnaire which were considered and noted. The questionnaire was finalized after an in-depth discussion among the authors. The modified version was administered to a sample of 50 students in a pilot study. K value for the inter-participants' agreement was calculated to as 0.91, indicating an "almost perfect agreement" according to Cohen [25].

2.5. Statistical Analysis

Descriptive Kolmogorov–Smirnov, and Shapiro–Wilks tests were applied to check the normal data distribution. The data was entered and analyzed using SPSS 24.0 version statistical software (IBM Inc., Chicago, IL, USA). Findings were presented through frequencies, percentages, mean, and standard deviation values. The following elements were evaluated: participants' demographic characteristics, most frequently used electronic resources/applications by students, the average duration of daily electronic resources/applications used for academic performance, students' observations of incorporation of e-learning by faculty members and the age of faculty members, and the relationship between faculty members' dependence on social media for communication and their age.

3. Results

3.1. Participants' Characteristics

In this study, health science students ($n = 211$; 134 females and 77 males) with a mean age of 21 years $\pm$ 3 years participated. About two-thirds of the participating students were enrolled in dentistry and the college of allied health sciences (Table 1). The majority of the study sample comprised of female students (63.5%).

Table 1. Participants' characteristics.

Characteristics	Frequency	Percentage
Specialty		
College of Dentistry	111	52.6

Table 1. Cont.

Characteristics	Frequency	Percentage
College of Medicine	24	11.4
College of Pharmacy	17	8.1
College of Applied Medical Sciences	32	15.2
College of Nursing	14	6.6
Prince Sultan Bin Abdul-Aziz College for Emergency Medical Services	13	6.2
Age		
18–20	70	33.2
21–23	125	59.2
24 and more	16	7.6
Gender		
Male	77	36.5
Female	134	63.5

3.2. Most Frequently Used E-Resources

Table 2 presents the descriptive summary of the item that required students to record their three most frequently used e-resources. Regarding preferred resources perceived by students to improve their academic performance, 16 different e-resources were identified. The four most frequently used were: Zoom (38%), followed by YouTube (31%), Google applications (29%), and Blackboard (27%) (Table 2). E.E.E., Saudi Digital Library, and Dropbox were the three least used electronics resources, with all the three being reported to be used by less than 1% of the participating students. More than one-third of the students identified 'others' as one of the resources.

Table 2. Frequency distribution of students' most frequently used electronic resources/applications in decreasing order.

Electronic Resources/Applications	Frequency	Percentage
Zoom	81	38.4
YouTube	66	31.3
Google applications	62	29.4
Blackboard	57	27.0
Notability	48	22.7
Microsoft Office applications	18	8.5
Telegram	12	5.7
Twitter	8	3.8
Adobe	7	3.3
WhatsApp	7	3.3
Flashcard applications	6	2.8
Instagram	4	1.9
Dropbox	1	0.5
EEE	1	0.5
Saudi Digital Library	1	0.5
Others	81	38.4

3.3. Electronic Resources: Daily Use by Students, Gender and Age Pattern among Faculty Members

About 65 respondents (30.8%) used e-resources for two to three hours every day (Table 3). Most of the participating students reported either no gender-related difference or 'I do not know' in incorporating e-resources by faculty members (74%). However, the biggest group of students recorded that faculty members who more prevalently used e-resources were under 50 years of age (Table 4). Similarly, almost half of the students replied that there was a relationship between faculty members' dependence on social media for communication and their age because it was more commonly seen in those under 50 years of age (Table 5).

Table 3. Students' average duration of daily electronic resources/applications for academic performance.

Average Duration	Frequency (n)	Percentage (%)
Less than 1 h	30	14.2
1–2 h	42	19.9
2–3 h	65	30.8
3–4 h	29	13.7
More than 4 h	45	21.4

Table 4. Students' observations of incorporation of e-learning by faculties and the age of faculties.

Incorporation of E-Learning by Faculty Members	Frequency (n)	Percentage (%)
More prevalent among male faculties	22	10.4
More prevalent among female faculties	33	15.6
There is no difference in the use	93	44.1
I do not know	63	29.9
Observed relation in using e-resources and age of faculty members		
More prevalent among faculties over 50 years of age	9	4.2
More prevalent among faculties under 50 years of age	103	48.8
There is no difference in use by age groups	59	28.0
I do not know	40	19.0

Table 5. Relationship between faculty's dependence on social media for communication and their age.

Relationship between Faculty Member's Dependence on Social Media and Their Age	Frequency (n)	Percentage (%)
More prevalent among faculties over 50 years of age	5	2.3
More prevalent among faculties under 50 years of age	103	48.8
There is no difference in use by age groups	63	29.9
I do not know	40	19.0

3.4. Online Applications/Animations: Student's Perceived Academic Performance and Reliance on Faculty Recommendations

Students regarded e-resources recommended by faculty members with a high level of credibility; this is indicated by a majority (58.2%) replying that they were greatly influenced by teachers' feedback on such matters (Figure 1). Organization/logic of the content, credibility of the video, and up-to-date "look and feel" of the video were the three most influential factors on the students' perceived academic performance with 64.5%, 64.5%, and 60.6%, respectively. While online presentation under 15 min was perceived to be least influential in academic performance, most students (55.9%) recorded a response of 'neutral' or 'least influence' for this factor (Table 6).

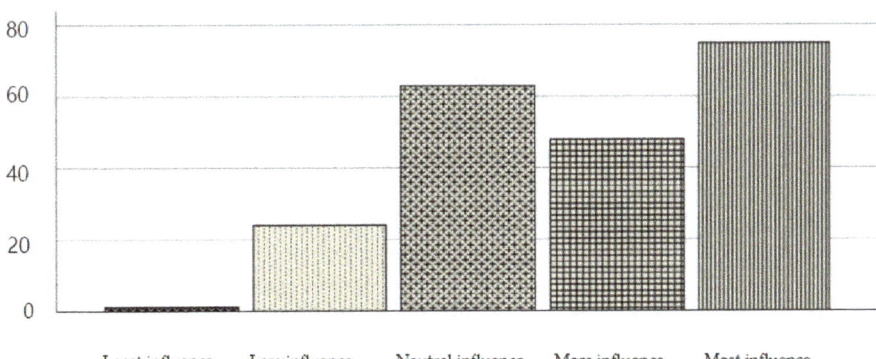

Figure 1. The "level of credibility" is given by students to e-resources recommended by faculty members.

Table 6. Influence of online applications/animations on the students' perceived academic performance.

Influence Level	Least Influence	Less Influence	Neutral Influence	More Influence	Most Influence
Scale	1	2	3	4	5
Factors					
Online presentation under 15 min	9.0	16.6	30.3	25.1	19.0
Mobile friendly	8.1	13.7	24.6	24.2	29.4
Up-to-date "look and feel" of the video	3.8	13.3	22.3	23.2	37.4
The credibility of the video	2.4	9.0	24.2	24.2	40.3
Organization/logic of the content	1.9	10.0	23.7	20.9	43.6

4. Discussion

The present study's results highlighted that e-learning resources significantly impacted education during the coronavirus pandemic (COVID-19) outbreak when used by health sciences students at King Saud University.

Findings revealed that the most frequently used e-resources were Zoom, followed by YouTube, Google applications, and Blackboard. This sequence in preference could be attributed to the increasing urge for a videoconferencing technology to augment online learning, which unfolded at the pandemic's peak when people were adjusting to the new normal. Zoom is one of the most helpful resources to enhance effective and synchronous e-learning since it allows visual interaction between the students and instructors. It was established that Zoom could accommodate 1000 participants in one meeting. This application can be downloaded and used for free (Ismawati, Iis, et al. 2021, Wibawanto, 2020) as cited by Kasman et al. [24,25] One could infer that due to its ability to accommodate a large number of participants, its simple interface and low cost explains the dominance of this e-resource compared to other applications.

In contrast, this result was supported by the findings from a previous study [14], we discovered that the second most used e-resource is YouTube. Before the pandemic,

YouTube was globally the go-to site for virtual learning. However, recent authors [26,27] established that the COVID-19 outbreak pushed all universities to incorporate the use of video conferencing technology (V.C.T.) to supplement learning management systems for e-learning, including YouTube.

When the students were asked about the duration spent on e-resources, most of the respondents reported using e-resources for at least 3 h at a time. This relatively long duration can be explained by the nature of health sciences lectures and seminars, which usually require a significant amount of time.

Regarding the observed relationship between using e-resources and faculty members' age, the majority of the respondents reported that the faculty members who prevalently used e-resources were more likely to be under the age of 50 years old. This may be due to the fact that the majority of this age category have been more exposed to recent technologies and more enthusiastic than the older age category. This result coincides with the results of the research work carried out by Turkyilmaz et al. [14], in which they discovered that faculty members that frequently used e-resources were under 50 years of age. They are more likely to have been exposed to technology in their education and early career stages. Therefore, they may be more inclined to use technology in learning settings and communication. Several investigators discovered that only a few faculty members use advanced online learning tools.

Faculty members hesitated to shift their teaching style to e-learning due to several reasons which included: low perceived benefit, difficulty in using these online resources, frequency of students' usage, and the time required to invest in the process [24]. However, even faculty members over 50 years of age were compelled to use the e-resources in a limited fashion. This observation can also be explained by the variation of exposure to e-resources by different generations and the ubiquity of computers and the internet in modern academic environments. Moreover, this trend will keep increasing as more educators bring technology-based activities into the classrooms [14].

Furthermore, when faculty members' gender was observed, results revealed that about 44% of the students did not perceive a gender-related pattern regarding incorporating e-resources. These findings were supported by a recent study where authors also discovered that the students in their study observed no gender-related pattern in incorporating distance learning [14].

Concerning students' perceived academic performance and reliance on faculty members' recommendations, the results indicated that most students viewed online applications recommended by faculty members with a high level of credibility. It was discovered that the organization/logic of the content, credibility and up-to-date "look and feel" of the video were the three most influential factors on the students' perceived academic performance. These findings were contrary to the results of previous studies that reported the e-learning system's efficacy on organization and attractiveness of the course content [12,13].

Several limitations have been observed in the present study, including statistical bias, as samples were not evenly distributed. Half of the sample size predominantly included dental students, while the other half contained medicine, nursing, pharmacy, and applied medical sciences. The present study is a cross-sectional study within one university which may limit the inference of the findings to other regions of the country or the world. Likewise, the study did not evaluate the students' actual academic performance but rather their perceived performance, which may be subjective rather than objective. It should be highlighted that present findings were based only on surveys without structured interviews with faculty members. Therefore, future studies with a well-controlled and improved methodology are recommended to confirm present study findings.

In summary, the findings of this study helped understand the perception of health science students in adopting E-learning resources, the effect of E-learning on their ability to comprehend academic topics, and its influence on their academic performance.

5. Conclusions

E-learning resources were frequently used during the present study and they had significant impact on the participating health science students' education. Most e-resources used were Zoom, followed by YouTube, Google applications, and Blackboard. The faculty members' age was a significant factor affecting their use and reliance on e-resources. Organization, credibility, and updated status of e-resources were also significant contributors to health sciences students' academic performance. In conclusion, incorporation of e-learning resources training and application in the schools' curriculum is essential to improve health sciences students' and faculty members' distance learning experience and outcomes.

Author Contributions: Conceptualization, R.A.; methodology, R.A., L.A., D.A. and S.A.; software, R.A.; validation R.A., L.A., S.A. and D.A.; formal analysis, M.D.M.; investigation, L.A., D.A. and S.A.; resources, R.A.; data curation, M.D.M.; writing—original draft preparation, All authors; writing—review and editing, All Authors; visualization, R.A.; supervision, A.A. project administration, R.A. and A.A.; funding acquisition, R.A. and A.A. All authors have read and agreed to the published version of the manuscript.

Funding: This research received no external funding.

Institutional Review Board Statement: Institutional review board approval was obtained from King Saud University, Riyadh, Saudi Arabia (E-20-5052).

Informed Consent Statement: Informed consent was required for the participants to answer the questionnaire. Therefore responses without the participant's consent were not recorded.

Data Availability Statement: The data presented in this study are available on request from the corresponding author. The data are not publicly available due to ethical and institutional restrictions.

Acknowledgments: The authors would like to thank the College of Dentistry Research Center at King Saud University, Riyadh, Saudi Arabia for all the support provided for this study in terms of revising the manuscript and distributing the surveys.

Conflicts of Interest: The authors declare no conflict of interest. The funder had no role in designing the study, data collection, analyses, interpretation, writing of the manuscript, or decision to publish the results.

References

1. Badia Gargante, A.; Meneses Naranjo, J.; García Tamarit, C. Technology use for teaching and learning. *Píxel-Bit. Rev. Medios Educ.* **2015**, *46*, 9–24.
2. Touro University Worldwide. Available online: https://www.tuw.edu (accessed on 30 August 2021).
3. UNESCO, United Nations Educational, Scientific and Cultural Organization. *COVID-19 Educational Disruption and Response*; SAGE: New York, NY, USA, 2020.
4. Belfi, L.M.; Dean, K.E.; Bartolotta, R.J.; Shih, G.; Min, R.J. Medical student education in the time of COVID-19: A virtual solution to the introductory radiology elective. *Clin. Imaging* **2021**, *75*, 67–74. [CrossRef]
5. U.S. Department of Education, Office of Planning, Evaluation and Policy Development. *Evaluation of Evidence-Based Practice in Online Learning; a Meta-Analysis and Review of Online Learning Studies*; American Department of Education: Washington, DC, USA, 2010.
6. Kim, S. The Future of E-Learning in medical education: Current trend and future opportunity. *J. Educ. Eval. Health Prof.* **2006**, *3*, 3. [CrossRef] [PubMed]
7. Sinclair, P.; Kable, A.; Levett-Jones, T. The effectiveness of internet-based e-learning on clinician behavior and patient outcomes: A systematic review protocol. *JBI Database Syst. Rev. Implement Rep.* **2015**, *13*, 52–64. [CrossRef]
8. Aloia, L.; Vaporciyan, A.A. E-learning trends and how to apply them to thoracic surgery education. *Thorac. Surg. Clin.* **2019**, *29*, 285–290. [CrossRef] [PubMed]
9. Wolbrink, T.A.; Burns, J.P. Internet-based learning and applications for critical care medicine. *J. Intensive Care Med.* **2012**, *27*, 322–332. [CrossRef]
10. Bond, S.E.; Crowther, S.P.; Adhikari, S.; Chubaty, A.J.; Yu, P.; Borchard, J.P.; Boutlis, C.S.; Yeo, W.W.; Miyakis, S. Evaluating the Effect of a Web-Based E-Learning Tool for Health Professional Education on Clinical Vancomycin Use: Comparative Study. *JMIR Med. Educ.* **2018**, *4*, e5. [CrossRef]
11. Sinclair, P.M.; Kable, A.; Levett-Jones, T.; Booth, D. The effectiveness of Internet-based e-learning on clinician behavior and patient outcomes: A systematic review. *Int. J. Nurs. Stud.* **2016**, *57*, 70–81. [CrossRef] [PubMed]

12. Nakanishi, H.; Doyama, H.; Ishikawa, H.; Uedo, N.; Gotoda, T.; Kato, M.; Nagao, S.; Nagami, Y.; Aoyagi, H.; Imagawa, A.; et al. Evaluation of an e-learning system for diagnosis of gastric lesions using magnifying narrow-band imaging: A multicenter randomized controlled study. *Endoscopy* **2017**, *49*, 957–967. [CrossRef]
13. Broudo, M.; Walsh, C. MEDICAL: Online learning in medicine and dentistry. *Acad. Med.* **2002**, *77*, 926–927. [CrossRef]
14. Turkyilmaz, I.; Hariri, N.H.; Jahangiri, L. Student's perception of the impact of E-learning on dental education. *J. Contemp. Dent. Pract.* **2019**, *20*, 616–621. [CrossRef]
15. O'Doherty, D.; Dromey, M.; Lougheed, J.; Hannigan, A.; Last, J.; McGrath, D. Barriers and solutions to online learning in medical education—An integrative review. *BMC Med. Educ.* **2018**, *18*, 130. [CrossRef] [PubMed]
16. Mojtahedzadeh, R.; Mohammadi, A.; Emami, A.H.; Rahmani, S. Comparing live lecture, internet-based & computer-based instruction: A randomized controlled trial. *Med. J. Islam Repub. Iran.* **2014**, *28*, 136.
17. Kearney, R.C.; Premaraj, S.; Smith, B.M.; Olson, G.W.; Williamson, A.E.; Romanos, G. Massive Open Online Courses in Dental Education: Two Viewpoints: Viewpoint 1: Massive Open Online Courses Offer Transformative Technology for Dental Education and Viewpoint 2: Massive Open Online Courses Are Not Ready for Primetime. *J. Dent. Educ.* **2016**, *80*, 121–127. [CrossRef] [PubMed]
18. Shintaku, W.H.; Scarbecz, M.; Venturin, J.S. Evaluation of interproximal caries using the IPad 2 and a liquid crystal display monitor. *Oral Surg. Oral Med. Oral Pathol. Oral Radiol.* **2012**, *113*, e40–e44. [CrossRef]
19. Link, T.M.; Marz, R. Computer literacy and attitudes towards e-learning among first-year medical students. *BMC Med. Educ.* **2006**, *6*, 34. [CrossRef]
20. Tan, P.L.; Hay, D.B.; Whaites, E. Implementing e-learning in a radiological science course in dental education: A short-term longitudinal study. *J. Dent. Educ.* **2009**, *73*, 1202–1212. [CrossRef]
21. Schulz, P.; Sagheb, K.; Affeldt, H.; Klumpp, H.; Taylor, K.; Walter, C.; Al-Nawas, B. Acceptance of e-learning devices by dental students. *Medicine 2.0* **2013**, *2*, e6. [CrossRef] [PubMed]
22. Lahaie, U. Web-based instruction: Getting faculty onboard. *J. Prof. Nurs.* **2007**, *23*, 335–342. [CrossRef]
23. Dhawan, S. Online learning: A panacea in the time of COVID-19 crisis. *J. Educ. Technol. Syst.* **2020**, *49*, 5–22. [CrossRef]
24. Kasman, K.; Hamdani, Z.; Lampung, U.M. The effect of Zoom App towards students' interest in learning on online learning. *DIJEMSS* **2021**, *2*, 404–408. [CrossRef]
25. Cohen, J. A coefficient of agreement for nominal scales. *Educ. Psychol. Meas.* **1960**, *20*, 37–46. [CrossRef]
26. Mukhopadhyay, S.; Kruger, E.; Tennant, M. YouTube: A new way of supplementing traditional methods in dental education. *J. Dent. Educ.* **2014**, *78*, 1568–1571. [CrossRef] [PubMed]
27. Mpungose, C.B. Lecturers' reflections on the use of Zoom video conferencing technology for E-learning at a South African university in the context of coronavirus. *Afr. Identities* **2021**, *7*, 113. [CrossRef]

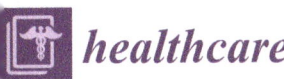

Article

Improving Humanization Skills through Simulation-Based Computers Using Simulated Nursing Video Consultations

Diana Jiménez-Rodríguez [1,*], Mercedes Pérez-Heredia [2], María del Mar Molero Jurado [3], María del Carmen Pérez-Fuentes [3,4] and Oscar Arrogante [5]

1 Department of Nursing, Physiotherapy and Medicine, University of Almería, 04120 Almeria, Spain
2 Research Management Department, Primary Care District Poniente of Almeria, Despacho: 29, 04120 Almeria, Spain; mmercedesph@yahoo.es
3 Department of Psychology, Faculty of Psychology, University of Almería, 04120 Almeria, Spain; mmj130@ual.es (M.d.M.M.J.); mpf421@ual.es (M.d.C.P.-F.)
4 Department of Psychology, Universidad Autónoma de Chile, Providencia 7500870, Chile
5 Red Cross University College of Nursing, Spanish Red Cross, Autonomous University of Madrid, Avenida Reina Victoria 28, 28003 Madrid, Spain; oscar.arrogante@cruzroja.es
* Correspondence: d.jimenez@ual.es

Citation: Jiménez-Rodríguez, D.; Pérez-Heredia, M.; Molero Jurado, M.d.M.; Pérez-Fuentes, M.d.C.; Arrogante, O. Improving Humanization Skills through Simulation-Based Computers Using Simulated Nursing Video Consultations. *Healthcare* 2022, 10, 37. https://doi.org/10.3390/healthcare10010037

Academic Editors: José João Mendes, Vanessa Machado, João Botelho and Luís Proença

Received: 2 December 2021
Accepted: 24 December 2021
Published: 26 December 2021

Publisher's Note: MDPI stays neutral with regard to jurisdictional claims in published maps and institutional affiliations.

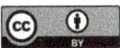

Copyright: © 2021 by the authors. Licensee MDPI, Basel, Switzerland. This article is an open access article distributed under the terms and conditions of the Creative Commons Attribution (CC BY) license (https://creativecommons.org/licenses/by/4.0/).

Abstract: During the COVID-19 confinement, we converted our clinical simulation sessions into simulated video consultations. This study aims to evaluate the effects of virtual simulation-based training on developing and cultivating humanization competencies in undergraduate nursing students. A quasi-experimental study was conducted with 60 undergraduate nursing students. A validated questionnaire was used to evaluate the acquisition of humanization competencies (self-efficacy, sociability, affection, emotional understanding, and optimism). The development of humanization competencies in this group composed of undergraduate nursing students was evaluated using virtual simulation-based training, comparing the levels obtained in these competencies at baseline (pre-test) and after the virtual simulation experience (post-test). After the virtual simulation sessions, students improved their levels in humanization total score and the emotional understanding and self-efficacy competencies, obtaining large effects sizes in all of them (rB = 0.508, rB = 0.713, and rB = 0.505 respectively). This virtual simulation modality enables training in the humanization of care with the collaboration of standardized patients in the form of simulated nursing video consultations and the performance of high-fidelity simulation sessions that comply with the requirements of best practices. Therefore, this methodology could be considered as another choice for virtual simulation. Additionally, this virtual modality could be a way to humanize virtual simulation.

Keywords: COVID-19; high fidelity simulation training; nursing education; remote consultation; telemedicine

1. Introduction

During the COVID-19 pandemic, governments around the world have declared social distancing measures to ensure the confinement of the population, including the closure of schools and universities. In this sense, this pandemic represents a challenge not only to health services but also to nursing education. In response to this exceptional situation, simulation-based education had to adapt through the use of virtual simulation modalities, thus highly increasing its use, leading to virtual simulation becoming a primary teaching strategy to provide simulated experiences [1] using online platforms, specific software or mobile devices [2,3]. Virtual simulation modalities comprise immersive simulation, screen-based simulation, serious games, virtual reality, virtual simulation/virtual patients, virtual reality simulation, and web-based simulation [4]. All these modalities provide students with near-reality, interactive virtual simulation learning experiences when face-to-face simulations are not possible [3].

To adapt our high-fidelity clinical simulation sessions to virtual simulation, we implemented simulated nursing video consultations in our university during the COVID-19 confinement [5,6]. Additionally, we considered that nursing students should practice simulated video consultations to train in this healthcare modality that has become both popular and necessary during this pandemic. In this sense, among the different telemedicine modalities, video consultations have been significantly increased [7,8], implementing them in many countries has been a digital health strategy to provide healthcare [9,10]. This modality of healthcare has multiple benefits such as avoiding agglomerations owing to social distancing restrictions, patient satisfaction, and cost reduction [11,12]. However, we were concerned about virtual interactions between nursing students and a standardized patient using virtual simulation sessions, since the distancing between them and the inability to perform an in-person consultation could lead to providing dehumanized and depersonalized nursing care training.

According to David Gaba, considered to be one of the fathers of clinical simulation, simulation is a technique not a technology [13], because simulation sessions must not be exclusively based on the use of technological equipment or devices. A simulation setting can help train students in nursing clinical skills, procedures, or techniques, and also the art of nursing generally [14]. Additionally, it can help students recognize the totality of the human being, providing patient-centered care [15]. This approach to healthcare is closely linked to the humanization of care construct [16].

Nowadays, humanization of care is a fashionable construct within healthcare services, possibly owing to society perceive they are dehumanized and depersonalized [16]. In short, humanizing healthcare means putting the human being at the center to promote and protect the health, cure diseases, or provide the best care [17]. However, there is not a consensus on the humanization of care definition to date, but most approaches to this construct offer a definition based on responding to patient's needs [16]. The humanization of care construct implies a set of personal competencies that healthcare professionals should have to care for patients effectively and humanely [18]. In this sense, Pérez-Fuentes et al. [18] have recently proposed a humanization of care model which comprises 5 competencies required in healthcare clinical practice: optimism (to generate positive future expectations), sociability (to relate to others appropriately with assertiveness and empathy), emotional understanding (to empathize cognitively with others, placing ourselves in their place), self-efficacy (to manage successfully complex and stressful situations), and affection (to empathize emotionally with the affective state of another person).

Previous studies have demonstrated the effectiveness of simulation-based training mainly in the self-efficacy [19] and empathy [20] competencies, but no research to date has studied the effects of simulation training in all competencies required to provide humanized nursing care. Specifically, this could represent a significant challenge if this training is conducted through a virtual simulation modality, owing to the virtual interaction and distancing between nursing students and virtual patients. Therefore, this study aimed to evaluate the effects of virtual simulation-based training on developing and cultivating humanization competencies in undergraduate nursing students.

2. Materials and Methods

2.1. Research Context and Setting

A quasi-experimental study was conducted using a single-group pre-test post-test design. The development of humanization competencies in this group composed of undergraduate nursing students was evaluated using virtual simulation-based training, comparing the levels obtained in these competencies at baseline (pre-test) and after the virtual simulation experience (post-test).

2.2. Setting and Sample

The study was performed in a public University between 20 April and 21 May 2020, including 3rd-year undergraduate students enrolled in nursing degree (66 students). These students performed virtual simulation sessions. A total of 60 nursing students participateD in the study (90.9% response rate).

2.3. Simulation Design Process

All simulated nursing video consultations followed the INACSL Standards of Best Practice: Simulation^{SM} [21–24]. During these simulated sessions, all stages included in high-fidelity clinical simulation were accomplished: pre-briefing, briefing, simulated scenario, and debriefing. A virtual platform of online video conferences provided by the university (Blackboard Collaborate Launcher^{TM}) was used to develop all simulation stages [5,6].

We designed six simulated scenarios related to basic healthcare at patients' homes who presented the following clinical cases: a patient diagnosed with arterial hypertension, a post-surgical patient (laparoscopic cholecystectomy), a woman with an anxiety disorder (potential case of gender-based violence), a bed-ridden patient with a pressure ulcer, a child diagnosed with attention deficit hyperactivity disorder (ADHD), and a child with a febrile syndrome.

Besides attending to each reason for consultation, adequate management and protection measures to COVID-19 were considered, since all patients were confined during this pandemic. Standardized patients played the role of patients' homes. These standardized patients were also facilitators during the simulated sessions, and they were changed during the different simulated scenarios. It should be noted a standardized patient played the role of caregiver in the clinical case of a bed-ridden patient with a pressure ulcer, and another played the role of mother when a child needed to be treated. To ensure a high-fidelity level of the simulation experience, we chose all standardized patients for their experience in clinical simulation methodology, and we trained them to play their roles according to recommendations by Lewis et al. [25].

All nursing students were divided into 4 groups of 12–16 students per group. In this sense, they formed 6 operational work teams of 2–3 students per group, performing a simulated scenario together and portraying the role of nursing professionals online. Meanwhile, the rest of the work teams were at home, observing their performance in their computer screen using the corresponding virtual platform for online video conferences. In this way, they could learn from the mistakes of their classmates who were performing a simulated scenario. Each simulated session lasted 4 h, and each student completed 3 simulation sessions (1 session of pre-briefing and 2 sessions where 6 simulated scenarios were performed), so each student completed a total of 12 h of simulation experience.

2.4. Data Collection Instrument

To evaluate the acquisition of humanization competencies, the Healthcare Professional Humanization Scale (HUMAS) [18] was used. This questionnaire consists of 19 items with a 5-point Likert response scale (from 1 = 'never' to 5 = 'always'). HUMAS comprises the 5 dimensions of humanization of care construct: self-efficacy (5 items), sociability (3 items), affection (5 items), emotional understanding (3 items), and optimism (3 items). To examine the humanization questionnaire reliability, the coefficient omega (ω) [26] was calculated. In this way, the internal consistency obtained by its creators for each dimension was satisfactory: optimism (pre-test: $\omega = 0.78$, post-test: $\omega = 0.84$), sociability (pre-test: $\omega = 0.81$, post-test: $\omega = 0.85$), emotional understanding (pre-test: $\omega = 0.74$, post-test: $\omega = 0.74$), self-efficacy (pre-test: $\omega = 0.79$, post-test: $\omega = 0.78$), affection (pre-test: $\omega = 0.88$, post-test: $\omega = 0.90$), and total score (pre-test: $\omega = 0.88$, post-test: $\omega = 0.88$). It should be noted, some items were minimally adapted since the participants were students, and not healthcare professionals (e.g., 'I feel nervous when I am caring for my patients' was changed by 'I feel nervous when I think about caring for patients during my clinical practices.' The humanization questionnaire was completed online pre- and post-virtual simulation sessions, through a link provided to the participating students.

2.5. Statistical Analysis

Descriptive statistics were calculated (minimal, maximal and mean scores, standard deviation, and percentages) to analyze the results obtained for demographic data and each item, subscale, and the total score obtained in HUMAS. Additionally, the coefficients omega (ω) were calculated to analyze the reliability of this questionnaire. Subsequently, the assumption of normality was tested using the Kolmogorov–Smirnov test, confirming that data did not follow a normal probability distribution. Consequently, to analyze the differences at baseline (pre-test) and after the virtual simulation experience (post-test), the Wilcoxon test was used. Additionally, to determine the effect size of the statistically significant differences obtained, the rank-biserial correlation (rB) was calculated, considering the following cut-off points: 0.10 (small), 0.30 (medium), and 0.50 (large) [27]. These data were analyzed using IBM SPSS Statistics version 24.0 software for Windows (IBM Corp., Armonk, NY, USA).

2.6. Ethical Considerations

This study was carried out following ethical principles for medical research of the international Declaration of Helsinki [28]. Additionally, this study was approved by the Research and Ethics Board of the Department of Nursing, Physiotherapy, and Medicine of A. University (Approval no. EFM-75/2020). All nursing students were informed about the study and who accepted to participate voluntarily, signed a written consent.

3. Results

A total of 60 nursing students participated in the study. The age of students ranged from 20 to 50 years (mean = 23.83; SD = 6.63). Most students were women (n = 52; 86.7%).

Descriptive data and reliabilities for each item, subscale, and the total score obtained in HUMAS at baseline (pre-test) and after virtual simulation sessions (post-test) are shown in Table 1. It should be noted that the reliability coefficients calculated for each subscale and the total score in HUMAS were quite similar to values obtained by its creators, indicating satisfactory reliability.

Table 1. Descriptive data (minimal, maximal and mean scores, and standard deviation) and reliabilities for each item, subscale and the total score obtained in HUMAS at baseline (pre-test) and after virtual simulation sessions (post-test) (N = 60).

Items and Subscales of HUMAS	Pre-Test					Post-Test				
	Min [1]	Max [2]	M [3]	SD [4]	ω	Min [1]	Max [2]	M [3]	SD [4]	ω
Subscale 1—Optimism	4.00	15.00	11.28	2.17	0.81	6.00	15.00	11.66	2.32	0.87
1. I await the future enthusiastically.	2.00	5.00	4.13	0.87		2.00	5.00	4.23	0.90	
2. In general, I am satisfied with myself.	1.00	5.00	3.61	0.90		2.00	5.00	3.75	0.85	
3. When faced with problems, I trust that everything will come out all right in the end.	1.00	5.00	3.53	0.79		2.00	5.00	3.68	0.85	
Subscale 2—Sociability	10.00	15.00	14.40	1.15	0.79	11.00	15.00	14.50	1.03	0.87
4. In the future, when I care for patients, I will try to put myself in their place.	3.00	5.00	4.70	0.53		3.00	5.00	4.78	0.45	
5. When I start my professional career, I will give the patients or their families close, personal attention, if they need it.	3.00	5.00	4.85	0.40		4.00	5.00	4.86	0.34	
6. I will try to calm down patients and families, as I consider it an important part of caregiving.	3.00	5.00	4.85	0.44		4.00	5.00	4.85	0.36	
Subscale 3—Emotional understanding	6.00	15.00	10.50	2.07	0.77	6.00	15.00	11.23	2.09	0.70
7. When someone disrespects me, I try to understand their reasons and continue to treat that person respectfully.	2.00	5.00	3.71	0.78		1.00	5.00	3.93	0.86	
8. When I don't like someone, I try to understand them and give them a chance for me to get to know them.	2.00	5.00	3.55	0.89		2.00	5.00	3.70	0.83	
9. When someone goes against me, I tend to analyze the situation to try and justify their behavior rationally.	1.00	5.00	3.23	0.89		1.00	5.00	3.60	0.96	
Subscale 4—Self-efficacy	5.00	24.00	17.75	2.97	0.81	11.00	25.00	19.13	2.57	0.79
10. I am able to differentiate the changes in mood in others and try to act consequently.	1.00	5.00	3.48	0.72		1.00	5.00	3.78	0.76	
11. I am satisfied with what I do and how I do it in my clinical practices.	1.00	5.00	3.80	0.75		2.00	5.00	4.01	0.59	
12. I am able to differentiate my own moods and act consequently.	1.00	5.00	3.71	0.86		1.00	5.00	3.88	0.73	
13. I think I will be prepared to cope successfully with any situation in my clinical practices.	1.00	5.00	3.15	0.79		2.00	5.00	3.53	0.72	

[1] Min.: minimal score; [2] Max.: maximal score; [3] M: mean score; [4] SD: standard deviation.

Table 1. Cont.

Items and Subscales of HUMAS	Pre-Test					Post-Test				
	Min [1]	Max [2]	M [3]	SD [4]	ω	Min [1]	Max [2]	M [3]	SD [4]	ω
14. I feel that I will have a great capacity for perceiving when a patient is nor receiving adequate care.	1.00	5.00	3.60	0.80		1.00	5.00	3.91	0.67	
Subscale 5—Affection	5.00	25.00	13.10	3.48	0.86	5.00	25.00	12.81	4.18	0.89
15. When I am performing my clinical practices or I plan perform in my future career, I usually feel anxiety.	1.00	5.00	3.33	0.79		1.00	5.00	3.31	0.93	
16. I feel nervous when I think about caring for patients during my clinical practices.	1.00	5.00	2.85	0.98		1.00	5.00	3.21	0.97	
17. When in my clinical practices I perform or I think about performing clinical activities related to my future career, sometimes I feel afraid.	1.00	5.00	3.06	0.80		1.00	5.00	3.18	0.91	
18. When in my clinical practices I perform or I think about performing clinical activities related to my future career, there are situations in which I feel guilty.	1.00	5.00	3.98	0.81		1.00	5.00	3.83	1.07	
19. I feel affected when I am performing my clinical practices or I think about caring patients,	1.00	5.00	3.66	0.89		1.00	5.00	3.63	1.08	
Total score	36.00	89.00	70.83	8.66	0.89	53.00	95.00	73.71	8.07	0.86

[1] Min.: minimal score; [2] Max.: maximal score; [3] M: mean score; [4] SD: standard deviation.

The mean scores obtained in each humanization dimension at baseline (pre-test) and after virtual simulation sessions (post-test) were compared (Table 2). Statistically significant differences were obtained in emotional understanding and self-efficacy dimensions, as well as in total score for the humanization scale applied, obtaining large effects sizes in all of them (rB = 0.505, rB = 0.713, and rB = 0.508 respectively).

Table 2. Differences in mean scores for each humanization dimension and the total score obtained in HUMAS at baseline (pre-test) and after virtual simulation sessions (post-test) (N = 60).

Humanization Dimensions	z	p
Optimism	−1.68	0.091
Sociability	−0.61	0.540
Emotional understanding	−3.16 [1]	0.002
Self-efficacy	1.39 [2]	0.000
Affection	−0.98	0.324
Total score	−3.28 [1]	0.001

[1] $p < 0.01$; [2] $p < 0.001$.

Figure 1 shows graphically the magnitude of the statistically significant differences in emotional understanding and self-efficacy dimensions, and the total score obtained in HUMAS at baseline (pre-test) and after virtual simulation sessions (post-test). It should be noted that the rest of the humanization dimensions are not shown in this figure since only non-statistically significant differences were obtained.

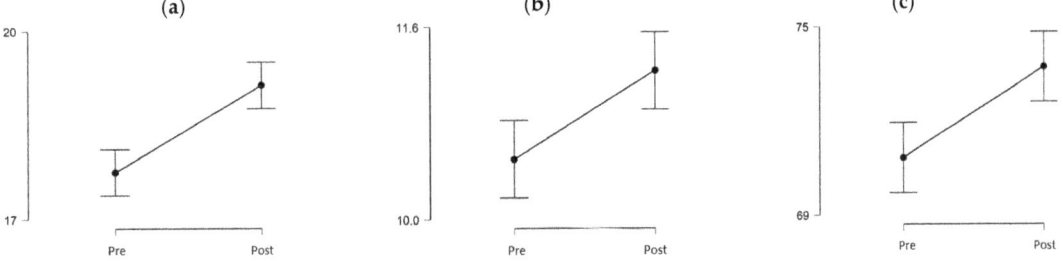

Figure 1. Statistically significant differences in self-efficacy and emotional understanding dimensions, and the total score obtained in HUMAS at baseline (pre-test) and after virtual simulation sessions (post-test). (a) Self-efficaccy, (b) Emotional understanding, (c) Total score.

4. Discussion

We converted our face-to-face simulated scenarios into a virtual format using simulated nursing video consultations in response to the closure of universities during the confinement due to the COVID-19 pandemic. We performed high-fidelity simulation sessions that complied with the requirements proposed by the INACSL Standards of Best Practice. In previous studies, nursing students expressed high satisfaction with this virtual simulation modality [5,6], perceiving that it was positively improving their learning process. However, we considered studying whether our conversion could lead nursing students to provide dehumanized and depersonalized nursing care, since virtual interactions are not the same as simulation sessions in a laboratory room.

Our results indicate the positive effects of virtual simulation-based training on developing and cultivating humanization competencies in undergraduate nursing students. After virtual simulation sessions, they improved their levels in humanization total score and the emotional understanding and self-efficacy competencies. It should be noted that emotional understanding is closely related to empathy [18]. Although there is a lack of studies analyzing the effects on the humanization of care of using clinical simulation methodology, improvements to empathy and self-efficacy in nursing students have been widely demonstrated [19,20,29].

Firstly, empathy is considered as the heart of all nurse-patient interactions [30], being a basic component of therapeutic relationships and a crucial factor in quality care [31]. Additionally, the positive impact of empathic healthcare interactions on patient outcomes has been widely demonstrated [31,32]. Numerous studies have demonstrated improvement to empathy levels using clinical simulation methodology [20]. Particularly, single-group studies have demonstrated a significant change in empathy between pre-test and post-test using standardized patients. However, the obtained effect sizes have been often low [30,33]. Notably, Strekalova et al. [34] used a virtual patient during simulated health history interviews and obtained empathic responses from nursing students. In our study, we obtained increases in empathy levels and a large effect size in this humanization competency using standardized patients during virtual simulation sessions.

Regarding self-efficacy, this competency consists of a future-oriented optimistic belief that increases motivation, equating to improved performance [35]. Self-efficacy is considered as a healthcare professional's skill in successfully managing complex and stressful situations [36]. In this sense, there is ample evidence in the literature to suggest simulation is effective at increasing this competency [19]. Specifically, single-group pre-test and post-test design studies have reported increases in self-efficacy after simulation sessions using standardized patients [37–39]. However, the effect sizes of simulation in self-efficacy reported by these studies are inconsistent and range from low to large. In contrast, we reported a large effect size in this humanization competence using not only standardized patients but also virtual simulation sessions.

Logically, simulated nursing video consultations mainly promote the development of non-technical skills (mainly communication skills, active listening, presence, empathy, and teamwork) [5,6]. In this sense, humanization of care and its related competencies could be included in these skills required to provide quality nursing care and decrease burnout [40]. However, while face-to-face simulation sessions usually improve technical skill performance [19,37,39], more studies are needed to analyze non-technical skill performance using virtual simulation modalities [41].

Lastly, although simulated nursing video consultations are not included among virtual simulation modalities in the evidence [3,4], this methodology could be considered as another choice for virtual simulation, according to their high level of fidelity in compliance with the requirements proposed by the INACSL Standards of Best Practice and the high satisfaction and positive perception expressed by nursing students in previous studies [5,6]. However, Cant et al. [3] consider clarification of the nomenclature of virtual simulation to be needed in terms of fidelity, since interactions between learners and virtual patients are different from face-to-face simulation experiences. Additionally, its use could be extended to other contexts, not only in the confinement due to the COVID-19 pandemic.

The main limitation of our study is related to the specific disadvantage of both simulated and real-life nursing video consultations: technical issues. Ensuring adequate network access and the correct functioning of virtual platforms could mitigate these potential problems [9,12]. Regarding methodological limitations, although our sample size was small, the response rate was high. Additionally, while our study did not analyze either self-efficacy or empathy using the specific validated scales, a validated scale that comprised both humanization competencies was utilized [18]. In this sense, the use of validated scales for evaluating these competencies is not consistent in the majority of the studies [19,20]. Finally, the positive effects of virtual simulation-based training on developing and cultivating humanization competencies should be confirmed by future research, so more studies are needed. These future studies should extend the sample recruited and compare it with a control group, using quasi-experimental or experimental designs and evaluating the outcomes obtained in follow-up periods (for instance, 3, 6 and/or 12 months later). Additionally, future research should also assess the acquisition of humanization of care competencies by nursing students or registered nurses using this virtual simulation modality and extend it to other settings and education centers.

5. Conclusions

This methodology allows nurses to be trained in the humanization of care using a virtual simulation format, in the form of simulated nursing video consultations by performing high-fidelity simulation sessions that comply with the requirements proposed by the INACSL Standards of Best Practice. Therefore, this methodology could be considered as another choice for virtual simulation. Additionally, this virtual modality allows the collaboration of standardized patients and, consequently, could be a way to humanize virtual simulation. Our results could be confirmed by future research projects using quasi-experimental or experimental designs and follow-up periods, recruiting more nursing students, including registered nurses, and extending this virtual simulation modality to other settings and education centers.

Author Contributions: Conceptualization, D.J.-R., M.d.M.M.J., M.d.C.P.-F. and O.A.; methodology, D.J.-R., M.d.M.M.J., M.d.C.P.-F. and O.A.; formal analysis, D.J.-R., M.d.M.M.J., M.d.C.P.-F. and O.A.; investigation, D.J.-R. and O.A.; data curation, D.J.-R., M.d.M.M.J., M.d.C.P.-F. and O.A.; writing—original draft preparation, D.J.-R., M.d.M.M.J., M.d.C.P.-F., M.P.-H. and O.A.; writing—review and editing, D.J.-R., M.P.-H. and O.A.; supervision, D.J.-R. and O.A.; project administration, D.J.-R., M.P.-H. and O.A. All authors have read and agreed to the published version of the manuscript.

Funding: This research received no external funding.

Institutional Review Board Statement: The study was conducted according to the guidelines of the Declaration of Helsinki and approved by the Research and Ethics Board of the Department of Nursing, Physiotherapy, and Medicine of the A. University (Approval no. EFM-75/2020).

Informed Consent Statement: Informed consent was obtained from all subjects involved in the study.

Data Availability Statement: The data presented in this study are available on request from the corresponding author.

Conflicts of Interest: The authors declare no conflict of interest.

References

1. Harder, N. Simulation amid the COVID-19 pandemic. *Clin. Simul. Nurs.* **2020**, *43*, 1–2. [CrossRef] [PubMed]
2. Bogossian, F.; Cooper, S.; Kelly, M.; Levett-Jones, T.; McKenna, L.; Slark, J.; Seaton, P. Best practice in clinical simulation education—Are we there yet? A cross-sectional survey of simulation in Australian and New Zealand pre-registration nursing education. *Clin. Simul. Nurs.* **2018**, *25*, 327–334. [CrossRef]
3. Cant, R.; Cooper, S.; Sussex, R.; Bogossian, F. What's in a name? Clarifying the nomenclature of virtual simulation. *Clin. Simul. Nurs.* **2017**, *27*, 26–30. [CrossRef]

4. Lioce, L.; Lopreiato, J.; Downing, D.; Chang, T.P.; Robertson, J.M.; Anderson, M.; Diaz, D.A.; Spain, A.E.; Terminology and Concepts Working Group. *Healthcare Simulation Dictionary*, 2nd ed.; Lioce, L., Lopreiato, J., Downing, D., Chang, T.P., Robertson, J.M., Anderson, M., Diaz, D.A., Spain, A.E., Eds.; Agency for Healthcare Research and Quality: Rockville, MD, USA, 2020. [CrossRef]
5. Jiménez-Rodríguez, D.; Arrogante, O. Simulated video consultations as a learning tool in undergraduate nursing: Students' perceptions. *Healthcare* **2020**, *8*, 280. [CrossRef] [PubMed]
6. Jiménez-Rodríguez, D.; Torres Navarro, M.D.M.; Plaza Del Pino, F.J.; Arrogante, O. Simulated nursing video consultations: An innovative proposal during COVID-19 confinement. *Clin. Simul. Nurs.* **2020**, *48*, 29–37. [CrossRef]
7. Contreras, C.M.; Metzger, G.A.; Beane, J.D.; Dedhia, P.H.; Ejaz, A.; Pawlik, T.M. Telemedicine: Patient-provider clinical engagement during the COVID-19 pandemic and beyond. *J. Gastrointes. Surg.* **2020**, *24*, 1692–1697. [CrossRef] [PubMed]
8. Hong, Y.R.; Lawrence, J.; Williams, D., Jr.; Mainous, A., III. Population-level interest and telehealth capacity of us hospitals in response to COVID-19: Cross-sectional analysis of google search and national hospital survey data. *JMIR Public Health Surveill.* **2020**, *6*, e18961. [CrossRef]
9. Greenhalgh, T.; Wherton, J.; Shaw, S.; Morrison, C. Video consultations for COVID-19. *BMJ* **2020**, *368*, m998. [CrossRef]
10. Ohannessian, R.; Duong, T.A.; Odone, A. Global telemedicine implementation and integration within health systems to fight the COVID-19 pandemic: A Call to Action. *JMIR Public Health Surveill.* **2020**, *6*, e18810. [CrossRef]
11. de la Torre-Diez, I.; López-Coronado, M.; Vaca, C.; Sáez Aguado, J.; de Castro, C. Cost-utility and cost-effectiveness studies of telemedicine, electronic, and mobile health systems in the literature: A systematic review. *Telemed. J. E Health* **2015**, *21*, 81–85. [CrossRef]
12. Ignatowicz, A.; Atherton, H.; Bernstein, C.J.; Bryce, C.; Court, R.; Sturt, J.; Griffiths, F. Internet videoconferencing for patient-clinician consultations in long-term conditions: A review of reviews and applications in line with guidelines and recommendations. *Digit. Health* **2019**, *5*, 2055207619845831. [CrossRef]
13. Gaba, D.M. The future vision of simulation in health care. *Qual. Saf. Health Care* **2004**, *13*, i2–i10. [CrossRef] [PubMed]
14. Tarnow, K.G. Humanizing the learning laboratory. *J. Nurs. Educ.* **2005**, *44*, 43–44. [CrossRef]
15. Cohen, B.S.; Boni, R. Holistic nursing simulation: A concept analysis. *J. Holist. Nurs.* **2018**, *36*, 68–78. [CrossRef] [PubMed]
16. Busch, I.M.; Moretti, F.; Travaini, G.; Wu, A.W.; Rimondini, M. Humanization of care: Key elements identified by patients, caregivers, and healthcare providers. A systematic review. *Patient* **2019**, *12*, 461–474. [CrossRef] [PubMed]
17. Heras, G.; Oviés, Á.A.; Gómez, V. A plan for improving the humanisation of intensive care units. *Intensive Care Med.* **2017**, *43*, 547–549. [CrossRef] [PubMed]
18. Pérez-Fuentes, M.C.; Herrera-Peco, I.; Molero, M.M.; Oropesa, N.F.; Ayuso-Murillo, D.; Gázquez, J.J. The development and validation of the healthcare professional humanization scale (HUMAS) for nursing. *Int. J. Environ. Res. Public Health* **2019**, *16*, 3999. [CrossRef]
19. Cant, R.P.; Cooper, S.J. Use of simulation-based learning in undergraduate nurse education: An umbrella systematic review. *Nurse Educ. Today* **2017**, *49*, 63–71. [CrossRef]
20. Levett-Jones, T.; Cant, R.; Lapkin, S. A systematic review of the effectiveness of empathy education for undergraduate nursing students. *Nurse Educ. Today* **2019**, *75*, 80–94. [CrossRef]
21. INACSL Standards Committee. INACSL standards of best practice: Simulation^{SM} Simulation design. *Clin. Simul. Nurs.* **2016**, *12*, 5–12. [CrossRef]
22. INACSL Standards Committee. INACSL standards of best practice: Simulation^{SM} Facilitation. *Clin. Simul. Nurs.* **2016**, *12*, 16–20. [CrossRef]
23. INACSL Standards Committee. INACSL standards of best practice: Simulation^{SM} Simulation glossary. *Clin. Simul. Nurs.* **2016**, *12*, 39–47. [CrossRef]
24. INACSL Standards Committee. INACSL standards of best practice: Simulation^{SM} Debriefing. *Clin. Simul. Nurs.* **2016**, *12*, 21–25. [CrossRef]
25. Lewis, K.L.; Bohnert, C.A.; Gammon, W.L.; Hölzer, H.; Lyman, L.; Smith, C.; Thompson, T.M.; Wallace, A.; Gliva-McConvey, G. The Association of Standardized Patient Educators (ASPE) Standards of Best Practice (SOBP). *Adv. Simul.* **2017**, *2*, 1–8. [CrossRef]
26. McDonald, R.P. *Test Theory: A Unified Approach*; Lawrence Erlbaum Associates: Mahwah, NJ, USA, 1999.
27. Coolican, H. *Research Methods and Statistics in Psychology*, 5th ed.; Hodder Education Group: London, UK, 2009.
28. World Medical Association. World Medical Association Declaration of Helsinki: Ethical Principles for Medical Research Involving Human Subjects. *JAMA* **2013**, *310*, 2191–2194. [CrossRef]
29. Li, J.; Li, X.; Gu, L.; Zhang, R.; Zhao, R.; Cai, Q.; Lu, Y.; Wang, H.; Meng, Q.; Wei, H. Effects of simulation-based deliberate practice on nursing students' communication, empathy, and self-efficacy. *J. Nurs. Educ.* **2019**, *58*, 681–689. [CrossRef] [PubMed]
30. Ward, J. The empathy enigma: Does it still exist? Comparison of empathy using students and standardized actors. *Nurse Educ.* **2016**, *41*, 134–138. [CrossRef]
31. Hojat, M.; Louis, D.Z.; Maio, V.; Gonnella, J.S. Empathy and health care quality. *Am. J. Med. Qual.* **2013**, *28*, 6–7. [CrossRef]
32. Trzeciak, S.; Roberts, B.W.; Mazzarelli, A.J. Compassionomics: Hypothesis and experimental approach. *Med. Hypotheses* **2017**, *107*, 92–97. [CrossRef]
33. Bas-Sarmiento, P.; Fernández-Gutiérrez, M.; Baena-Baños, M.; Romero-Sánchez, J.M. Efficacy of empathy training in nursing students: A quasi-experimental study. *Nurse Educ. Today* **2017**, *59*, 59–65. [CrossRef]

34. Strekalova, Y.A.; Krieger, J.L.; Kleinheksel, A.J.; Kotranza, A. Empathic communication in virtual education for nursing students: I'm sorry to hear that. *Nurse Educ.* **2017**, *42*, 18–22. [CrossRef]
35. Bandura, A. *Self-Efficacy: The Exercise of Control*; W.H. Freeman and Company: New York, NY, USA, 1997.
36. Orgambídez, A.; Borrego, Y.; Vázquez-Aguado, O. Self-efficacy and organizational commitment among Spanish nurses: The role of work engagement. *Int. Nurs. Rev.* **2019**, *66*, 381–388. [CrossRef] [PubMed]
37. Foronda, C.; Liu, S.; Bauman, E.B. Evaluation of simulation in undergraduate nurse education: An integrative review. *Clin. Simul. Nurs.* **2013**, *9*, e409–e416. [CrossRef]
38. Franklin, A.E.; Lee, C.S. Effectiveness of simulation for improvement in self-efficacy among novice nurses: A meta-analysis. *J. Nurs. Educ.* **2014**, *53*, 607–614. [CrossRef] [PubMed]
39. Oh, P.J.; Jeon, K.D.; Koh, M.S. The effects of simulation-based learning using standardized patients in nursing students: A meta-analysis. *Nurse Educ. Today* **2015**, *35*, e6–e15. [CrossRef]
40. Pérez-Fuentes, M.C.; Molero, M.M.; Gázquez, J.J.; Simón, M.M. Analysis of Burnout Predictors in Nursing: Risk and Protective Psychological Factors. *Eur. J. Psychol. Appl. Leg. Context* **2019**, *11*, 33–40. [CrossRef]
41. Bracq, M.S.; Michinov, E.; Jannin, P. Virtual Reality Simulation in Nontechnical Skills Training for Healthcare Professionals: A Systematic Review. *Simul. Healthc.* **2019**, *14*, 188–194. [CrossRef]

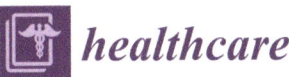

Article

Development of an Online Asynchronous Clinical Learning Resource ("Ask the Expert") in Dental Education to Promote Personalized Learning

Rohit Kunnath Menon [1,*] and Liang Lin Seow [2]

1 Restorative Dentistry, School of Dentistry, International Medical University, Kuala Lumpur 57000, Malaysia
2 Division Clinical Dentistry, School of Dentistry, International Medical University, Kuala Lumpur 57000, Malaysia; lianglin_seow@imu.edu.my
* Correspondence: rohitkunnath@imu.edu.my

Abstract: This article describes the development and testing of an online asynchronous clinical learning resource named "Ask the Expert" to enhance clinical learning in dentistry. After the resource development, dental students from years 3 and 4 were randomly allocated to two groups (Group A—"Ask the Expert" and L—"lecturer-led"). All the students attempted a pre-test related to replacement of teeth in the anterior aesthetic zone. Group A (33 students) underwent an online case-based learning session of 60 minutes' duration without a facilitator, while Group L (27 students) concurrently underwent a case-based learning session of 60 minutes' duration with a lecturer facilitating the session. An immediate post-test was conducted followed by a retention test after one week. Student feedback was obtained. There was a significant increase in the test scores (maximum score 10) for both groups when comparing the pre-test (Group A—5.61 ± 1.34, Group L—5.22 ± 1.57) and immediate post-test scores (Group A—7.42 ± 1.34, Group L—8.04 ± 1.22; paired t-test, $p < 0.001$). However, no significant difference was observed in the test scores when comparing Group A to Group L for both the immediate post-test as well as the retention test (Group A—5.36 ± 1.29, Group L—5.33 ± 1.39 (independent sample t-test, $p > 0.05$). To conclude, adequately structured online asynchronous learning resources are comparable in their effectiveness to online synchronous learning in the undergraduate dental curriculum.

Keywords: e-learning; online learning; dentistry; dental education

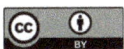

1. Introduction

Learning from clinical cases or case-based learning provides an opportunity for students to demonstrate application of knowledge, thus augmenting the relevance of their learning [1]. Case-based learning promotes inherent motivation to learn, encourages self-directed learning and enhances clinical decision making abilities by repeated experiences [2,3], leading to a profounder understanding and reflection [4]. However, clinical case discussions are usually conducted between a clinical supervisor or lecturer and a group of students in a clinical setting. Clinical learning from clinical cases may also occur during case-based learning sessions conducted by a lecturer for a cohort. In view of the current pandemic, these sessions are routinely being conducted as online synchronous sessions between a lecturer and a group of students. These discussions are usually isolated bundles of learning between a faculty and a group of students. This approach provides restricted opportunity for feedback from other faculty who are not involved in the primary discussion and also precludes the participation from students who are undergoing clinical learning in other cohorts.

Harden and Hart have explained the benefits of e-learning in removing constraints for learning and expanding possibilities [5]. Computer-assisted learning (CAL) provides flexibility for students and teachers by enabling students to choose the time for learning and freeing the time for teachers to focus on topics needing more close supervision [6]. Enhanced accessibility, diminished costs and effective time management have been cited as significant advantages that e-learning may offer as compared to other modes of learning [7,8]. Educational benefits of e-learning have been previously demonstrated in multiple areas including knowledge acquisition, assessment, development of professionalism and also acquisition of physical skills [9–12]. The concept of developing a "reusable learning package" [13,14] is advantageous in clinical learning, since it provides collaborative learning (learning across semesters/years and disciplines) available anytime and anywhere.

In addition to the development of new e-learning resource to enhance learning, evaluation and comparison of these resource to conventional/traditional methods of learning is equally important. In dentistry, e-learning has been previously found to be equally [6,15–17] or more effective [18–20] than traditional methods. However, some studies have significant limitations with respect to the method of assessment employed [18], and none of the aforementioned studies have investigated the impact of clinical case-based learning in dentistry on the knowledge acquisition and retention among dental students by employing methodology with minimal bias, thus ensuring reproducibility.

This study describes the development and evaluation of an asynchronous online clinical learning resource and the subsequent evaluation of its effectiveness by a randomized study. This study aimed to compare the knowledge acquisition and retention amongst dental students who utilized the online asynchronous clinical learning resource to those who underwent a lecturer-led learning session with the same content.

2. Materials and Methods

Development of the Online Asynchronous Learning Resource: "Ask the Expert"

We developed an online clinical learning resource named "Ask the Expert". The portal contains video-recorded clinical case discussions between a clinical supervisor/lecturer and a student. Students are encouraged to contribute clinical cases of interest in a previously provided case template. The case template is a PowerPoint presentation where the areas to enter the relevant patient details and the required photographs and radiographs are indicated. This is provided to ensure a relatively standardized format for case presentations in the learning resource (Supplementary Material Figure S1). The student is required to prepare the case as per the template and store it in a mobile device. Each clinical case is discussed with a clinical supervisor/lecturer using the student's mobile device (with screen recording) with two additional cameras capturing the discussion (Figure 1a). One camera focuses on the conversation between the student and the lecturer, whereas the other camera focuses on any study models used during the discussion. The discussion between the student and the lecturer is enhanced with the capability to draw on the clinical images and radiographs shown in the student's mobile device. Upon completion of discussion, the editing team combines the data from the two cameras and the student's recording on the mobile device to create an interactive video-based learning resource (Figure 1b). Self-assessment components are incorporated into each clinical case in the form of single best answer questions (Figure 1c). At the end of each recorded session, the student is asked to reflect briefly on the discussion with the expert with respect to what they learned. This is included at the end of each video. Further, a forum is created for each case, which is accessible to other students and internal experts for review and discussion. Students and faculty are able to access this anywhere and anytime by scanning a QR code.

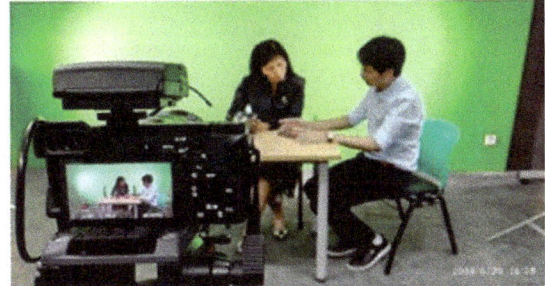
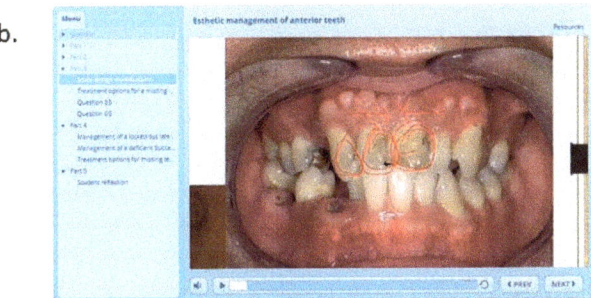
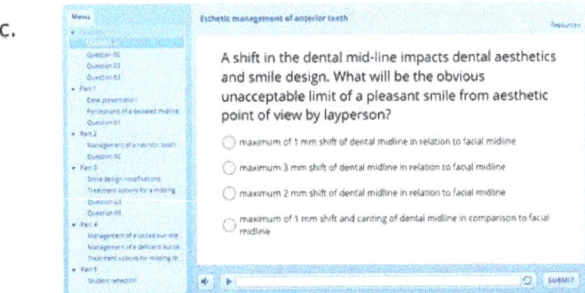

Figure 1. (a) Video recording of the case discussion; (b) interactive video-based learning resource; (c) self-assessment.

At the preliminary phase, the videos are shared with a group of 20 students to acquire preliminary feedback. The videos are re-edited as per student feedback into shorter segments of 1–5 min each. Self-assessment questions are provided in the initial segment before the clinical case discussion commences for each case. When answered incorrectly, students are directed to the section of the video where the correct answer is discussed. The learning resource is a learning bank for clinical cases covering a variety of cases in restorative dentistry. Each case has different learning outcomes, and the self-assessment questions are created from the recorded discussion and then incorporated into the resource.

To evaluate the educational impact of this learning resource, students in years 3 and 4 at the School of Dentistry at the International Medical University, Kuala Lumpur, Malaysia, were invited to participate in the study. The primary outcome of the study was to identify any difference in test scores between the two modes of learning. Ethical approval for the study was obtained from the Joint Committee on Research and Ethics at the International Medical University (Project ID: IMU 480/220). A study information sheet was provided to the students, and the students were given a period of one week to carefully study the information sheet. Students who participated in the creation of the online content were excluded from the study.

The topic covered for the clinical learning session was "Aesthetic restorative dentistry" and, specifically, restoration/replacement of teeth in the anterior aesthetic zone. The learning levels of both the year 3 and year 4 students were assumed to be similar for this topic.

Step 1: Pre-Test

A pre-test comprised of 10 one best answers (OBAs) of one mark each (based on the learning outcomes) were answered by the students who gave written informed consent to participate in the study.

Step 2: Randomization

Subsequently, the students were randomized into two groups, namely Group A (Ask the Expert group) and Group L (Lecturer-led group), by a simple cluster randomization technique. The allocation ratio was 50:50; however, only students who were interested in participating were asked to enroll. The random sequence was computer generated from a random number table. Hence, there was a difference in the number of groups. Consent to participate is an important consideration, especially in education research where students are vulnerable, which was maintained in this context. The learning outcomes and content for the topic were kept standard for both groups to eliminate bias.

Step 3: Intervention

Both the groups underwent the test concurrently during a commonly scheduled time.

Group "Ask the Expert" (A; Online asynchronous learning)—30 students

Students in this group were able to access the online asynchronous learning resource "Ask the Expert" by using a login ID and password, which were provided for each student in the group for 60 min. The resource was uploaded with three clinical cases for the test. The students used the source independently and were not facilitated by a lecturer.

Group "Lecturer" (L; Lecturer-led learning)—27 students

An online synchronous session over Microsoft TEAMs was conducted by a single lecturer with the same clinical cases and content as for Group A for 60 min. The lecturer shared the cases as static PowerPoint slides with the group. After the case was presented, the lecturer instructed the students to answer questions in an OBA format for self-assessment (same as those included in the self-assessment for Group A). This was followed by a discussion between the students and the lecturer regarding the clinical case. The lecturer maintained the discussion similar to the content in Group A, ensuring that the content delivery was standardized. The session was recorded.

Both the online asynchronous session for Group A and the online synchronous session for Group L were conducted concurrently.

Step 4: Immediate post-test

Upon completion of the sessions, an online test was conducted for both groups concurrently, where 10 OBAs were to be answered in 20 min. This was the immediate knowledge acquisition test. The questions used in the immediate knowledge acquisition test were the same as in the pre-test.

Step 5: Retention Test

Both groups were provided with additional reading material including journal articles related to the topic covered. One week after the immediate test, a retention test was conducted for both groups (10 OBAs in 20 min). The questions in the retention test were new questions that included content discussed in the earlier session and information from the shared reading material. However, the newly prepared questions were aligned with the learning outcomes. The primary outcome of the study was to identify any difference in test scores between the two modes of learning.

After the completion of the retention test, all the students were provided access to the asynchronous clinical learning resource "Ask the Expert" and the recorded synchronous sessions to ensure fairness.

Step 6: Student feedback and evaluation of the "Ask the Expert" resource

Student feedback was obtained using a previously validated questionnaire [16]. Various Likert scales were used to test the students' beliefs about acceptability (Q1), effectiveness (Q2–5) and learning preferences (Q6–7). A section was provided for open comments.

3. Results

The average time taken for the development of a clinical case as a learning resource was calculated to be 180 min. The time calculated included the contribution by the student, the lecturer and the personnel involved in editing and uploading the content (Supplementary Material, Figure S2).

The mean and standard deviation of the scores in the pre-test, immediate post-test and the retention test obtained by the students with the pertinent analysis are depicted in Table 1.

Table 1. Test scores from the pre-test, immediate post-test and retention test.

Test	Group	Mean	Standard Deviation	p Value, t test
Pre-Test	A	5.61	1.34	0.406
	L	5.22	1.57	
Immediate Post-Test	A	7.42	1.34	0.395
	L	8.04	1.22	
Retention Test	A	5.36	1.29	0.788
	L	5.33	1.39	

The distribution of the scores for both groups are provided in Supplementary Material, Figures S3 and S4.

There was no significant difference in the test scores at baseline (pre-test) between the two groups (Group A—5.61 ± 1.34, Group L—5.22 ± 1.57; independent sample t-test, $p = 0.406$). There was a significant increase in the test scores for both groups when comparing the pre-test and immediate post-test scores (Group A—7.42 ± 1.34, Group L—8.04 ± 1.22; paired t-test, $p < 0.001$). No significant difference was observed in the test scores when comparing Group, A to Group L for the immediate post-test scores (independent sample t-test, $p = 0.395$).

We did not find a significant difference when comparing the pre-test scores to the scores of the retention test (Group A—5.36 ± 1.29, Group L—5.33 ± 1.39; paired t-test, $p > 0.05$). No significant difference was observed in the test scores when comparing Group A to Group L for the scores in the retention test (independent sample t-test, $p = 0.788$). The distribution of the scores for both groups for the pre-test and immediate post-test are depicted in (Supplementary Material Figures S1 and S2).

The questions used for all the tests are provided as Supplementary Material, Figure S5.

Student feedback was obtained in the domains of acceptability of the learning resource, and its effectiveness and the learning preferences of the students are depicted in Table 2. A total of 52% of the students (30/57) responded to the questionnaire. All the respondents found the method to be acceptable; 93% of the respondents rated the resource as good/very good, and 87% of the respondents indicated that the resource stimulated them to explore the topic further. A total of 60% of the respondents found the method to be time-efficient, 30% were neutral in relation to this question and 10% did not find the resource to be time-efficient.

Table 2. Student feedback.

Domain	Question	Possible Responses	No. of Respondents/Student Response
Acceptability	Was the method acceptable to you?	Yes No	30, 100% 0
Effectiveness	How would you rate this method?	Very Good Good Neither Bad Very Bad	7, 23% 21, 70% 2, 7% 0 0
	The method was time-efficient?	Strongly Agree Agree Neutral Disagree Strongly Disagree	3, 10% 15, 50% 9, 30% 3, 10% 0
	The method stimulate you to look up the topic further	Strongly Agree Agree Neutral Disagree Strongly Disagree	3, 10% 23, 77% 4, 13% 0 0
	Would you recommend this method?	Yes No Maybe	19, 63% 0 11, 37%
Learning preferences	Which method do you usually use to learn?	Books Journals E-learning Internet Others	18, 60% 4, 13% 1, 3.5% 6, 20% 1, 3.5%
	Which method do you prefer the most?	Lecture Seminar E-learning Private study Other	21, 70% 0 1, 3% 5, 17% 3, 10%
Student feedback	Open comments and feedback	Open comments	"Good and effective" "Good intervention" "Proper guidance"

A total of 63% of the respondents indicated that they would recommend the resource, while the rest remained neutral on this question; 60% of the respondents mentioned that they prefer learning from books, while 37% indicated online resources as the preferred method. A total of 70% of the respondents mentioned lectures as the preferred method, with the remaining indicating private study, e-learning and other methods.

4. Discussion

The need for the development of an online asynchronous clinical learning resource emerged from the inability of faculty and students who were not participants in a clinical case discussion to learn from and more importantly contribute to the discussion. A key factor which dictated the demand was feedback from students regarding lack of opportunities to learn from clinical cases being treated by their peers in different cohorts.

Provision of a standard case template was deemed necessary to enable standardization of presentation of cases and minimize preparation time. The students were encouraged to volunteer and share their own cases for discussion. Clinical learning may become more meaningful for dental students when they delve into their own experiences or clinical cases and learn from the content. This approach aligns with the theory of constructivism initially worked on by John Dewey, which proposes that learning is inherently related to action-knowledge, and when students extract learning from their own experiences, it may provide more meaning and significance to the learning [21]. Moreover, learning from one's own cases and cases treated by peers and faculty in the institution may lend a dimension of authenticity to the learning process, which may be absent in routine learning from the internet or textbooks.

The video-recorded case discussion with the expert marks the next step in the development of resource for clinical case learning. Interaction with the experts contributes to the learning process, where students are exposed to the thinking process of the expert during decision making. This mode of learning aligns with the concept of social constructivism emphasized by Jean Piaget and Lev Vygotsky. Profounder understanding may be achieved by the discussion, increasing the ability of the students to test their own ideas and synthesize and analyses the ideas of others [22,23]. Expert–student dialogue has been previously shown to enhance retention of knowledge and stimulate thinking in undergraduate dental students [24]. With respect to competency assessment in dentistry, expert–student dialogue has been previously shown to result in higher confidence and preparedness, leading to diminished uncertainty and stress. The aforementioned have been reported to contribute to the development of higher-order thinking and a broader clinical experience [25].

Self-assessment in the form of one best answers was incorporated at the commencement of each clinical case, and the same questions re-appeared after the segment of the video in which the answer to the question was discussed by the expert. Self-assessment has been previously established as an integral component of student learning through various studies conducted in dentistry [26–32]. Self-assessment may enable the students to understand and gauge their thinking and devise strategies to improve in this domain.

Another key element of each clinical case recording was a section on student reflection, where the student reflects on the learning after the completion of the discussion with the expert. After the video recording, the student summarizes and reflects on the discussion with the expert briefly. Reflective learning enables the student to critically review their own experience [33] and connect their current experience with previous learning and build on deeper learning. The incorporation of reflection as a component in the video segment is likely to facilitate deeper learning and critical thinking [34]. Observing a peer performing a reflective discourse (when other students watch the video) gives an opportunity for other students to reflect on and compare their own thought process while critically evaluating the clinical case. Further, the students and faculty may utilize the interactive forum to contribute to a discussion on the clinical case and share their views and experience. This helps to create an avenue for transparency in decision making in the institution and sharing of evidence-based resources in support of the decision or otherwise. Apart from internal faculty, external faculty when visiting as external examiners were also invited to participate in the clinical case discussion. This facilitated collaborative learning with faculty from an external university and hence provided a unique opportunity for the students.

It takes time, effort and money to generate computer-assisted learning (CAL) tools [35,36]. The development of a completed clinical case video takes 3 h. This includes contribution time from all the contributors, students, faculty and the e-learning department. The reusable learning object thus developed can be used by students and faculty anywhere and at any time and provides unique advantages. Sharing of learning resources and co-operation between universities can lead to economic advantage in the long run. CAL enables standardization of learning material delivery as compared to traditional methods of teaching, which involve different lecturers. Further, improving the interactivity, repeatability and feedback in the CAL program may increase their effectiveness. Real-time feedback and increased interactivity has previously been shown to enhance learning [37,38]. Interactivity incorporated into a CAL program might even be better in holding a student's attention when compared to traditional methods. Considering the advantages of CAL, new strategies to incorporate these into the curriculum and hence augment/replace conventional teaching should be deliberated.

The randomized study was conducted to evaluate the effectiveness of the current resource in teaching a topic in aesthetic restorative dentistry: "Replacement of teeth in the anterior aesthetic zone". Two cohorts were invited to participate in the study, and the current learning levels of both the cohorts were assumed to be similar for the specified learning outcome. There may be differences in the knowledge levels of year 3 and 4 students; however, the scope of the learning resource is aligned for all clinical semesters and hence addresses topics with considerable overlap. The scores from the pre-test were not significantly different for both groups, and hence the assumption of baseline comparability was confirmed. Previous studies in dentistry comparing an e-learning intervention to a traditional method of learning have practiced this approach of conducting a pre-test to ensure homogeneity between the groups being compared [15,19,20,39], and out of these three studies used the same questions for the pre-test and immediate post-test as in the current study [15,20,39]. Ensuring the comparability between the groups at baseline is important to ensure homogeneity, particularly since the students belong to two different cohorts. Clinical learning during year 3 and year 4 involve topics which may be of interest and aligned with the learning outcomes for students across the semesters/years. Conventionally, clinical learning may inadvertently be restricted to a particular semester/year due to the allotment of clinical sessions or case-based learning sessions as per the scheduled timetable. This creates a situation where learning may occur in isolated bundles with inaccessibility for the other cohorts, even though the learning may be relevant to them. The creation of an online asynchronous learning resource was hence aimed at creating unbundled learning, which spans across faculty/students in the institution and beyond. There was a significant increase in the test scores at the immediate post-test, which was conducted immediately upon completion of the session for both groups. Hence, we concluded that both the asynchronous learning resource and the synchronous session with a lecturer were equally effective in delivering the learning outcomes for the session. However, no significant difference was found when comparing the scores between the two groups. Previous studies that have evaluated the effectiveness of e-learning and compared it with other forms of learning have yielded mixed results. Overall, e-learning is either equally [6,15–17] or more [18–20] effective than traditional methods of teaching. However, the use of different methods of assessment for the two groups as undertaken by Eitner et al. is a significant limitation of the study [18]. It is interesting to note that two [18,20] out of three studies in which e-learning had significantly better outcomes than traditional learning had an element of enhanced interactivity in the e-learning tool in the form of assessments and feedback. It is beneficial to assess both short-term knowledge acquisition and long-term retention in the same cohort, as the examinations and real test of what the student has learned is spaced out by time [6,19,39]. The finding from the study conducted by Silveira is also significant, as it indicates that knowledge retention regarding identification of cephalometric landmarks are significantly better after two weeks when compared to conventional learning [19]. Contrary to this finding, we did not find a significant increase in test scores for both groups at the retention test, which was conducted after one week. This may be explained by the fact that we used newly framed questions that were also based on the reading material provided to both groups after the immediate post-test. Nevertheless, the key finding was that there was no significant difference between the two groups when comparing the scores of the retention test, hence suggesting that the online asynchronous learning resource performed at par with the online synchronous learning session. It is interesting to note that the retention test scores were almost the same as the pre-test scores. This can be attributed to the fact that the questions in the retention test were formulated from topics included in the additional learning material shared with both groups. The students may not have adequately covered the learning material provided, leading to the drop in scores. This may reflect the real-life situation in education, where students need to fortify their learning with additional reading; however, they seldom do so. Over-dependence on content from learning tools alone or lecture notes may not be the best way to develop life-long learning skills. This could be considered as a limitation of the study, and in the future, reminders to refer to the additional learning material and feedback based on the exam performance may be used to motivate the learner to refer to the material.

The response rate for the feedback survey was low and may be attributed to survey fatigue for e-learning courses and other feedback requested by the school. The feedback on the e-learning resource was taken after the resource was made available to both groups after the completion of the study to ensure fairness. Hence, intergroup comparisons were not made. The online asynchronous resource was acceptable and received good ratings from the respondents to the feedback survey. Most of the students gave feedback that the resource stimulated the students to explore the topic further. There is previous evidence that structured educational resources may develop desirable habits, linking curiosity and inquisitiveness in the minds of learners, leading to reflection and mindfulness [40]. Interestingly, when queried about learning preferences, most students still prefer to learn from books and through lectures. This may explain the fact that 63% of the respondents indicated that they would recommend the learning resource and the remaining remained neutral in their response. There is previous evidence on the superior effectiveness of lectures over e-learning in dental education [39]. Even though significant effort is being put into the development and validation of digital and e-learning resources, students may use these resources more when employed as augmentation to conventional methods of teaching and learning.

5. Conclusions

The online asynchronous clinical learning resource "Ask the Expert" was as effective as online synchronous teaching by a lecturer for clinical case discussions in restorative dentistry. The resource augments other modes of teaching in delivering learning outcomes related to clinical dentistry. This offers a "reusable learning environment" that provides unbundled learning, self-assessment, opportunity for reflection, discussion among peers and opportunity for collaboration with collaborating universities.

Supplementary Materials: The following are available online at https://www.mdpi.com/article/10.3390/healthcare9111420/s1, Figure S1: Case template, Figure S2: Time distribution for video resource generation, Figure S3: Distribution of test scores for Group A, Figure S4: Distribution of test scores for Group L, Figure S5: Questions used for pre-, post- and retention test.

Author Contributions: R.K.M. contributed to conception, design, data acquisition and interpretation and drafted the manuscript; L.L.S. contributed to conception and data interpretation and critically revised the manuscript. All authors gave final approval and agreed to be accountable for all aspects of the work. All authors have read and agreed to the published version of the manuscript.

Funding: The APC was funded by IMU.

Institutional Review Board Statement: The study was approved by the Institutional Review Board (or Ethics Committee) of the International Medical University (Project ID: IMU 480/220).

Informed Consent Statement: Informed consent was obtained from all subjects involved in the study.

Data Availability Statement: The data presented in this study are available on reasonable request from the corresponding author.

Acknowledgments: We would like to acknowledge the support from the e-learning department at the International Medical University, Malaysia, for their support in the development of the learning resource in the form of video recording and editing.

Conflicts of Interest: The authors declare no conflict of interest.

References

1. Thistlethwaite, J.E.; Davies, D.; Ekeocha, S.; Kidd, J.M.; MacDougall, C.; Matthews, P.; Purkis, J.; Clay, D. The Effectiveness of Case-Based Learning in Health Professional Education. A BEME Systematic Review: BEME Guide No. 23. *Med. Teach.* **2012**, *34*, e421–c444. [CrossRef]
2. Schwartz, P.L.; Egan, A.G.; Heath, C.J. Students' Perceptions of Course Outcomes and Learning Styles in Case-Based Courses in a Traditional Medical School. *Acad. Med.* **1994**, *69*, 507. [CrossRef]
3. Richards, P.S.; Inglehart, M.R. An Interdisciplinary Approach to Case-Based Teaching: Does It Create Patient-Centered and Culturally Sensitive Providers? *J. Dent. Educ.* **2006**, *70*, 284–291. [CrossRef]
4. Dupuis, R.E.; Persky, A.M. Use of Case-Based Learning in a Clinical Pharmacokinetics Course. *Am. J. Pharm. Educ.* **2008**, *72*, 29. [CrossRef] [PubMed]

5. Harden, R.M.; Hart, I.R. An International Virtual Medical School (IVIMEDS): The Future for Medical Education? *Med. Teach.* **2002**, *24*, 261–267. [CrossRef] [PubMed]
6. Bissell, V.; McKerlie, R.A.; Kinane, D.F.; McHugh, S. Teaching Periodontal Pocket Charting to Dental Students: A Comparison of Computer Assisted Learning and Traditional Tutorials. *Br. Dent. J.* **2003**, *195*, 333–336; discussion 329. [CrossRef] [PubMed]
7. Wong, G.; Greenhalgh, T.; Pawson, R. Internet-Based Medical Education: A Realist Review of What Works, for Whom and in What Circumstances. *BMC Med. Educ.* **2010**, *10*, 12. [CrossRef] [PubMed]
8. Ozuah, P.O. Undergraduate Medical Education: Thoughts on Future Challenges. *BMC Med. Educ.* **2002**, *2*, 8. [CrossRef]
9. Wilson, A.S.; Goodall, J.E.; Ambrosini, G.; Carruthers, D.M.; Chan, H.; Ong, S.G.; Gordon, C.; Young, S.P. Development of an Interactive Learning Tool for Teaching Rheumatology—A Simulated Clinical Case Studies Program. *Rheumatology* **2006**, *45*, 1158–1161. [CrossRef]
10. Choules, A.P. The Use of Elearning in Medical Education: A Review of the Current Situation. *Postgrad. Med. J.* **2007**, *83*, 212–216. [CrossRef]
11. Bernardo, V.; Ramos, M.P.; Plapler, H.; De Figueiredo, L.F.P.; Nader, H.B.; Anção, M.S.; Von Dietrich, C.P.; Sigulem, D. Web-Based Learning in Undergraduate Medical Education: Development and Assessment of an Online Course on Experimental Surgery. *Int. J. Med. Inform.* **2004**, *73*, 731–742. [CrossRef]
12. Davis, M.H.; Harden, R.M. E Is for Everything-e-Learning? *Med. Teach.* **2001**, *23*, 441–444. [CrossRef] [PubMed]
13. Greenhalgh, T. Computer Assisted Learning in Undergraduate Medical Education. *BMJ* **2001**, *322*, 40–44. [CrossRef]
14. Lau, F.; Bates, J. A Review of E-Learning Practices for Undergraduate Medical Education. *J. Med. Syst.* **2004**, *28*, 71–87. [CrossRef] [PubMed]
15. Aly, M.; Elen, J.; Willems, G. Instructional Multimedia Program versus Standard Lecture: A Comparison of Two Methods for Teaching the Undergraduate Orthodontic Curriculum. *Eur. J. Dent. Educ.* **2004**, *8*, 43–46. [CrossRef] [PubMed]
16. Bains, M.; Reynolds, P.A.; McDonald, F.; Sherriff, M. Effectiveness and Acceptability of Face-to-Face, Blended and e-Learning: A Randomised Trial of Orthodontic Undergraduates. *Eur. J. Dent. Educ.* **2011**, *15*, 110–117. [CrossRef] [PubMed]
17. Howerton, W.B.; Enrique, P.R.T.; Ludlow, J.B.; Tyndall, D.A. Interactive Computer-Assisted Instruction vs. Lecture Format in Dental Education. *J. Dent. Hyg.* **2004**, *78*, 10.
18. Eitner, S.; Holst, S.; Wichmann, M.; Karl, M.; Nkenke, E.; Schlegel, A. Comparative Study on Interactive Computer-Aided-Learning and Computer-Aided-Testing in Patient-Based Dental Training in Maxillofacial Surgery. *Eur. J. Dent. Educ.* **2008**, *12*, 35–40. [CrossRef]
19. Silveira, H.L.D.; Gomes, M.J.; Silveira, H.E.D.; Dalla-Bona, R.R. Evaluation of the Radiographic Cephalometry Learning Process by a Learning Virtual Object. *Am. J. Orthod. Dentofac. Orthop.* **2009**, *136*, 134–138. [CrossRef]
20. Shapiro, M.C.; Anderson, O.R.; Lal, S. Assessment of a Novel Module for Training Dental Students in Child Abuse Recognition and Reporting. *J. Dent. Educ.* **2014**, *78*, 1167–1175. [CrossRef]
21. Silva, D. John Dewey: Implications for Schooling. *Am. J. Occup. Ther.* **1977**, *31*, 40–43.
22. Scott, H.K.; Cogburn, M. Piaget. In *StatPearls*; StatPearls Publishing: Treasure Island, FL, USA, 2021.
23. Vasileva, O.; Balyasnikova, N. (Re)Introducing Vygotsky's Thought: From Historical Overview to Contemporary Psychology. *Front. Psychol.* **2019**, *10*, 1515. [CrossRef]
24. Botelho, M.G.; Chan, A.K.M. A Microanalysis of Expert-Student Dialogue Videos: Supporting Preparation and Learning for Clinical Competence Assessment. *Eur. J. Dent. Educ.* **2021**. [CrossRef]
25. Botelho, M.; Gao, X.; Bhuyan, S.Y. Mixed-Methods Analysis of Videoed Expert-Student Dialogue Supporting Clinical Competence Assessments. *Eur. J. Dent. Educ.* **2020**, *24*, 398–406. [CrossRef] [PubMed]
26. Wiener, R.C.; Waters, C.; Doris, J.; McNeil, D.W. Comparison of Dental Students' Self-Evaluation and Faculty Evaluation of Communication Skills During a Standardized Patient Exercise. *J. Dent. Educ.* **2018**, *82*, 1043–1050. [CrossRef]
27. Habib, S.R.; Sherfudhin, H. Students' Self-Assessment: A Learning Tool and Its Comparison with the Faculty Assessments. *J. Contemp. Dent. Pract.* **2015**, *16*, 48–53. [CrossRef] [PubMed]
28. Emam, H.A.; Jatana, C.A.; Wade, S.; Hamamoto, D. Dental Student Self-Assessment of a Medical History Competency Developed by Oral and Maxillofacial Surgery Faculty. *Eur. J. Dent. Educ.* **2018**, *22*, 9–14. [CrossRef] [PubMed]
29. McKenzie, C.T.; Tilashalski, K.R.; Peterson, D.T.; White, M.L. Effectiveness of Standardized Patient Simulations in Teaching Clinical Communication Skills to Dental Students. *J. Dent. Educ.* **2017**, *81*, 1179–1186. [CrossRef] [PubMed]
30. Kim, A.H.; Chutinan, S.; Park, S.E. Assessment Skills of Dental Students as Peer Evaluators. *J. Dent. Educ.* **2015**, *79*, 653–657. [CrossRef] [PubMed]
31. Quick, K.K. The Role of Self- and Peer Assessment in Dental Students' Reflective Practice Using Standardized Patient Encounters. *J. Dent. Educ.* **2016**, *80*, 924–929. [CrossRef]
32. Bitter, K.; Rüttermann, S.; Lippmann, M.; Hahn, P.; Giesler, M. Self-Assessment of Competencies in Dental Education in Germany—A Multicentred Survey. *Eur. J. Dent. Educ.* **2016**, *20*, 229–236. [CrossRef] [PubMed]
33. Schwoegl, E.N.; Rodgers, M.E.; Kumar, S.S. Reflective Journaling by Second-Year Dental Students During a Clinical Rotation. *J. Dent. Educ.* **2020**, *84*, 157–165. [CrossRef] [PubMed]
34. Boyd, L.D. Reflections on Clinical Practice by First-Year Dental Students: A Qualitative Study. *J. Dent. Educ.* **2002**, *66*, 710–720. [CrossRef] [PubMed]

35. Lowe, C.I.; Wright, J.L.; Bearn, D.R. Computer-Aided Learning (CAL): An Effective Way to Teach the Index of Orthodontic Treatment Need (IOTN)? *J. Orthod.* **2001**, *28*, 307–311. [CrossRef]
36. Bahrami, M.; Deery, C.; Clarkson, J.E.; Pitts, N.B.; Johnston, M.; Ricketts, I.; MacLennan, G.; Nugent, Z.J.; Tilley, C.; Bonetti, D.; et al. Effectiveness of Strategies to Disseminate and Implement Clinical Guidelines for the Management of Impacted and Unerupted Third Molars in Primary Dental Care, a Cluster Randomised Controlled Trial. *Br. Dent. J.* **2004**, *197*, 691–696; discussion 688. [CrossRef]
37. Brezis, M.; Cohen, R. Interactive Learning with Voting Technology. *Med. Educ.* **2004**, *38*, 574–575. [CrossRef]
38. Uhari, M.; Renko, M.; Soini, H. Experiences of Using an Interactive Audience Response System in Lectures. *BMC Med. Educ.* **2003**, *3*, 12. [CrossRef]
39. Peroz, I.; Beuche, A.; Peroz, N. Randomized Controlled Trial Comparing Lecture versus Self Studying by an Online Tool. *Med. Teach.* **2009**, *31*, 508–512. [CrossRef]
40. Dyche, L.; Epstein, R.M. Curiosity and Medical Education. *Med. Educ.* **2011**, *45*, 663–668. [CrossRef]

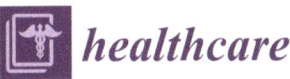

Article

Social Media Usage among Dental Undergraduate Students—A Comparative Study

Eswara Uma [1], Pentti Nieminen [2,*], Shani Ann Mani [3], Jacob John [4], Emilia Haapanen [5], Marja-Liisa Laitala [6], Olli-Pekka Lappalainen [7], Eby Varghase [1], Ankita Arora [1] and Kanwardeep Kaur [1]

1. Faculty of Dentistry, Manipal University College Malaysia, Melaka 75150, Malaysia; eswara.uma@manipal.edu.my (E.U.); eby.varghese@manipal.edu.my (E.V.); ankita.arora@manipal.edu.my (A.A.); kanwardeep.kaur@manipal.edu.my (K.K.)
2. Medical Informatics and Data Analysis Research Group, University of Oulu, 90014 Oulu, Finland
3. Department of Paediatric Dentistry and Orthodontics, Faculty of Dentistry, University of Malaya, Kuala Lumpur 50603, Malaysia; shani@um.edu.my
4. Department of Restorative Dentistry, Faculty of Dentistry, University of Malaya, Kuala Lumpur 50603, Malaysia; drjacob@um.edu.my
5. Research Unit of Oral Health Sciences, Faculty of Medicine, University of Oulu, 90014 Oulu, Finland; emilia.haapanen@student.oulu.fi
6. Research Unit of Oral Health Sciences, Faculty of Medicine, University of Oulu and Medical Research Centre Oulu, Oulu University Hospital, 90014 Oulu, Finland; marja-liisa.laitala@oulu.fi
7. Faculty of Medicine, University of Helsinki, 00014 Helsinki, Finland; olli.pekka.lappainen@helsinki.fi
* Correspondence: pentti.nieminen@oulu.fi

Abstract: Social media use among students has infiltrated into dental education and offers benefits but may also cause problems. The aim of this study was to explore and compare current social media usage among dental undergraduate students from two countries—Malaysia and Finland. A self-administered structured online questionnaire was used. WhatsApp, YouTube, Instagram, Facebook and Snapchat were the services that were most familiar to the respondents from both countries. There were differences between the students from the two countries among the most preferred platforms. The most frequently used applications were WhatsApp (91.1% of students in Malaysia and 96.1% in Finland used it very frequently) and Instagram (74.3% of students in Malaysia and 70.0% in Finland used it very frequently). Students in Malaysia spent significantly more hours per week using the platforms as study tools than students in Finland. Over 80% of the Finnish dental students reported that lack of knowledge was not an issue in social media usage, while 85% of Malaysian students felt that lack of knowledge prevented them from using social media platforms frequently. The findings offer evidence that dental students used social media extensively.

Keywords: social media use; dental students; social media platforms; dental training; Malaysia; Finland

1. Introduction

In today's digital world, most people are logged in perpetually and always connected. Our devices have ensured that technology is "always on us and always on"! Never has it become so easy to access information, and social media has become a major tool for communication and seeking information. We have a multitude of interactions with others, on topics that can be varied, and this has fused our professional and personal lives [1].

Social media is defined as "websites and applications that enable users to create and share content or to participate in social networking." Social media includes social networking platforms including Facebook and Twitter and media sharing sites, for example, YouTube and Instagram. In addition, there are other platforms like blog sites and microblogging sites. Healthcare professionals use social media extensively and it was reported that up to 90% of practicing doctors use Facebook accounts for professional or personal use [2]. Social media platforms offer different approaches to content sharing, and this has wide-ranging uses in dentistry. Social media is useful not only for education and networking, but also for marketing and recruitment. Studies in health professionals' education have found benefits in the use of social media tools in clinical education [3]. Social media has become pervasive in society and is playing an important role in the personal and professional lives with dentistry being no exception.

In remote study conditions during the COVID-19 pandemic, the use of digital tools and social media platforms became imperative for medical and dental medical education for information retrieval, sharing of learning materials, and video meetings and discussions [4,5]. These tools were often used for both academic and non-academic purposes among students and teachers. Social media platforms were found to enhance ways of studying, allow for learning new skills, enhance performance, foster social relationships and social support and strengthen organizational identification [6,7].

Reports indicate that dental students use more than one social media application with Facebook being the most used platform among students in the United States and the United Kingdom [2–8]. The second most favored platforms were YouTube and Instagram. Skype and YouTube were used to improve dental skills while Twitter and blogging sites for interactions with the faculty and also to enhance communication [9].

A bibliometric study of articles published in journals indexed by the Web of Science database found 41 studies related to social media and dentistry during the period of 2010–2016 [10]. Most of these studies focused on the impact of social media on dental education and professional practice. These studies emphasized the extension of the dental curriculum to involve the teaching and learning using social media platforms. However, these studies also highlighted the concern towards educational preparedness of future generations in the academic community, and understand the limitations of discourse produced by social media platforms. These studies also noted the concern regarding information mediation through social media platforms and its impact on dental education [10].

Significant differences in social trends, cultural beliefs and perceptions between Asian and European countries can affect the use of different social media applications and other technologies. This may also influence how these technologies are utilised by undergraduate students in their academics.

There are some previous studies about social media and dentistry in Malaysia [11–14]. Rani et al. [13] have described how dental undergraduates were trained to use social media for promoting oral health in the community, while Affendi et al. [11] evaluated the use of social media for marketing by dentists. See et al. [14] investigated the support, exposure and use of social media technologies among students, academics and administrators from both informatics and non-informatics undergraduate programs in Malaysia. In addition, internet addiction among dental students was also studied [12]. To our knowledge, there are no published studies about social media usage among Finnish dental or medical students.

The main purpose of our study was to compare the social media usage among dental undergraduate students from two countries Malaysia and Finland. This comparative study between similar cohorts of students from two different countries from two continents will help to estimate the extent and nature of social media use among undergraduate dental students. In addition, the study will provide suggestions for social media training in the dental curriculum. In this article, empirical data focused on the following research questions: How familiar are students with social media platforms? How often do students use social media services? How competent are the students at using social media services? How many hours do students spend using social media platforms as part of dental education? What factors encourage or prevent students to use social media?

2. Materials and Methods

2.1. Study Design and Data Collection

This was a cross-sectional online questionnaire survey conducted among dental undergraduates of the academic year 2020–2021 from two dental schools in Malaysia (Manipal Melaka Medical College and University of Malaya) and Finland (the University of Helsinki and University of Oulu) each. Ethical approval to conduct this study was obtained for the institutions in Malaysia; Medical Ethics Committee, Faculty of Dentistry, University of Malaya [DF CD2105/0015 (L)] and Research Ethics committee, Faculty of Dentistry, Melaka Manipal Medical college [MMMC/FOD/AR/E C-2021(F-01)] prior to commencement of the study. According to the guidelines of the Ministry of Education and Culture in Finland, survey studies with anonymous questionnaires do not need approval from an ethics committee.

The instrument used was a questionnaire modified from a previous study among dental students in the USA [15]. The validated questionnaire assesses social media usage among medical undergraduates. Twelve items from the questionnaire were used to assess social media usage and the perceptions of social media usage in relation to dentistry/dental practice. Questionnaire items had three sections; Part A consisted of five questions regarding the demographic characteristics of the participants. Part B had six items regarding their familiarity, competence, time spent on various social media platforms and factors that encouraged and discouraged students from using social media. Part C had one item which addressed practice and perceptions regarding social media use in dentistry. Most questions required responses on a 4-point or 5-point Likert scale. The updated version of the questionnaire is included as the Supplementary Materials.

In Malaysia, the English questionnaire was pre-tested on a sample of five students in different years of the dental undergraduate programme at the Manipal Melaka Medical College and University of Malaya to check for semantic comprehension. Only minor modifications were made to the questionnaire following feedback from the pre-test. The questionnaire was translated into Finnish. In Finland, five dental students also pretested the first Finnish version. Based on their feedback, minor changes were made to improve the language and to clarify the purpose of the questions. The final questionnaire was administered using Google Forms from March 23rd, 2021, to April 11th, 2021, in both countries, the link being circulated via email and WhatsApp to student representatives of each year of study who then forwarded it to their classmates.

All dental undergraduates who received the online survey link were invited to participate in this study. In the online Google form, all the participants were asked to declare that they had read the participant information sheet (PIS) and voluntarily give consent for data collection and processing. If they refused consent, the questionnaire was closed. Inclusion and exclusion criteria were specified in the PIS. The survey was anonymous and did not include personal sensitive data.

For the estimation of sample sizes, we selected the time spent using social media as the outcome variable. The following formulas with finite population correction for proportions were used to estimate the minimum sample sizes in Malaysia and Finland:

$$n_0 = \frac{z_{\alpha/2}^2 p(1-p)}{e^2} \qquad (1)$$

and

$$n = \frac{n_0 N}{n_0 + (N-1)} \qquad (2)$$

where n = required minimum sample size, n_0 = Cochran's sample size for large populations, N = available number of students (years 1–5) (population size), e = maximum error in estimation, p = proportion of the outcome variable (more than 15 h a week), $p(1-p)$ = variance of the outcome variable, $z^2_{\alpha/2}$ = 1.96 for 95% confidence limit [16,17].

Setting maximum error to 5%, presuming that 50% of the student population have the outcome proportion of using more than 15 h a week social media and estimating that the population size N = 3250 in Malaysia, the minimum number of participating students should be at least 344 in Malaysia. Currently, there are about 1000 dental students (years 1–5) in Finland. So, the required sample size was 278 students in Finland.

2.2. Data Analysis

Tabular and graphical displays of data were used as the main tools of data presentation and analysis. The frequency and percentage distributions of participant characteristics (age, sex, year of study, and hours a week using social media) were presented for students from Malaysia and Finland. Percentage distributions were used to estimate the proportions of responses to questions "How familiar are you with each of the following social media services?", "How often do you use each of the following social media services?", "Approximately how many hours a week do you spend using the following social media services as part of your dental education?", and to question "How competent are you with each of the following social media services?" by country. We also compared the percentage distributions of students using very frequently the five most popular social media platforms and how competent they felt using these platforms by age, sex and year of dental school. In addition, frequency and percentage distributions of factors that encouraged or prevented students to use social media platforms were presented. Statistical significance of differences between Malaysian and Finnish student groups and basic characteristics were evaluated using a chi-square test with exact p-values. Among applications, we also evaluated the relationship between overall high use, competence at using and use in dental education using Spearman's rank correlation coefficient (rho). The data satisfactorily fulfilled the underlying assumptions and preconditions of the applied analysis methods. All statistical analyses were performed using IBM SPSS Statistics software (version 26) and Origin 2020 graphing software.

3. Results

3.1. Participants

A total of 613 students participated in this study. Table 1 shows the distribution of age, sex, year of dental school and hours per week using social media by country. Most of the participants were female in both countries. The student groups were quite different in terms of age and year of dental school. In particular, the Malaysian students were younger than the Finnish dental students. Most of the students spent more than 11 h per week using social media. Almost 75% of the Finnish dental students reported that they used social media at least 11 h per week.

Table 1. The frequency and percentage distributions of basic characteristics among dental students from Malaysia ($n = 440$) and Finland ($n = 203$).

Characteristics	Malaysia n (%)	Finland n (%)	All n (%)	p-Value of Exact Chi-Square Test
Age				<0.001
20 years or younger	70 (17.0)	12 (5.9)	87 (13.5)	
21–23 years	250 (56.8)	56 (27.6)	306 (47.6)	
24–26 years	114 (25.9)	69 (34.0)	183 (28.5)	
27–29 years	1 (0.2)	38 (18.7)	39 (6.1)	
30 years or above	0	28 (13.8)	28 (4.4)	
Sex				>0.999
Male	103 (23.4)	47 (23.2)	150 (23.3)	
Female	337 (76.6)	156 (76.7)	493 (76.7)	
Year of dental school				0.038
First	70 (15.9)	39 (19.2)	109 (17.0)	
Second	78 (17.7)	54 (26.6)	132 (20.5)	
Third	79 (18.0)	33 (16.3)	112 (17.4)	
Fourth	108 (24.5)	42 (20.7)	150 (23.3)	
Fifth	105 (23.9)	35 (17.2)	140 (21.8)	
Hours a week using social media				<0.001
Do not use	1 (0.2)	2 (1.0)	3 (0.5)	
Less than 5 h	51 (11.6)	7 (3.4)	58 (9.0)	
6–10 h	114 (25.9)	42 (20.7)	156 (24.3)	
11–15 h	81 (18.4)	62 (30.5)	143 (22.2)	
16–20 h	76 (17.3)	44 (21.7)	120 (18.7)	
More than 20	117 (26.6)	46 (22.7)	163 (25.3)	

3.2. Familiarity with Social Media Platforms

Most of the students were familiar with several applications (Figure 1). WhatsApp, YouTube, Instagram, Facebook and Snapchat were the most familiar services to the respondents from both countries. All Malaysian and Finnish students were familiar or very familiar with WhatsApp. In addition, all Finnish students were at least familiar with YouTube and Facebook. The number of students not familiar with YouTube or Instagram was also minimal. Only two students from Malaysia reported that they were not familiar with YouTube. Seven Malaysian students and one Finnish student reported that they had heard about Instagram but were not sure of its purpose. Students in Malaysia were more aware of Telegram, WeChat and Weibo than students in Finland. Respectively, the Finnish students were more familiar with Facebook, Snapchat, Jodel and LinkedIn.

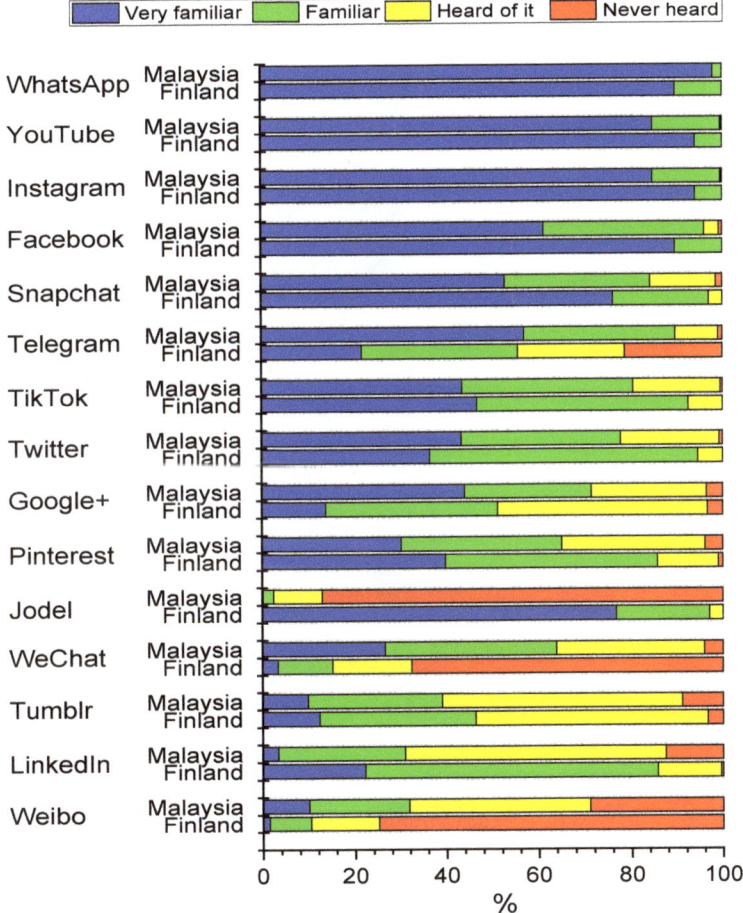

Figure 1. Percentage distributions of responses to question "How familiar are you with each of the following social media services?" by country. Data include dental undergraduate students from Malaysia ($n = 440$) and Finland ($n = 203$). Statistical significances between countries evaluated by exact chi-square test are as follows: 0.059 (Instagram), 0.054 (Tumblr), 0.002 (YouTube), <0.001 (all other services).

3.3. Reported Frequency of Social Media Use

Figure 2 shows that all students reported using more than one social media platform at least regularly. WhatsApp was the most commonly used, all students used it at least regularly, 91.1% very frequently in Malaysia and 96.1% in Finland. Instagram was the second most frequently used platform, 74.3% used it very frequently in Malaysia and 70.0% in Finland. Students in Malaysia were more likely to use YouTube, Telegram, Twitter, Google+ frequently or regularly than those in Finland. The Finnish students were more likely to use Snapchat and Jodel compared to students from than in Malaysia. Most of the respondents in our survey had never used WeChat, Tumblr, LinkedIn, or Weibo.

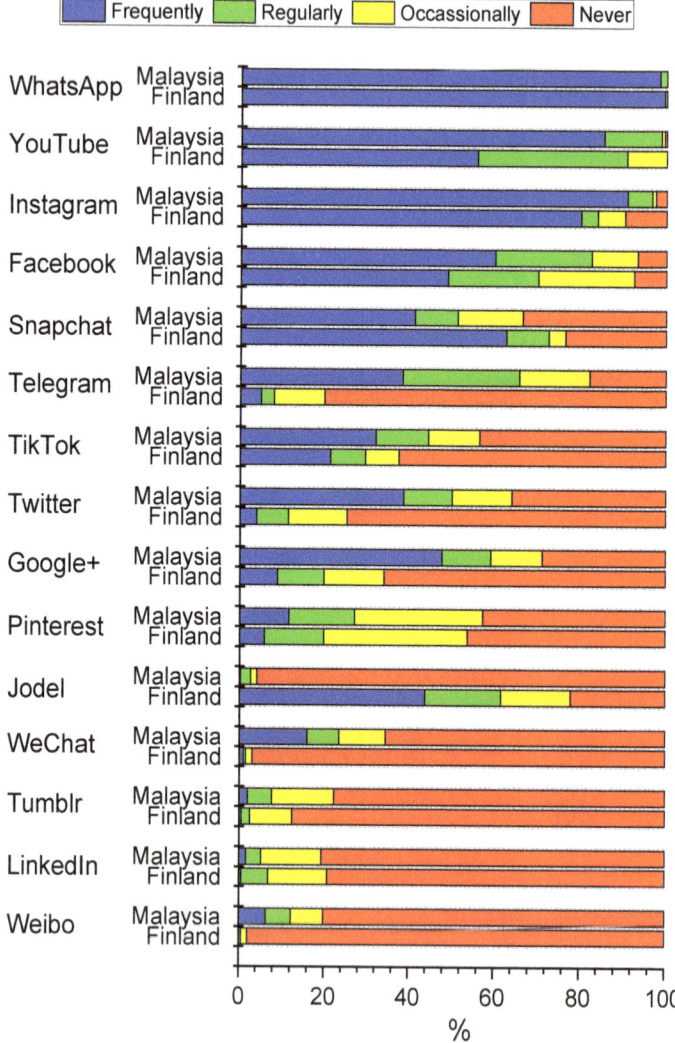

Figure 2. Percentage distributions of responses to question "How often do you use each of the following social media services?" by country. Data include dental undergraduate students from Malaysia ($n = 440$) and Finland ($n = 203$). Statistical significances between countries evaluated by exact chi-square test are as follows: 0.304 (LinkedIn), 0.294 (WhatsApp), 0.118 (Pinterest), 0.014 (Tumblr), 0.002 (Facebook), <0.001 (all other services).

We also analysed the associations of background characteristics with the frequency of social media usage. For this analysis, we included only the five most popular platforms presented in Figure 2 and the analyses were stratified by country. Table 2 shows the proportions of respondents using frequently these basic student characteristics. The age of students was not associated with the frequent use of these services in Malaysia. However, younger students used Instagram and Snapchat more frequently than older students in Finland.

In Malaysia, male participants were more likely to report very frequent use of Facebook than female participants (45.6% vs. 27.9%). In Finland, male students were more likely to report using very frequently YouTube than females (51.1% vs. 12.8%) and female students used Instagram (77.6% vs. 44.7%) or Snapchat (55.1% vs. 38.1%) more often than males. Year of study was not associated in either country with the very frequent use of the platforms (Table 2).

Table 2. Percentage of students using very frequently the five most popular social media platforms by age, sex and year of dental school. Data include dental undergraduate students from Malaysia ($n = 440$) and Finland ($n = 203$).

Characteristics	WhatsApp %	YouTube %	Platform Instagram %	Facebook %	Snapchat %	Number of Students
Malaysia						
Age	$p = 0.725$	$p = 0.556$	$p = 0.778$	$p = 0.333$	$p = 0.185$	
20 years or younger	90.7	66.7	77.3	26.7	33.3	75
21–23 years	90.4	59.6	72.8	32.4	26.0	250
24–26 years	93.0	57.9	75.4	34.2	24.6	114
27–29 years	100.0	100.0	100.0	100.0	100.0	1
30 years or above	-	-	-	-	-	0
Sex	$p = 0.073$	$p = 0.135$	$p = 0.369$	$p = 0.001$	$p > 0.999$	
Male	86.4	67.0	70.9	45.6	27.2	103
Female	92.6	58.5	75.4	27.9	27.0	337
Year of dental school	$p = 0.462$	$p = 0.109$	$p = 0.304$	$p = 0.629$	$p = 0.524$	
First	92.9	65.7	77.1	27.1	30.0	70
Second	92.3	70.5	76.9	37.2	21.8	78
Third	88.6	59.5	64.6	30.4	22.8	79
Fourth	88.0	51.9	75.9	29.6	31.5	108
Fifth	94.3	59.0	76.2	35.2	27.6	105
Finland						
Age	$p = 0.184$	$p = 0.214$	$p = 0.025$	$p = 0.860$	$p < 0.001$	
20 years or younger	83.3	16.7	83.3	16.7	75.0	12
21–23 years	98.2	14.3	78.6	32.1	82.1	56
24–26 years	97.1	24.6	63.8	33.3	49.3	69
27–29 years	94.7	18.4	78.9	31.6	39.5	38
30 years or above	96.4	35.7	50.0	32.1	0.0	28
Sex	$p > 0.999$	$p < 0.001$	$p < 0.001$	$p = 0.107$	$p = 0.047$	
Male	95.7	51.1	44.7	21.3	38.3	47
Female	96.2	12.8	77.6	34.6	55.1	153
Year of dental school	$p = 0.131$	$p = 0.285$	$p = 0.509$	$p = 0.400$	$p = 0.155$	
First	89.7	23.1	66.7	23.1	56.4	39
Second	98.1	14.8	66.7	27.8	61.1	54
Third	93.9	18.2	75.8	30.3	48.5	33
Fourth	100.0	21.4	78.6	35.7	50.0	42
Fifth	97.1	34.3	62.9	42.9	34.3	35

Statistical significances evaluated by exact chi-square test for each platform.

3.4. Perceived Competence of Social Media Use

Both Malaysian (99.6%) and Finnish (100.0%) students reported that they were highly competent or competent in using WhatsApp (Figure 3). We found some substantially significant differences in the reported competencies between students from Malaysia and Finland. More Malaysian students declared that they were highly competent in using YouTube, Instagram, Telegram, TikTok, Twitter and Google+. On the other hand, the Finnish respondents declared more often than they were highly competent using Facebook, Snapchat and Jodel. Figure 3 also shows that the majority of the students do feel that they are beginners or not at all competent in using Tumblr, LinkedIn or Weibo.

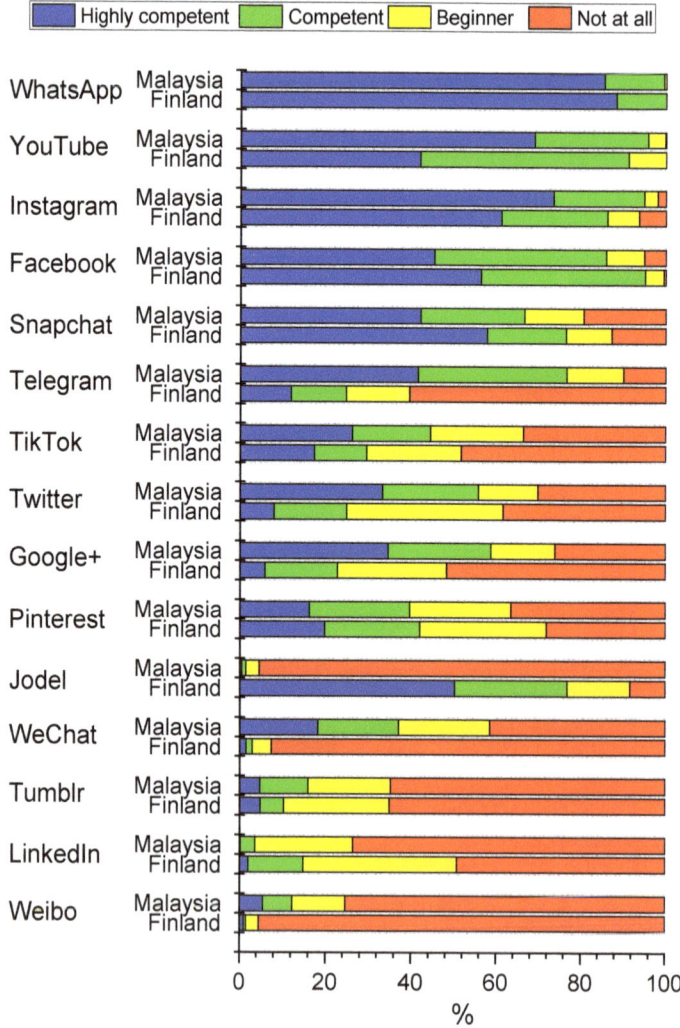

Figure 3. Percentage distributions of responses to question "How competent are you with each of the following social media services?" by country. Data include dental undergraduate students from Malaysia ($n = 440$) and Finland ($n = 203$). Statistical significances between countries evaluated by exact chi-square test are as follows: 0.426 (WhatsApp), 0.105 (Pinterest), 0.080 (Tumblr), 0.003 (Snapchat), <0.001 (all other services).

Table 3 shows the proportions of self-reported high competence in using the most preferred social media platforms by basic student characteristics and stratified by country. Sex was associated with the reported competence of using the most commonly used applications. Female students in both countries are more likely reported to be highly competent using popular social networking sites than males. In Malaysia, no substantial difference between males and females was found only in the self-reported skill of using Facebook. In Finland, males and females reported similar highly competent only in the use of YouTube. Year of study had little influence on the self-reported competence of using the most common platforms (Table 3). However, our analysis indicated that age was associated with the perceived high competence differently in Malaysia and Finland. In Malaysia, younger dental students felt less often highly competent with YouTube and Facebook. In Finland, younger students reported more likely that they were highly competent in applying Instagram and Snapchat.

Table 3. Percentage of students reporting high competence in using the five most commonly used social media platforms by age, sex and year of dental school. Data include dental undergraduate students from Malaysia ($n = 440$) and Finland ($n = 203$).

Characteristics	WhatsApp %	YouTube %	Instagram %	Facebook %	Snapchat %	Number of Students
Malaysia						
Age	$p = 0.774$	$p = 0.040$	$p = 0.537$	$p = 0.009$	$p = 0.294$	
20 years or younger	88.0	78.7	78.7	32.0	49.3	75
21–23 years	84.4	69.6	73.6	44.8	40.8	250
24–26 years	86.0	60.5	69.3	54.4	39.5	114
27–29 years	100.0	100.0	100.0	100.0	100.0	1
30–35 years	-	-	-	-	-	0
Sex	$p = 0.001$	$p = 0.010$	$p < 0.001$	$p > 0.999$	$p = 0.255$	
Male	74.8	58.3	56.3	45.6	36.9	103
Female	88.7	72.1	78.6	45.1	43.6	337
Year of dental school	$p = 0.347$	$p = 0.013$	$p = 0.313$	$p = 0.142$	$p = 0.430$	
First	88.6	81.4	80.0	32.9	45.7	70
Second	88.5	78.2	79.5	46.2	44.9	78
Third	84.8	64.6	68.4	41.8	34.2	79
Fourth	79.6	63.9	71.3	50.0	46.3	108
Fifth	87.6	61.9	70.5	50.5	39.0	105
Finland						
Age	$p = 0.015$	$p = 0.079$	$p = 0.009$	$p = 0.322$	$p < 0.001$	
20 years or younger	75.0	50.0	66.7	41.7	66.7	12
21–23 years	91.1	44.6	71.4	55.4	78.6	56
24–26 years	94.2	50.7	65.2	63.8	66.7	69
27–29 years	89.5	23.7	57.9	57.9	42.1	38
30–35 years	71.4	35.7	32.1	42.9	10.7	28
Sex	$p = 0.009$	$p = 0.867$	$p < 0.001$	$p = 0.001$	$p = 0.019$	
Male	76.6	40.4	31.9	34.0	42.6	47
Female	91.7	42.3	69.9	62.8	62.2	156
Year of dental school	$p = 0.568$	$p = 0.659$	$p = 0.339$	$p = 0.529$	$p = 0.311$	
First	87.6	38.5	61.5	43.6	56.4	39
Second	87.0	44.4	61.1	59.3	59.3	54
Third	97.0	51.5	75.8	60.6	72.7	33
Fourth	85.7	40.5	52.4	57.1	52.4	42
Fifth	85.7	34.3	57.1	60.0	48.6	35

Statistical significances evaluated by exact chi-square test for each platform.

3.5. Reported Frequency of Social Media Use for Dental Education

Participants were also asked about the time (hours per week) they spent using social media sites as part of their dental education (Table 4). Frequency and percentage distributions by country show that there were statistically significant differences between the countries among the most preferred platforms. For most applications, students in Malaysia spent more hours per week using the platforms as study tools than students in Finland. Jodel was the only social media application where the Finns spent more hours per week to manage their study assignments or tutorials.

Table 4. Frequency and percentage distributions of responses to question "Approximately how many hours a week do you spend using the following social media services as part of your dental education?" by country. Data include dental undergraduate students from Malaysia ($n = 440$) and Finland ($n = 203$).

Platform	Country	Do Not Use n (%)	Less than 1 h n (%)	1–5 h n (%)	6–10 h n (%)	More than 11 h n (%)	p-Value of Exact Chi-Square test
WhatsApp	Malaysia	26 (5.9)	63 (14.3)	155 (35.2)	91 (20.7)	105 (23.9)	<0.001
	Finland	6 (3.0)	77 (37.9)	101 (49.8)	14 (6.9)	5 (2.5)	
YouTube	Malaysia	19 (4.3)	104 (23.6)	204 (46.4)	71 (16.1)	42 (9.5)	<0.001
	Finland	35 (17.2)	101 (49.8)	53 (26.1)	10 (4.9)	4 (2.0)	
Instagram	Malaysia	31 (7.0)	146 (33.2)	157 (35.7)	50 (11.4)	56 (12.7)	<0.001
	Finland	77 (37.9)	78 (38.4)	36 (17.7)	7 (3.4)	5 (2.5)	
Facebook	Malaysia	187 (42.5)	140 (31.8)	75 (17.0)	22 (5.0)	16 (3.6)	<0.001
	Finland	62 (30.5)	124 (61.1)	16 (7.9)	1 (0.5)	0	
Snapchat	Malaysia	334 (75.9)	51 (11.6)	34 (7.7)	7 (1.6)	14 (3.2)	0.006
	Finland	141 (69.5)	44 (21.7)	15 (7.4)	1 (0.5)	2 (1.0)	
Telegram	Malaysia	260 (59.1)	99 (22.5)	42 (9.5)	21 (4.8)	18 (4.1)	<0.001
	Finland	187 (92.1)	16 (7.9)	0	0	0	
TikTok	Malaysia	304 (69.1)	58 (13.2)	38 (8.6)	18 (4.1)	22 (5.0)	<0.001
	Finland	173 (85.2)	24 (11.8)	3 (1.5)	2 (1.0)	1 (0.5)	
Twitter	Malaysia	281 (63.9)	88 (20.0)	48 (10.9)	9 (2.0)	14 (3.2)	<0.001
	Finland	183 (90.1)	19 (9.4)	1 (0.5)	0	0	
Google+	Malaysia	197 (44.8)	59 (13.4)	91 (20.7)	49 (11.1)	44 (10.0)	<0.001
	Finland	172 (84.7)	20 (9.9)	10 (4.9)	1 (0.5)	0	
Pinterest	Malaysia	349 (79.3)	65 (14.8)	22 (5.0)	2 (0.5)	2 (0.5)	0.007
	Finland	175 (86.2)	29 (13.8)	0	0	0	
Jodel	Malaysia	435 (98.9)	1 (0.2)	2 (0.5)	0	2 (0.5)	<0.001
	Finland	112 (55.2)	66 (32.5)	23 (11.3)	2 (1.0)	0	
WeChat	Malaysia	402 (91.4)	18 (4.1)	12 (2.7)	5 (1.1)	3 (0.7)	0.036
	Finland	192 (94.6)	11 (5.4)	0	0	0	
Tumblr	Malaysia	414 (94.1)	17 (3.9)	6 (1.4)	1 (0.2)	2 (0.5)	0.275
	Finland	192 (94.6)	11 (5.4)	0	0	0	
LinkedIn	Malaysia	409 (93.0)	19 (4.3)	11 (2.5)	0	1 (0.2)	<0.001
	Finland	176 (86.7)	27 (13.3)	0	0	0	
Weibo	Malaysia	419 (95.2)	13 (3.0)	6 (1.4)	1 (0.2)	1 (0.2)	0.003
	Finland	185 (91.1)	18 (8.9)	0	0	0	

We also analysed whether students used the same social media platforms for their personal use as well as for their educational purposes and if their perceived competence correlated with the use of these specific platforms for dental education. Figure 4 shows a strong association between personal and educational use of platforms in both countries. In addition, perceived knowledge of the use of the applications was associated with their use in educational purposes.

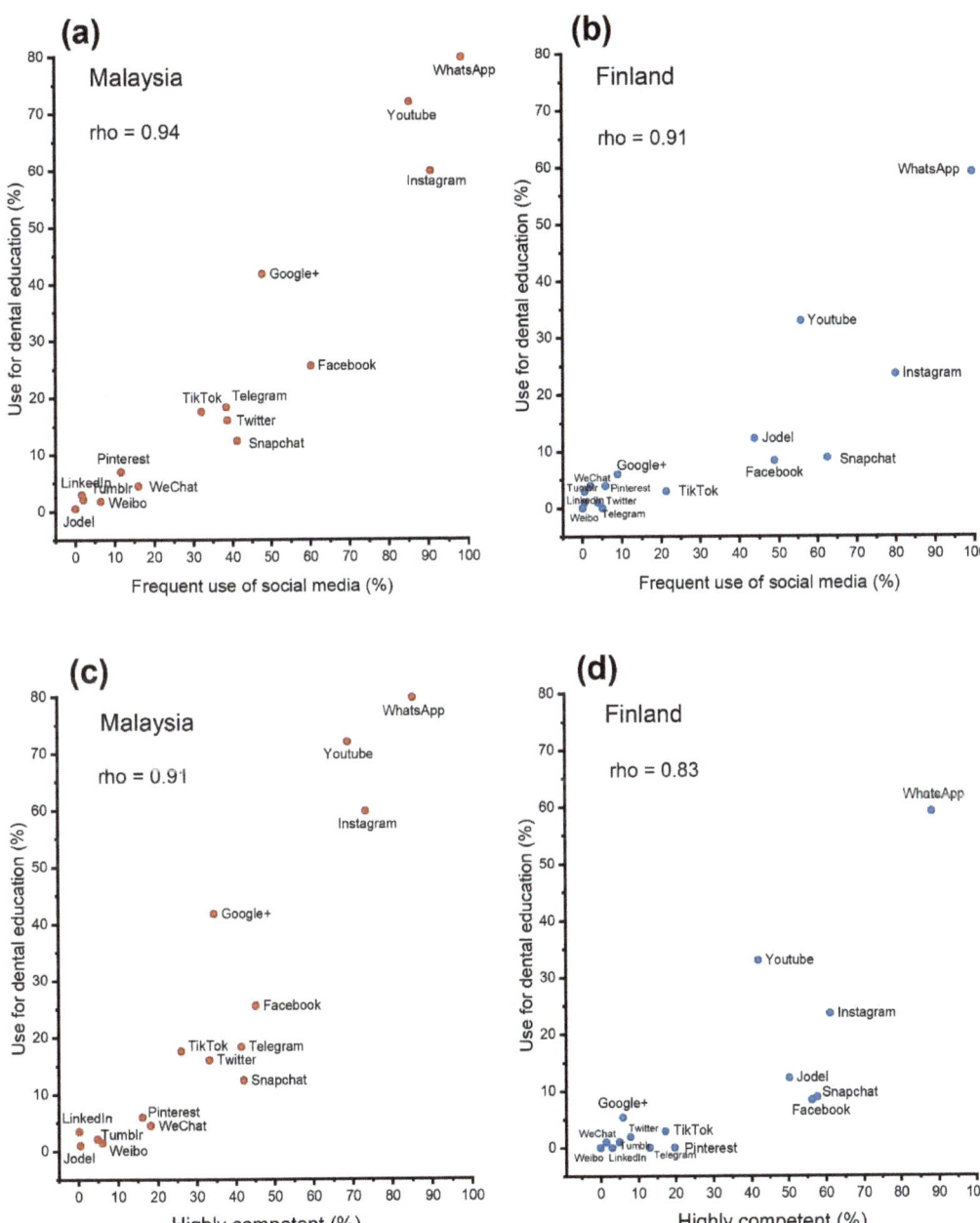

Figure 4. (a) Scatter plot showing correlation between percentage frequency of use of social media platforms (frequent and very frequent) for personal use vs. use in dental education in Malaysia and (b) in Finland; (c) Scatter plot showing correlations between perceived competence (highly competent) of use of social media platforms vs. use in dental education in Malaysia, and (d) in Finland. Data include dental undergraduate students from Malaysia (n = 440) and Finland (n = 203). rho = Spearman's rank correlation coefficient.

3.6. Encouraging or Preventing Factors to Use Social Media

Table 5 reports factors that encouraged students to use social media platforms. To stay in touch with friends and family members was very important in both countries (77.0% in Malaysia vs. 86.2% in Finland). However, Malaysian students valued platforms more in connecting with old friends they had lost touch with than Finnish students. Malaysian students found social media platforms also more encouraging in communicating about issues related to dental training (Table 5).

Table 5. Frequency and percentage distributions of responses to questions "How important is each of the following factors in encouraging you to use social media?" by country. Data include dental undergraduate students from Malaysia (n = 440) and Finland (n = 203).

Factor	Country	Not at All Important n (%)	Somewhat Important n (%)	Very Important n (%)	I Don't Use Social Media n (%)	p-Value of Exact Chi-Square Test
To stay in touch with current friends and family members	Malaysia	5 (1.1)	91 (20.7)	339 (77.0)	5 (1.1)	0.006
	Finland	5 (2.5)	23 (11.3)	175 (86.2)	0	
To connect with old friends, I have lost touch with	Malaysia	20 (4.5)	195 (44.3)	219 (49.8)	6 (1.4)	<0.001
	Finland	44 (21.7)	113 (55.7)	42 (20.7)	4 (2.0)	
To connect around a shared hobby	Malaysia	61 (13.9)	200 (45.5)	166 (37.7)	13 (3.0)	0.884
	Finland	33 (16.3)	89 (43.8)	75 (36.9)	6 (3.0)	
To communicate about issues relating to dental training	Malaysia	13 (3.0)	198 (45.0)	217 (49.3)	12 (2.7)	<0.001
	Finland	27 (13.3)	97 (47.8)	79 (38.9)	0	

We also asked students about factors that prevented them from using social media. Students from Malaysia reported more often reasons that they experienced important not to use social media than students from Finland (Figure 4). Over 80% of the Finnish dental students reported that lack of knowledge was not an issue in social media usage, while 85% of Malaysian students felt that lack of knowledge prevented them from using social media platforms somewhat or very much. Similar differences were observed with lack of time, lack of interest, lack of perceived value and concern about harm to professional image (Figure 5).

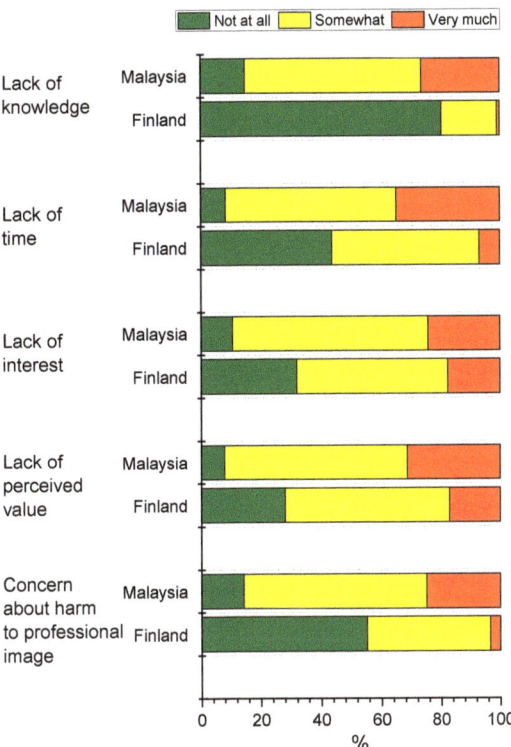

Figure 5. Percentage distributions of responses to question "How much the following reasons (factors) prevent you from using social media?" by country. Data include dental undergraduate students from Malaysia ($n = 440$) and Finland ($n = 203$). There were statistically significant differences ($p < 0.001$) between the countries among all reasons (factors). Significances were evaluated by chi-square test.

4. Discussion

The present comparative study between Malaysian and Finnish universities was conducted to evaluate the social media usage among dental undergraduate students. We found that the same top five platforms (WhatsApp, YouTube, Instagram, Facebook and Snapchat) were the most familiar services to the respondents from both countries. There were country-specific differences among students in the familiarity and usage of the other platforms. For most applications, students in Malaysia spent more hours per week using the platforms as study tools than students in Finland. Malaysian students found social media platforms more encouraging in communicating about issues related to dental training. Finnish dental students reported more often that lack of knowledge was not an issue in social media usage, while the majority of Malaysian students felt that lack of knowledge prevented them from using social media platforms somewhat or very much. Age and year of dental studies were not clearly associated in either country with the frequent use of the platforms.

Most students from both countries used social media for more than eleven hours per week. In addition, 25.3% of the respondents used social media more than twenty hours per week. This is not surprising but reflects the current habits of communication among young adults. Recent studies from different fields of study have reported that undergraduate students spent on average about three to four hours per day using social media platforms [18–21]. These services include mainly entertainment and communication, but also learning and searching for general information.

Our findings reflect the global popularity of the same platforms in contemporary society and show that most students are now heavy users of these platforms in the two culturally different countries. Most of the participants from both countries were familiar with WhatsApp, YouTube, Instagram, and Facebook. In a global world, students are also aware of other several social media services, but do not necessarily use all of them. There was a difference in the familiarity with some of the social media applications by the students in both countries. Malaysian students were more familiar with Telegram, WeChat, and Weibo while Finnish students were more familiar with Snapchat, Jodel and LinkedIn. This difference could be attributed to the students being familiar with the social media applications that are more commonly used in their region. Probably most of the students use those applications that their peers use so that there is an ease in communication and sharing. Jodel is a community-based social media application and is limited to its use in Europe and part of the Middle East [22]. LinkedIn is a social platform that mainly caters to people involved in business and has so far been very popular with the older age group [23] and among dental professionals looking to develop connections [24]. Finnish students being slightly older could account for their greater familiarity with LinkedIn. Familiarity with Telegram and its usage has grown exponentially in Malaysia as it is a popular medium to disseminate official information from Government [25]. There was no statistically significant difference in the usage of social media based on age, sex, and years of study in both the groups of students, though female students showed a greater tendency to use Instagram than the male which is similar to the worldwide data [26].

When considering the prevalence of using social media services among dental students, it is worth noting that these services have different purposes and target audiences. For example, the students in our sample may be too old to use Snapchat, a popular chat and communication channel for children and young people, for daily communication. On the other hand, they are still too young and without sufficient work experience to seek new work contacts through LinkedIn. The popularity of WhatsApp among study participants reflects the importance of keeping in touch with friends, family members or members of other restricted messaging groups in a convenient way (whether by text, picture or voice). Instagram and Twitter offer channels to increase internet online visibility. Using YouTube involves sharing your own videos and watching and commenting on other users' videos.

It was observed that all the students had greater competency in the social media applications they used most frequently which was primarily WhatsApp. Between both the groups of students, the difference observed regarding competence in using social media was the same as observed related to social media usage. Application usage by individual increases as he/she becomes more familiar with its features and thereby feels competent in using the application. Age of the student, year of study did not show any significance regarding the perception of competence for using social media applications, though females showed statistically significant competence in using Instagram, which seems to be very popular among females [26].

Our research clearly showed that students prefer to use for educational purposes the same platforms as they use for personal communication and online visibility. An interesting finding was spending a greater number of hours per week on the most popular social media applications like WhatsApp, YouTube, Instagram, and Facebook by the Malaysian students for purposes related to their dental education. This was statistically significant compared to Finnish students who used more hours on Jodel for the assignments or tutorials. This contrasts with a study from Saudi where dental students preferred to use Facebook for their learning [21].

The literature is not conclusive about the effects of social media on healthcare education. Some studies have reported a positive impact of social media on education while some have mentioned the reluctance of students to use social media for their education due to perceived negative impacts [27–30]. There is a study on the use of social media for dental health promotion [13], for dental marketing [11] and for dental education [31], as well as a review on what has been carried out so far in literature [10]. Literature also has studies on the usage of social media by dental students and its effects [21,29,32], however, in Malaysia and Finland, it is not known how dental students are using social media. It is known that the dental students of the present cohort are digital natives, they use social media universally and their dental education includes information retrieval studies using online platforms [33]. In Finland, all study programs in the participating faculties require the use of social media in different forms now. Social media is an integral part of modern pedagogy along with other methods. The dental schools of this study in Malaysia (Manipal Melaka Medical College and the University of Malaya) and Finland (the University of Helsinki and the University of Oulu) follow the official guidelines for social media use and learning these is also an elementary study content of every dental student.

Dental students from both countries considered keeping in touch with family and friends as a very important factor that encouraged them to use social media. This is probably why WhatsApp as a communication tool is so popular. It should be noted that the effect of social media tools may affect soft skills such as communication and confidence in spoken language in the future among these students.

For Malaysian students, the reasons for refraining from the use of social media applications such as lack of knowledge about a particular application of interest, lack of time, lack of interest, lack of perceived value and concern about harmful effects on professional image, were more important than to Finnish students. In Malaysia, as per the MCMC report, one of the top reasons for Malaysians not using the internet in 2020 was a lack of interest [25]. The same report also mentioned that while the majority of Malaysians' online activity is sending text messages to communicate and visit social media sites, sharing of content using social media has gone up since 2018.

The extensive use of social media may have several drawbacks. Dental students should be made aware of the quality of information that they obtain from social media [33,34]. Social media content related to education may not be evidence-based or referenced from reliable sources since anyone can upload content that can affect not only their learning but also the profession [21]. Using social media can be time-consuming, addictive and distract from studying [19–21]. The social media activity of some healthcare students has also resulted in unanticipated ethical consequences [6]. In our study, questions were not specific to dental education and most of the questions were regarding the general use of social media. So, it would be inappropriate to extrapolate the questions of our study to social media use in dental learning. We will explore the disadvantages of using social media, long-term consequences, and perceptions of e-professionalism among dental students in our further study.

The present study used only a self-completed questionnaire and may suffer from the disadvantages of a cross-sectional online survey. The questionnaire failed to explain the underlying reasons for using specific platforms. In addition, the cross-sectional nature of our study made it impossible to assess possible rapid changes in students' use and preferences of social media. We did not study how social media communication has affected study engagement before and during the COVID-pandemic. Thus, we do not know whether and how the pandemic changed students' social media use. Future studies will need to study trends and priorities of social media use among dental students. Another limitation of this study should be noted. It was performed in local settings in Malaysia and Finland. Each regional setting is unique. Despite its limited scope, our findings might be helpful in considering the use of social media in different forms, and especially when considering students' attitudes, preferences, and experiences with various platforms.

5. Conclusions

This multi-institutional study provides useful information on the usage of social media during the COVID-pandemic among dental students in two culturally different countries. The findings offer evidence that dental students used social media extensively in both countries. A few apps, which are popular worldwide, are widely used by students for both personal communication and education. Regionally popular platforms bring variety to the social media toolbox of dental students. Extensive use of social media can also be a distraction, especially when used for non-educational purposes. Students should be guided if they have specific interests or lack knowledge in some respects.

Supplementary Materials: The following are available online at https://www.mdpi.com/article/10.3390/healthcare9111408/s1, Questionnaire.

Author Contributions: Conceptualization, E.U., P.N. and S.A.M.; methodology, E.U., P.N. and S.A.M.; formal analysis, P.N.; data curation, P.N. and E.H.; writing—original draft preparation, E.U.; writing—review and editing, P.N., S.A.M., J.J., E.H., M.-L.L., O.-P.L., E.V., A.A. and K.K.; supervision, P.N. All authors have read and agreed to the published version of the manuscript.

Funding: This research received no external funding.

Institutional Review Board Statement: Ethical approval to conduct this study was obtained for the institutions in Malaysia; Medical Ethics Committee, Faculty of Dentistry, University of Malaya [DF CD2105/0015 (L)] and Research Ethics committee, Faculty of dentistry, Melaka Manipal Medical college [MMMC/FOD/AR/E C-2021(F-01)] prior to commencement of the study. According to the guidelines of the Ministry of Education and Culture in Finland, survey studies with anonymous questionnaires do not need an approval from an ethics committee.

Informed Consent Statement: Informed consent was obtained from all students involved in the study.

Data Availability Statement: The data presented in this study are available on request from the corresponding author.

Conflicts of Interest: The authors declare no conflict of interest.

References

1. Oakley, M.; Spallek, H. Social media in dental education: A call for research and action. *J. Dent. Educ.* **2012**, *76*, 279–287. [CrossRef]
2. Kenny, P.; Johnson, I.G. Social media use, attitudes, behaviours and perceptions of online professionalism amongst dental students. *Br. Dent. J.* **2016**, *221*, 651–655. [CrossRef]
3. De Peralta, T.L.; Farrior, O.F.; Flake, N.M.; Gallagher, D.; Susin, C.; Valenza, J. The use of social media by dental students for communication and learning: Two viewpoints. *J. Dent. Educ.* **2019**, *83*, 663–668. [CrossRef]
4. Oksa, R.; Kaakinen, M.; Savela, N.; Hakanen, J.J.; Oksanen, A. Professional Social Media Usage and Work Engagement AmongProfessionals in Finland Before and During the COVID-19 Pandemic: Four-Wave Follow-Up Study. *J. Med. Internet Res.* **2021**, *23*, e29036. [CrossRef]
5. Desta, M.A.; Workie, M.B.; Yemer, D.B.; Denku, C.Y.; Berhanu, M.S. Social Media Usage in Improving English Language Proficiency from the Viewpoint of Medical Students. *Adv. Med. Educ. Pract.* **2021**, *12*, 519–528. [CrossRef]
6. Dobson, E.; Patel, P.; Neville, P. Perceptions of E-Professionalism among Dental Students: A UK Dental School Study. *Br. Dent. J.* **2019**, *226*, 73–78. [CrossRef]
7. Sharka, R.; San Diego, J.P.; Nasseripour, M.; Banerjee, A. Identifying Risk Factors Affecting the Usage of Digital and Social Media: A Preliminary Qualitative Study in the Dental Profession and Dental Education. *Dent. J.* **2021**, *9*, 53. [CrossRef] [PubMed]
8. Arnett, M.R.; Christensen, H.L.; Nelson, B.A. A School-Wide Assessment of Social Media Usage by Students in a US Dental School. *Br. Dent. J.* **2014**, *217*, 531–535. [CrossRef] [PubMed]
9. Aboalshamat, K.; Alkiyadi, S.; Alsaleh, S.; Reda, R.; Alkhaldi, S.; Badeeb, A.; Gabb, N. Attitudes toward Social Media among Practicing Dentists and Dental Students in Clinical Years in Saudi Arabia. *Open Dent. J.* **2019**, *13*, 143–149. [CrossRef]
10. Pereira, C.A. Dentistry and the Social Media. *RGO-Rev. Gaúcha Odontol.* **2017**, *65*, 229–236. [CrossRef]
11. Affendi, N.H.K.; Hamid, N.F.A.; Razak, M.S.A.; Nudin, I.I.I. The Pattern of Social Media Marketing by Dentist in Malaysia. *Malays. Dent. J.* **2020**, *1*, 24–42.
12. Radeef, A.S.; Faisal, G.G. Internet Addiction among Dental Students in Malaysia. *J. Int. Dent. Med. Res.* **2019**, *12*, 1452–1456.
13. Rani, H.; Yahya, N.A.; Rosli, T.I.; Mohd-Dom, T.N. Preparing Dental Students to Use Social Media as a Platform to Promote Oral Health. *J. Dent. Educ.* **2020**, 1–2. [CrossRef] [PubMed]
14. Lim, J.S.Y.; Agostinho, S.; Harper, B.; Chicharo, J.F. Investigating the use of social media by university undergraduate informatics programs in Malaysia. In *International Conference on Educational Technologies Proceeding Book*; 2013; pp. 143–147. ISBN 978-972-8939-99-1.
15. Kitsis, E.A.; Milan, F.B.; Cohen, H.W.; Myers, D.; Herron, P.; McEvoy, M.; Weingarten, J.; Grayson, M.S. Who's Misbehaving? Perceptions of Unprofessional Social Media Use by Medical Students and Faculty. *BMC Med. Educ.* **2016**, *16*, 1–7. [CrossRef]
16. Bartlett, J.E.; Kotrlik, J.W.; Higgins, C.C. Organizational Research: Determining Appropriate Sample Size in Survey Research. *Inform. Technol. Learn. Perform. J.* **2001**, *19*, 43–50.
17. Cochran, W.G. *Sampling Techniques*, 3rd ed.; John Wiley & Sons: New York, NY, USA, 1977; ISBN 978-0-471-16240-7.

18. Chaklader, M.A.; Zahir, Z.; Yasmeen, S. Original article effects of social media on academic performance of medical students of a selected tertiary medical college. *Bangladesh Med. Coll. J.* **2021**, *26*, 30–35.
19. Eriş, H.; Havlioğlu, S.; Kaya, M. The Effect of Mobile Phone Use of Universty Students on Their Academic Success. *Eur. J. Sci. Technol.* **2021**, *27*, 433–438. [CrossRef]
20. Kircaburun, K.; Alhabash, S.; Tosuntaş, Ş.B.; Griffiths, M.D. Uses and gratifications of problematic social media use among university students: A simultaneous examination of the big five of personality traits, social media platforms, and social media use motives. *Int. J. Ment. Health Addict.* **2020**, *18*, 525–547. [CrossRef]
21. Rajeh, M.T.; Sembawa, S.N.; Nassar, A.A.; Al Hebshi, S.A.; Aboalshamat, K.T.; Badri, M.K. Social media as a learning tool: Dental students' perspectives. *J. Dent. Educ.* **2021**, *85*, 513–520. [CrossRef]
22. Jodel. About Us. Available online: https://about.jodel.com/#numbers (accessed on 21 July 2021).
23. Hootsuite. Top LinkedIn Demographics That Matter to Social Media Marketers. Available online: https://blog.hootsuite.com/linkedin-demographics-for-business/#general (accessed on 21 July 2021).
24. Dentistry Today. Use LinkedIn to Promote Your Dental Practice. Available online: https://www.dentistrytoday.com/news/todays-dental-news/item/2858-use-linkedin-to-promote-your-dental-practice (accessed on 21 July 2021).
25. Malaysian Communications and Multimedia Comission. Internet Users Survey. Available online: https://www.mcmc.gov.my/en/resources/statistics/internet-users-survey (accessed on 21 July 2021).
26. Farsi, D. Social Media and Health Care, Part i: Literature Review of Social Media Use by Health Care Providers. *J. Med. Internet Res.* **2021**, *23*. [CrossRef]
27. Lahiry, S.; Choudhury, S.; Chatterjee, S.; Hazra, A. Impact of social media on academic performance and interpersonal relation: A cross-sectional study among students at a tertiary medical center in east india. *J. Educ. Health Promot.* **2019**, *8*. [CrossRef]
28. Spallek, H.; Turner, S.P.; Donate-Bartfield, E.; Chambers, D.; McAndrew, M.; Zarkowski, P.; Karimbux, N. Social Media in the Dental School Environment, Part B: Curricular Considerations. *J. Dent. Educ.* **2015**, *79*, 1153–1166. [CrossRef]
29. Saadeh, R.A.; Saadeh, N.A.; de la Torre, M.A. Determining the Usage of Social Media for Medical Information by the Medical and Dental Students in Northern Jordan. *J. Taibah Univ. Med. Sci.* **2020**, *15*, 110–115. [CrossRef] [PubMed]
30. Deogade, S.C.; Saxena, S.; Mishra, P. Adverse Health Effects and Unhealthy Behaviors among Dental Undergraduates Surfing Social Networking Sites. *Ind. Psychiatry J.* **2017**, *26*, 207. [CrossRef] [PubMed]
31. Seo, C.W.; Cho, A.R.; Park, J.C.; Cho, H.Y.; Kim, S. Dental Students' Learning Attitudes and Perceptions of YouTube as a Lecture Video Hosting Platform in a Flipped Classroom in Korea. *J. Educ. Eval. Health Prof.* **2018**, *15*, 24. [CrossRef] [PubMed]
32. Naguib, G.H. Social Media Usage and Self Perception among Dental Students at King Abdulaziz University, Saudi Arabia. *J. Med. Educ.* **2018**, *17*, 109–119. [CrossRef]
33. Nieminen, P.; Uma, E.; Pal, S.; Laitala, M.-L.; Lappalainen, O.-P.; Varghese, E. Information Retrieval and Awareness about Evidence-Based Dentistry among Dental Undergraduate Students — A Comparative Study between Students from Malaysia and Finland. *Dent. J.* **2020**, *8*, 103. [CrossRef]
34. Nieminen, P.; Virtanen, J.I. Information Retrieval, Critical Appraisal and Knowledge of Evidence-Based Dentistry among Finnish Dental Students. *Eur. J. Dent. Educ.* **2017**, *21*, 214–219. [CrossRef]

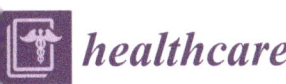

Article

Pharmacy Student Challenges and Strategies towards Initial COVID-19 Curriculum Changes

Luyao Liu, Suzanne Caliph, Claire Simpson, Ruohern Zoe Khoo, Geenath Neviles, Sithira Muthumuni and Kayley M. Lyons *

Faculty of Pharmacy and Pharmaceutical Sciences, Monash University, Parkville, VIC 3052, Australia; lliu0007@student.monash.edu (L.L.); Suzanne.Caliph@monash.edu (S.C.); csim0005@student.monash.edu (C.S.); rkho0002@student.monash.edu (R.Z.K.); gnev0001@student.monash.edu (G.N.); smut0004@student.monash.edu (S.M.)
* Correspondence: Kayley.lyons@monash.edu

Abstract: Due to COVID-19, tertiary institutions were forced to deliver knowledge virtually, which proposed challenges for both institutions and students. In this study, we aimed to characterize pharmacy students' challenges and strategies during COVID-19 curriculum changes, therefore developing a comprehensive understanding of students' learning, wellbeing, and resilience in the ever-changing situation. Data were collected from student written reflections across four year levels at one school of pharmacy from March–May 2020. In addition, data were collected from written responses of second-year pharmacy students responding to prompted questions. The data were qualitatively analyzed inductively by five coders using NVivo 12. For each piece of data, two coders independently coded the data, calculated the inter-rater agreement, and resolved discrepancies. The most coded challenges were 'negative emotional response' and 'communication barrier during virtual learning'. The most coded strategies were 'using new technology' and 'time management'. This study allows researchers and education institutions to gain an overview of pharmacy students' experiences during COVID-19, therefore helping universities to provide students with necessary support and techniques on how to self-cope with COVID-19 as well as stressful events in the future.

Keywords: e-learning; healthcare education; clinical teaching

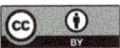

1. Introduction

At the beginning of the COVID-19 global crisis, healthcare education institutions and their students underwent transformative change. Overnight, institutions cut placements, moved small-group learning to Zoom®, and delivered education virtually. The self-isolation and new virtual learning systems influenced students' study and daily life, potentially resulting in negative impacts on some students' well-being [1,2]. For example, a recent study in China reported that 24.9% of their medical student cohort experienced anxiety to some degree due to social distancing and a lack of interpersonal communication during the COVID-19 pandemic [3]. Students have reported several challenges and low satisfaction with engaging in virtual learning during COVID-19 [1,4]. In contrast, other authors have reported that health professions students have adapted well from the challenges and virtual learning has resulted in better attendance, engagement, and feedback as both teaching staff and students have created various ways to cope [5,6].

Due to these varied responses to online learning, scholars have been interested in exploring the factors that influence student satisfaction during COVID-19. Chen and colleagues have found that student satisfaction with online learning during COVID-19 was explained by the quality of the online platform, emotional changes, and communication with students [4]. Chiu proposes that self-determination theory can help explain student engagement during COVID-19 [7]. Self-determination theory encourages educators to support student autonomy, competence, and relatedness in online learning. Satisfaction of three basic needs will, therefore, improve students' behavioural, emotional, and cognitive engagement [7,8].

The purpose of this study is to gain a comprehensive understanding of pharmacy student benefits, challenges and strategies during the first few months of the COVID-19 pandemic. By examining the fallout from the immediate transition from face-to-face learning to distance virtual learning, this study contributes to a better understanding healthcare students' adaptability and well-being throughout the pandemic. There is limited research on what types of strategies students have implemented in response to COVID-19's effect on their learning, well-being, and motivation. For example, we are extending the work by Chiu into higher education. Additionally, this study will add to the emerging literature of the types of benefits that COVID-19 has had on their learning and development as future health care professionals. Insights from this study will allow healthcare education institutions to identify necessary student supports for this current pandemic and any future interruptions. This study will also provide an insight for future researchers during this time of unprecedented stress on the students.

Research questions for this study as follows:

RQ1: What types of benefits did pharmacy students experience during COVID-19?
RQ2: What types of challenges did pharmacy students experience during COVID-19?
RQ3: What types of strategies did pharmacy students use during COVID-19?

2. Materials and Methods

2.1. Study Design

The study design was a qualitative case study at one university institution. Our aim was to characterize pharmacy students' experience during the first few months of the COVID-19 pandemic. The study was conducted through the analysis of students' written reflections relevant to COVID-19 curriculum changes. In total, 774 responses from March 2020 to May 2020 were analyzed using Nvivo 12. Our six coders were guided by the research questions to independently code students' written responses, and a codebook was developed based on several theories.

Previous studies have utilized software log data, questionnaires, interviews, and more [3,4,6,7]. Though these data sources are beneficial for understanding our studied phenomenon, we add a new perspective by analyzing students' naturally occurring reflections. We mined students' written reflections for what they spontaneously say affected them during COVID-19. These responses may differ than if we asked students directly in a questionnaire or interview. Other researchers have also mined written reflections for insights on the effects of COVID-19 but these were conducted with a focus on educators [9] and graduate students [10]. Findyartini and colleagues also explored health professions students' written reflections by looking at medical students in Indonesia [11]. Our study provides another case-study in this area to triangulate Finyartini and colleagues' results.

2.2. Participants and Study Context

The participants of this study included first, second, third, and fourth-year pharmacy students studying a Bachelor of Pharmacy (Honors) and/or Master of Pharmacy at Monash University in Melbourne, Australia. The program follows the Pharmaceutical Society of Australia's National Competency Standards Framework for Pharmacists in Australia [12].

The data collection occurred from March to May in 2020 following emergency education changes due to COVID-19. A summary of changes we made are outlined in a recent commentary [13]. Overall, the curriculum followed a standardized flipped classroom model explained in recent investigations of our program [14,15]. For on-campus learning, each week the students complete the following activities: (1) one day of self-directed online learning, (2) a day of large-class interactive lectures, (3) two days of small group workshops (one facilitator for 30 students in teams of five), and (4) a final day of "close-the-loop" lectures to answer any question and solidify the material. Before the first few months of COVID-19, the students attended large lectures and small group workshops in person.

After COVID-19, these activities were shifted to Zoom conferencing technology. Some of the lectures and workshops were shortened or replaced with interactive online modules [10]. Before COVID-19, students attended placements in hospitals and community pharmacies, taking more responsibility each year they progressed in the program. After the first few months of COVID-19, some placements were shifted to virtual placements and others granted students more responsibility to assist with the increased workload at the pharmacy.

At Monash University, all pharmacy students complete a skills coaching program. The data for this study were collected in the context of a skills coaching program. The purpose of the skills coaching program is for students to develop their professional skills by discussing and reflecting upon eight professional skills: problem-solving, oral communication, written communication, empathy, reflective practice, integrity, teamwork, and inquiry. Students are required to attend skill coach meetings every few weeks. Before every skill coach meeting, students write Personalized Learning Plans (PLPs) on an ePortfolio. After submitting to the ePortfolio, a skill coach (e.g., faculty member, practicing pharmacist) provides feedback on the students' PLP.

2.3. Data Collection

Data were collected from two sources. The first data source was the students' PLPs across all year levels. The second source of data was second-year students' written answers to written prompts during a skill coach meeting discussing student challenges and strategies related to COVID-19.

For the PLPs, students have the liberty to talk about incidents that have affected their skills, and therefore COVID-19 was a frequent and naturally emerging topic. The PLPs were collected from March 2020 to May 2020, following the start of the COVID-19 outbreak. From all available PLPs, we only selected PLPs which contained the following words for this study: 'corona', 'COVID-19', 'online', 'zoom', 'virtual', 'virus', 'lockdown', 'quarantine', and 'pandemic.' Of the many written PLPs, there were a total of 879 PLPs that met this inclusion criteria (i.e., contained certain words). A further 67 PLPs were excluded by coders due to the lack of relevance with our study. Each PLP varied in length from 100 to 400 words.

In addition to the PLPs, we collected data from an in-class learning activity. During a skills coach meeting, second-year pharmacy students were asked prompts on a shared Google Doc® to facilitate discussion in groups of 10-12 students and a skills coach. The prompts were "What impacts are you seeing from COVID19?" and "How are you supporting your well-being during this time?" We collected all available student responses—197 responses from the first prompt and 97 responses from the second prompt.

2.4. Ethical Considerations

The Monash University Human Ethics Low Risk Review Committee approved this study (Project ID 24477). At the Monash Faculty of Pharmacy and Pharmaceutical Sciences, the pharmacy students are enrolled in an education research registry. Each year all students were informed of education research projects and presented with the opportunity to opt out of having their student data used for education research. For this study, we removed any PLPs from students who have opted-out of the education research registry.

2.5. Data Analysis

To analyze the data, we used a directed content analysis approach according to our three research questions [16,17]. First, we developed a codebook based on relevant theoretical frameworks and previous literature on self-determination theory, motivational strategies, learning strategies, and time management [18–21]. Research question two was guided by self-determination theory. Research question three was guided by frameworks in motivational, learning, and time management strategies. We open-coded responses for research question one.

Self-determination theory. Self-determination theory (SDT) is an empirically based theory of human motivation, development and wellness [18]. In our research, SDT served as the primary theoretical framework for coding students' challenges, investigating how the pandemic has been causing frustration on their three basic needs: competence, relatedness, and autonomy [22].

Motivational strategies. Motivation refers to a student's willingness to engage and persist in a task. Motivational regulation strategies may be triggered when students experience problems with their ongoing level of motivation, learning, and performance [19]. The coding was developed based on seven motivation regulation strategies identified by Maenpaa including environment structuring, self-consequating, goal-oriented self-talk, efficacy management, emotion regulation, regulation of value, and interest enhancement [19].

Learning strategies. The codes for learning strategies were primarily developed from ten different types of learning strategies examined by Dunlosky and colleagues including elaborative interrogation, self-explanation, summarization, highlighting (or underlining), the keyword mnemonic, imagery use for text learning, rereading, practice testing, distributed practice, and interleaved practice [20]. Ten learning techniques were either summarized from literature indicating they might improve student performance or surveys that students reported using them most frequently. As we aimed to identify strategies in virtual learning, the techniques were intentionally selected as students should be able to practice them without assistance and supervision.

Time management. Self-learning regulation models mainly focus on three perspectives of managing time: planning, monitoring, and regulating [23]. Uzir et al. clearly demonstrated that students who actively and consistently use time management strategies were associated with higher academic performance, established the relationship between the use of time management strategies and learning performance in blended learning of a health science course [21].

Six coders (LL, CS, RK, GN, SM, and KL) applied the codebook to the data using Nvivo12®. First, the six coders underwent a calibration phase by coding the data together. During the calibration phase, the coders added emerging codes and built group agreement for accurately coding the data. Then, five coders coded all of the second-year pharmacy student written responses together. After the calibration phase, the PLP data set (879 PLPs) were divided into teams of two coders. For each PLP, two coders independently coded the PLP. During this process, pairs of coders met to calculate inter-coder reliability and resolve their coding disagreements. The overall team of six coders met frequently to discuss changes to the codebook and KL frequently audited all of the team's coding output.

After coding 480 out of the 879 PLPs, the team decided it had reached a saturation point and ceased coding. The saturation point was defined as the time when coding did not produce any new codes and the data coded under each code was often redundant [24]. After coding had ceased, the team calculated a final inter-rater agreement rate. Following coding, we identified themes and categories according to the established research questions. Frequent and salient themes were reported.

3. Results

The simple inter-rater agreement rate for all codes was 80.3%. The final codebook is included in Table 1. The results are organized according to research question.

3.1. What Types of Benefits Did Pharmacy Students Experience during COVID-19?

Although to a lesser extent than the challenges, many students discussed how COVID-19 had resulted in positive impacts on their studies and lives. Although we did not originally plan to investigate the benefits of COVID-19, it became an important and emerging research question. The benefits pharmacy students gained during COVID-19 depended on their experiences. In general, students on placement during COVID-19 shared positive practice experiences, whereas students completing remote learning benefited from 'more time for themselves, family, friends, and Uni' and 'less travel commuting'.

Table 1. The types of benefits that pharmacy students experienced during initial COVID-19 changes.

Theme	Number of References (n =)	Student Quotes
Having satisfying placement experiences	n = 27	"As such, I was able to see the positive impact of a level-headed and knowledgeable health professional on an anxious patient" "This position has given me great exposure, learning to dispense in a hospital, understand how our healthcare system is adapting to flatten the curve and even given me a chance to work on a COVID ward"
Less travel commuting	n = 14	"I can manage my study at my own time" "I can catch up with Uni work because I spent less time travelling to Uni"
More family time	n = 14	"Getting to spend more time at home with family members" "Calling my family and friends back in Malaysia more often"
Feeling valued and helpful during the pandemic	n = 13	"I felt a sense of responsibility in being able to juggle assisting and being of value to the pharmacy team during this demanding time"

Overall, of the benefit codes, having positive placement experiences was the most frequently coded theme (n = 27 instances). For some students, their placements during COVID-19 were the most experiential of their learning experiences. For example, one student said, "in my time at [hospital] amidst the COVID-19 pandemic, I had my most productive & growth-driven placement that has fundamentally changed how I approach my patients even as a student pharmacist." Students discussed various reasons for why their placements were valuable during this time. Several students said they were "contributing", "helping the pharmacy" and "a part of the team". Students also thought their placements were interesting as they witnessed firsthand how pharmacies handled the fallout from pandemic.

The second most frequently coded theme was less travel commuting (n = 14). Transitioning to virtual learning meant some students "can manage [their] study at [their] own time" and "catch up with uni work" because they "spend less time travelling to uni". Some students appreciated staying at home to enjoy more family time (n = 14), more friend time (n = 4) and more self-time (n = 7).

3.2. What Types of Challenges Did Pharmacy Students Experience during COVID-19?

Similar to the benefits, the challenges of COVID-19 depended on the setting. We identified three main themes under challenges using SDT: Autonomy frustration, relatedness frustration, competence frustration. However, challenges also varied whether students were participating in virtual learning, placements, part-time pharmacy job, and a group inquiry (i.e., research) project (See Table 2).

Autonomy frustration refers to the feeling of no choice when students are carrying out an activity [22]. For example, students discussed in their reflections about how they were negatively impacted by the travel ban. The travel restriction (n = 12) has particularly impacted on the students coming from/planning to travel to the regions on the travel ban list, resulting in ending their trips early or cancelling their future trips, especially international students.

Competence frustration refers to feeling incapable of carrying out an activity [22]. For example, some students were struggling with managing their time (n= 22) and keeping up to date with their study (n = 22). Without the accountability of physically attending lectures and workshops, some of them "found [themselves] tend to procrastinate the work and the work [kept] piling up day by day", and sometimes even worse, "[they] tend to forget that [they] actually still have classes and accidentally plan [ned] something on the time slot when [they] should be attending classes". Students who were unable to manage their time generally felt "rushed", "stagnant", "overwhelmed" and eventually "lost in [their] study".

Table 2. The types of challenges that pharmacy students experienced during initial COVID-19 changes.

Theme	Number of References (n =)	Student Quotes
Challenges of working in community pharmacy (part-time job and placement)	n = 256	"Felt overwhelmed by extra workload" "The pharmacy I work at has become 10 times busier than usual to the point where I have to work overtime unpaid, and get feverish from trying to remain calm with patients whilst maintaining empathy for our patients" "Some customers are frustrated, unwilling to wait and abusive to staff members"
Emotional responses	n = 147	"It has caused a lot of anxiety and frustration" "I have also continued to maintain professionalism in my work place as well as volunteer at the COVID-19 screening but it can be very mentally draining" "I found it quite disheartening and confronting, as this virus shows no rate of slowing down and its only getting worse and worse"
Communication barrier in virtual learning	n = 68	"Due to workshops occurring online, it was much more difficult for students to openly communicate with one another." "No one really wants to talk unless asked a question"
Social isolation	n = 49	"Being by myself has been a struggle because I can't meet my friends on weekends" "This has been hard for me as I live alone so I feel like I have lost all of my human interaction"
Difficulty adapting to online environment	n = 43	"I was completely lost with the new virtual learning environment" "I felt very uncomfortable and distracted to study with my camera on me as it creates a feeling of under surveillance"
Technical issues during virtual learning	n = 26	"I saw a message on top of my screen, stating that my "connection is lost" and this was when I freaked out even more."

Relatedness frustration refers to a lack of sense of belonging and connection to others [22]. As one of most coded themes, social isolation was coded 49 times (n = 49). Students were upset with entertainment restriction (n = 5) and travel restriction (n = 12). As one student illustrated, "while I love my alone time, finding anything to look forward to is a challenge". Unfortunately, a few students reported observing or personally experiencing racism (n = 6) during their part-time job in pharmacies. Students described "unfair", "feel attacked", and "upset" about the distressing incidents.

Emotional responses (n = 147). As one of the most coded themes, emotional responses refer to any negative emotions such as stress and anxiety. The emotional responses were related to curriculum changes, social isolation, placement and working environment changes and the risk of getting infected during the pandemic. Some students "lost [a] sense of routine" in virtual learning; some students "[felt] terrible about staying at home only"; some students were "overwhelmed to attend the placement during a pandemic" and some students were worried about serving an infected patient.

For those students participating in virtual learning, the most frequently coded theme was communication barriers (n = 68), followed by difficulty adapting to the virtual environment (n = 43). For some students, communication with their peers via virtual meetings was much more difficult than face-to-face communication. One of the barriers was the lack of body language (n = 11). The students said they "can't see visual cues" and it was "hard to make eye contact", making it harder to communicate virtually. Lack of engagement (n = 26), motivation (n = 26), and teammate contribution (n = 19) have worsened students' virtual learning experiences, especially with group assignments. Students complained that they "[feel] oddly disconnected during group meetings because people tend to stay silent" and "[they] don't feel like [they] are learning or contributing".

For the students that were undertaking a placement at the time, many challenges were posed against them. This mostly included fourth-year pharmacy students who were assigned two 4-week placement blocks. Many other students also reflected on their part-time job in the pharmacy. The most frequently coded challenge was a busy pharmacy (n = 63) and angry and difficult customers (n = 61). An example of a busy pharmacy response from a student includes "this was the most busiest and strangest experience for me in pharmacy". In addition, they were required to supply limited stock to patients who tried to stockpile medications (n = 45) due to stock shortage (n = 32). Many students witnessed "the rush of medication hoarding", which raised their concern for continuing care as "regular elderly patients [unable] to get their medications due to low stock". In addition, some placement students had very limited placement exposure (n = 37) due to COVID-19.

3.3. What Types of Strategies Did Pharmacy Students Use during COVID-19?

We identified four main categories under strategies: mental and physical wellbeing, learning strategies, time management, and motivational strategies (See Table 3).

Table 3. The types of strategies that pharmacy students used during initial COVID-19 changes.

Theme	Number of References (n =)	Student Quotes
Mental and physical well-being	n = 362	"I feel like that it is a very normal thought to have after talking to all my friends and opening up to them about my feelings" "Furthermore, practices of mindfulness that develop skills of resilience to help students to alleviate stress and objectively review the situation." "I will also try to reach out to a friend everyday and see how they are doing and offer support and relief the best I can"
Learning strategies	n = 285	"Eventually, I came up with the idea to work on the project via zoom, so we worked together, tapping in and out of the document and zoom when we needed to. This was far more efficient than working separately and waiting for the rest of the group members to see changes to the document and were able to complete and submit the report a day early" "We decided to make a group chat on messenger, making it easier for all group members to keep updates and to communicate with each other.'
Time management	n = 172	"Given the challenge of being at home and trying to keep on top of everything, I am going to make a timetable, that will separate my day into blocks, one block per subject." "I will reflect on how effective my timetable was at the end of each day. I will also make modifications to my timetable every Sunday until the timetable is suitable with my current lifestyle" "By doing this, my stress levels will decrease since I am more organized and I can also avoid completing my assignments at the very last minute."
Motivational strategies	n = 61	'It also acts as a way of keeping myself accountable in terms of studying, as we check up on each other's progress daily, and it has also made me more motivated to study and stay on top of coursework as it is the only time we get to see each other."

Physical and mental well-being. In terms of mental and physical wellbeing, COVID-19 preventative measures was the most coded theme (n = 84). Students emphasize that they have been practicing preventative and one student reflected, "As a pharmacist in training, this is an important lesson to be particularly vigilant and be role models for other students, friends and families". Following by COVID-19 preventative measures, virtual social activities (n = 55) and leisure activities (n = 51) were the next two most coded themes. Some students have planned to "reach out family and friends" every day because they believe "stay connected" is very important during the 'isolation period'. Meanwhile, doing leisure activities such as "pick[ing] a new hobby", "baking", and "watch[ing] TV shows" took students' attention away from the current situation and their stress.

Learning strategies. Not every one of Dunlosky's learning strategies was coded from students' reflection [20]. However, students have developed their own learning strategies in response to virtual learning. The most frequently coded strategy from Dunlosky was distributed practice (n = 25); implementing a schedule to spare their learning activities evenly over time. For example, one student commented, "I just have to get into a routine of studying during study time, while giving myself breaks so that I don't wear out too soon." Most students have also employed their own learning strategies to assist with their continued learning. Most coded strategy was the use of new technology (n = 169) (e.g., Google Calendar) to adapt themselves to the virtual learning environment, especially for group communication and collaboration.

Time management. Most of the students acknowledged the importance of managing their time appropriately, especially in independent learning. Planning time ahead (n = 107) was one of the most coded themes in the codebook. Students implemented different tactics of planning their time ahead of study to help them keep on track. However, only one student mentioned evaluating use of time after the task was completed (n = 1).

Motivational strategies. Out of motivational strategies, the most frequently coded theme was goal-oriented self-talk (n = 21), which refers to the process that students think about various reasons for persisting or completing a task. For example, one student said, "If I ever get into a low head space with little motivation, I will remember my goal of wanting to help people which will put me back on track." Students also reported that they were motivated by peer support. Students appreciated the support from friends and team members, motivating them to "keep [themselves] accountable in studying". On the other hand, some students have also employed the same strategy to encourage their team members by "sharing how well [they] have worked so far and appreciating each member's contribution to the team.

4. Discussion

Our study characterized pharmacy students' benefits, challenges and strategies during the COVID-19 pandemic. Although previous literature has focused on students' mental and learning challenges during pandemic [1–3], our research results provide an overview of both positive and negative pharmacy students' experiences in specific contexts (e.g., placement, virtual learning). Overall, the transition to virtual learning was welcomed by some students and challenging for others. In placements, students experienced novel situations. However, students working and learning at community pharmacies experienced work demands, racism and difficult patient encounters. Nonetheless, students have implemented various strategies in order to overcome these difficulties and adapt to the new learning environment.

Similar to previous research [1], we found that the emergency implementation of virtual learning created new dynamics and posed new challenges for the students. In terms of self-determination theory, many students experienced competence frustration due to the abrupt transition to virtual learning. The competence frustration may have been attributed to a lack of structure [25]. In this case, students no longer have the structure of the campus, going to the library, starting their day, and hallway conversations with peers. As a potential result, many students described their struggles with personal accountability, procrastination, and time management. Deci and Ryan also outlined that the frustration of basic psychological needs can thwart the autonomous motivation therefore negatively affect the academic performance and achievement [18,26,27]. In addition to motivational strategies, the educators might consider implementing strategies to support students' basic psychological needs in virtual learning. For example, educators might consider including students in decision-making of emergency changes to encourage student empowerment.

In particular, students cited poor-quality teamwork in virtual settings due to a lack of effective communication, motivation, and active engagement of all team members. The overwhelming descriptions of poor-quality teamwork is especially important considering that these students will work in healthcare in their career. These poor-quality teamwork experiences may discourage students from working collaboratively in the future. Therefore, educators may need to modify their approach. Just as multiplayer games and sport teams, group assignments requiring a strong team spirit can enhance students' relatedness satisfaction [8]. For example, educators may design the virtual group assignments to be more competitive to ensure effective engagement and contribution. Additionally, it might be necessary to consider liaising with students regarding expectations of active engagement in a virtual learning environment, such as switching on the webcam during lessons. Although previous researchers have shown that the characteristics of educators do not significantly influence students' learning outcomes in computer supported collaborative learning, they are still pivotal in relieving students' anxiety therefore improving students' academic performance [28].

Our research findings suggest that the majority of pharmacy students did not tend to employ learning strategies that were summarized from previous literature [20]. In a study conducted by Wolters et al., focusing on motivational regulation strategies, Wolters also found out that "students do not use all the types of motivational strategies equally" [29]. Although it is inspiring to see many students report developing their own strategies to overcome challenges and adapt to the new learning environment, this may reveal the need to educate the students on evidence-based approaches and introduce more advanced learning and motivational strategies. Due to the nature of the data source, the effectiveness of these self-developed strategies was not assessed. Therefore, future research that evaluates these strategies in the context of pandemic may be required.

In contrast, some students perceived some aspects of virtual learning as advantageous due to ease of accessibility and flexibility. Universities should apply what they learned from the emergency delivery of virtual learning to their future offerings. For example, our results suggest that students may prefer a combination of virtual learning on-campus learning. However, our research did not explore the correlation between virtual learning and academic learning outcomes and future research should continue to explore the affordance, effectiveness and barriers of blended learning models in the new post-COVID-19 reality. Specifically, future researchers could explore the impacts on educators, resources, and other types of students.

In addition to the findings that are corresponding to previous literature, our results provide an insight into the exclusive challenges faced by pharmacy students who went on placement or were participating in part-time jobs at local pharmacies. During the COVID-19 pandemic, some pharmacy students encountered limited placement exposure due to COVID-19 regulations in hospitals. On the other hand, students in community pharmacies felt that they were expected to handle excessive and unreasonable demands from customers in community pharmacy. In these cases, students may require individualized support from the faculty, in response to the rapidly changing placement and working environment. For example, educators might consider assigning additional assessment to students with limited exposure or providing additional training to students regarding how to handle these tough situations [13]. Our research is only limited to students' experiences, and future research might explore faculties' and preceptors' perspectives.

However, some students reported only the benefits of COVID-19 on their placement experience. These future pharmacists were able to contribute more in their placements than if COVID-19 had never occurred. This increased participation in practice may then contribute to students' professional identity formation [30] and sense of belonging [31]. When students participate in real-world communities of practice, they learn theories and skills in ways that are more readily applied in future careers [32].

Pharmacy students in our study reported heightened negative feelings and emotions during the pandemic, similar to a recent study by Zhai and colleagues involving medical students [?]. Factors that contributed to the negative emotions might be related to unfamiliar learning environments and placement experience and universal uncertainty during the pandemic. Many students have employed different tactics to support their mental health throughout the hard time. However, our results show that only a handful of students have self-reported utilizing the counselling service available at the University. Accordingly, it may be seen as an opportunity for the educators to encourage the pharmacy students to take advantage of the supporting services provided by the tertiary institutions. In addition to current existing services, educators may consider developing new programs to support students' mental health during COVID-19 pandemic.

Our research finding suggests that autonomy and relatedness frustrations were related to the international students and students who live far away from their families. It is well established that the fulfilment of each basic psychological need is determinative with regard to an individual's daily well-being [8]. While a large number of students reported experiencing negative emotion towards the pandemic as per our research results, specific plans may be tailored for individuals, specifically for international students and those who live far away from home. For example, the educators may consider scheduling group meetings for those students and a sense of belonging can be enhanced by sharing their experience with people in similar situations [33].

Our study was not without limitations. A limitation of our study was that we were unable to identify the year level of each student from the data source. To better aid student development, future researchers could evaluate the impacts and needs for each stage of student development. Although this research provides an in-depth view of one pharmacy cohort, any national or international policies should also account for related research in other cohorts, professions, institutions, and countries. Further, the data source used in this study is limited. Although analyzing student reflections reveals topics of central importance to students, some students may have written their reflections as an academic exercise, thereby "going through the motions" while writing their PLPs. In addition, it is possible that some students may be more challenged to express themselves in writing than in an interview or focus group study, whereas others may be more apt to express themselves through written reflections. Furthermore, the research provides first-hand information on pharmacy students' experience in the early stage of the pandemic. However, due to the time constraint, we were not able to follow up any possible changes over time. The future research might compare students' experiences in the early stage and the experiences in the later stage to better understand how students adapt to the COVID-19 pandemic. In addition, since the data were collected for other purposes (i.e., teaching and learning), there was a missed opportunity to comprehensively address all of the theoretical frameworks. For example, we were unable to explore social support factors for self-determination theory.

5. Conclusions

This study provides a high-level overview of pharmacy students' benefits, challenges and strategies during the initial months of the COVID-19 pandemic. Our result demonstrated that the most coded challenges were "negative emotional response" and "communication barrier during virtual learning". The most coded strategies were "using new technology" and "time management". These research findings may help researchers and educators better understand students' well-being and adaptability during the COVID-19 pandemic. Future researchers should investigate the long-term effects of COVID-19 on health professions students. Overall, tertiary institutions and educators may use the research findings to provide support that better suits the pharmacy students' needs in the ongoing pandemic and any future emergency events.

Author Contributions: Conceptualization, K.M.L.; methodology, K.M.L.; formal analysis, C.S., R.Z.K., G.N., S.M., K.M.L.; writing—original draft preparation, L.L., C.S., R.Z.K., G.N., S.M., K.M.L.; writing—review and editing, S.C.; supervision, K.M.L., S.C. All authors have read and agreed to the published version of the manuscript.

Funding: This research received funding from the Faculty of Pharmacy and Pharmaceutical Sciences at Monash University.

Institutional Review Board Statement: The study was conducted according to the guidelines of the Declaration of Helsinki, and approved by the Monash University Human Ethics Low Risk Review (Project ID 24477, 2020).

Informed Consent Statement: Participant consent followed an opt-out consent process due to the low-risk study. At the Monash University Faculty of Pharmacy and Pharmaceutical Sciences, the pharmacy program runs an education research registry. Each year all students are informed of education research projects and presented with the opportunity to opt-out of having their student data used for education research. For this study, we removed any PLPs from students who have opted-out of the education research registry.

Conflicts of Interest: The authors declare no conflict of interest.

References

1. Jowsey, T.; Foster, G.; Cooper-Ioelu, P.; Jacobs, S. Blended learning via distance in pre-registration nursing education: A scoping review. *Nurse Educ. Pract.* **2020**, *44*, 102775. [CrossRef]
2. Zhai, Y.; Du, X. Mental health care for international Chinese students affected by the COVID-19 outbreak. *Lancet. Psychiatry* **2020**, *7*, e22. [CrossRef]
3. Cao, W.; Fang, Z.; Hou, G.; Han, M.; Xu, X.; Dong, J.; Zheng, J. The psychological impact of the COVID-19 epidemic on college students in China. *Psychiatry Res.* **2020**, *287*, 112934. [CrossRef]
4. Chen, T.; Peng, L.; Yin, X.; Rong, J.; Yang, J.; Cong, G. Analysis of user satisfaction with online education platforms in China during the COVID-19 pandemic. *Healthcare* **2020**, *8*, 200. [CrossRef]
5. Bowen, M. Covid-19 has changed how we teach students. *Vet. Rec.* **2020**, *186*, 461. [CrossRef]
6. Morgado, M.; Mendes, J.J.; Proença, L. Online problem-based learning in clinical dental education: Students' self-perception and motivation. *Healthcare* **2021**, *9*, 420. [CrossRef] [PubMed]
7. Chiu, T.K. Applying the self-determination theory (SDT) to explain student engagement in online learning during the COVID-19 pandemic. *J. Res. Technol. Educ.* **2021**, 1–17. [CrossRef]
8. Ryan, R.M.; Deci, E.L. Self-determination theory and the facilitation of intrinsic motivation, social development, and well-being. *Am. Psychol.* **2000**, *55*, 68–78. [CrossRef] [PubMed]
9. Erlich, D.; Armstrong, E.; Gooding, H. Silver linings: A thematic analysis of case studies describing advances in health professions education during the Covid-19 pandemic. *Med. Teach.* **2021**, 1–6. Available online: https://www.tandfonline.com/doi/abs/10.1080/0142159X.2021.1958174 (accessed on 10 August 2021).
10. Kee, C.E. The impact of COVID-19: Graduate students' emotional and psychological experiences. *J. Hum. Behav. Soc. Environ.* **2021**, *31*, 476–488. [CrossRef]
11. Findyartini, A.; Anggraeni, D.; Husin, J.M.; Greviana, N. Exploring medical students' professional identity formation through written reflections during the COVID-19 pandemic. *J. Public Health Res.* **2020**, *9*, 4–10. [CrossRef]
12. Pharmacy Practitioner Development Committee. *National Competency Standards Framework for Pharmacists in Australia 2016*; Pharmaceutical Society of Australia Ltd.: Deakin West, Australia, 2017.
13. Lyons, K.M.; Christopoulos, A.; Brock, T.P. Sustainable pharmacy education in the time of COVID-19. *Am. J. Pharm. Educ.* **2020**, *84*, 667–672. [CrossRef]
14. Lyons, K.M.; Brock, T.P.; Malone, D.T.; Freihat, L.; White, P.J. Predictors of Pharmacy Student Performance on Written and Clinical Examinations in a Flipped Classroom Curriculum. *Am. J. Pharm. Educ.* **2020**, *84*, 8038. [CrossRef] [PubMed]
15. Forrester, C.A.; Lee, D.S.; Hon, E.; Lim, K.Y.; Brock, T.P.; Malone, D.T.; Furletti, S.G.; Lyons, K.M. Preceptor Perceptions of Pharmacy Student Performance Before and After a Curriculum Transformation. *Am. J. Pharm. Educ.* **2021**, 8575. [CrossRef]
16. Hsieh, H.-F.; Shannon, S.E. Three approaches to qualitative content analysis. *Qual. Health Res.* **2005**, *15*, 1277–1288. [CrossRef]
17. Vaismoradi, M.; Turunen, H.; Bondas, T. Content analysis and thematic analysis: Implications for conducting a qualitative descriptive study. *Nurs. Health Sci.* **2013**, *15*, 398–405. [CrossRef] [PubMed]
18. Deci, E.L.; Ryan, R.M. Self-determination theory: A macrotheory of human motivation, development, and health. *Can. Psychol./Psychol. Can.* **2008**, *49*, 182. [CrossRef]
19. Mäenpää, K.; Järvenoja, H.; Peltonen, J.; Pyhältö, K. Nursing students' motivation regulation strategies in blended learning: A qualitative study. *Nurs. Health Sci.* **2020**, *22*, 602–611. [CrossRef] [PubMed]

20. Dunlosky, J.; Rawson, K.A.; Marsh, E.J.; Nathan, M.J.; Willingham, D.T. Improving Students' Learning With Effective Learning Techniques: Promising Directions From Cognitive and Educational Psychology. *Psychol. Sci. Public Interest* **2013**, *14*, 4–58. [CrossRef]
21. Uzir, A.; Gašević, D.; Matcha, W.; Jovanović, J.; Pardo, A.; Lim, L.-A.; Gentili, S. Discovering time management strategies in learning processes using process mining techniques. In Proceedings of the European Conference on Technology Enhanced Learning, Delft, The Netherlands, 16–19 September 2019; pp. 555–569.
22. Ryan, R.M.; Deci, E.L. *Self-Determination Theory: Basic Psychological Needs in Motivation, Development, and Wellness*; Guilford Publications: New York, NY, USA, 2017.
23. Cicchinelli, A.; Veas, E.; Pardo, A.; Pammer-Schindler, V.; Fessl, A.; Barreiros, C.; Lindstädt, S. Finding traces of self-regulated learning in activity streams. In Proceedings of the 8th International Conference on Learning Analytics and Knowledge, Sydney, Australia, 7–9 March 2018; pp. 191–200.
24. Faulkner, S.L.; Trotter, S.P. Theoretical saturation. In *The International Encyclopedia of Communication Research Methods*; John Wiley & Sons, Inc.: Hoboken, NJ, USA, 2017; pp. 1–2. [CrossRef]
25. Jang, H.; Reeve, J.; Deci, E.L. Engaging students in learning activities: It is not autonomy support or structure but autonomy support and structure. *J. Educ. Psychol.* **2010**, *102*, 588–600. [CrossRef]
26. Boggiano, A.K.; Flink, C.; Shields, A.; Seelbach, A.; Barrett, M. Use of techniques promoting students' self-determination: Effects on students' analytic problem-solving skills. *Motiv. Emot.* **1993**, *17*, 319–336. [CrossRef]
27. Eisenberg, N.; Emde, R.; Hartup, W.W.; Hoffman, L.; Maccoby, E.E.; Monks, F.J.; Parke, R.; Rutter, M.; Zahn-Waxler, C. *Achievement and Motivation: A Social-Developmental Perspective*; Cambridge University Press: Cambridge, UK, 1992.
28. Solimeno, A.; Mebane, M.E.; Tomai, M.; Francescato, D. The influence of students and teachers characteristics on the efficacy of face-to-face and computer supported collaborative learning. *Comput. Educ.* **2008**, *51*, 109–128. [CrossRef]
29. Wolters, C.A.; Benzon, M.B. Assessing and predicting college students' use of strategies for the self-regulation of motivation. *J. Exp. Educ.* **2013**, *81*, 199–221. [CrossRef]
30. Birden, H.; Glass, N.; Wilson, I.; Harrison, M.; Usherwood, T.; Nass, D. Teaching professionalism in medical education: A Best Evidence Medical Education (BEME) systematic review. BEME Guide No. 25. *Med. Teach.* **2013**, *35*, e1252–e1266. [CrossRef] [PubMed]
31. Kern, A.; Montgomery, P.; Mossey, S.; Bailey, P. Undergraduate nursing students' belongingness in clinical learning environments: Constructivist grounded theory. *J. Nurs. Educ. Pract.* **2014**, *4*, 133. [CrossRef]
32. Lave, J.; Wenger, E. Legitimate peripheral participation in communities of practice. *Supporting Lifelong Learn.* **2002**, *1*, 111–126.
33. St-Amand, J.; Girard, S.; Smith, J. Sense of belonging at school: Defining attributes, determinants, and sustaining strategies. *IAFOR J. Educ.* **2017**, *5*, 105–119. [CrossRef]

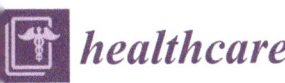

Article

AI for Doctors—A Course to Educate Medical Professionals in Artificial Intelligence for Medical Imaging

Dennis M. Hedderich [1,*], Matthias Keicher [2], Benedikt Wiestler [1], Martin J. Gruber [1], Hendrik Burwinkel [2], Florian Hinterwimmer [2,3], Tobias Czempiel [2], Judith E. Spiro [4], Daniel Pinto dos Santos [5], Dominik Heim [2], Claus Zimmer [1], Daniel Rückert [3], Jan S. Kirschke [1] and Nassir Navab [2]

[1] Department of Neuroradiology, Klinikum rechts der Isar, School of Medicine, Technical University of Munich, D-81675 Munich, Germany; b.wiestler@tum.de (B.W.); martin.gruber@tum.de (M.J.G.); claus.zimmer@tum.de (C.Z.); jan.kirschke@tum.de (J.S.K.)
[2] Computer Aided Medical Procedures, Technical University of Munich, D-81675 Munich, Germany; matthias.keicher@tum.de (M.K.); hendrik.burwinkel@tum.de (H.B.); Florian.Hinterwimmer@tum.de (F.H.); tobias.czempiel@tum.de (T.C.); dominik.heim@tum.de (D.H.); nassir.navab@tum.de (N.N.)
[3] Institute for Artificial Intelligence and Informatics in Medicine, Technical University of Munich, D-81675 Munich, Germany; daniel.rueckert@tum.de
[4] Department of Radiology, University Hospital, LMU Munich, D-80336 Munich, Germany; judith.spiro@med.uni-muenchen.de
[5] Department of Radiology, University Hospital Cologne, D-50937 Cologne, Germany; daniel.pinto-dos-santos@uk-koeln.de
* Correspondence: dennis.hedderich@tum.de

Abstract: Successful adoption of artificial intelligence (AI) in medical imaging requires medical professionals to understand underlying principles and techniques. However, educational offerings tailored to the need of medical professionals are scarce. To fill this gap, we created the course "AI for Doctors: Medical Imaging". An analysis of participants' opinions on AI and self-perceived skills rated on a five-point Likert scale was conducted before and after the course. The participants' attitude towards AI in medical imaging was very optimistic before and after the course. However, deeper knowledge of AI and the process for validating and deploying it resulted in significantly less overoptimism with respect to perceivable patient benefits through AI (p = 0.020). Self-assessed skill ratings significantly improved after the course, and the appreciation of the course content was very positive. However, we observed a substantial drop-out rate, mostly attributed to the lack of time of medical professionals. There is a high demand for educational offerings regarding AI in medical imaging among medical professionals, and better education may lead to a more realistic appreciation of clinical adoption. However, time constraints imposed by a busy clinical schedule need to be taken into account for successful education of medical professionals.

Keywords: artificial intelligence; medical imaging; machine learning; clinical translation; continuing medical education

1. Introduction

Artificial intelligence (AI) has become one of the dominant topics in medical research, especially in processing and analysis of medical imaging data [1,2]. This is documented by an ever-increasing number of research studies on AI in medical imaging, and various start-ups and established companies entering the medical-imaging market [3,4]. However, clinical adoption of AI algorithms for medical imaging is lagging behind for various reasons, such as a lack of clinical validation of AI algorithms, regulatory burdens, hesitance of patients to accept AI for individual clinical decisions, and as of yet, often unsatisfactory reimbursement for AI algorithms [3–6].

Another important reason may be that educational programs on AI in medical imaging tailored to the needs of medical professionals are lacking, which may lead to hesitance to use new algorithmic tools in clinical practice [7,8]. Very recently, some training programs for residents have been implemented into the formal radiology curriculum [9]. However, educational programs, which are open to a broader audience of medical professionals working with medical-imaging data, such as ophthalmologists or pathologists, are very rare.

To fill this gap, we created a 12-week, online-only course on AI in medical imaging and offered it for free to medical doctors (MDs) at our institution, and also to medical students and non-MD researchers. The overall goal of the course was to offer educational material on AI in medical imaging to healthcare professionals to give them a better appreciation of the underlying principles and so they could understand the potential pitfalls of using AI in clinical practice. The second point especially should lead to a better translation of imaging AI into clinical practice by reducing the commonly observed reservations of healthcare professionals to use AI in practice. Thus, the course material comprised the theoretical basics of AI in general, special challenges in medical imaging, basics of Python programming, and special-focus lessons highlighting particularly interesting fields of AI in medical imaging and its translation into clinical practice.

In this article, we report on our initial experience with this educational program and how the participants perceived it. Furthermore, we assessed the participants' opinions on AI in medical imaging, as well as their self-rated skills pertaining to the topic in order to inform other institutions seeking to develop educational programs for MDs in medical imaging.

2. Materials and Methods

2.1. Course Curriculum

The course was designed as a 12-week, online-only curriculum, consisting of two six-week blocks plus live online meetings before, during, and after the course. In the first block, the objective was to teach basics of AI in general and its applications in medical imaging. The study material was presented to the participants through an online teaching platform (Moodle) in a synchronous (i.e., live online lectures) and asynchronous manner (e.g., pre-recorded screencasts, reading assignments, and multiple-choice questions). Furthermore, there was an introduction to the concepts of Python programming, with dedicated examples based on Google Colab notebooks. Live lectures were held weekly at a fixed time, and were recorded for those who could not attend. The content was produced mostly by medical and non-medical researchers and lecturers from our institution in a standardized format. Topics of the first six weeks included "Introduction to Machine Learning: Historical Context, Systematic Considerations and Basics of Linear Algebra (part 1)" (week 1), "Introduction to Artificial Neural Networks: What Can AI Learn? and Basics of Linear Algebra (part 2)" (week 2), "Applying AI to Imaging: Special Considerations for Medical Imaging" (week 3), "Advanced Learning Methods with Artificial Neural Networks: Unsupervised Learning" (week 4), "Generative Adversarial Networks and Medical Image Formats" (week 5), and "Critical Appraisal of AI studies in Radiology: Reporting Metrics and Paper Analysis" (week 6).

The second block consisted of one special-focus lesson per week, highlighting a particular topic of applied AI. These lessons were prepared following a flipped-classroom concept with pre-recorded lectures, reading assignments, and a live question-and-answer session with the lecturer. The topics were the following: "Structured Reporting in Radiology" (week 7), "Explainable AI in Medical Imaging" (week 8), "Computational Pathology" (week 9), "AI in Dermatology" (week 10), "AI in Imaging Neuroscience: Ethical, Legal, and Societal Aspects" (week 11), and "Ethics in AI" (week 12). Accompanying the second half of the course, the participants were asked to perform a group work task, which consisted of the detailed analysis and presentation of a current research publication in the field of medical imaging AI. Numbers of participants per group before and after the course can be found in Table 1 and in Figure 1.

Table 1. A list of the course participants according to group before and after the course.

Participant Group	MD	Medical Student	PhD Student	Non-MD Researcher
At course start	40	35	7	11
Successful course completion	13	9	4	2

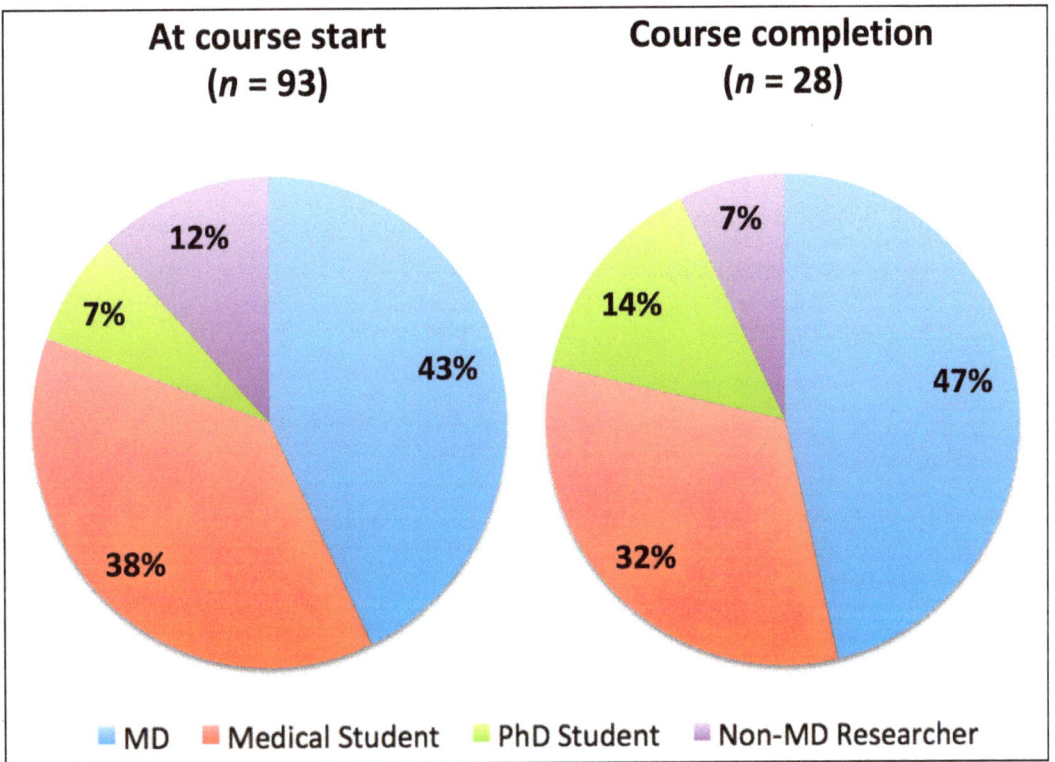

Figure 1. Pie chart diagrams showing the percentages of professional groups at course start (**left**) and after successful course completion (**right**).

2.2. Pre- and Post-Course Questionnaires

Pre- and post-course questionnaires were individually administered to the participants through the online learning system. Answers were given either in a yes/no manner, based on a five-point Likert-scale evaluation or as free text. The input was saved anonymously. The questionnaires and survey results are depicted in Tables 2–4.

2.3. Statistical Analysis

Descriptive and comparative statistics were performed using SPSS version 26.0 (SPSS, IBM Corp. 2019, Armonk, NY, USA). Pre- and post-course evaluations were compared using Wilcoxon's signed-rank test. Statistical significance was assumed for $p < 0.05$.

Table 2. Questionnaire on the participants' opinions on artificial intelligence in medical imaging and its clinical adoption. Results of the pre-course survey were given on a five-point Likert scale ranging from 1 = strong disagreement to 5 = complete agreement.

Question (Answers Ranging from 1 = Strongly Disagree to 5 = Completely Agree)	Median	Minimum	Maximum	25th Percentile	75th Percentile
Using AI in medical imaging will benefit patients in the foreseeable future.	5	3	5	4	5
It is important to understand how an AI algorithm works in order to use its results in clinical decision making.	5	2	5	4	5
I would use an AI algorithm in medical decision making if it has been thoroughly evaluated by others with good performance, although I don't understand how it works.	4	1	5	3	4
I will not use AI in medical imaging algorithms unless I can fully explain them to my patients.	3	1	5	2	4
Education about AI must be integrated in medical training in university.	4	1	5	4	5
Education about AI must be integrated in medical training in residency.	4	1	5	4	5
Using AI in medical imaging will reduce the workload of physicians.	4	2	5	3	4
Clinical adoption of AI in medical imaging will replace physicians e.g., radiologists in the next 10 years.	2	1	5	1	3
Image-analysis tasks in general can be performed by an AI algorithm today at medical-expert level.	3	1	5	2	4
Some particular tasks can be performed by an AI algorithm today at medical-expert level.	4	2	5	4	5
Clinical adoption of AI algorithms in medical imaging is mostly hindered by regulatory barriers and traditions, not by the performance of the developed algorithms.	3	1	5	3	4
Doctors should have basic programming skills.	3	1	5	2	4

Table 3. Self-assessment of AI-related skills before and after the course shows significant improvement in all domains after the course.

Timepoint		Before Course			After Course		
Areas of self-Assessment (Ranging from 1 = No Skills to 5 = Expert Skills)	Median	25th Percentile	75th Percentile	Median	25th Percentile	75th Percentile	p
Understanding Python code when reading it.	1	1	2	2.5	2	3	0.001
Creating Python code for statistical analysis.	1	1	2	2	2	3	0.002

Table 3. Cont.

Timepoint	Before Course			After Course			
Areas of self-Assessment (Ranging from 1 = No Skills to 5 = Expert Skills)	Median	25th Percentile	75th Percentile	Median	25th Percentile	75th Percentile	p
Understanding concepts in linear algebra pertaining to machine learning.	2	1.5	2	3	2	3.25	0.006
Assessing a machine-learning paper validating AI algorithms for medical imaging.	2	1	2	2.5	2	3.25	0.005
Applying a ML algorithm in a clinical setting.	1	1	2	2	2	2.25	0.013
Incorporating decisions made by a ML algorithm into clinical decision making.	1	1	3	2.5	2	3.25	0.042

Table 4. General course evaluation results given on a five-point Likert scale ranging from 1 = strong disagreement to 5 = complete agreement.

Question (Answers Ranging from 1 = Strongly Disagree to 5 = Completely Agree)	Median	Minimum	Maximum	25th Percentile	75th Percentile
The course was well organized	5	2	5	4	5
Overall, the study material was well prepared	5	3	5	4	5
The content of the course was important for my work as a clinician	3,5	2	5	3	4
The content of the course was important for my work as a scientist	4	2	5	4	5
The course could easily be taken alongside clinical work	3	1	5	2	3
I expected the workload to participate in the course to be	3	2	3	2	3
I missed in-person lectures and meetings with teachers and other students.	4	1	5	2	4
I feel more competent at dealing with AI in medical imaging than before the course	4	1	5	4	5

2.4. Ethics Statement

Participants consented to the statistical evaluation and potential publication of the evaluation results. Evaluation results were submitted anonymously. No confidential medical information was used in this study.

3. Results

3.1. Course Participants

In total, 93 participants (46 female (49.5%), 47 male (50.5%), mean age 29.6 ± 7.1 years) enrolled into the course and filled in the pre-course evaluation form. For post-graduates (n = 52), median time since graduation was 4.00 years (interquartile range: 2.00–8.75 years). The group of participants consisted of 40 medical doctors (MDs) (43.0%), 35 medical students (37.6%), 7 PhD students (7.5%), and 11 postgraduate researchers without an MD degree (11.8%). Within the group of medical doctors, eight specialized in neuroradiology, six in pathology, and three each in radiology, ophthalmology, nuclear medicine, neurology, internal medicine and dermatology. Two participating medical doctors specialized in psychiatry and surgery, and one each in pediatrics, neurosurgery, nephrology, and anesthesiology. Most participating medical doctors were residents (30; 75.0%), next to eight participating consultants (22.5%) and one head of department (2.5%). The majority of participants stated that they currently do not use AI in their daily work (77; 82.8%) and half of them had previous programming experience (46; 49.5%); 36 participants (39.2%) stated that they had no previous education in the field of artificial intelligence, while 40 (43.0%) had read some articles, and 16 (17.2%) had previously taken a course related to the topic. Overall, the participants planned to spend a median of 4.00 h per week on the course (IQR: 3.00–5.00).

A total of 47 (25 female (53.2%), 22 male (46.8%)) participants filled in the post-course evaluation, and 28 completed the course (16 female (57.1%) and 12 male (42.9%)), including 13 MDs, 9 medical students, 4 PhD students and 2 non-MD researchers (see Table 1).

3.2. Opinions towards AI in Medical Imaging

As part of the evaluation, we asked the course participants about their opinions and attitudes towards AI in medical imaging (see Table 2). Summarizing the results, the participants highly supported the statements that AI in medical imaging will benefit patients in the foreseeable future, that it will reduce the workload of physicians, and that it is already capable of performing particular, well-defined tasks at an expert-physician level. The majority of participants had the opinion that education about AI should be integrated into medical school and into residency, and that the doctor must understand how an algorithm works in order to use it on patients. Participants opposed the notion that AI will replace doctors, and were undecided on whether AI can perform image-analysis tasks in general at an expert-physician level. When it comes to obstacles for clinical adoption, there was a trend towards attributing this more to regulatory processes than to algorithmic performance per se.

In order to explore whether opinions on these topics changed after successful course completion, we analysed the participants' answers before and after the course. There was a significant difference regarding their opinion on whether AI will lead to patient benefit in the foreseeable future, with less overoptimistic but still very positive answers after the course (pre-course evaluation: 5 ("I completely agree"); IQR (4.5–5.0); post-course evaluation: 4 ("I rather agree"); IQR (4.0–5.0); $p = 0.020$) (see Figure 2). With regard to the other questions, no significant change could be noted, other than a trend towards a slightly more affirmative opinion regarding the question "Some particular tasks can be performed by an AI algorithm today at medical-expert level" ($p = 0.096$).

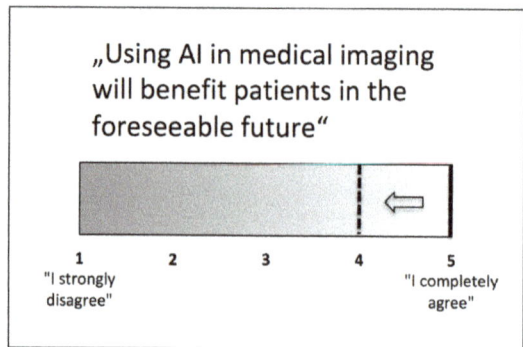

Figure 2. Median agreement with the statement "Using AI in medical imaging will benefit patients in the foreseeable future" changed from full to partial after the course.

3.3. Self-Perceived Skills Relating to AI and Medical Imaging

In order to assess whether the course impacted on skills regarding AI in medical imaging, we evaluated self-rated skills of those who successfully completed the course. For results in the particular areas of self-assessment, please see Table 3. In summary, self-perceived skills improved in all areas, for understanding Python code as well as for understanding concepts of linear algebra pertaining to AI. Furthermore, participants felt more confident to analyse a research paper in the field, to implement an AI algorithm in a clinical environment and to incorporate the decisions given by an algorithm into their clinical decision making.

3.4. Overall Appraisal of the Course

The participants were overall very satisfied with the study material and the organization of the course, and deemed the content of the course important for their work as a clinician or scientist. There was a small tendency to underestimate the time effort necessary for the course and towards the notion that taking the course alongside clinical work might be problematic. Most of the participants felt more competent at dealing with AI in medical imaging after the course. A majority of participants missed in-person events (which were not held due to the online-only character of the course). Please see Table 4 for details.

4. Discussion

When evaluating this pilot educational program for medical professionals who wanted to study AI in medical imaging, we found that the interest in the medical community was very high. Furthermore, education about AI has the potential to change the opinions of medical professionals with regard to AI, and to improve their competencies pertaining to the topic. However, time constraints due to a busy schedule of clinical work impose a substantial hurdle for thorough education of medical doctors.

The interest in our educational offering was very high among MDs and medical students from our institution, as expressed by the high number of enrolled participants at the beginning of the study. This was supported by results from recent surveys among radiologists: three-quarters of all participants in a survey ($n = 270$) from 2019 stated that they had received insufficient information about AI tools, and more than 90% would participate in continuing medical education offers on this topic [10]. The need for advanced teaching courses on AI in medical imaging was emphasized by results from a recent global survey among radiologists, in which only around 11% stated that they had advanced knowledge in the field [7]. In summary, our experience corroborated the high demand and need for educational offers for medical professions in the field of AI.

Our course participants had a rather positive opinion about AI in medical imaging, embracing its potential to perform defined tasks in image analysis, and thus to take workload off the current physician workforce. This could be explained by a positive selection bias, and fits with previous reports that openness for AI tools resulted in a more optimistic view on the topic and its impact on medicine [7].

Despite this optimism with respect to the impact of AI in medical imaging, most participants did not believe that AI would eventually replace physicians in a clinical environment. This was in line with a survey among medical students, who largely refuted the impression that radiologists would be replaced in the future [11]. The fear of replacement through new, AI-related technologies seemed more relevant in the largest currently available survey among radiologists, which found this to be of importance to almost 40% of participants [7]. Interestingly, this survey also proposed a potential explanation through an inverse correlation between AI-specific knowledge and fear of replacement through AI [7].

Although the attitude of MDs towards AI in medical imaging seems quite consolidated, we did find a significant change with respect to the question regarding whether AI will lead to patient benefits in the foreseeable future, with less-optimistic attitudes after the course. However, the answer to that question left room for interpretation, and did not differentiate whether the participants did not believe in patient benefits through AI at all, or just not in the foreseeable future. We interpreted this change in opinions as an indicator that our course and increased knowledge about AI among medical professionals impacts their attitude and judgment of clinical practicability, by highlighting not only the potential of AI (which is heavily discussed), but also discussing and teaching about the challenges and limitations of AI.

Underlining the impact of the described course, we saw a significant increase in the self-assessed ratings of the participants' skills pertaining to AI in medical imaging. Although this was an encouraging finding, and was also assessed in a similar way in previous studies [9], the subjective nature of these self-assessed ratings left room for some uncertainty. Future courses and educational programs should define a clear list of skills and capacities that participants will possess after the course, and (most importantly) a clear way to test those [12]. At best, these learning objectives will incorporate theoretical and practical skills based on broad consensus by medical schools, resident programs, and professional associations.

A clear downside of our course experience was the rather high drop-out rate. Based on the participants' feedback, we did not attribute this to the quality of our course and the study material, but rather to the tight schedules of clinicians and medical students, which do not allow for easy integration of additional five to 10 working hours per week. However, as drop-out rates were comparable among the different participant groups, a busy schedule may not have been the only reason for participants to quit the course. Particularly for medical students, the fact that the course was not part of the regular curriculum and no mandatory credits had to be earned may have been of importance. For PhD students and non-MD researchers, a reason might be that the clinical orientation of course content did not fit their focus, as it was most likely unrelated to their work. We hypothesized that the drop-out rate could be reduced by integrating the course into a mandatory curriculum; e.g., in medical school or by setting a participation fee for doctors. These two measures could potentially increase the participants' adherence to the schedule and their motivation to finish the course. Another aspect would be that the course curriculum could be adapted in order to avoid large leaps in complexity and to ensure step-wise learning without asking too much of the participants. Future studies should address how topics related to computer science and AI are best taught to medical professionals. Another point with a potential negative effect on the participants' motivation was the online-only character of the course, which was mostly due to the current COVID-19 pandemic and restrictions on in-person meetings. We hypothesized that in-person meetings and the establishment of tighter personal relationships between students and teachers could also decrease the drop-out rate substantially.

5. Conclusions

In summary, we found that educational offerings on AI in medical imaging were regarded very well by medical professionals, leading to improved skills and (in part) to a less-optimistic perception of AI in medical imaging. In our opinion, this also showed that educating medical professionals on AI is feasible and may potentially contribute to a successful implementation of AI in clinical practice. However, time constraints of medical professionals may hinder successful course completion. Future efforts should aspire to clearly define learning objectives for medical professionals, and ideally to harmonize curricula integrated in medical schools and/or residency programs.

Author Contributions: Conceptualization, M.K., B.W., M.J.G., H.B., T.C., J.E.S., D.P.d.S., D.H., D.R. and J.S.K.; data curation, B.W.; formal analysis, D.M.H., F.H. and T.C.; investigation, D.M.H., F.H., D.P.d.S., D.H. and J.S.K.; methodology, D.M.H., B.W., T.C. and J.E.S.; project administration, D.M.H., M.K., B.W., M.J.G., H.B., F.H., T.C. and J.S.K.; resources, C.Z., J.S.K. and N.N.; supervision, C.Z., D.R. and N.N.; writing—original draft, D.M.H.; writing—review and editing, D.M.H., M.K., B.W., M.J.G., H.B., F.H., T.C., J.E.S., D.P.d.S., D.H., C.Z., D.R., J.S.K. and N.N. All authors have read and agreed to the published version of the manuscript.

Funding: This research received no external funding.

Institutional Review Board Statement: Evaluation results were submitted anonymously. No confidential medical information was used in this study, thus IRB approval was not obtained.

Informed Consent Statement: Participants consented to the statistical evaluation and potential publication of the evaluation results.

Data Availability Statement: Original data are stored by the authors and available upon reasonable request.

Acknowledgments: We thank Simon Eickhoff, Alexander Zink, Peter Schüffler, Mauricio Reyes, Amelia Fiske, and Stuart McLennan for providing the special-focus lectures during the course. We thank Paul Eichinger, Timo Löhr, Christoph Baur, Johannes Paetzold, Malek El-Husseini, Anjany Sekuboyina, Claudio von Schacky, and Michael Dieckmeyer for producing the educational screencasts for the course. We thank all participants for taking part in and evaluating the course.

Conflicts of Interest: The authors declare no conflict of interest.

References

1. Hinton, G. Deep Learning—A Technology With the Potential to Transform Health Care. *JAMA* **2018**, *320*, 1101–1102. [CrossRef] [PubMed]
2. Jha, S.; Topol, E.J. Adapting to Artificial Intelligence: Radiologists and Pathologists as Information Specialists. *JAMA* **2016**, *316*, 2353–2354. [CrossRef] [PubMed]
3. Liu, X.; Faes, L.; Kale, A.U.; Wagner, S.K.; Fu, D.J.; Bruynseels, A.; Mahendiran, T.; Moraes, G.; Shamdas, M.; Kern, C.; et al. A comparison of deep learning performance against health-care professionals in detecting diseases from medical imaging: A systematic review and meta-analysis. *Lancet Digit. Health* **2019**, *1*, e271–e297. [CrossRef]
4. Nagendran, M.; Chen, Y.; Lovejoy, C.A.; Gordon, A.C.; Komorowski, M.; Harvey, H.; Topol, E.J.; Ioannidis, J.P.A.; Collins, G.S.; Maruthappu, M. Artificial intelligence versus clinicians: Systematic review of design, reporting standards, and claims of deep learning studies. *BMJ* **2020**, *368*, m689. [CrossRef]
5. Singh, R.P.; Hom, G.L.; Abramoff, M.D.; Campbell, J.P.; Chiang, M.F. Current Challenges and Barriers to Real-World Artificial Intelligence Adoption for the Healthcare System, Provider, and the Patient. *Transl. Vis. Sci. Technol.* **2020**, *9*, 45. [CrossRef]
6. Pesapane, F.; Volonté, C.; Codari, M.; Sardanelli, F. Artificial intelligence as a medical device in radiology: Ethical and regulatory issues in Europe and the United States. *Insights Imaging* **2018**, *9*, 745–753. [CrossRef] [PubMed]
7. Huisman, M.; Ranschaert, E.; Parker, W.; Mastrodicasa, D.; Koci, M.; Pinto dos Santos, D.; Coppola, F.; Morozov, S.; Zins, M.; Bohyn, C.; et al. An international survey on AI in radiology in 1041 radiologists and radiology residents part 1: Fear of replacement, knowledge, and attitude. *Eur. Radiol.* **2021**, *31*, 7058–7066. [CrossRef] [PubMed]
8. Jungmann, F.; Jorg, T.; Hahn, F.; Pinto dos Santos, D.; Jungmann, S.M.; Düber, C.; Mildenberger, P.; Kloeckner, R. Attitudes Toward Artificial Intelligence Among Radiologists, IT Specialists, and Industry. *Acad. Radiol.* **2020**. [CrossRef] [PubMed]
9. Lindqwister, A.L.; Hassanpour, S.; Lewis, P.J.; Sin, J.M. AI-RADS: An Artificial Intelligence Curriculum for Residents. *Acad. Radiol.* **2020**. [CrossRef] [PubMed]
10. Waymel, Q.; Badr, S.; Demondion, X.; Cotten, A.; Jacques, T. Impact of the rise of artificial intelligence in radiology: What do radiologists think? *Diagn. Interv. Imaging* **2019**, *100*, 327–336. [CrossRef] [PubMed]
11. Pinto Dos Santos, D.; Giese, D.; Brodehl, S.; Choon, S.H.; Staab, W.; Kleinert, R.; Maintz, D.; Baeßler, B. Medical students' attitude towards artificial intelligence: A multicentre survey. *Eur. Radiol.* **2019**, *29*, 1640–1646. [CrossRef] [PubMed]
12. Neri, E.; de Souza, N.; Brady, A.; Bayarri, A.A.; Becker, C.D.; Coppola, F.; Visser, J. What the radiologist should know about artificial intelligence—An ESR white paper. *Insights Imaging* **2019**, *10*, 44. [CrossRef]

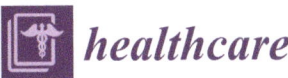

Article

Social Media Improves Students' Academic Performance: Exploring the Role of Social Media Adoption in the Open Learning Environment among International Medical Students in China

Muhammad Azeem Ashraf [1], Muhammad Naeem Khan [2,*], Sohail Raza Chohan [3,4], Maqbool Khan [5], Wajid Rafique [6], Muhammad Fahad Farid [2] and Asad Ullah Khan [3]

1. Research Institute of Educational Science, Hunan University, Changsha 410082, China; azeem@hnu.edu.cn
2. School of Social and Behavioral Sciences, Nanjing University, Nanjing 210023, China; muhammadfahad@smail.nju.edu.cn
3. School of Information Management, Nanjing University, Nanjing 210023, China; sohail@smail.nju.edu.cn (S.R.C.); DG1714502@smail.nju.edu.cn (A.U.K.)
4. Department of Information Sciences, University of Education, Lahore 54770, Pakistan
5. Department of IT and Computer Science, Pak-Austria Fachhochschule Institute of Applied Sciences and Technology, Haripur 22621, Pakistan; maqbool.khan@fecid.paf-iast.edu.pk
6. Department of Computer Science and Operational Research, University of Montreal, Montreal, QC H3C 3J7, Canada; wajid.rafique@umontreal.ca
* Correspondence: naeem@smail.nju.edu.cn

Abstract: Numerous studies have examined the role of social media as an open-learning (OL) tool in the field of education, but the empirical evidence necessary to validate such OL tools is scant, specifically in terms of student academic performance (AP). In today's digital age, social media platforms are most popular among the student community, and they provide opportunities for OL where they can easily communicate, interact, and collaborate with each other. The authors of this study aimed to minimize the literature gap among student communities who adopt social media for OL, which has positive impacts on their AP in Chinese higher education. We adopted social constructivism theory (SCT) and the technology acceptance model (TAM) to formulate a conceptual framework. Primary data containing 233 questionnaires of international medical students in China were collected in January 2021 through the survey method. The gathered data were analyzed through structural equation modeling techniques with SmartPLS 3. The results revealed that perceived usefulness, perceived ease of use, and interactions with peers have positive and significant influence on OL. In addition, OL was found to have positive and significant influence on students' AP and engagement. Lastly, engagement showed a positive impact on students' AP. Thus, this study shows that social media serves as a dynamic tool to expedite the development of OL settings by encouraging collaboration, group discussion, and the exchange of ideas between students that reinforce their learning behavior and performance.

Keywords: open learning; engagement; collaboration; communication; electronic-learning

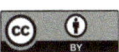

1. Introduction

The term social media (SM) is considered as a form of communication through electronic platforms, which intends to make online communities for users to share knowledge, information, opinions, messages, and other content [1]. In the 21st century, SM became an essential part of human life, while the use of SM has spread across the world. In 2020, almost 3.06 billion individuals from all walks of life used at least one SM platform, such as WeChat, Facebook, Twitter, Weibo, WhatsApp, and Instagram, in their daily life [2]. The use of SM has become an integral part of intellectual work, and students posting study-related material on SM platforms is considered a reliable source of information that is important to each community, such as those of students, customers, and employees [3]. The users of SM (computational technology that helps to develop and share ideas, perceptual knowledge, professional interests, information, and other expressions through social network platforms) may read or see their friends' activities online without direct contact with them [4]. Furthermore, SM networking sites utilize features, such as comments, postings, digital photographs, video-sharing, and data about online interactions, that provide vitality for SM users [4]. People who use SM are called netizens. Netizens often access online platforms using the internet or other web technologies on their computers or laptops, or they download programs to the mobile devices (such as smartphones or tablets) that expand the functionality of SM networks [4]. The use of SM platforms in educational activities is increasing day by day. Because of the engagement of SM users with such services, they usually develop highly interactive platforms wherein students may create or exchange ideas and discuss information or previously published online content in user-created groups. SM promotes interactions between teachers, subject specialists, students, communities, and major companies. This revolution is the focus of new and creative information technology (IT) areas [3].

SM has been used in medicine extensively, as almost one-third of the adults with internet access have viewed different social media sites concerning the medical experience of other people, while almost 6% of these people have participated through text messages, comments, replies, photos, recorded files, and personal assessments of health conditions by professionals [5]. SM has provided opportunity for individuals with specific illnesses to take part in online communities to share their personal experiences, contact other people to learn from their experiences, and contact medical specialists to glean comprehensive knowledge about their illnesses. Similarly, healthcare workers including doctors and nurses are also using SM significantly in their professional lives, where they exchange information regarding their professional problems as well as clinical experiences [6]. Likewise, current medical students are also using SM broadly as a tool of communication among their educational and professional lives. In medical education literature, communication, peer feedback, collaboration, material sharing, and social media ability are reflected as the major aspects essential for SM usage among medical students [7]. Since SM holds massive importance in educational settings, Davis, Ho, and Last suggested that medical schools revise their syllabi by integrating social media in their instruction in ways that are innovative, timely, and evidence-based to meet the demands of this dynamic learning landscape [8]. Thus, studies on the role of SM use in medical education would enhance and improve the teaching and learning environments for both medical students and medical practitioners [3].

In addition, SM (characterized by user-generated content (UGC)) enables students "to create, circulate, share, and exchange information in a variety of formats and with multiple communities" [9]. WhatsApp, WeChat, Facebook, Instagram, Pinterest, Linked In, Snap Chat, Twitter, Telegram, Baidu, Google+, SlideShare, Weibo, Tumblr, and related websites are the most popular platforms among SM users [1]. Google+, which provides a single destination to students to easily and quickly communicate and discuss their problems, is widely used all around the world. WeChat is widely used by people in China for social networking [1]. Thus, social media has now become a popular platform for knowledge sharing between medical students and teachers [7]. SM platforms have enabled students to work together, interact with colleagues and classmates, and acquire the latest knowledge, which has positive impacts on their AP [10]. One constructive effect of using SM platforms is the introduction of the public to consumer data, ideas, and programming, which has promoted further technical advances and increased knowledge in educational institutions [9].

OL is a terminology that indicates that "an inner feeling conveyed in this technique through external actions involving students in existing, continuous learning groups or teams" [11]. Rapid expansions of information communication technology (ICT) have led to pragmatic practices. Many terms such as online learning, blended learning, web-based learning, m-learning, and computer-mediated learning have been used in the literature to show the importance of technology in academic learning. All these terms have distinct features, but they are linked to each other through the ability to use a computer that is connected to a network, which provides the opportunity to study from any place at any time [6,11]. OL can be characterized as an instrument that has made knowledge-learning practices more innovative, student-centered, and flexible [4]. OL is a procedure of reciprocity, communication, and collaboration within student communities in which students share their difficulties with other group members and receive solutions, guidance, and advice; it also improves their learning processes, enhances abilities such as collaboration and social abidance, and creates productive interplay as a potential tool for learning [11]. Additionally, OL makes it easier to elaborate and develop critical thinking, materials interchange, and proficient knowledge on online platforms [12]. SM has become the essential tool for OL in student communities and others [3], and SM use is widely used as the main communication platform for student learning [11] because some of its associated tools are not too costly to enable their utilization and growth in acceptable and satisfactory settings for OL. SM has led to the wide distribution of several group exercises, such as sharing knowledge and information, communications, and interactions, in education, thus enhancing students' learning potential.

Several scholars have examined the link between SM and AP, and they have highlighted many mixed results when using such platforms. For example, according to Ktoridou and Eteokleous [13], SM platforms allow students to interact with group members to find help in solving learning problems. Moreover, using SM platforms may enhance learning achievement in OL environments [11]; however, some studies have shown that students' use of SM platforms for study (assignment) does not improve learning outcomes [14]. Hence, students must monitor and analyze the patterns of collaboration that emerge throughout OL on SM, where motivating cognitive skills, reflection, and metacognition is crucial for learning [11]. Nevertheless, earlier research revealed that students have negative attitudes regarding social media, as they believe that most SM platforms do not help them achieve AP [15,16]. According to Anderson and Jiang, the use and availability of SM platforms have led to a decline in AP [17]. However, other studies have found that there is no link between SM use and AP [18].

Alenazy, Mugahed Al-Rahmi, and Khan explained that students are suspicious of the idea that using SM platforms can aid them in measuring education sustainability [19]. Other scholars have claimed that while students prefer face-to-face contact with peers and lecturers, they have a favorable attitude toward learning activities integrated with SM platforms [20]. Therefore, more research is required in the field of attitude regarding SM platform use for OL and AP [11]. Cyberstalking and cyberbullying via SM platforms have been linked to psychological and emotional issues such as discomfort, anxiety, and insecurity [21,22]. However, the better integration of SM in academic courses has provided positive effects on students' AP, such as improving motivation in learning and encouraging students to communicate with their teachers [20].

Despite having reached many countries, there remains a scarcity of studies on the use of SM platforms in higher education, especially in China. Thus, the authors of the current study sought to fill in this literature gap by investigating the use of SM platforms to achieve the goal of OL, positively affecting AP, and positively affecting student engagement (ENG). Following the literature gap, our study's main objectives were:

1. To explore the factors that influence the use of SM platforms among international medical students throughout their studies.
2. To explore the effect of SM-based OL that promotes student AP.
3. To explore how medical students use SM to maintain their ENG with peers and their performance.

This research aimed to provide new opportunities to include SM platforms in progressive education in medicine, and to take advantage of the exciting benefits of OL tools in medical training. The present research model was based on two theories: SCT by Vygotsky [23] and the TAM by Davis [24]. The TAM is known as one of the most widely used models for analyzing attitudes about the use of SM platform technology, and SCT addresses interactions and their effect on the OL and ENG of students. These two theories were utilized to assess students' AP, which is still seriously unexplored. Furthermore, there is a lack of research models for OL, AP, and ENG, including the use of SM platforms in the context of higher education in China. Hence, the goal of this research was to fill in the gaps in the literature by examining SM platforms' characteristics utilized for OL and ENG that affect students' AP.

2. Literature Review

Through the alteration of our social standards, values, and culture, SM has progressively become an important part of human society [25]. Information and content dissemination are becoming significant for people. The learning processes at education institutions have transformed the lives of individuals, including university students and (especially) women, by changing method of communication and engagement in learning [26]. These new media platforms play essential roles in the exchange of material between university students and society. Students now have the opportunity to share their routine life through photographs, comments, and the dissemination of ideas in social and academic discussions [27,28], and SM affects the everyday life of young people and especially university students [29]. Digital and social networking have revolutionized daily ways of communication by developing content, exchanging information, and consuming information [30].

SM platforms allow for social interaction and communication between users by exchanging knowledge and transforming monologues into dialogues between consumers [31]. SM, based on a specific philosophical worldview and technological underpinnings and functionalities, encompasses numerous internet-based tools and apps [32] that have enabled its users to distribute material across digital media and internet spaces [33]. It has provided chances for the inexpensive and viable online advertising of goods and services, it offers new ways of dealing with and coordinating interactions amongst users [34], and many SM users consistently disseminate and share their articles, images, videos, and records on different SM apps [35].

SM offers venues for students and the public to exchange ideas and information by discussing information with each other, as well as to build up relationships through social networking [13,36]. In today's society, SM platforms and education are inextricably linked [37] because they work as central spaces for debate, discussion, and feedback among students and teachers [38]. SM platforms can be a valuable tool to enhance learning behavior [39] by allowing people to organize content; share information, movies, photos, communication, and coordination; and build social links with others based on collaborative efforts [13,40]. SM platforms include websites, wireless internet connections, and video or photo-sharing sites. At the moment, it is not just advantageous to participate in digital media sharing and social networking—it also enables social contact and communication through the development of brands and professional possibilities [41,42]. According to Wodzicki, Schwämmlein, and Moskaliuk, social networking offers a variety of resources that may be used for instant access to learning and information [43]. For instance, students of higher academic levels extensively use SM platforms for educational purposes [13]. In addition, these platforms have several other uses, such as entertainment and interactions with others [44].

Joachim, Geert, and Soetaert stated that the trustworthiness of these webpages is typically based on demonstrated taste and expertise, rather than on the institution's association and recognition [45]. According to academics, SM platforms comprise a technology that is used to facilitate social relationships, facilitate collaborations, and enable negotiations among large populations [46]. SM platforms have allowed for the promotion of personalized learning environments as an educational strategy for enhancing self-regulated learning [47]. According to educational experts, SM platforms provide the majority of the characteristics of an excellent educational technology in terms of peer reaction, scholar mentoring, and matching the social circumstances of electronic learning (e-learning) [29].

3. Research Model and Hypotheses

In the current research, we incorporated two core theories (TAM and SCT) to develop a conceptual model to attain the research objectives. Firstly, Davis conceived a TAM to regulate the causal relationships between the internal views, perspectives, and intentions of users to adopt computer technology [24]. Scholars have extensively used the TAM to study information systems (ISs) and computer technologies (CTs). For instance, Chandra applied the TAM to investigate the adoption of online auctions by users [48].

The SCT defines knowledge as constructed in a collaborative way within a social context. It considers learning as a condition wherein individuals construct their personal meaning from the content and materials presented to them, rather than simply memorizing the information [23]. In addition, SCT is based on the idea that learning can be enhanced and made to be more constructive within the orbit of social process in cognition groups. Moreover, knowledge is an ongoing process that needs improvements with time, and learning is best accomplished when it follows social perspective in effective and constructive process [49–53]. According to Bhattacharjee [54], the emergence of constructivism research in the recent era has enhanced the tools and focus of media technologies for the fast transfer of information and knowledge to the next generation. Similarly, as suggested by Ershler and Stabile, learning is a process that results in the transmission of culture, which may attract constructivists to reconsider the influence of social media on culture [55]. The recent emergence of social media has massively affected attitudes towards education by changing the landscape of information availability.

In SCT, teaching and learning ought to focus on consuming content to develop means of understanding, and these contents have become abundant and easily reachable through social media. The effects of social media for SCT involves significant changes to the ways students often communicate, and how they acquire basic understandings. Thus, as social media permits the alteration, integration, and distribution of information, it has massive influence on the learning of individuals. The strengths of SM platforms follow the principles espoused by constructivists [56]. For instance, Churcher showed that SM platforms lead to online communities of learning practice [57]. Other studies have shown that SM platforms facilitate participation, communication, social interactions, the use of modern technologies, the use of online applications, collaboration, and the construction of personal meaning that satisfies the learning condition of constructivism [58,59]. Likewise, SCT suggests that information on OL activities, personal activities, and social interactions can be gathered through the use of modern tools of technology [60]. Figure 1 illustrates the conceptual model of this research.

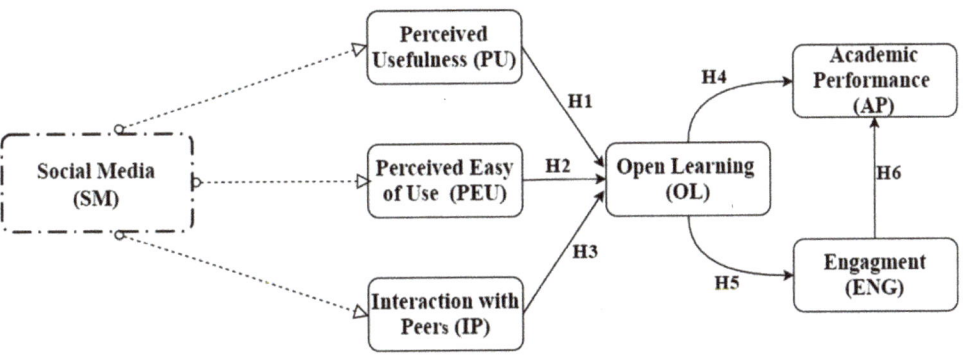

Figure 1. Conceptual model based on TAM and SCT.

3.1. Perceived Usefulness

PU refers the level to which a student thinks that using a specific technology would increase their job performance [61]. In our study, PU was defined as how much a user feels that SM platforms can be used for OL to enhance their AP. The current research provides evidence that PU affects the attitudes and intentions of those using technology [21,62]. Since PU has a direct impact on attitudes, it was assumed to have an indirect impact on intention to use technology. Hence, the following hypothesis was formulated:

Hypothesis 1. *PU is positively related to OL.*

3.2. Perceived Ease of Use

PEU refers to the level a student perceives that the use of a specific technology is effortless [24]. In this research, PEU refers to the extent to which an individual believes that using SM platforms for OL will increase their AP. Al-Rahmi et al. [11] stated that PEU has significant impacts on e-learning acceptance and adoption. Several studies have shown that PEU affects PU, though both have positive impacts on the behavioral intention of adopting technological systems [63]. In addition, several studies have shown that the intention of continuing to use SM platforms for OL is largely influenced by PEU [11,19]. Accordingly, we formulated the following hypothesis:

Hypothesis 2. *PEU is positively related to OL.*

3.3. Interact with Peers

SM platforms allow students to communicate, share content with classmates, and connect with others [64]. In today's world, most students are regular users of SM platforms to remain aware of and updated on current events [65]. Utilizing SM platforms in academic-related activities such as discussions allows students to participate in subject discussions and interact with content [66]. This single destination of conversation paves the way for communication and enhances students' learning strengths, which can move beyond the subject raised by teachers or hosts [67]. SM platforms are the best resource for improving communication, promoting positive learning attitudes, encouraging students to seriously consider learning and learning activities, and maximizing social capital through virtual communications. It has been noticed that students or scholars in online settings spend time on SM platforms to work through the learning process [68]. It is believed that the use of SM platforms in educational institutions enhances the level of interaction between instructors and students [69]. According to Alamri et al. [68], learning tools are just as essential as learning objectives because they encourage social interaction, entail interactive learning, and aid open learning. Thus, we proposed the following hypothesis:

Hypothesis 3. *IP is positively related to OL.*

3.4. Open Learning

OL can be defined as a learning process in which an individual has opportunities to work in a team or group so that learning is fostered through interpersonal interaction, group collaboration, and active learning [68]. Dumford and Miller observed that OL and student ENG through the use of SM platforms have significant relationships with team member interactions [70]. Balakrishnan and Gan used an SM platform adoption model to investigate the various factors that affect students' intentions to use SM for learning based on, for instance, the commitment, competitive, and autonomous styles [71]. In addition, according to a study by Ratneswary and Rasiah, the use of SM platforms improves OL and establishes a strong and engaging bond between students and teachers [72]. Thus, the authors of this study claim that OL improves student AP. Based on earlier studies, we posited the following hypotheses:

Hypothesis 4. *OL is positively related to AP.*

Hypothesis 5. *OL is positively related to ENG.*

3.5. Engagement

In the context of SM platforms, ENG creates a learning atmosphere characterized by discussion and interaction among colleagues that foster closer collaboration and communication [73]. Furthermore, research has shown that the use of SM platforms leads to positive AP and ENG experiences [74]. SM platforms are seen as online learning tools that offer significant benefits for better results and experiences through cognitive participation and social ENG [68]. To this end, OL enables the expansion of ENG in curriculum activities and knowledge-sharing systems [75]. According to Blasco-Arcas et al., students learn more effectively when they participate in appropriate cognitive processes, so student ENG is a significant explanatory variable for academic performance. In addition, SM platforms enable students to engage in knowledge construction, which ultimately involves a higher level of perceived learning. When students are engaged with learning activities, their AP improves [68]. Following prior studies, we proposed the following hypothesis:

Hypothesis 6. *ENG is positively related to AP.*

3.6. Academic Performance

This study applied the concept of academic performance as the achievement of educational objectives in terms of knowledge acquisition and skills development [68]. Social media refers to the electronic platforms which allow their users to interact with other user users to share information [76]. Previous studies have observed some forms of impact of SM on AP [18,47,68], but there is very little research on SM and AP in the Chinese context, particularly on international students. Therefore, this study aimed at finding the impact of SM on students AP in open learning environments through the SCT and TAM models. In this research, perceived usefulness (PU), perceived ease of use (PEU), and interactions with peers (IP) were independent variables, and OL was chosen as the mediator variable. The dependent variables were ENG and AP (Figure 1).

4. Methodology

This study was part of a large project funded by the National Natural Science Foundation of China (grant no. 71950410624) to investigate the role of internet and technology in improving teaching and learning practices in Chinese higher education. As indicated in previous sections, social media holds great impact in all aspects of teaching and learning, including in the medical field [3–7]. It has been debated in terms of its use as a tool of communication among individuals, ease of use, improvement in learning, and better professional development. Considering these outcomes, more evidence on educational usage of social media has yet to arise to evaluate to what extent medical practitioners can yield educational benefits from these resources. Therefore, the purpose of the current study is to explore the role of social media use as a tool of OL among international medical students in China. The population of this study comprised 231 international undergraduate and graduate medical students between the ages of 20 and 40 from universities in the Jiangsu province of China. This study focused on SM as an OL tool; learning platforms other than SM were not included. Prior to conducting this research, we analyzed the complexity of the term social media, because it has been defined and used differently in the previous literature. We considered all web-based tools that allow users to create and exchange content and enable them to interact with other people, as explained by Miller et al. [76].

As the study was located in China, we considered the most commonly used SM platforms in China, such as WeChat, Weibo, QQ, Tencent Meeting, and others [77]. WeChat is considered a super version of Facebook and is the most popular social media platform among people in China, and it provides many different services such as instant personal and group messaging, sharing of information/videos/news through WeChat Moments, payment services, marketing services, and many other services all in one app [77].

All participants gave their informed consent before they participated in the study, which was conducted in accordance with the Declaration of Helsinki 1975, revised in 2013. The period of data collection was from January to March 2021. We investigated the driving factors behind SM platform adoption for OL and its impact on student AP.

4.1. Constructs Development and Pilot Study

A structured online survey questionnaire was used to collect data because the online data collection method is considered appropriate, fast, inexpensive, and able to minimize incorrect data and incomplete responses [78,79], as well as suitable to overcome difficult physical access due to long travel times and/or COVID-19 [80]. The study constructs of PEU and PU were defined based on work by Davis [24], and OL, IP, ENG, and AP were defined and measured following the works of Al-Rahmi et al. [81] and Alamri et al. [68]. AP was measured through the students' self-reporting on their academic performance in the 2020–2021 fall semester. Each construct (multiple items) was measured on a five-point Likert scale (i.e., from strongly disagree to strongly agree). At the start of the survey, all respondents were informed that their participation was voluntary and were provided a brief overview of the purpose of the study. The respondents were assured that their information would be kept strictly confidential and used for research purposes only. Before the actual study, a pilot test or pilot study was carried out with 33 respondents to ensure the legibility of the survey questionnaire [13]. Based on feedback, small changes, such as to questionnaire terminology, were made. Detailed information regarding constructs and item measurements are listed in the Appendix A.

4.2. Formal Survey

To test the hypotheses, we distributed a revised questionnaire (Appendix A) through WeChat, QQ, and email. Before filling out the questionnaire, the respondents were informed that this questionnaire was only for those who use SM platforms for educational purposes for at least two hours a day. We used two pieces of software for analysis: Jamovi for the organization of demographic data and SmartPLS 3 for the data analysis model.

4.3. Descriptive Analysis

The respondents' demographic information is shown in Table 1. The authors received a total of 297 responses, and the final sample contained 233 respondents, which is valid for data analysis. In the dataset, N = 104 were female students and N = 129 were male students.

Table 1. Respondents' demographic information.

Items		Percentage
Gender	Male	55.4
	Female	44.6
Education	Under Graduate	69.95
	Masters	21.03
	Doctoral	9.01
Social Media Use Frequency for Educational Purposes	2 h	10.1
	Almost 3 h	15.5
	Almost 5 h	27.9
	More than 5 h	46.5
	Pakistan	38.19
	Bangladesh	16.73
International Medical Student Home Country	India	24.2
	Malaysia	11.58
	Afghanistan	9.3

4.4. Common Method Variance

We applied Harman's single-factor test to assess the potential for common method variance (CMV) in our data [82]. The results demonstrated that the first factor's value was 37.97%, which was lower than the recommended minimum value of 50%. In the data, we found no common method bias and no CMV issue.

5. Data Analysis

We used "structural equation modeling (SEM)" to test the research hypotheses (Figure 1) with SmartPLS 3 software. We divided the structural equation model into two stages. In the first stage, we analyzed the measurement model to test the reliability and validity of the data, and in the second stage, we analyzed the relationships hypothesized by the structural model.

5.1. Measurement Model

The results of Table 2 demonstrate the constructs' reliability and validity. The factor loadings, Cronbach's alpha (CA), composite reliability (CR), and rho_A of each construct were found to be greater than the value of 0.70 recommended by Hair, Hollingsworth, Randolph, and Chong in all cases [83]. The values of average variance extracted (AVE) of all constructs were higher than the value of 0.5 suggested by Fornell and Larcker [84]. An appropriate discriminant validity (defined as the degree that one construct differs from another construct [85]) was achieved because all correlations between dimensions were less than the square root of the AVE [84] (Table 3) and the heterotrait–monotrait (HTMT) relationship of the correlations between two constructs was less than 0.9 [86] (Table 3). Lastly, we examined variance inflation factors (VIFs) to analyze collinearity problem; they were found to be lower than 5 [87,88], which indicated that common method variance was not an issue in this study, as shown in Table 2.

Table 2. Factor loadings, Cronbach's alpha, rho_A, CR, AVE, and VIF.

Constructs	PU	PEU	IP	OL	ENG	AP	Cronbach's a	rho_A	CR	AVE	VIF
PU							0.878	0.883	0.916	0.732	
PU1	0.817										1.806
PU2	0.836										2.184
PU3	0.867										2.491
PU4	0.901										2.836
PEU							0.833	0.865	0.892	0.680	
PEU1		0.832									1.232
PEU2		0.904									3.004
PEU3		0.873									2.524
PEU4		0.897									3.532
IP							0.871	0.876	0.912	0.722	
IP1			0.848								2.096
IP2			0.801								1.847
IP3			0.902								2.963
IP4			0.847								2.184
OL							0.896	0.896	0.928	0.762	
OL1				0.829							2.017
OL2				0.881							2.810
OL3				0.887							2.662
OL4				0.894							3.008
ENG							0.888	0.889	0.922	0.748	
ENG1					0.854						2.438
ENG2					0.870						2.632
ENG3					0.882						2.626
ENG4					0.853						2.364
AP							0.900	0.903	0.930	0.770	
AP1						0.859					2.245
AP2						0.899					3.060
AP3						0.878					2.796
AP4						0.872					2.439

Table 3. Discriminant validity.

Constructs	PU	PEU	IP	OL	ENG	AP
PU	**0.855**	0.867	0.845	0.883	0.886	0.773
PEU	0.433	**0.824**	0.857	0.853	0.841	0.826
IP	0.521	0.607	**0.849**	0.873	0.821	0.786
OL	0.489	0.547	0.623	**0.873**	0.858	0.650
ENG	0.333	0.631	0.573	0.577	**0.864**	0.814
AP	0.525	0.589	0.625	0.596	0.669	**0.877**

Note: Diagonal elements in bold represent Fornell and Larcker criteria, and those in italics represent heterotrait–monotrait (HTMT).

5.2. Structural Model

To check the structural model, we examined the significant relationships among exogenous and endogenous variables. To examine the significance of the path coefficients, a bootstrapping procedure with 5000 resamples was performed [89]. Figure 2 illustrates the results of the structural model assessment, showing that all our hypotheses had significant relationships and that the overall model fit following bootstrapping allowed for significant values. Furthermore, Figure 2 shows that the three endogenous variables had substantial R^2 values. The effect size (f^2) of a structural model relationship measures the contribution of exogenous constructs in endogenous constructs. Following the work of Cohen [90], we found f^2 values of PU -> OL 0.064, PEU -> OL 0.078, PE -> OL 0.194, OL -> SAT 1.329, OL -> AP 0.208, and SAT -> AP 0.451, all of which were greater than zero. In addition, to further test the predictive relevance of the model, we obtained Stone–Geisser's Q^2 (the measure of cross-validated redundancy for all endogenous constructs) via the blindfolding algorithm of SmartPLS [91], which is shown in Figure 2. All Q^2 values were found to be greater than 0, indicating that constructs had predictive relevance [89]. Finally, to test our research hypotheses regarding the significance of the paths, we obtained the standardized path coefficient (β) values and the coefficients of determination (R^2) of the endogenous constructs in the research model; see Figure 2.

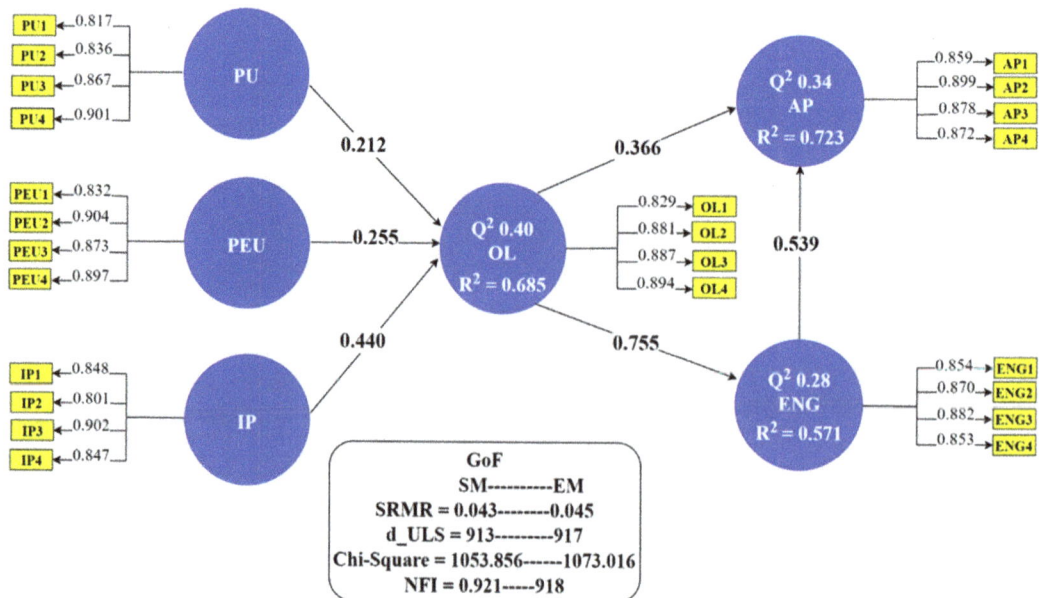

Figure 2. Results of proposed model.

6. Discussion

The use of SM platforms has become a key part of education, and it has grown increasingly significant in both course delivery and course evaluations. The work by Stathopoulou et al. showed a beneficial effect of the integration of SM in education on the profound learning experience of students [29]. SM can be used as a tool to support students and help instructors during their learning processes. Research has illustrated that the significant role of using SM platforms in the concepts of OL can be observed globally because these technologies increase learning, cooperation, and information sharing among students, teachers, and subject professionals as they are crucial for learning and training. The authors of this paper aimed to examine the real motives behind the use of SM in an international medical student community. We proposed a conceptual model that utilizes TAM and SCT. According to Rauniar, Rawski, Yang, and Johnson, the use of SM platforms to promote interpersonal interactions, communication, entertainment, and social bonding among users has become a global phenomenon [92]. In the context of OL, our results also provide important contributions to SCT and TAM [93]. Thus, we recommend the use of SM platforms for OL in higher education because they provide opportunities to students for interaction, ENG, and collaboration with peers, all of which improve their AP. Over time, we hope that many advisors will integrate SM platforms into educational programs in order to aid modern students and encourage OL [4,94]. The use of the most well-liked SM platform applications, such as WeChat, Weibo, Tencent Meeting, Twitter, Facebook, WhatsApp, and Google Classroom, for online class sessions is becoming more functional. Simultaneously, the widespread use of technology such as laptops, mobiles, and tablets (which allow for easy access to SM) can enhance students' educational activities.

The present study has revealed that SM platforms aid the creation of learning environments by enhancing student cooperation, communication, and articulation. The findings of the study show that there is a significant and positive relationship between H1, H2, and H3 with OL. Most of the students reported that using SM platforms for OL is a good idea. In other words, the use of social media affects OL, which, in turn, has a significant impact on students' AP through information sharing, material exchange, and peer discussion. When students engage in OL and enjoy using SM platforms, they also participate in discussions with subject specialists and peers while engaging with their own social presence. These findings are in line with those of earlier studies [11,13], which support the idea that SM platforms are useful for OL. We also identified that student collaboration could be promoted via the use of SM platforms in learning and teaching; consequently, adequate learning results and student AP can be increased through interactions with virtual communities. Similar results were also reported by Tarantino, McDonough, and Hua [95]. Another study showed that recently created apps have inspired students to utilize SM to learn in diverse educational environments [71]. Though SM has larger implications for classroom students, scholars have also investigated SM for use by technicians [96,97]. In her case study on technology, Bernadette Longo said that SM is an important element of the broad and complex social networks that comprise human technology [98].

OL was found to show significant relationships with H4 and H5. Through SM, OL improves the AP of students by enhancing the communication skills and knowledge exchange among fellow learners. Our analysis also indicated an essential correlation between OL and AP because students reported having confidence in improving their learning outcomes with greater accomplishments, greater productivity, and lower research workloads by using social media, and they expect to use it in the future. We believe that incorporating SM platforms into traditional blogging could positively increase the academic outcomes of students. Furthermore, according to the results of this study, regarding H6, the use of SM platforms can contribute to the creation of a supportive and learning-conducive atmosphere, which is invaluable for student ENG, student learning, lecturer teaching experiences, and academic supervision. SM can improve learning settings by encouraging interaction and ENG among students, as well as promoting team discussions and the completion of projects. Overall, this study and previous studies have shown that students may use SM platforms for engagement to increase their AP [65]. Related to this result, Balakrishnan and Gan reported that SM platforms could change educational methods and provide space for students to directly communicate and collaborate with different people around the world [71]. This idea is supported via two theoretical perspectives: SCT and computer-mediated learning (CML). SCT's main emphasis is on social contact and collaboration, and CML advocates the omnipresent stresses of topographical hurdles. Hence, to gain useful learning experiences related to OL, it is necessary to develop social groups to apply and use OL abilities via SM platforms.

7. Conclusions

This research contributes to the field of knowledge on the student adoption of SM platforms for the benefit of OL; it also emphasizes the role of SM in the worldwide adoption of collaborative working and OL principles. Such resources are beneficial to studying and teaching because they help students understand, collaborate, and share knowledge. These conclusions were reached by developing and empirically evaluating a conceptual framework based on the TAM and SCT. The applications of internet resources and SM platforms as sources of learning are enormously important and essential for students and scholars. Our findings revealed that studying in a group of peers is advantageous to researchers and students because it can enhance group output. In this manner, students can efficiently propose new ideas and sentiments in group debates and collaborations with each other. Furthermore, using SM platforms for OL and ENG can enrich students' learning experiences while facilitating team discussions. This study has shown that the PEU, PU, and IP of SM platforms positively effects students' OL, ENG, and, ultimately, AP. Particularly in a time of growing focus on expediently delivering coursework through digital technologies, students, higher educational institutions, and policymakers may see positive impacts of SM platform adoption by students on OL. However, this research had limitations, such as its sample size of N = 233 and its focus on international medical students in Jiangsu province universities of China, both of which make it difficult to draw conclusive inferences about the conceptual model's effectiveness; therefore, the replication of this study in other countries with different economic and cultural conditions is crucial.

7.1. Implications

The present research has a few significant implications for students, higher educational institutes, and policymakers. Understanding the link between the use of SM platforms and their beneficial impacts on student performance is critical to comprehend the function of SM during their studies. The findings may be useful for those who are interested in improving online learning or using SM platforms to facilitate OL. This research endorses the idea that students should be welcomed, rather than forced, by their learning institutions to make use of SM to achieve OL in order to improve their AP in higher education. Additionally, lecturers and supervisors must help students with any questions they might have regarding the use of SM or information sharing. Students' knowledge-seeking experiences and research expertise can be enhanced through the provision of useful knowledge by lecturers and supervisors. Following our results, interventions to stop or at least diminish cyberstalking and bullying should be adopted by legislators in universities to avoid their detrimental impacts on student academic achievement. These measures may lead to the development of a blueprint for recognising the variables that are expected to have significant impacts on the use of SM platforms for open learning to improve AP. The authors of this study implemented a variety of theoretical and empirical analyses, but the ideas of the research emerged from practice and will serve as the foundation for the implementation of new theories and approaches in the framework of China's adoption of OL. This could be the first time that SCT and TAM have been applied to higher education in China, specifically to investigate the effect of SM platforms on OL and student AP, and our findings showed that SCT, when combined with the TAM, was an important theory for examining the impact of SM use on students' OL and AP in Chinese higher education.

7.2. Future Perspective and Limitations

Further research can be conducted to fill in the gaps caused by the limitations of this study. This research was quantitative; data were collected with online survey questionnaires and were cross-sectional. The sample size was small and only included international medical students studying in universities located in the Jiangsu province of China. Results could be different in other provinces or geographical locations, even in the same country. In this research, AP was collected through participants' self-reported construct, which may add limitations to the outcome. Thus, future studies may consider including students' grades as students' actual reported performance and achievement. For this research, we used specific social networks such as WeChat, QQ, Tencent Meeting, and Weibo; however, future studies can consider other social networks sites such as Facebook, LinkedIn, Twitter, and blogs. Furthermore, in future studies, mixed research approaches can be used, and the model could be expanded to include other variables such as enjoyment, satisfaction, interactions with teachers, and knowledge sharing.

Author Contributions: Conceptualization, M.N.K. and M.A.A.; methodology, M.N.K. and M.A.A.; software, M.N.K.; formal analysis, M.N.K. and M.A.A.; resources, M.N.K., S.R.C. and M.K.; writing—original draft preparation, M.N.K., M.A.A., M.K., W.R. and M.F.F.; writing—review and editing, M.N.K., M.A.A., A.U.K. and S.R.C. All authors have read and agreed to the published version of the manuscript.

Funding: This research was supported by the National Natural Science Foundation of China (The Research Fund for International Young Scientists, grant no. 71950410624). Opinions reflect those of the authors and do not necessarily reflect those of the grant agencies.

Institutional Review Board Statement: The study was conducted in accordance with the Declaration of Helsinki, and the protocol was approved by the Ethics Committee of Hunan University.

Informed Consent Statement: Informed consent was obtained from all subjects involved in the study.

Data Availability Statement: The data analyzed in this study are available from the corresponding author on reasonable request: naeem@smail.nju.edu.cn.

Conflicts of Interest: The authors declare no conflict of interest.

Appendix A

Questionnaire

Perceived Usefulness

PU1: Using social media for open learning can help me to make my learning more efficient.

PU2: Using social media for open learning can be helpful for my learning needs.

PU3: Using social media for open learning can increase my assignment productivity.

PU4: Using social media for open learning allows me to communicate with more people in short periods.

Perceived Ease of Use

PEU1: Using social media for open learning enables flexible interactions with others.

PEU2: I find it easy to use social media to do what I want to do.

PEU3: It is easy to become skillful at using social media.

PEU4: I find social media easy to use for open learning.

Interaction with peers

IP1: Social media facilitates interactions with my peers.

IP2: Social media gives me the opportunity to engage in discussion with my peers.

IP3: Social media allows for the exchange of information with my peers.

IP4: Social media facilitates dialogue with my peers.

Open learning

OL1: Open learning builds strong and engaging connections between students and tutors.

OL2: Open learning offers opportunity for interaction and communication with instructors, other students, and content experts.

OL3: Open learning provides opportunities to students for team cooperation (collaboration), which has a direct impact on their performance.

OL4: Students have a positive attitude toward the use of social media for open learning and academic purposes.

Engagement

ENG1: By using social media, I engage in interactions with my peers.

ENG2: By using social media, I engage in interactions with my lecturers.

ENG3: By using social media, I have learned how to work with others effectively.

ENG4: By using social media, I have become satisfied with my engagement with studies.

Academic Performance

AP1: Social media has led to a better learning experience in this module.

AP2: Social media has allowed me to better understand my studies.

AP3: Social media is helpful in my studies and makes it easy to learn.

AP4: Social media improves my academic performance.

References

1. Avcı, K.; Çelikden, S.G.; Eren, S.; Aydenizöz, D. Assessment of medical students' attitudes on social media use in medicine: A cross-sectional study. *BMC Med. Educ.* **2015**, *15*, 1–6. [CrossRef]
2. Statista. Number of Social Network Users Worldwide from 2017 to 2025. Available online: https://www.statista.com/markets/424/topic/540/social-media-user-generated-content/#overview (accessed on 12 September 2021).
3. Pekkala, K.; van Zoonen, W. Work-related social media use: The mediating role of social media communication self-efficacy. *Eur. Manag. J.* **2021**. [CrossRef]
4. Sutherland, S.; Jalali, A. Social media as an open-learning resource in medical education: Current perspectives. *Adv. Med. Educ. Pract.* **2017**, *8*, 369–375. [CrossRef]
5. Fox, S. Peer-to-Peer Healthcare. Pew Internet & American Life Project. 2011. Available online: http://pewinternet.org/Reports/2011/P2PHealthcare.aspx (accessed on 16 September 2021).
6. Mansfield, S.J.; Morrison, S.G.; Stephens, H.O.; Bonning, M.A.; Wang, S.; Withers, A.H.J.; Olver, R.C.; Perry, A.W. Social media and the medical profession. *Med. J. Aust.* **2011**, *194*, 642–644. [CrossRef] [PubMed]
7. Liu, Q.; Peng, W.; Zhang, F.; Hu, R.; Li, Y.; Yan, W. The Effectiveness of Blended Learning in Health Professions: Systematic Review and Meta-Analysis. *J. Med. Internet Res.* **2016**, *18*, e2. [CrossRef] [PubMed]
8. Davis, W.M.; Ho, K.; Last, J. Advancing social media in medical education. *Can. Med. Assoc. J.* **2015**, *187*, 549–550. [CrossRef] [PubMed]
9. Leonard, P.M.; Vaast, E. Social media and their affordances for organizing: A review and agenda for research. *Acad. Manag. Ann.* **2017**, *11*, 150–151. [CrossRef]
10. Wakefield, J.; Frawley, J.K. How does students' general academic achievement moderate the implications of social networking on specific levels of learning performance? *Comput. Educ.* **2020**, *144*, 103694. [CrossRef]
11. Al-Rahmi, W.M.; Yahaya, N.; Alamri, M.M.; Aljarboa, N.A.; Kamin, Y.B.; Saud, M.S.B. How Cyber Stalking and Cyber Bullying Affect Students' Open Learning. *IEEE Access* **2019**, *7*, 20199–20210. [CrossRef]
12. Bylieva, D.; Bekirogullari, Z.; Kuznetsov, D.; Almazova, N.; Lobatyuk, V.; Rubtsova, A. Online Group Student Peer-Communication as an Element of Open Education. *Future Internet* **2020**, *12*, 143. [CrossRef]
13. Khan, M.N.; Ashraf, M.A.; Seinen, D.; Khan, K.U.; Laar, R.A. Social Media for Knowledge Acquisition and Dissemination: The Impact of the COVID-19 Pandemic on Collaborative Learning Driven Social Media Adoption. *Front. Psychol.* **2021**, *12*, 648253. [CrossRef] [PubMed]
14. Ertmer, P.A.; Newby, T.J.; Liu, W.; Tomory, A.; Yu, J.H.; Lee, Y.M. Students' confidence and perceived value for participating in cross-cultural wiki-based collaborations. *Educ. Technol. Res. Dev.* **2011**, *59*, 213–228. [CrossRef]
15. Meishar-Tal, H.; Kurtz, G.; Pieterse, E. Facebook groups as LMS: A case study. *Int. Rev. Res. Open Distrib. Learn.* **2012**, *13*, 33–48. [CrossRef]
16. Al-Maatouk, Q.; Othman, M.S.; Aldraiweesh, A.; Alturki, U.; Al-Rahmi, W.M.; Aljeraiwi, A.A. Task-Technology Fit and Technology Acceptance Model Application to Structure and Evaluate the Adoption of Social Media in Academia. *IEEE Access* **2020**, *8*, 78427–78440. [CrossRef]
17. Anderson, M.; Jiang, J. Teens, social media & technology. *Pew Res. Cent.* **2018**, *31*, 1673–1689.
18. Krasilnikov, A.; Smirnova, A. Online social adaptation of first-year students and their academic performance. *Comput. Educ.* **2017**, *113*, 327–338. [CrossRef]
19. Alenazy, W.M.; Al-Rahmi, W.M.; Khan, M.S. Validation of TAM Model on Social Media Use for Collaborative Learning to Enhance Collaborative Authoring. *IEEE Access* **2019**, *7*, 71550–71562. [CrossRef]

20. Ryane, I.; El Faddouli, N.-E. A Case Study of Using Edmodo to Enhance Computer Science Learning for Engineering Students. *Int. J. Emerg. Technol. Learn.* **2020**, *15*, 62–73. [CrossRef]
21. Al-Rahmi, W.M.; Yahaya, N.; Alturki, U.; Alrobai, A.; Aldraiweesh, A.A.; Alsayed, A.O.; Kamin, Y.B. Social media—Based collaborative learning: The effect on learning success with the moderating role of cyberstalking and cyberbullying. *Interact. Learn. Environ.* **2020**, 1–14. [CrossRef]
22. Rasheed, M.I.; Malik, M.J.; Pitafi, A.H.; Iqbal, J.; Anser, M.K.; Abbas, M. Usage of social media, student engagement, and creativity: The role of knowledge sharing behavior and cyberbullying. *Comput. Educ.* **2020**, *159*, 104002. [CrossRef]
23. Vygotsky, L.S. *Mind in Society: The Development of Higher Psychological Processes*; Harvard University Press: Cambridge, MA, USA; London, UK, 1978.
24. Davis, F.D. Perceived Usefulness, Perceived Ease of Use, and User Acceptance of Information Technology. *MIS Q. Manag. Inf. Syst.* **1989**, *13*, 319–339. [CrossRef]
25. Chukwuere, J.E.; Chukwuere, P.C. The Impact of Social Media on Social Lifestyle: A Case Study of University Female Students. *Gend. Behav.* **2017**, *15*, 9966–9981.
26. Terzi, B.; Bulut, S.; Kaya, N. Factors affecting nursing and midwifery students' attitudes toward social media. *Nurse Educ. Pract.* **2019**, *35*, 141–149. [CrossRef] [PubMed]
27. Kim, T.T.; Karatepe, O.M.; Lee, G.; Demiral, H. Do Gender and Prior Experience Moderate the Factors Influencing Attitude toward Using Social Media for Festival Attendance? *Sustainability* **2018**, *10*, 3509. [CrossRef]
28. Brinkman, C.S.; Gabriel, S.; Paravati, E. Social achievement goals and social media. *Comput. Hum. Behav.* **2020**, *111*, 106427. [CrossRef]
29. Stathopoulou, A.; Siamagka, N.-T.; Christodoulides, G. A multi-stakeholder view of social media as a supporting tool in higher education: An educator–student perspective. *Eur. Manag. J.* **2019**, *37*, 421–431. [CrossRef]
30. Tulin, M.; Pollet, T.V.; Lehmann-Willenbrock, N. Perceived group cohesion versus actual social structure: A study using social network analysis of egocentric Facebook networks. *Soc. Sci. Res.* **2018**, *74*, 161–175. [CrossRef]
31. Hansen, D.T. *The Teacher and the World: A Study of Cosmopolitanism as Education*; Routledge: Milton Park, UK, 2017; ISBN 1136632972.
32. Penni, J. The future of online social networks (OSN): A measurement analysis using social media tools and application. *Telemat. Inform.* **2017**, *34*, 498–517. [CrossRef]
33. Baccarella, C.V.; Wagner, T.F.; Kietzmann, J.; McCarthy, I.P. Social media? It's serious! Understanding the dark side of social media. *Eur. Manag. J.* **2018**, *36*, 431–438. [CrossRef]
34. Dong, J.K.; Saunders, C.; Wachira, B.W.; Thoma, B.; Chan, T.M. Social media and the modern scientist: A research primer for low- and middle-income countries. *Afr. J. Emerg. Med.* **2020**, *10*, S120–S124. [CrossRef]
35. Salmeron, L.; García, A.; Vidal-Abarca, E. The development of adolescents' comprehension-based Internet reading activities. *Learn. Individ. Differ.* **2018**, *61*, 31–39. [CrossRef]
36. Berkani, L. A semantic and social-based collaborative recommendation of friends in social networks. *Softw. Pract. Exp.* **2020**, *50*, 1498–1519. [CrossRef]
37. Fuse, A.; Lanham, E.A. Impact of social media and quality life of people who stutter. *J. Fluen. Disord.* **2016**, *50*, 59–71. [CrossRef]
38. Tess, P.A. The role of social media in higher education classes (real and virtual)—A literature review. *Comput. Hum. Behav.* **2013**, *29*, A60–A68. [CrossRef]
39. Rahman, S.; Ramakrishnan, T.; Ngamassi, L. Impact of social media use on student satisfaction in Higher Education. *High. Educ. Q.* **2020**, *74*, 304–319. [CrossRef]
40. Richey, M.; Ravishankar, M. The role of frames and cultural toolkits in establishing new connections for social media innovation. *Technol. Forecast. Soc. Chang.* **2019**, *144*, 325–333. [CrossRef]
41. Berezan, O.; Krishen, A.S.; Agarwal, S.; Kachroo, P. The pursuit of virtual happiness: Exploring the social media experience across generations. *J. Bus. Res.* **2018**, *89*, 455–461. [CrossRef]
42. Rozgonjuk, D.; Sindermann, C.; Elhai, J.D.; Montag, C. Fear of Missing Out (FoMO) and social media's impact on daily-life and productivity at work: Do WhatsApp, Facebook, Instagram, and Snapchat Use Disorders mediate that association? *Addict. Behav.* **2020**, *110*, 106487. [CrossRef]
43. Wodzicki, K.; Schwämmlein, E.; Moskaliuk, J. "Actually, I Wanted to Learn": Study-related knowledge exchange on social networking sites. *Internet High. Educ.* **2012**, *15*, 9–14. [CrossRef]
44. Greenhow, C.; Galvin, S.M.; Willet, K.B.S. What Should Be the Role of Social Media in Education? *Policy Insights Behav. Brain Sci.* **2019**, *6*, 178–185. [CrossRef]
45. Vlieghe, J.; Vandermeersche, G.; Soetaert, R. Social media in literacy education: Exploring social reading with pre-service teachers. *New Media Soc.* **2016**, *18*, 800–816. [CrossRef]
46. López-Yáñez, I.; Yanez-Marquez, C.; Camacho-Nieto, O.; Aldape-Pérez, M.; Argüelles-Cruz, A.-J. Collaborative learning in postgraduate level courses. *Comput. Hum. Behav.* **2015**, *51*, 938–944. [CrossRef]
47. Alwagait, E.; Shahzad, B.; Alim, S. Impact of social media usage on students academic performance in Saudi Arabia. *Comput. Hum. Behav.* **2015**, *51*, 1092–1097. [CrossRef]
48. Chandra, C.P. The adoption of e-auction in Indonesia: The extended technology acceptance model study. *iBuss Manag.* **2015**, *3*, 423–433.

49. Bruner, J. *Acts of Meaning*; Harvard University Press: Cambridge, MA, USA, 1990.
50. Gaytan, J. Integrating social media into the learning environment of the classroom: Following social constructivism principles. *J. Appl. Res. Bus. Instr.* **2013**, *11*, 1.
51. Mishra, R.K. Social Constructivism and Teaching of Social Science. *J. Soc. Stud. Educ. Res.* **2014**, *5*, 1–13. [CrossRef]
52. Slavin, R.E. Cooperative learning and intergroup relations. In *Handbook of Research on Multicultural Education*; Banks, J.A., Banks, C.A.M., Eds.; Macmillan: New York, NY, USA, 1995; pp. 628–634.
53. Brown, J.S.; Collins, A.; Duguid, P. Situated cognition and the culture of learning. *Educ. Res.* **1989**, *18*, 32–42. [CrossRef]
54. Bhattacharjee, J. Constructivist approach to learning—An effective approach of teaching learning. *Int. Res. J. Interdiscip. Multidiscip. Stud.* **2015**, *1*, 23–28.
55. Stabile, C.; Ershler, J. (Eds.) *Constructivism Reconsidered in the Age of Social Media: New Directions for Teaching and Learning*; John Wiley & Sons: Hoboken, NJ, USA, 2015.
56. Kelm, O.R. Social media: It's what students do. *Bus. Commun. Q.* **2011**, *74*, 505–520. [CrossRef]
57. Churcher, K. "Friending" Vygotsky: A Social Constructivist Pedagogy of Knowledge Building through Classroom Social Media Use. *J. Eff. Teach.* **2014**, *14*, 33–50.
58. Lee, M.J.W.; McLoughlin, C. *Web 2.0-Based E-Learning: Applying Social Informatics for Tertiary Teaching: Applying Social Informatics for Tertiary Teaching*; IGI Global: Hershey, PA, USA, 2010; ISBN 160566295X.
59. McLoughlin, C.; Lee, M.J.W. Personalised and self regulated learning in the Web 2.0 era: International exemplars of innovative pedagogy using social software. *Australas. J. Educ. Technol.* **2010**, *26*, 28–43. [CrossRef]
60. Golub, J. *Focus on Collaborative Learning*; National Council of Teachers of English: Urbana, IL, USA, 1988; ISBN 0814117538.
61. Min, G.; Yan, X.; Yuecheng, Y. An Enhanced Technology Acceptance Model for Web-Based Learning. *J. Inf. Syst. Educ.* **2004**, *15*, 365–374.
62. Teo, T.; Zhou, M. Explaining the intention to use technology among university students: A structural equation modeling approach. *J. Comput. High. Educ.* **2014**, *26*, 124–142. [CrossRef]
63. Abdullah, F.; Ward, R.; Ahmed, E. Investigating the influence of the most commonly used external variables of TAM on students' Perceived Ease of Use (PEOU) and Perceived Usefulness (PU) of e-portfolios. *Comput. Hum. Behav.* **2016**, *63*, 75–90. [CrossRef]
64. Cain, J. Online Social Networking Issues within Academia and Pharmacy Education. *Am. J. Pharm. Educ.* **2008**, *72*, 10. [CrossRef]
65. Ansari, J.A.N.; Khan, N.A. Exploring the role of social media in collaborative learning the new domain of learning. *Smart Learn. Environ.* **2020**, *7*, 1–16. [CrossRef]
66. Patera, M.; Draper, S.; Naef, M. ExploringMagic Cottage: A virtual reality environment for stimulating children's imaginative writing. *Interact. Learn. Environ.* **2008**, *16*, 245–263. [CrossRef]
67. Hurt, N.E.; Moss, G.; Bradley, C.; Larson, L.; Lovelace, M.; Prevost, L.; Riley, N.; Domizi, D.; Camus, M. The 'Facebook' Effect: College Students' Perceptions of Online Discussions in the Age of Social Networking. *Int. J. Sch. Teach. Learn.* **2012**, *6*. [CrossRef]
68. Alamri, M.; Almaiah, M.; Al-Rahmi, W. Social Media Applications Affecting Students' Academic Performance: A Model Developed for Sustainability in Higher Education. *Sustainability* **2020**, *12*, 6471. [CrossRef]
69. Greenhow, C.; Gleason, B. Twitteracy: Tweeting as a New Literacy Practice. *Educ. Forum* **2012**, *76*, 464–478. [CrossRef]
70. Dumford, A.D.; Miller, A.L. Online learning in higher education: Exploring advantages and disadvantages for engagement. *J. Comput. High. Educ.* **2018**, *30*, 452–465. [CrossRef]
71. Balakrishnan, V.; Gan, C.L. Students' learning styles and their effects on the use of social media technology for learning. *Telemat. Inform.* **2016**, *33*, 808–821. [CrossRef]
72. Rasiah, R.R.V. Transformative Higher Education Teaching and Learning: Using Social Media in a Team-based Learning Environment. *Procedia Soc. Behav. Sci.* **2014**, *123*, 369–379. [CrossRef]
73. Jacobsen, W.C.; Forste, R. The Wired Generation: Academic and Social Outcomes of Electronic Media Use Among University Students. *Cyberpsychol. Behav. Soc. Netw.* **2011**, *14*, 275–280. [CrossRef]
74. Junco, R.; Heiberger, G.; Loken, E. The effect of Twitter on college student engagement and grades. *J. Comput. Assist. Learn.* **2011**, *27*, 119–132. [CrossRef]
75. Baird, D.E.; Fisher, M. Neomillennial User Experience Design Strategies: Utilizing Social Networking Media to Support "Always on" Learning Styles. *J. Educ. Technol. Syst.* **2005**, *34*, 5–32. [CrossRef]
76. Miller, D.; Sinanan, J.; Wang, X.; McDonald, T.; Haynes, N.; Costa, E.; Spyer, J.; Venkatraman, S.; Nicolescu, R. *How the World Changed Social Media*; Duke University Press: Durham, NC, USA, 2016.
77. Statista. Social Networks in China-Statistics & Facts. Available online: https://www.statista.com/topics/1170/social-networks-in-china (accessed on 16 September 2021).
78. Bhattacherjee, A. Social science research: Principles, methods, and practices. In *Global Text Project*; University of South Florida: Tampa, FL, USA, 2012.
79. Dutot, V.; Bhatiasevi, V.; Bellallahom, N. Applying the technology acceptance model in a three-countries study of smartwatch adoption. *J. High Technol. Manag. Res.* **2019**, *30*, 1–14. [CrossRef]
80. Kavota, J.K.; Kamdjoug, J.R.K.; Wamba, S.F. Social media and disaster management: Case of the north and south Kivu regions in the Democratic Republic of the Congo. *Int. J. Inf. Manag.* **2020**, *52*, 102068. [CrossRef]
81. Al-Rahmi, W.M.; Alias, N.; Othman, M.S.; Marin, V.I.; Tur, G. A model of factors affecting learning performance through the use of social media in Malaysian higher education. *Comput. Educ.* **2018**, *121*, 59–72. [CrossRef]

82. Podsakoff, P.M.; MacKenzie, S.B.; Podsakoff, N.P. Sources of Method Bias in Social Science Research and Recommendations on How to Control It. *Annu. Rev. Psychol.* **2012**, *63*, 539–569. [CrossRef]
83. Hair, J.; Hollingsworth, C.L.; Randolph, A.B.; Chong, A.Y.L. An updated and expanded assessment of PLS-SEM in information systems research. *Ind. Manag. Data Syst.* **2017**, *117*, 442–458. [CrossRef]
84. Fornell, C.; Larcker, D.F. Evaluating Structural Equation Models with Unobservable Variables and Measurement Error. *J. Mark. Res.* **1981**, *18*, 39–50. [CrossRef]
85. Hair, J.F., Jr.; Sarstedt, M.; Hopkins, L.; Kuppelwieser, V.G. Partial least squares structural equation modeling (PLS-SEM): An emerging tool in business research. *Eur. Bus. Rev.* **2014**, *26*, 106–121. [CrossRef]
86. Henseler, J.; Ringle, C.M.; Sarstedt, M. A new criterion for assessing discriminant validity in variance-based structural equation modeling. *J. Acad. Mark. Sci.* **2015**, *43*, 115–135. [CrossRef]
87. Becker, J.-M.; Ringle, C.M.; Sarstedt, M.; Völckner, F. How collinearity affects mixture regression results. *Mark. Lett.* **2015**, *26*, 643–659. [CrossRef]
88. Mason, C.H.; Perreault, W.D. Collinearity, Power, and Interpretation of Multiple Regression Analysis. *J. Mark. Res.* **1991**, *28*, 268. [CrossRef]
89. Hair, J.F.; Ringle, C.; Sarstedt, M.; Hult, G.T.M. *A Primer on Partial Least Squares Structural Equation Modeling (PLS-SEM)*; Sage: Thousand Oaks, CA, USA, 2014.
90. Cohen, J. *Statistical Power Analysis for the Behavioral Sciences*, 2nd ed.; Lawrence Erlbaum Associate: Hillsdale, NJ, USA, 2013; ISBN 08058028395. [CrossRef]
91. Ringle, C.M.; Wende, S.; Becker, J. *SmartPLS 3*; SmartPLS: Boenningstedt, Germany, 2015.
92. Rauniar, R.; Rawski, G.; Yang, J.; Johnson, B. Technology acceptance model (TAM) and social media usage: An empirical study on Facebook. *J. Enterp. Inf. Manag.* **2014**, *27*, 6–30. [CrossRef]
93. Alamri, M.M. Undergraduate Students' Perceptions toward Social Media Usage and Academic Performance: A Study from Saudi Arabia. *Int. J. Emerg. Technol. Learn.* **2019**, *14*, 61. [CrossRef]
94. Depietro, P. Social media and collaborative learning. *Counterpoints* **2013**, *435*, 47–62.
95. Tarantino, K.; McDonough, J.; Hua, M. Effects of Student Engagement with Social Media on Student Learning: A Review of Literature. *J. Technol. Student Aff.* **2013**, *1*, 1–8.
96. Hea, A.C.K. Social Media in Technical Communication. *Tech. Commun. Q.* **2013**, *23*, 1–5. [CrossRef]
97. Kaufer, D.; Gunawardena, A.; Tan, A.; Cheek, A. Bringing Social Media to the Writing Classroom: Classroom Salon. *J. Bus. Tech. Commun.* **2011**, *25*, 299–321. [CrossRef]
98. Longo, B. Using Social Media for Collective Knowledge-Making: Technical Communication Between the Global North and South. *Tech. Commun. Q.* **2014**, *23*, 22–34. [CrossRef]

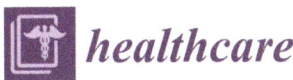

Article

E-Learning as a Factor Optimizing the Amount of Work Time Devoted to Preparing an Exam for Medical Program Students during the COVID-19 Epidemic Situation

Magdalena Roszak [1,†], Bartosz Sawik [2,3,4,*,†], Jacek Stańdo [5] and Ewa Baum [6]

1. Department of Computer Science and Statistics, Poznan University of Medical Sciences, 60-806 Poznan, Poland; mmr@ump.edu.pl
2. Department of Business Informatics and Engineering Management, AGH University of Science and Technology, 30-059 Krakow, Poland
3. Haas School of Business, University of California at Berkeley, Berkeley, CA 94720, USA
4. Department of Statistics, Computer Science and Mathematics, Public University of Navarra, 31006 Pamplona, Spain
5. Centre of Mathematics and Physics, Lodz University of Technology, 90-924 Lodz, Poland; jacek.stando@p.lodz.pl
6. Department of Social Sciences and the Humanities, Poznan University of Medical Sciences, 60-806 Poznan, Poland; ebaum@ump.edu.pl
* Correspondence: B_Sawik@cal.berkeley.edu
† Magdalena Roszak and Bartosz Sawik are both the first authors and these authors contributed equally to this work as the first authors.

Citation: Roszak, M.; Sawik, B.; Stańdo, J.; Baum, E. E-Learning as a Factor Optimizing the Amount of Work Time Devoted to Preparing an Exam for Medical Program Students during the COVID-19 Epidemic Situation. *Healthcare* 2021, 9, 1147. https://doi.org/10.3390/healthcare9091147

Academic Editors: José João Mendes, Vanessa Machado, João Botelho and Luís Proença

Received: 25 June 2021
Accepted: 30 August 2021
Published: 2 September 2021

Publisher's Note: MDPI stays neutral with regard to jurisdictional claims in published maps and institutional affiliations.

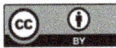

Copyright: © 2021 by the authors. Licensee MDPI, Basel, Switzerland. This article is an open access article distributed under the terms and conditions of the Creative Commons Attribution (CC BY) license (https://creativecommons.org/licenses/by/4.0/).

Abstract: The COVID-19 pandemic had a huge impact on the learning and teaching processes, particularly in healthcare education and training, because of the principal position of the cutting-edge student–patient interaction. Replacing the traditional form of organization and implementation of knowledge evaluation with its web-based equivalent on an e-learning platform optimizes the whole didactic process not only for the unit carrying it out but, above all, for students. This research is focused on the effectiveness of the application of e-learning for computer-based knowledge evaluation and optimizing exam administration for students of medical sciences. The proposed approach is considered in two categories: from the perspective of the providers of the evaluation process, that is, the teaching unit; and the recipients of the evaluation process, that is, the students.

Keywords: e-learning; digital training; healthcare education; innovation in teaching; clinical teaching; e-exams

1. Introduction

During the COVID-19 pandemic and mandatory lockdown, academic institutions have shifted to distance learning. This pandemic had a massive impact on the learning and teaching processes, especially in healthcare education, due to the predominant role of the current student–patient interaction. Replacing the traditional form of organization and implementation of knowledge evaluation with its web-based equivalent on an e-learning platform optimizes the whole didactic process not only for the unit carrying it out but, above all, for students. This research is focused on the effectiveness of the application of e-learning for computer-based knowledge evaluation and optimizing exam administration for students of medical sciences. The proposed approach is considered in two categories: from the perspective of the providers of the evaluation process, that is, the teaching unit; and the recipients of the evaluation process, that is, the students. Worldwide higher education institutions were forced to accelerate the introduction of web-based learning methodologies in areas where this was not the main core, such as clinical teaching. This paper presents the current trends and new challenges that emerge from this new e-learning environment, focusing on its potential to revolutionize healthcare education and exploring how it may help to better prepare future healthcare professionals for their daily practice. The process of optimization through e-learning should become a natural part of the didactic process conducted in every subject at all types of higher education institutions, including medical universities.

For more than a decade, medical schools have been working to transform pedagogy by eliminating/reducing lectures; using technology to replace/enhance anatomy and laboratories; implementing team-facilitated, active, and self-directed learning; and promoting individualized and interprofessional education [1–3]. The situation of the spread of the novel Severe Acute Respiratory Syndrome Coronavirus 2 (SARS-CoV-2) accelerated the application of online teaching and examination in medical schools around the world. Many authors recently considered these issues, for instance, as in a recently published paper by Bianchi et al. about the effects of the SARS-CoV-2 pandemic on medical education [4]. Bianchi et al. presented considerations and tips for the Italian medical education system under the new circumstances of COVID-19 [4]. While the COVID-19 outbreak has been one of the most significant challenges faced in the history of medical education, it has also provided an impetus to develop innovative teaching practices, bringing unprecedented success in allowing for medical students to continue their education, for instance, in ophthalmology, despite these challenges [5]. Different types of online courses are provided at present to develop and implement an effective learning process for medical students. Paper [3], by Rose, presents and discusses the challenges in medical students' education in the time of COVID-19. This author also pointed out that additional unknown academic issues will require attention, including standardized examinations when testing centers are closed, the timeline for residency applications for current third-year students, and the ability to meet the requirements for certain subspecialties prior to applying to residency [3]. Another interesting example of the educational challenges during this pandemic can be found in medical and surgical nursing, with a core course in baccalaureate nursing programs that requires active and effective teaching and learning strategies to enhance students' engagement [6]. The unprecedented, abrupt shift to remote online learning within the context of the national lockdown due to the 2019 coronavirus disease (COVID-19) highlights the importance of addressing students' preparedness in managing their first experiences with online learning [7]. Many authors have tried to explore the medical students' and faculty members' perspectives of online learning during the COVID-19 era [8]. As examples, two recent papers by Varvara et al. [9] and by Iurcov et al. [10] consider the impact of this pandemic on academic activity and health status among medical dentistry students in Romania [9], and also in general dental education challenges during COVID-19 for dentistry undergraduate students in Italy [10]. At present, during the COVID-19 pandemic, e-learning has become a potential approach to technology in education that provides contemporary learners with authentic knowledge acquisitions. As a practical contribution, electronic examination (e-exam) is a novel approach to e-learning, designed to solve traditional examination issues. It is a combination of assorted questions designed by specialized software to detect an individual's performance. Despite the intensive research carried out in this area, the completion of e-exams brings challenges, such as authentication of the examinee's identity and answered papers [11]. It is important to explore the factors affecting students' preference for remote e-exams, methods of course assessment/evaluation, factors related to students' exam dishonesty/misconduct during remote e-exams and measures that can be considered to reduce this behavior [12]. This type of research has been carried out in many medical schools around the world to evaluate the experience of students at faculties of Medicine, Dentistry, Pharmacy, Nursing and Applied Medical Sciences regarding remote e-exams preferences and academic dishonesty during the pandemic [12].

2. Technologies in Education

Technology has always changed methods of learning and knowledge transfer. Generalized access to the Internet has brought about a revolution in learning and teaching. In one new method, a technologically new way of publishing educational content, we now have previously known methods along with new elements that had no equivalent in the past [13–16]. Their emergence in education is determined by the application of modern digital technologies of sound and image recording and their integration with traditional text-based instruction [17,18]. The instant sharing of e-materials for education participants and their prompt updating by teachers is also of crucial significance. The evaluation of student knowledge and the learning process has also been revolutionized [19]. Online tests including a broad interface of questions and automatic verification of answers are now available, as well as self-study tests with explanations and decision-making labyrinths which encourage creative thinking [20–22]. The authors of papers [23–26] have published very interesting recent examples of the usage of technological innovation in medicine. In paper [23] by Guiter et al., the authors present the development of remote online collaborative medical school pathology and explain how students across several international sites, throughout the COVID-19 pandemic, could control the digital slides and offer their own diagnoses, followed by group discussions. In publication [24] by Guadalajara et al., the authors demonstrate whether it is possible to create a technological solution to flexibly self-manage undergraduate general surgery practices within hospitals. In this interesting research study, it was proven that the usage of innovative educational technology could be efficient. The use of mobile-learning application designed to be an educational opportunities' manager tool might be very helpful in promoting self-directed learning, flexible teaching, and bidirectional assessments. The authors also show some limitations for teachers who employ a personal teaching style, which may not need either checkerboards or a tool. Presented solution [24] supports teaching at hospitals in a pandemic without checkerboards. In paper [25], by Bianchi et al., the authors concentrated on an evaluation of the effectiveness of digital technologies during anatomy learning in nursing school. Nicholson et al. also considered anatomy in paper [26], but as an interactive, multi-modal anatomy workshop. The authors proved that an interactive workshop improved attendees' examination performance and promoted engaged enquiry and deeper learning. This tool accommodates varied learning styles and improves self-confidence, which may be a valuable supplement to traditional anatomy teaching [26].

3. Changes and Challenges in the Process of Education at an Academic Level

At present, students take full advantage of new digital technologies in both their daily lives and in the process of formal and informal education [27,28]. In higher education institutions, where teaching and learning are pursued only in the form of traditional practical and laboratory classes held in classrooms, learners do not find the means of information transfer that they know from the Internet. This contributes to a decrease in effective memorizing and generally reduced motivation to learn [29–31]. Distance education is a new method of working with students, which is becoming more crucial in current academic education, particularly in the face of the COVID-19 epidemic [32–34].

Technological progress inevitably leads to the implementation of up-to-date technologies in distance education at every level, including continuing education [17,35–37]. Students particularly favour interactive online courses, as they seem to produce better effects than traditional methods in terms of knowledge acquisition [38–41]. The numerous advantages that online learning offers leads students to turn to the Internet and multimedia sources of knowledge more than they turn to traditional textbooks [42,43]. Therefore, it seems appropriate to implement online learning and provide access to multimedia materials that include reliable educational content, which can replace traditional classes. The application of the methods and techniques of distance learning can be a source of competitive advantage for the school. It can considerably contribute to the quality and efficiency of contemporary student education [44,45].

The methods and techniques of distance education are commonly applied in medical schools, and scientific reports confirm their comparable or even greater effectiveness in comparison with traditional forms [16,37,38,44]. Acquiring skills in virtual reality will translate to a higher quality of medical procedures being administered to patients.

To date, most online trainings were intended for doctors (58%) and also for nurses, pharmacists and stomatologists [46]. It should be remembered that e-learning is not exclusive to higher education [47–49] but is also used for courses or training that the future graduates of medical schools will attend, broadening their knowledge after their medical studies [50]. A lack of experience with participating in online education is a burden for a graduate, as there is no easy way to gain such skills outside of school. Thus, distance learning allows the students to develop additional competences; not just digital ones but also soft competences [51]. All of this facilitates the development of skills such as collaborative work, time management and problem-solving, as well as encouraging creativity and flexibility. Consequently, embracing state-of-the-art technologies may result in a growing number of better-educated graduates who can adapt to the changing labour market and are interested in positions that present nontypical professional and scientific challenges.

Before the pandemic, distance education in medical universities, due to its character, was pursued mainly as part of a hybrid system, in which part of the learning process takes place in direct contact with the teacher in the classroom, and the other part takes place online [39,40,48]. In the case of practical classes, virtual education is combined with supervised hands-on practice, performed on patients in a hospital or medical simulation centres. Such is the nature of most courses taught at medical universities.

Additionally, education through simulation is becoming increasingly popular in the medical academic environment. This is the best teaching method, enabling the creation of real situations in risk-free conditions. Decision-making games can be used successfully in the educational process of future medical staff. The aim of this work was to create a didactic computer program "Trauma", analyze its impact on students' knowledge of the direction of medical rescue and evaluate the attractiveness of classes conducted using this method. The results show that the use of the "Trauma" program in didactics has allowed for improvements in the knowledge and skill levels of students taking part in the study in the field of trauma patients' treatment. In the assessment of students, the classes in which the program was used were interesting. The vast majority of respondents would like to participate in such classes again [52].

There are few reports concerning distance education in medical schools in Poland, especially its application in teaching and learning, as well as in evaluation, comprising credits and examinations [19–21,39,40,53]. It can, therefore, be concluded that, prior to the outbreak of the COVID-19 pandemic, distance learning was not common or its scope was limited. The present paper is a contribution to an academic discussion on e-learning for basic sciences and particularly its use to optimize the amount of time devoted to preparing an exam for medical programs. It looks at two categories: its usefulness for the educational institution and the recipients of the process—in this case, medical university students. The scope of the article involves a comparison of the amount of work time is needed before an examination administered entirely in a computer-based form and how much work time is needed before one given in a traditional paper-based form.

4. Data and Methods

The data collected in the article present the results of research into the working time and organization of electronic (in an e-learning portal) and traditional version of the evaluation of medical knowledge (without e-learning technologies) expressed in minutes (clock hours). The statistical analysis is based on descriptive statistics with the use of Excel [54] and R language [55]. The analysis shows the sum of the working time (clock hours) according to own formulas describing the same process, including a way to build databases for knowledge evaluation. There was no need to statistically analyze the collected data using statistical tests, as the complete data were compared.

The research conducted by the authors is very demanding, due to the labor-intensive preparation of databases, level of technology competence, slower implementation of e-learning in medical education, which is significantly different from education in other fields, and its use by a large group of students from one year. For this reason, standard educational theories were insufficient and could not fully meet all the conditions for the study and the stated goal of the authors' analyses. It was necessary to develop own procedures, accounting for the e-learning methodology.

The research necessary to carry out an analysis of the optimization of knowledge evaluation was conducted in the Department of Pathophysiology in cooperation with the Department of Computer Science and Statistics of Poznan University of Medical Sciences, Poland (PUMS) in the academic years of 2009–2019. Academic teachers (knowledge supply), technical and administrative staff (organizational support) and medical e-learning experts were involved in this research. An electronic evaluation of knowledge was conducted on the Online Learning and Training (OLAT) e-learning portal under an open source license.

The analysis of working time and the organization of electronic knowledge evaluation was carried out on 333 students in their second year of medical studies in the preclinical subject of pathophysiology in the 2018–2019 academic year. These students were studying for one year, and completed the subject at the same time.

The analysis of teachers' working time in the preparation of substantive content in pathophysiology, including the database of international standards for testing and assessment [19,20], the Question and Test Interoperability (QTI), was carried out in the 2015–2016 academic year. The same team of teachers and employees supporting the work participated in the organization and implementation of the evaluation of the delivered traditionally and with the use of an e-learning portal. It was necessary to compare both versions, implementing the evaluation of knowledge in pathophysiology for a large group of students at the same time.

5. Preliminary Conditions for the Analysis of Work Time Devoted to Administering Examinations in Medical Sciences

The analysis of the amount of time devoted to the evaluation of students' performance requires data on the distribution of tasks necessary to set regular exam and paper-based credit test in comparison with its electronic counterpart on an e-learning platform. The organization of the evaluation of students' knowledge usually involves teachers, supported by administrative and/or technical-engineering staff. Student evaluation, conducted in large groups in the traditional form, requires cooperation between these staff members in the auditorium hall or a lecture hall in which the exam or credit test is held; their work is purely organizational, not substantive.

The analysis of the amount of time devoted to the evaluation of students' knowledge in the medical program was conducted using the subject of pathophysiology as an example. This subject is taught in the 2nd year of studies, where the number of students is very high and often varies between 200 and 400. This serves to demonstrate the usefulness of e-learning for the evaluation of students' knowledge. The example presents how it is carried out on an e-learning platform, which complies with the international standards for testing and assessment [19,20], Question and Test Interoperability (QTI).

The study was conducted on a sample of one grade-level group, comprising 333 students taking the course over one semester of an academic year at the Department of Pathophysiology in PUMS [53].

6. Implementation of Evaluation of Knowledge in Pathophysiology

Continuous assessment tests (benchmark tests) given throughout the course, as well as the final test, had to be administered on the premises of the university, according to the act on studies pre-COVID [56].

The course in pathophysiology includes three tests:
1. An introductory test in physiology, beginning the subject;
2. A test on clinical cases, summarizing practical classes;
3. A final test covering the substantive knowledge provided during practical courses and seminars.

Lectures in the subject also end with a summative test, which constitutes either part of the final exam or the credit required for course completion.

The analysis of the process of knowledge evaluation does not account for retakes (two additional attempts) to which students who fail continuous assessment are entitled. Similarly, the report does not consider retake final exams, which are available to people who fail the final exam. Sometimes a need arises to organize a committee course crediting for students who do not pass the course according to the above rules, or a committee exam granted by the Dean, following the consideration of an individual application submitted by the student or teacher.

Following the School Regulations, there must be two dates for the exam, settled by the student representative and the examiner. Additionally, the so-called pre-term exam date may be established, which increases the number of exam dates. Consequently, the minimum number of dates scheduled for the first-attempt examination is three. Every student independently decides on which day he or she wants to take the exam, considering his or her credit and exam calendar. Still, other individual cases have to be noted when a student or a group of students requests a different date to those already scheduled, which may be due to a fortuitous event or the individual organization of studies. As is apparent from the above, the evaluation of knowledge is somewhat burdensome for the unit responsible for the teaching process and the exam session. It requires excellent organization and flexibility, the fixing of teachers' dates with the students' requests and the availability of the halls where the evaluation is to take place. Accommodating all these aspects is a tough challenge for those coordinating the teaching process in a given department.

The university runs a continuous examination session, comprising a period of one or more years of study, during which the exams can be taken at any date. A regular two-week exam session, held directly after the end of the term for all subjects, is unworkable here, not least for organizational reasons. Such a session is hardly feasible, especially for students of medical programs, where groups are enormous.

7. Traditional Examination vs. an E-Exam on an E-Learning Platform

Table 1 presents a comparison of the organization and implementation of knowledge evaluation, using a traditional paper version and an online evaluation. This is a complement to earlier classifications and comparisons, compiled at Poznan University of Medical Sciences in the years 2009–2013 [19], using the example of courses in pathophysiology, medical didactics and andragogy, biostatistics, mathematics or information technology, for different study programs.

Requirements that have to be met to conduct a computer-based evaluation of knowledge on an e-learning platform include:

1. Information technology facilities in the university. An increasing number of universities are now equipped with advanced facilities such as examination centers, medical simulation centers, libraries and computer labs for the Chair of Computer Science, fitted with a sufficient number of computers. An online exam can be held on the school's e-learning platform. Another solution is to deploy smaller seminar rooms on the campus, each equipped with 20–25 computers, where online exams can be held with the support of administrative or technical-engineering staff. Benchmark tests throughout the course are run in classrooms where desktop computers or laptops can easily be installed without changing the arrangement or intended use of the room. To optimize the effective use of computer rooms and help examinees schedule their tests more conveniently, different exams can be administered in one place at one time. Some students can make their first attempt, others can retake, and those with an individual organization of studies might take their summative credit test.
2. Information technology facilities of the participants of the evaluation. Currently, every student has a few electronic devices with Internet access at their disposal. Consequently, online evaluation during the course can be conducted using students' own equipment.

3. Testing out of school. According to an ordinance of the Minister of Science and Higher Education [49], an examination can be held outside of school under conditions that allow for supervision and recording of the exam.
4. Support from the experienced. The departments conducting online evaluation should receive technical support from the IT units responsible for the computer infrastructure of the university. The help provided by experienced teams, which develop and implement e-learning tools or educational research technologies, is vital [18,35,45,57]. These tasks are assigned to university e-learning centers, specialized research units, research departments or other larger academic departments, where e-learning specialists are employed part-time or for the duration of a project, supporting knowledge evaluation processes.

Table 1. A comparison of tasks necessary for the implementation of student evaluation.

No.	Task	Method of Testing	
		Paper-Based	Computer-Based
1.	Preparing test questions	For a single exam	Question bank sufficient for a few years of testing
2.	A few sets of questions for a test	Preparing new versions of questions is necessary	A unique collection of questions for each student from the existing question bank
3.	Preparing questions for the retake	New versions necessary	Preparation of new questions; unnecessary questions are drawn from the existing question bank
4.	Graphic- and multimedia-based questions	Difficult and rarely used. The projector is available in halls with Internet access. Difficult to manage with large groups of examinees.	Easy to manage and increasingly used.
5.	Copying and distributing	Printing paper version. Confidentiality necessary	None. Confidentiality unnecessary
6.	Duration of the test	Difficult to enforce a timeframe with large groups of examinees.	Automated and individual time control for each student
7.	Independence of work	Dubious. A few (2–3) versions of the test with the same order of questions and answers. Difficult to manage with large groups of examinees.	Independent work of the student. Each student gets a (randomly selected) set of questions with a random order of answers.
8.	Assessment	Necessary. Work after the exam	None. Automated instant assessment on the platform
9.	Exam results	After some time. Within five working days	Immediately after the test
10.	Issuing the results	Necessary. Sending the results by e-mail or entering an e-form of student achievement (virtual student office)	None. Automated information in student account on the platform
11.	Exam archiving	Necessary. Labelled sets of tests must be stored in an indicated place in an arranged class/group order	None. Automated, with access to tests by any search criteria for every class
12.	Course evaluation/ participation in evaluation surveys	Rarely used. Requires additional preparation (printing) and organization of the exam.	Easy to administer. Fills the free time before or after taking the exam.
13.	Exam paper score review (assessment feedback) for students and teachers	Appointment in the storage room requires searching for the exam paper.	Instant review in any place with Internet access.

8. The Amount of Time Devoted to Preparing a Computer-Based Exam, on the School Premises, Compared to Its Traditional (Paper-Based) Version

Table 2 presents a sample application of the above comparison, including the analysis of the work time and tasks necessary to evaluate the basic science knowledge (pathophysiology) of 333 students attending the course on the school premises. The set comprises one final exam and three benchmark tests throughout the course: four tests in total. Benchmark tests are scheduled to be taken on predetermined dates during the classes. For some of the tasks, the amount of time is difficult to estimate, so they are described without a determined duration. However, staff members are able to state duration on an individual basis depending on the department in which they work.

Table 2. The amount of time devoted to preparing and administering knowledge evaluation using traditional paper-based tests vs. online tests on an e-learning platform.

No.	Task	Method of Testing	
		Paper-Based	Computer-Based
1.	People involved in the evaluation	T: teachers and A: assistants, administrative staff or technical-engineering staff	A: assistants, administrative staff or technical-engineering staff and T: teachers.
2.	Preparing test versions	T. prepares and sends the A. 2–3 electronic versions of tests by e-mail	0 min. Question bank sufficient for a few years. The time needed to create it currently under analysis
3.	Copying and printing	(60–120 min) A's work with four tests. Preparation of tests divided by group, printing paper versions. Assumed time: 15–30 min per test.	0 min. None
4.	Registration for an exam.	A. Collecting lists of students, coordinated by A. via e-mail or in person with group representatives.	Online, on the platform. The student registers with a convenient date, time, place. The choice can be cancelled.
5.	Order of questions and answer choices in the test	The same, 2–3 versions of the test. Independence of students' work difficult to oversee.	Different, random set of questions and answers—multiple versions. Independent student work
6.	The Time required to administer one exam on the premises. Benchmark tests are held during classes.	(100–200 min) T and/or A: two supervisors simultaneously 100 min each (auditorium hall), or in two rounds on one day with two supervisors × 100 min = 200 min (lecture hall).	(400 min) A and/or T: four supervisors in four computer rooms simultaneously. Exam carried out in four rounds at four times on one day: 4 × 100 min = 400 min. Department can accommodate 84 students per round.
7.	Assessment. (marking students' work).	(3996 min) A: We assume 3 min. Is necessary to mark one student paper with a template. 333 papers × 4 tests × 3 min = 3996 min = 66.6 h equals 8 working days One test: 333 papers × 3 min = 999 min = 16.7 h (approx. 2 working days).	0 min.
8.	Test results	Students receive the results a few days later—up to 5 working days.	The student knows the result immediately after the test.
9.	Marking (grading) errors	(30 min) A: Highly probable. Time is required for re-marking, counting the points again and sending explanations to students.	None.

Table 2. Cont.

No.	Task	Method of Testing	
		Paper-Based	Computer-Based
10.	Test result delivery	(44.4 min) A: Entering the results to an e-form of student achievement (virtual student office) and notifying students. We assume a required time of 2 s per result. 333 papers per test × 2 s = 666 s, with four tests this amounts to 4 × 666 s = 2664 s = 44.4 min. There is a likelihood of committing errors while entering the results.	0 min.
11.	Archiving test papers on the premises	A. 333 papers per test For 4 tests, 1332 papers are stored in cabinets on the premises.	None. All works are available online—see the example below.
12.	Calculating the average score for crediting after three benchmark tests	(15–30 min) A. Advanced use of spreadsheets required. Result analysis concerning retakes and preparing a list of people who failed the course.	0 min. Automated scores on the platform. Result lists can be imported as an .xls file.
13.	Access to current and past results and papers	A. Searching for paper-based tests in department archives and/or in files on a computer disc—is time-consuming	A/T. Full access on the platform (example—figure)
14.	Result availability for students	None.	Yes. All test results are available in one place on the platform (example—figure)
15.	Course evaluation/ study surveys	A. Difficult to conduct—rarely practised. (1) Survey/questionnaire printout necessary. (2) Significant amount of time required to enter hand-written answers in the file. (3) Poor hand-writing legibility.	Frequently practised—guarantees close to 100% student participation. (1) Automated process. (2) 0 min. time required to enter hand-written answers to the file. (3) Everything is instantly recorded in a file on the platform, ready to be imported to an external data storage device.
	Total of work time to preparation and implementation of knowledge evaluation:	4245.4–4420.4 min. equals 70.8–73.7 h Assumed average = 72.2 h	400 min = 6.7 h
	Recapitulation of significant aspects of the organization of knowledge evaluation:	(1) printout of large numbers of test papers, (2) required space for archiving thousands of test papers, (3) score review possible only on the premises, during the school's working time, (4) T. needs support from A./staff for distributing, assessing and archiving tests, (5) T. creates a few test versions for every course edition. Work is demanding, taking place under time and deadline pressure.	(1) more people physically involved in conducting the exam, (2) access to computer rooms, (3) labour-intensive creation of question bank in the first year of testing, which is a capital for the future. Subsequent editions of the course require minor corrections, updating the database. New questions created by T. are continually supplied over the whole year, without the time and deadline pressure.

Symbol h in the table stands for *one hour*—60 min.

9. The Analysis of the Amount of Time Needed to Create an Examination Question Bank

The creation of an electronic database of questions used for exams and credit tests consists of two stages of work, carried out by teachers alone or teachers supported by administrative or technical-engineering staff. The preparation of questions involves the time spent working on the actual substantive content and then the time needed to save them in the QTI format. This is a standard format used in computer-based knowledge evaluation held on e-learning platforms [19,20].

Studies conducted in the years 2015–2016 [58] demonstrated that teacher working time devoted to writing 20 pathophysiology test questions, with 4–5 answer choices in an electronic form, varied between 40 and 150 min. Therefore, the time needed by pathophysiology teachers to develop a bank of 200 questions is 18.5 h of work and an additional 8 h to export the questions in QTI format. This is performed by entering the questions from a document created by the author (teacher), followed by parameterization. This relates to, for example, answer keys, the random selection of answers, ways of displaying the question on the screen, or a random selection of questions from the bank. This work is performed once, and it serves its purpose for many years in the future.

Preparing a question bank of 200 questions for use in e-testing on an e-learning platform thus takes 26.5 h of work time. The analysis of the results in the above table for a computer-based test shows a calculated work time of 6.7 h, plus 26.5 h to create a question bank in QTI standard format. The summative result is 33.2 h. Traditional testing takes longer, approximately 72.2 h. This is the result of the analysis of the testing process presented in Table 2, plus the time spent composing the actual test questions (item 3, Table 2). We assume that 200 questions have to be developed for the paper-based test versions, which takes teachers about 18.5 h. Work time required in the case of a traditional test amounts to 90.7 h. Comparing the conventional form with the computer-based form, we can conclude that the latter is much more effective and beneficial for the educational institution, as it takes 37% of the time necessary to conduct a traditional form of testing. The time saved can be allotted to other teaching assignments, such as expanding the question bank at any time that they see fit.

The substantive content, depending on the nature of the subject, has a predicted lifespan of from 5 to 7 years from teaching the course [19,58,59]. The amount of time required to create an electronic question bank in the first year of e-testing and evaluation is more significant than that required for paper-based test versions, but it is spread over 5 to 7 years of use. The obtained values then have to be divided by at least 5, which provides the real hourly workload needed to develop an electronic question bank for a given academic year.

The size of the question bank developed for a given unit should depend on the number of groups, in which credit tests are administered as well as the number of course editions over one academic year. It is also important that a few test/exam dates are available per attempt, which is typical of the continuous examination session. The more students, test dates and course editions there are, the larger the base should be, to ensure an objective evaluation of student knowledge.

The amount of time required to expand the question bank in a database was also analyzed, and the results were calculated with regard to the work time needed for its development, along with the work time needed to prepare and carry out the testing process, comparing paper- and computer-based forms (Table 3).

Examining the results obtained in Table 3, we can see that, in the case of a question bank comprising 1600 test questions, the amount of time needed to organize and prepare the process of knowledge evaluation is similar for both paper-based and computer-based testing. When the number is increased to 2000 questions, the computer-based form requires more time than the traditional version. Work time is longer by 14.5 h, which is an increase in time of 5.6% compared with the traditional form. Plans to develop a base of 3000 questions or even 5000 questions leads these values to rise to 15.6%. This is, respectively, 54.5 h of work time for a 3000-question database and 134.5 h for a 5000-question database, which is the extra time required in comparison with the traditional form of testing.

Therefore, it seems legitimate to ask whether computer-based evaluation, which requires a database of over 1000 questions, is, in fact, as useful as previous studies have suggested.

Table 3. The analysis of work time devoted to developing a question bank for paper-based and computer-based knowledge evaluation.

Number of Questions in the Base	Work Time in Hours (60 min) [h]			
	Developing a Question Bank (Item 2 in Table 2)		Organization and Implementation of the Knowledge Evaluation Process (All Items from Table 2)	
	Paper-Based Test [I]	Computer-Based Test [III]	Traditional Testing [II]	Computer-Based Testing [IV]
1 × 200 = 200	18.5	26.5	90.7	33.2
2 × 200 = 400	37	53	109.2	59.7
4 × 200 = 800	74	106	146.2	112.7
5 × 200 = 1000	92.5	132.5	164.7	139.2
8 × 200 = 1600	148	212	220.2	218.7
10 × 200 = 2000	185	265	257.2	271.7
30 × 200 = 3000	277.5	397.5	349.7	404.2
50 × 200 = 5000	462.5	662.5	534.7	669.2

[I] time for developing the content of 200 questions—18.5 h; [II] the result of adding the amount of time from the *paper-based test* column and the time calculated in Table 2: 72.2 h; [III] time for composing 200 questions and saving them in QTI format—26.5 h; [IV] the result of adding the amount of time from the *computer-based test* column and the time calculated in Table 2: 6.7 h.

To answer this question, other variables of the evaluation process must be analyzed, which influence the development of a question bank. These include a deadline for composing new questions, the number of teachers involved in the task and their IT competencies, and cooperation between units implementing e-evaluation. These aspects make it apparent that the traditional, paper-based form has severe limitations and are less useful when conducted on large groups of students, despite the reduced work time. When these aspects are added to the workload and organization time of the computer-based form, the difference is leveled for the excess time in the case of databases of over 1000 questions.

9.1. Time Pressure, Question Reusability

The sets of questions composed for paper-based tests form a base, which has to contain different or updated questions in every exam session. Paper-based test versions used with large groups of students in a given academic year are quickly known, so in order for them to be used again in the next academic year, they have to be revised and adjusted, which is as time-consuming as composing new questions. The work of writing questions for traditional tests has to be completed every year, and the deadline is determined by the pre-established schedule of tests. Consequently, the work is completed under time pressure, irrespective of the other assignments that teachers may have. That is why the development of question banks is sometimes abandoned, or too few questions are provided for the evaluation to be conducted properly. This stems from the ease of making the questions banks public, or a lack of randomness in test versions. For computer-based evaluation, the bank of questions can be enlarged as they can be supplied at any given time in the academic year, and combined with other activities. Inspiration for a valuable question could be derived from a discussion with students during a lecture or a clinical case study in a seminar. New test questions often appear as a result of the analysis of students' work on the e-learning platform or their self-test scores. Then, the teacher enters the new questions in the QTI format to the database at a convenient time. The work is calmer and more thoughtful, which translates into valuable testing material, which will serve well in the verification of learning outcomes.

9.2. Cooperation between Units

It is rare for a unit to have a question bank of over 1000 questions. Composing such a large number of questions is a challenge in terms of time expenditure and content-related effort. To support the process of developing substantial content, a collaboration of a team of experts from a given unit or a whole school would be advantageous, as the time devoted to creating questions would be spread. Such a question bank saved in the international QTI standard format can easily be relocated to another e-learning platform, which implements computer-based evaluation standards. This, in turn, allows for different universities to share their databases, which naturally enlarges the pool of proven test questions. As a result, the time needed to develop questions for a single unit, calculated in Table 3, is significantly reduced. Such resources are invaluable to units collaborating in their creation for particular courses whose learning outcomes are the same in respective institutions. Such cooperation between teams of experts enables the workload to be significantly reduced. Writing exam questions is a complex and difficult process, so databases of over 1000 questions are an asset for many years to come, and clearly worth investing in.

9.3. A Further Period of Use

A question bank of the right size gradually reduces the amount of time necessary for creating substantive content and restricts the work to revising and updating the questions. This is not as time-intensive, and levels the excess time seen inn Table 3 for pools containing over 1000 questions. In the case of paper-based exams, the amount of time taken to develop the substantive content of questions is always the same, which is a strain for teachers.

9.4. Experience Backed by Statistics

Another important aspect concerns the analysis of the usefulness of test questions in the utilized database. Keeping the statistics and assessment of the question bank after the conducted evaluation in a given year seems to be a necessity. It allows the user to investigate the content, paying attention to the elimination of flawed test questions, ones that did not work or those at the wrong level of difficulty. It also serves to objectively analyze suggestions from students, who can express their reservations about questions after the exam or credit test. Questions should be thoroughly verified, with an emphasis on the scores achieved by all students taking the test. This will contribute to a reduction in the work time needed to supply new questions in future, and will definitely shorten the time spent on the substantive content of questions for banks containing over 1000 items.

9.5. ICT Competences of the Teaching Staff

A computer-based evaluation of student knowledge encourages the development of ICT competences in its participants, both students and teachers. Online testing will help the teachers improve their computer proficiency and develop their competences in this field, which will also contribute to a reduction in the work time needed in future concerning the conversion of questions to the QTI standard.

9.6. Summary of Work Time Analysis

The calculations made for databases of over 1000 questions demonstrate a longer work time needed for computer-based testing than paper-based testing; however, in the long term, the overall workload for a unit is reduced. It can thus be concluded that the electronic form is more advantageous and efficient than the traditional form.

Determining the labour cost and time involved in the process of knowledge evaluation in a particular teaching unit in one academic year must also consider the gains derived from the switch to an automated process. These include exempting assistants, administrative and technical-engineering staff from organizational duties connected with preparing and implementing the evaluation. The time devoted to preparing paper-based versions of tests, marking them using a template and archiving the results can be saved, and invested in developing their ICT competences. Their work on the e-learning platform will become more proficient and guarantee support to the authors of test questions in the creation and updating of items on the platform.

10. Discussion

The research was performed at the Department of Pathophysiology in cooperation with the Department of Computer Science and Statistics of Poznan University of Medical Sciences, Poland (PUMS). Academic teachers attended the research, as well as technical and administrative staff, and also e-learning experts. In 2009, this team introduced an e-learning portal for the entire university, further conducting its own research on the effectiveness and optimization of medical e-learning.

The research presented in the article was conducted by the Department of Pathophysiology, Poznan University of Medical Sciences, Poland on the ESTUDENT portal for remote education, which is an installation of the OLAT applications developed by the University of Zurich under an open-source license. The ESTUDENT portal is a proprietary LCMS application adapted to e-learning in the field of pathophysiology.

The described analysis of working time and the organization of electronic knowledge evaluation was carried out using an example of a large year of students in their second year of medicine in the preclinical subject of pathophysiology.

The working time of the analyzed knowledge evaluation through the e-learning portal is about 10% of the working time needed to carry out the evaluation in a traditional way. Electronic knowledge testing requires a greater amount of work time in the first year of application, due to the preparation of a larger database of questions compared to the number of questions required for the evaluation of knowledge conducted in the traditional (paper) version. However, teachers' working time is spread over 5–7 years of using the electronic question base. As part of the research, an analysis of the working time of building the database from 200 to 5000 test questions for the evaluation of knowledge in e-learning and the evaluation carried out in the traditional version was performed.

The data presented in the article are the result of pioneering research conducted by the authors in the field of the evaluation of preclinical knowledge of very numerous generations of medical students using the e-learning portal, which was carried out in 2009–2019. The described electronic realization used the example of the academic year of 2018–2019, when 333 students were studying medicine. On the basis of our own research, in 2015–2016, the time spent by teachers on exam questions was measured for those participating in traditional education and the e-learning portal. To conduct this research, the same team of academic teachers must participate, and the same conditions must be met for the implementation of both traditional knowledge evaluation and evaluation using e-learning methods.

The confirmation of the usefulness of e-learning in medical education is in the comparison of the benefits and limitations of the electronic evaluation of knowledge and the didactic process and evaluation using the traditional implementation. The work contains such analyses, also indicating the different stages of conducting these components of education in the e-learning portal. An important element of the research was the analysis of the work time needed for the preparation and implementation of electronic knowledge evaluation. The results clearly indicate the advantage of e-learning over traditional organization in terms of the implementation of examinations and surveys.

11. Summary of Study Results

The application of e-learning for computer-based knowledge evaluation and optimizing the administration of exams for students of medical sciences should be considered in two categories: from the perspective of the providers of the evaluation process, that is, the teaching unit, and from the recipients of the evaluation process, that is, the students.

The advantages to computer-based evaluation providers, that is, the teaching unit, include:

1. Automated test marking and information about the result (course credits, passing an exam).
2. Exporting test scores as a spreadsheet with the possibility of importing scores to a statistical package for quick analysis of the obtained data.

3. Full archiving of all evaluation results, including practice tests (self-tests) and papers submitted as project work or group work during the course or as a credit requirement
4. Online access to current and archived results of evaluations, broken down by group, date or type of test, with full information about the test results for each student.
5. Web-based questionnaire administration. The excess time during the evaluation can be used to administer course evaluation questionnaires or study surveys. This encourages student participation in research projects and ensures a high questionnaire return rate, which cannot be said for paper questionnaire distribution.
6. Developing a question bank without time or deadline pressure, except for the first year of e-evaluation, which requires a heavier workload and more time for preparation. An extensive database is more cost-effective in the long term.
7. Random selection of test questions from a large database with a random order of possible answers, providing a more objective assessment of a student's knowledge.
8. An opportunity to use questions based on graphic or multimedia elements. In paper-based evaluation, such possibilities cannot be used efficiently; an exam could be held in a room with Internet access and projector but, in the case of a large group of examinees, this is organizationally difficult.
9. Investment in the development of the staff's ICT competences, resulting in a higher proficiency in work on the e-learning platform and its full application in the organization and realization of the didactic process. The time saved can be devoted to composing new test questions.

The advantages to computer-based evaluation recipients, that is, the students, include:
1. Test results are delivered immediately after the test. In the case of practice tests, the student receives detailed results accompanied by correct answers, explanations and hints.
2. Access to all evaluation results from the course in one place, on the e-learning platform.
3. Automated and individual control of each test-writing time.
4. Independence of students' work during a test or examination. Each examinee has an individual, random selection of questions, drawn from an extensive database, with a random order of answer choices and a time limit depending on the need and test parameters.
5. Comprehensive communication regarding the organization of evaluation via the e-learning platform. This includes enrollment for test dates with the possibility of cancelling and changing them, without the necessity to contact the unit or group representatives, who often compile lists of students and deliver them to teachers. It also includes the submission of complaints or remarks concerning test questions online after the test.
6. Computer-based evaluation saves students' time and improves their participation. The time saved can be dedicated to additional study and revision before the exam.

12. Limitations

The authors' research indicates several factors common to the evaluation of knowledge in large groups of students completing a subject at one time, and the factors significantly influencing the optimization of this process. This includes the labor-intensive preparation of databases with questions, the competence level of suppliers (teachers) and recipients (students) of knowledge in the field of e-learning technologies, ensuring conditions for independent work (parameterization of tests or examination rooms), archiving results or the speed of feedback after evaluation knowledge.

Certain elements of this process are changeable and difficult to standardize, depending on the university's IT infrastructure. The differences may be related to the type of e-learning application or technical service support, which can be expanded on, and is at the full disposal of the candidates (university-wide center) or available locally (unit's own resources).

In order to optimize the implementation of the process, both traditional and e-learning variants should be carefully analyzed with the same human team, as shown in the diagram from the university, paying attention to its individual conditions (limitations, possibilities during a pandemic) and the specificity of issues. The final calculations may, therefore, differ slightly from those presented in the article. The analysis presented by the authors, as an example, indicates the superiority of the evaluation using e-learning technologies compared to the traditional evaluation. It proposes solutions to the optimal direction of this process, paying attention, for example, to cooperation between units, and sharing resources that will minimize the time spent working on question databases. The presented analysis is typical of universities working on open-source portals with limited funding, which is common in Eastern and Central Europe. It allows for a successful, remote execution, quickly, in one's own unit, over times such as the SARS-CoV-2 pandemic.

There are no complete, detailed analyses with the work time for all stages of work and the organization of medical evaluation for groups of more than 300 students. In order to be perform such analyses, the same team of academic teachers should be involved, and the same requirements should be met in the implementation of both traditional and remote application knowledge evaluation. Research also requires time and experience in the field of e-learning, which significantly affects the effectiveness of the process. There is no well-established educational theory for e-medical education, as remote methods contain parameters that are not known in traditional medical education. Research and discussion on the standardization of e-education and the development of patterns into which medical universities and schools are forced by the pandemic, testing of existing solutions, indications of limitations and addition of new variables are necessary in the important process of evaluation of the knowledge of medical students, who will become doctors (physicians).

13. Conclusions

Replacing the traditional form of organizing and implementing knowledge evaluation with a web-based equivalent on an e-learning platform optimizes the whole didactic process, not only for the unit carrying this out but, above all, for students. Due to this innovation, course participants have the opportunity to take full advantage of all the technological solutions that e-learning provides, with an implementation that can start from computer-based evaluation. The process of optimization through e-learning should become a natural part of the didactic process, conducted in every subject at all types of higher education institutions, including medical universities. The obtained results encourage their implementation, considering the nature and conditions of medical training, which is a key program in medical universities.

Author Contributions: Conceptualization, M.R., B.S., J.S. and E.B.; methodology, M.R., B.S., J.S. and E.B.; software, M.R., B.S., J.S. and E.B.; validation, M.R., B.S., J.S. and E.B.; formal analysis, M.R., B.S., J.S. and E.B.; investigation, M.R., B.S., J.S. and E.B.; resources, M.R., B.S., J.S. and E.B.; data curation, M.R., B.S., J.S. and E.B.; writing—original draft preparation, M.R., B.S., J.S. and E.B.; writing—review and editing, M.R. and B.S.; visualization, M.R., B.S., J.S. and E.B.; supervision, M.R., B.S., J.S. and E.B.; project administration, M.R., B.S., J.S. and E.B.; funding acquisition, M.R., B.S., J.S. and E.B. All authors have read and agreed to the published version of the manuscript.

Funding: This research was partly supported by Lodz University of Technology in Poland, Poznan University of Medical Sciences in Poland and AGH University of Science and Technology in Krakow, Poland.

Institutional Review Board Statement: Not applicable.

Informed Consent Statement: Not applicable.

Data Availability Statement: Department of Pathophysiology, Poznan University of Medical Sciences, Poland; www.estudent.ump.edu.pl (accessed on 29 August 2021).

Acknowledgments: The authors are grateful to anonymous reviewers for their comments. The authors acknowledge the teachers, assistants, administrative staff and technical-engineering staff that agreed to participate in these study.

Conflicts of Interest: The authors declare no conflict of interest. The funders had no role in the design of the study; in the collection, analyses, or interpretation of data; in the writing of the manuscript, or in the decision to publish the results.

References

1. Irby, D.M.; Cooke, M.; O'brien, B.C. Calls for Reform of Medical Education by the Carnegie Foundation for the Advancement of Teaching: 1910 and 2010. *Acad. Med.* **2010**, *85*, 220–227. [CrossRef]
2. Skochelak, S.E.; Stack, S.J. Creating the Medical Schools of the Future. *Acad. Med.* **2017**, *92*, 16–19. [CrossRef] [PubMed]
3. Rose, S. Medical Student Education in the Time of COVID-19. *JAMA* **2020**, *323*, 2131–2132. [CrossRef] [PubMed]
4. Bianchi, S.; Gatto, R.; Fabiani, L. Effects of the SARS-CoV-2 pandemic on medical education in Italy: Considerations and tips. *Euromediterr. Biomed. J.* **2020**, *15*, 100–101. [CrossRef]
5. Succar, T.; Beaver, H.A.; Lee, A.G. Impact of COVID-19 pandemic on ophthalmology medical student teaching: Educational innovations, challenges, and future directions. *Surv. Ophthalmol.* **2021**. [CrossRef]
6. Lin, C.-C.; Han, C.-Y.; Wu, M.-L.; Hsiao, P.-R.; Wang, L.-H.; Chen, L.-C. Enhancing reflection on medical and surgical nursing among nursing students: A participatory action research study. *Nurse Educ. Today* **2021**, *102*, 104935. [CrossRef]
7. Suliman, W.A.; Abu-Moghli, F.A.; Khalaf, I.; Zumot, A.F.; Nabolsi, M. Experiences of nursing students under the unprecedented abrupt online learning format forced by the national curfew due to COVID-19: A qualitative research study. *Nurse Educ. Today* **2021**, *100*, 104829. [CrossRef]
8. Bdair, I.A. Nursing students' and faculty members' perspectives about online learning during COVID-19 pandemic: A qualitative study. *Teach. Learn. Nurs.* **2021**, *16*, 220–226. [CrossRef]
9. Varvara, G.; Bernardi, S.; Bianchi, S.; Sinjari, B.; Piattelli, M. Dental Education Challenges during the COVID-19 Pandemic Period in Italy: Undergraduate Student Feedback, Future Perspectives, and the Needs of Teaching Strategies for Professional Development. *Healthcare* **2021**, *9*, 454. [CrossRef]
10. Iurcov, R.; Pop, L.-M.; Iorga, M. Impact of COVID-19 Pandemic on Academic Activity and Health Status among Romanian Medical Dentistry Students; A Cross-Sectional Study. *Int. J. Environ. Res. Public Health* **2021**, *18*, 6041. [CrossRef] [PubMed]
11. Ahmed, F.R.A.; Ahmed, T.E.; Saeed, R.A.; Alhumyani, H.; Abdel-Khalek, S.; Abu-Zinadah, H. Analysis and challenges of robust E-exams performance under COVID-19. *Results Phys.* **2021**, *23*, 103987. [CrossRef]
12. Elsalem, L.; Al-Azzam, N.; Jum'Ah, A.A.; Obeidat, N. Remote E-exams during COVID-19 pandemic: A cross-sectional study of students' preferences and academic dishonesty in faculties of medical sciences. *Ann. Med. Surg.* **2021**, *62*, 326–333. [CrossRef]
13. Ren-Kurc, A.; Roszak, M.; Mokwa-Tarnowska, I.; Kołowska-Gawiejnowicz, M.; Zych, J.; Kowalewski, W. E-Textbook Technologies for Academics in Medical Education. *Stud. Log. Gramm. Rhetor.* **2018**, *56*, 161–176. [CrossRef]
14. Kołowska-Gawiejnowicz, M.; Kołodziejczak, B.; Siatkowski, I.; Topol, P.; Zych, J. Infografiki—Nowy trend wizualizacji informacji wspomagający procesy edukacyjne. *Edukac. Tech. Inform.* **2018**, *9*, 138–148. [CrossRef]
15. Topol, P.; Kołodziejczak, B.; Roszak, M.; Dutkiewicz, A.; Zych, J.; Januszewski, M.; Bręborowicz, A. Światy wirtualne 3D w edukacji akademickiej. *Edukac. Tech. Inform.* **2017**, *19*, 205–216. [CrossRef]
16. Kleinsorgen, C.; Kankofer, M.; Gradzki, Z.; Mandoki, M.; Bartha, T.; von Köckritz-Blickwede, M.; Naim, H.Y.; Beyerbach, M.; Tipold, A.; Ehlers, J.P. Utilization and acceptance of virtual patients in veterinary basic sciences—The vetVIP-project. *GMS J. Med. Educ.* **2017**, *34*, Doc19. [CrossRef] [PubMed]
17. Kowalewski, W.; Kołodziejczak, B.; Roszak, M.; Ren-Kurc, A. Gesture recognition technology in education. In Proceedings of the Distance Learning, Simulation and Communication 2013, Proceedings (Selected Papers), Brno, Czech Republic, 21–23 May 2013; pp. 113–120, ISBN 978-80-7231-919-0.
18. Kowalewski, W.; Roszak, M.; Kołodziejczak, B.; Ren-Kurc, A.; Bręborowicz, A. Computational Fluid Dynamics Methods, and Their Applications in Medical Science. Studies in Logic, Grammar and Rhetoric. *Issue Log. Stat. Comput. Methods Med.* **2016**, *47*, 61–84. [CrossRef]
19. Ren-Kurc, A.; Roszak, M. Ewaluacja procesu dydaktycznego. Organizacja egzaminów testowych i ankietowania. In *Technologie Informacyjne w Warsztacie Nauczyciela. Nowe Wyzwania Edukacyjne*; Migdałek, J., Stolińska, A., Eds.; Wydawnictwo Naukowe Uniwersytetu Pedagogicznego: Kraków, Poland, 2011; pp. 253–260.
20. Roszak, M.; Kołodziejczak, B.; Kowalewski, W.; Ren-Kurc, A. Standard Question and Test Interoperability (QTI)—The evaluation of student's knowledge (Title in Polish: Standard Question and Test Interoperability (QTI)—Ewaluacja wiedzy studenta). *E-mentor* **2013**, *2*, 35–40. Available online: http://www.e-mentor.edu.pl/artykul/index/numer/49/id/1005 (accessed on 25 June 2021).
21. Gotlib, J.; Zarzeka, A.; Panczyk, M.; Gębski, P.; Iwanow, L.; Malczyk, M.; Belowska, J. Questions Quality Analysis of the Final Test in the 'Law in Medicine' Course for Nursing Students on The E-Exam Ask System Platform. *Pielęgniarstwo Pol.* **2016**, *3*, 332–339. [CrossRef]
22. BBC. The Spending Maze—Try—Activities © BBC | British Council 2004. Available online: https://www.teachingenglish.org.uk/sites/teacheng/files/million.pdf (accessed on 29 August 2021).

23. Guiter, G.E.; Sapia, S.; Wright, A.I.; Hutchins, G.G.A.; Arayssi, T. Development of a Remote Online Collaborative Medical School Pathology Curriculum with Clinical Correlations, across Several International Sites, through the COVID-19 Pandemic. *Med. Sci. Educ.* **2021**, *31*, 549–556. [CrossRef]
24. Guadalajara, H.; Palazón, Á.; Lopez-Fernandez, O.; Esteban-Flores, P.; Garcia, J.M.; Gutiérrez-Misis, A.; Baca-García, E.; Garcia-Olmo, D. Towards an Open Medical School without Checkerboards during the COVID-19 Pandemic: How to Flexibly Self-Manage General Surgery Practices in Hospitals? *Healthcare* **2021**, *9*, 743. [CrossRef]
25. Bianchi, S.; Bernardi, S.; Perilli, E.; Cipollone, C.; Di Biasi, J.; Macchiarelli, G. Evaluation of Effectiveness of Digital Technologies During Anatomy Learning in Nursing School. *Appl. Sci.* **2020**, *10*, 2357. [CrossRef]
26. Nicholson, L.L.; Reed, D.; Chan, C. An interactive, multi-modal Anatomy workshop improves academic performance in the health sciences: A cohort study. *BMC Med. Educ.* **2016**, *16*, 7. [CrossRef]
27. Cox, M. Formal to informal learning with IT: Research challenges and issues for e-learning. *J. Comput. Assist. Learn.* **2012**, *29*, 85–105. [CrossRef]
28. Alrefaie, Z.; Al-Hayani, A.; Hassanien, M.; Hegazy, A. Implementing group research assignment in undergraduate medical curriculum; impact on students' performance and satisfaction. *BMC Med. Educ.* **2020**, *20*, 229. [CrossRef] [PubMed]
29. Ebbinghaus, H. *Memory: A Contribution to Experimental Psychology*; Teachers College, Columbia University: New York, NY, USA, 1885. Available online: https://ia802605.us.archive.org/15/items/memorycontributi00ebbiuoft/memorycontributi00ebbiuoft.pdf (accessed on 25 June 2021).
30. Mokwa-Tarnowska, I. *E-Learning i Blended Learning w Nauczaniu Akademickim: Zagadnienia Metodyczne*; Wydawnictwo Politechniki Gdańskiej: Gdańsk, Poland, 2017.
31. Kushik, N.; Yevtushenko, N.; Evtushenko, T. Novel machine learning technique for predicting teaching strategy effectiveness. *Int. J. Inf. Manag.* **2016**, *53*, 101488. [CrossRef]
32. Favalea, T.; Soroa, F.; Trevisana, M.; Dragob, I.; Melliaa, M. Campus traffic and e-Learning during COVID-19 pandemic. *Comput. Netw.* **2020**, *176*, 107290. [CrossRef]
33. Vazquez, A.G.; Verde, J.M.; Mas, F.D.; Palermo, M.; Cobianchi, L.; Marescaux, J.; Gallix, B.; Dallemagne, B.; Perretta, S.; Gimenez, M.E. Image-Guided Surgical e-Learning in the Post-COVID-19 Pandemic Era: What Is Next? *J. Laparoendosc. Adv. Surg. Tech.* **2020**, *30*, 993–997. [CrossRef]
34. Warnecke, J.M.; Wang, J.; Deserno, T.M. Lessons Learned: Implementation of a Nationwide Innovative E-Learning Module for Health Enabling. *Technologies* **2020**, *272*, 39–42.
35. Kołodziejczak, B.; Mokwa-Tarnowska, I.; Roszak, M. Directions of the Evolution of Higher Education. In *E-Learning Volume 10: E-Learning and Smart Learning Environment for the Preparation of New Generation Specialists*; Smyrnova-Trybulska, E., Śląski, U., Eds.; Studio NOA for University of Silesia in Katowice: Katowice, Poland, 2018; Volume 10, pp. 135–152.
36. Noskova, T.; Yakovleva, O.; Pavlova, T.; Kołodziejczak, B.; Roszak, M. Information Behaviour and Attitude to Lifelong Learning: A Comparative Study for Students of Person-Oriented Specialties. In Proceedings of the DiVAI 2018, 12th International Scientific Conference on Distance Learning in Applied Informatics, Štúrovo, Slovakia, 2–4 May 2018; Wolters Kluwer: Prague, Czech Republic, 2018; pp. 139–150.
37. Takenouchi, A.; Otani, E.; Sunaga, M.; Toyama, T.; Uehara, H.; Akiyama, K.; Kawashima, T.; Ito, K.; Izuno, H.; Kinoshita, A. Development and evaluation of e-learning materials for dental hygiene students in six schools: Using smartphones to learn dental treatment procedures. *Int. J. Dent. Hyg.* **2020**, *18*, 413–421. [CrossRef]
38. Habib, M.N.; Jamal, W.; Khalil, U.; Khan, Z. Transforming universities in interactive digital platform: Case of city university of science and information technology. *Educ. Inf. Technol.* **2020**, *26*, 517–541. [CrossRef]
39. Leszczyński, P.; Charuta, A.; Łaziuk, B.; Gałązkowski, R.; Wejnarski, A.; Roszak, M.; Kołodziejczak, B. Multimedia and interactivity in distance learning of resuscitation guidelines: A randomised controlled trial. *Interact. Learn. Environ.* **2017**, *26*, 151–162. [CrossRef]
40. Leszczyński, P.; Charuta, A.; Kołodziejczak, B.; Roszak, M. Evaluation of virtual environment as a form of interactive resuscitation exam. *New Rev. Hypermedia Multimed.* **2017**, *23*, 265–276. [CrossRef]
41. Wang, T.H. What strategies are effective for formative assessment in an e-learning environment? *J. Comput. Assist. Learn.* **2007**, *23*, 171–186. [CrossRef]
42. Gutmann, J.; Kühbeck, F.; Berberat, P.O.; Fischer, M.R.; Engelhardt, S.; Sarikas, A. Use of Learning Media by Undergraduate Medical Students in Pharmacology: A Prospective Cohort Study. *PLoS ONE* **2015**, *10*, e0122624. [CrossRef] [PubMed]
43. Wynter, L.; Burgess, A.; Kalman, E.; Heron, J.E.; Bleasel, J. Medical students: What educational resources are they using? *BMC Med. Educ.* **2019**, *19*, 36. [CrossRef]
44. Faisal, C.M.N.; Fernandez-Lanvin, D.; De Andrés, J.; Gonzalez-Rodriguez, M. Design quality in building behavioral intention through affective and cognitive involvement for e-learning on smartphones. *Internet Res.* **2020**, *30*, 1631–1663. [CrossRef]
45. Khanal, S.S.; Prasad, P.; Alsadoon, A.; Maag, A. A systematic review: Machine learning based recommendation systems for e-learning. *Educ. Inf. Technol.* **2019**, *25*, 2635–2664. [CrossRef]
46. Frehywot, S.; Vovides, Y.; Talib, Z.; Mikhail, N.; Ross, H.; Wohltjen, H.; Bedada, S.; Korhumel, K.; Koumare, A.K.; Scott, J. E-learning in medical education in resource constrained low- and middle-income countries. *Hum. Resour. Health* **2013**, *11*, 4. [CrossRef]

47. Warriner, D.R.; Bayley, M.; Shi, Y.; Lawford, P.V.; Narracott, A.; Fenner, J. Computer model for the cardiovascular system: Development of an e-learning tool for teaching of medical students. *BMC Med. Educ.* **2017**, *17*, 220. [CrossRef]
48. Dhir, S.K.; Verma, D.; Batta, M.; Mishra, D. E learning in medical education in India. *Indian Pediatr.* **2017**, *54*, 871–877. [CrossRef]
49. Vance, S.R.; Lasofsky, B.; Ozer, E.; Buckelew, S.M. Using E-Learning to Enhance Interdisciplinary Pediatric Learners' Transgender-Related Objective Knowledge, Self-Perceived Knowledge and Clinical Self-Efficacy. *J. Adolesc. Health* **2018**, *62*, S104–S105. [CrossRef]
50. Patel, B.K.; Chapman, C.G.; Luo, N.; Woodruff, J.N.; Arora, V.M. Impact of Mobile Tablet Computers on Internal Medicine Resident Efficiency. *Arch. Intern. Med.* **2012**, *172*, 436–438. [CrossRef] [PubMed]
51. Mokwa-Tarnowska, I.; Roszak, M.; Kołodziejczak, B. Online Collaborative Projects to Enhance Soft Skills. In *E-Learning Volume 10: E-Learning and Smart Learning Environment for the Preparation of New Generation Specialists*; Smyrnova-Trybulska, E., Śląski, U., Eds.; Studio NOA for University of Silesia in Katowice: Katowice, Poland, 2018; Volume 10, pp. 443–464.
52. Trzepizur, M.; Statowski, W.; Myrcik, D.; Makarska, J.; Syrkiewicz-Świtała, M. Original educational computer program "Trauma" and its application in education of paramedic students—Preliminary results. *J. Med. Sci.* **2019**, *88*, 163–170. Available online: https://jms.ump.edu.pl/index.php/JMS/article/view/366 (accessed on 30 July 2021). [CrossRef]
53. Roszak, M. *Ocena Przydatności E-Learningu w Kształceniu Medycznym z Zakresu Patofizjologii*; Wydawnictwo Naukowe Uniwersytetu Medycznego im. Karola Marcinkowskiego w Poznaniu: Poznań, Poland, 2019.
54. Descriptive Statistics Tools in Excel. Available online: https://www.real-statistics.com/descriptive-statistics/descriptive-statistics-tools/ (accessed on 29 August 2021).
55. The R Project for Statistical Computing. Available online: https://www.r-project.org (accessed on 29 August 2021).
56. Rozporządzenie Ministra Nauki i Szkolnictwa Wyższego z Dnia 27 Września 2018 r. w Sprawie Studiów. Poz. 1861, Warszawa, Dnia 28 Września 2018 r. Rozdział 5—Kształcenie na Odległość. Available online: http://eli.sejm.gov.pl/eli/DU/2018/1861/ogl (accessed on 25 June 2021).
57. Chen, H.-J. Clarifying the impact of surprise in e-learning system design based on university students with multiple learning goals orientation. *Educ. Inf. Technol.* **2020**, *25*, 5873–5892. [CrossRef]
58. Roszak, M.; Kołodziejczak, B. Building a course with multimedia resources—The working time analysis on the example of the pathophysiology course. In Proceedings of the Distance Learning, Simulation and Communication 2017, Proceedings (Selected Papers), Brno, Czech Republic, 31 May–2 June 2017; pp. 161–170.
59. Roszak, M.; Mokwa-Tarnowska, I.; Kołodziejczak, B. E-learning Competencies for University and College Staff. In *Universities in the Networked Society. Critical Studies of Education*; Smyrnova-Trybulska, E., Kommers, P., Morze, N., Malach, J., Eds.; Springer: Cham, Switzerland, 2019; Volume 10. [CrossRef]

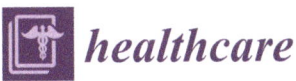

Article

Lessons Learned from Developing Digital Teaching Modules for Medical Student Education in Neurosurgery during the COVID-19 Pandemic

Rosita Rupa, Mirza Pojskic, Christopher Nimsky and Benjamin Voellger *

Department of Neurosurgery, University Hospital Marburg, Baldingerstr., 35033 Marburg, Germany; rupar@med.uni-marburg.de (R.R.); mirza.pojskic@uk-gm.de (M.P.); nimsky@med.uni-marburg.de (C.N.)
* Correspondence: voellger@med.uni-marburg.de; Tel.: +49-6421-5866447

Abstract: Background: The coronavirus 2019 (COVID-19) pandemic forced students and teachers to rapidly adopt digital education methods. Proper guidance for and refinement of such methods is continuously required. Here, we report on the educational experience students and academic staff at the neurosurgical department of a German university hospital made with digital teaching modules (DTMs) that were newly developed due to the transition to digital teaching during the first year of the COVID-19 pandemic and on the insights gained therefrom. Methods: Nine newly created DTMs provided students the option to anonymously evaluate each module by assigning a score from 0 (worst value) to 5 (best value) to it. Access count, evaluation count, average evaluation, number of included (interactive) figures, number of presented cases, number of linked publications, and number of included multiple-choice questions for each DTM were recorded retrospectively. For each DTM, we aimed to correlate access count, evaluation count, and average evaluation with the number of included (interactive) figures, number of presented cases, number of linked publications, and number of included multiple-choice questions. E-mail responses from individual students as to the DTMs were collected. Among students, an anonymous, voluntary online survey regarding the DTMs was conducted. Results: Number of figures and average evaluation per DTM were significantly positively correlated (Spearman's rho = 0.85; p = 0.0037). Number of figures and number of evaluations per DTM were also significantly positively correlated (Spearman's rho = 0.78; p = 0.0137). Responses from individual students indicated that illustrative cases and interactive figures might further increase DTM popularity. Conclusion: As a valuable adjunct in medical student education, DTMs should contain (interactive) figures, illustrative cases, a scoring option, and the option to give individual feedback towards the academic staff.

Keywords: COVID-19; digital teaching modules; feedback; learning management system; medical student education; neurosurgery

Citation: Rupa, R.; Pojskic, M.; Nimsky, C.; Voellger, B. Lessons Learned from Developing Digital Teaching Modules for Medical Student Education in Neurosurgery during the COVID-19 Pandemic. *Healthcare* **2021**, *9*, 1141. https://doi.org/10.3390/healthcare9091141

Academic Editors: Luís Proença, José João Mendes, João Botelho and Vanessa Machado

Received: 25 July 2021
Accepted: 28 August 2021
Published: 1 September 2021

Publisher's Note: MDPI stays neutral with regard to jurisdictional claims in published maps and institutional affiliations.

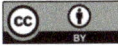

Copyright: © 2021 by the authors. Licensee MDPI, Basel, Switzerland. This article is an open access article distributed under the terms and conditions of the Creative Commons Attribution (CC BY) license (https://creativecommons.org/licenses/by/4.0/).

1. Introduction

Coronavirus disease 2019 (COVID-19) is an infectious condition caused by severe acute respiratory syndrome coronavirus type 2 (SARS-CoV-2) [1]. COVID-19 has an incubation period of up to 14 days during which the virus may already be transmitted [1]. For COVID-19, a basic reproduction number (R_0) of 2.5 has been estimated [1]. COVID-19 case fatality rates (CFR) of approximately 4 per cent have been encountered in some highly developed countries, such as Denmark and Germany, and much higher CFR have been observed elsewhere [2]. In a systematic meta-analysis, the infection fatality rate during the first wave of COVID-19 was found to be 0.68 per cent [3]. Since the end of 2019, COVID-19 has evolved into a pandemic [1] that made governments worldwide implement unprecedented non-pharmacological interventions in order to respond to the rapid spread of this new, life-threatening disease [4]. One of these measures, namely the enforcement of social distancing, resulted in fast transition from traditional teaching to digital teaching where feasible [5–7].

Prior to the emergence of COVID-19, we had already had access to a server hosting a derivative of the open-source digital learning management system (LMS) ILIAS (https://www.ilias.de) (accessed on 27 June 2021) [8] tailored for medical education ("Knowledge-Based Medical Education" (k-MED)) (https://www.kmed.uni-giessen.de) (accessed on 27 June 2021) [9] at our university. At that time, medical student education at our neurosurgical department had mainly consisted of traditional lectures and seminars and with daily changing attendees, bedside, and operating room (OR) teaching. In March 2020, the first lockdown in Germany (https://www.bundesregierung.de/breg-de/themen/coronavirus/beschluss-zu-corona-1730292) (accessed on 27 June 2021) [10] prompted us to implement contact tracing and social distancing measures, including digital teaching and changed schedules for approximately 160 students per term: lectures were thenceforth made available as moving picture experts group 4 (.mp4) files on the ILIAS server, while bedside and OR teaching necessarily continued with attendees changing weekly or biweekly in order to facilitate contact tracing. For the seminars, a hybrid approach was chosen: the option to attend traditional seminars as long as regulations allowed this (with mandatory enrolment prior to each event in order to facilitate contact tracing) was complemented with 9 ILIAS digital teaching modules (DTMs, Table 1) that authors B.V. and R.R. had developed from scratch after the first lockdown. The content of the DTMs matched the educational aims of the fourth year medical students' course in neurosurgery at our university. At the beginning of each term, all students—each at the same level of experience—were provided with a catalogue of the educational aims. Each DTM was designed to be followed independently from other DTMs, with prerequisites, i.e., recommended book chapters or video lectures, clearly defined. Numbers of figures, interactive figures (i.e., figures with additional information, such as the names of anatomical landmarks revealed by a hovering mouse pointer), cases, linked publications, and multiple-choice questions varied between DTMs (Table 1).

Table 1. Characteristics of 9 digital teaching modules.

Topic	Average Evaluation	Number of Evaluations	Number of Accesses	Number of Figures	Number of Inter-Active Figures *	Number of Questions	Number of Cases	Number of Linked Papers
Aneurysmal Subarachnoid Hemorrhage	4.5	13	90	4	0	2	1	1
Impairment of Consciousness	4.5	11	162	4	0	5	1	2
Elective Neurosurgery During the COVID-19 Pandemic	4.0	7	77	3	0	2	1	1
Fluorescence-Guided Glioma Surgery	1.0	5	85	0 **	0	2	1	3
Intracranial Pressure	5.0	13	98	7	0	6	1	0
Brain Death	4.0	7	126	2	0	4	0	2
Hydrocephalus	4.5	11	134	8	3	1	1	0
Lumbar Disc Hernia	4.0	8	109	3	0	4	2	0
Cervical Disc Hernia	5.0	7	91	4	1	2	1	0

* Subset of the number of figures; ** the papers linked to this module contained several figures.

Each DTM contained the e-mail address of an academic staff member (author B.V. or R.R.) responsible for collecting individual feedback from students and for clarifying any questions regarding the content of the DTM. In addition, students were given the opportunity to discuss any open issues during two online revision courses held by author B.V. at the end of the winter term 2020/2021.

During the COVID-19 pandemic, educational institutions worldwide have faced a similar need for transition to digital teaching [5–7], while students, particularly in low- or middle-income countries, may encounter new or increasing barriers complicating educational access [11–14]. Maity et al. [14] reported that university students, probably due to their overall higher maturity and commitment, appear to be less affected by the difficulties that arise from the pandemic-driven transition to digital education than students at school or at college. In their analysis of data on user experience collected among students after the onset of the pandemic, Chen et al. [15] found that the quality of the technical framework and of the content as well as the design of the user interface determine students' satisfaction with online education platforms. In 2021, Ramos et al. [16] published a review on works from the pre-COVID-19 era assessing video-based learning (VBL) methods. They conclude that VBL may improve students' and teachers' educational experience when going beyond one-way video lecturing [16]. Suggested methods include collaborative VBL, collaborative video analysis, collaborative video authoring, and the use of video annotation tools [16]. Katz et al. [17] recently reviewed numerous examples of how social media platforms (SMPs) were successfully deployed for the transfer of medical knowledge to professionals, students, and patients. With SMPs, however, caution must be taken to avoid the spread of misinformation [17].

As a consequence, digital literacy is, more than ever, considered a prerequisite for students and teachers [12,14,17]. Future publications in the field of digital education are expected to provide guidance for, to evaluate, and to refine recently adopted methods [17,18]. Here, we would like to report on the educational experience students and academic staff at our neurosurgical department made with the newly developed DTMs during the first year of the COVID-19 pandemic and on the insights we have gained therefrom.

2. Materials and Methods

Each student had the option to anonymously evaluate each DTM by assigning a score of 0 (worst value) to 5 (best value) to it. We retrospectively recorded access count, evaluation count, average evaluation, number of included (interactive) figures, number of presented cases, number of linked publications, and number of included multiple-choice questions for each DTM on 6 March 2021 (Table 1). For each DTM, we aimed to correlate access count, evaluation count, and average evaluation with the number of included (interactive) figures, number of presented cases, number of linked publications, and number of included multiple-choice questions (Tables 1 and 2).

Table 2. Correlation between design and popularity of 9 digital teaching modules.

Module Popularity Measure	Number of Figures per Module	Number of Interactive Figures per Module	Number of Cases per Module	Number of Questions per Module	Number of Linked Papers per Module
Number of accesses per module	0.4 (0.286)	0.25 (0.5147)	−0.09 (0.8153)	0.34 (0.3692)	−0.13 (0.7354)
Number of evaluations per module	0.78 (0.0137) *	−0.01 (0.9762)	0.19 (0.6294)	0.29 (0.4465)	−0.43 (0.2449)
Average evaluation per module	0.85 (0.0037) *	0.45 (0.2232)	0 (1)	0.17 (0.6653)	−0.62 (0.0743)

Spearman's *rho* served as statistical test. Data are presented as *rho* (*p* value). * Statistically significant.

Until 6 March 2021, e-mail responses from individual students regarding the DTMs were collected by authors B.V. and R.R. From 8 February 2021 to 1 March 2021, we conducted among our students an anonymous, voluntary online survey as to the DTMs (Supplementary Table S1). We placed the survey at the top of our DTM list and advertised the survey through our ILIAS weblog.

Statistical analysis was conducted, and figures were created using RStudio version 1.3.959 running R version 4.0.2 (https://www.r-project.org) (accessed on 30 June 2021) [19] on a Mac OS X 10.14.6. Spearman's rank correlation coefficient, *rho*, was estimated. Statistical significance was assumed with *p* values less than 0.05.

3. Results

Up to 13 scores per DTM were obtained (Table 1) A significant positive correlation was found between the number of figures included in a DTM and the average evaluation of the DTM (Spearman's rho = 0.85; p = 0.0037; Table 2; Figure 1).

An arc tangent curve (Figure 1) was manually fitted to the data representing the number of figures (x) and the average evaluation per DTM (y) by author B.V. as follows:

$$y = 3.4 * \arctan(x)$$

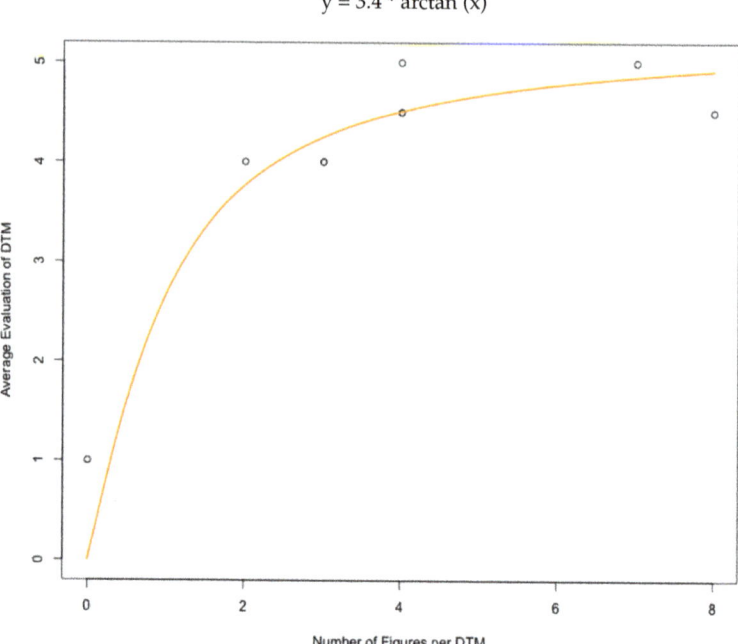

Figure 1. Number of figures per digital teaching module (DTM) and average evaluation (0: worst value; 5: best value) of the respective module.

A significant positive correlation was also found between the number of figures included in a DTM and the number of evaluations per DTM (Spearman's rho = 0.78; p = 0.0137; Table 2; Figure 2). Using the "lm" function in R, a regression line (Figure 2) was automatically fitted to the data representing the number of figures (x) and the number of evaluations per DTM (y) as follows:

$$y = 5.5355 + 0.9194 * x$$

One student answered solely to the open question in our online survey, indicating agreement with e-mail responses that we had received from two individual students stating that illustrative cases and interactive figures were found particularly helpful in the transfer of knowledge through DTMs. Eight students responded to the closed questions (Supplementary Table S1) but skipped the open question in our online survey.

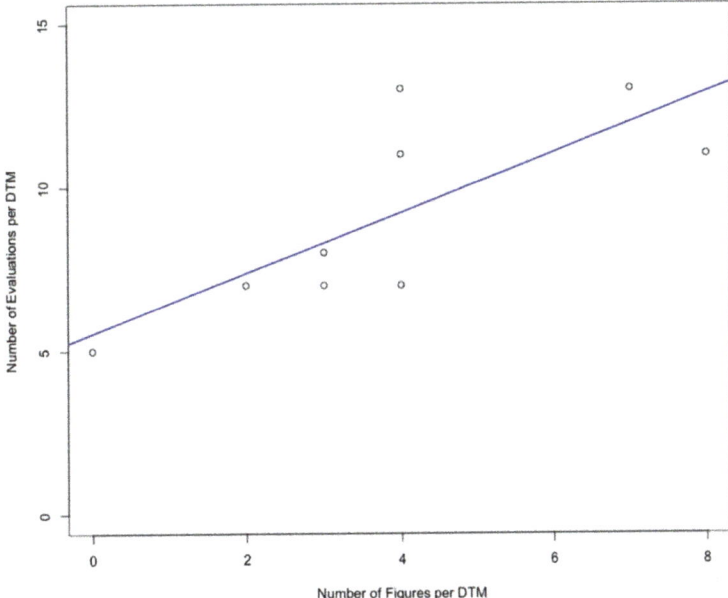

Figure 2. Number of figures per digital teaching module (DTM) and average number of evaluations of the respective module.

4. Discussion

There is an abundance of literature on feedback mechanisms in traditional medical student education. Comprehensive reviews on this topic have been provided by Keifenheim et al. and by Lerchenfeldt et al. [20,21]. Such feedback mechanisms, however, are based upon the principles of direct, hurdle-free verbal and non-verbal communication between two or more individuals. By contrast, video conferences, lecture videos, DTMs, and all other digital education channels contain a more or less permeable barrier to the direct interaction between participants [22].

While there is reason to believe that digital teaching will never replace bedside teaching [23], medical student education during the pandemic may certainly become more interesting through pre-made DTMs or similar digital collections of clinical case presentations, such as Capsule (https://www.capsule.ac.uk) (accessed on 27 June 2021) [24,25] or Eurorad (https://www.eurorad.org) (accessed on 27 June 2021) [26]. It remains the responsibility of the teacher to develop DTMs of high quality and to make the content of digital lessons as attractive and comprehensible as possible for medical students, and there is a demand for further research on this topic [23,27]. We believe that carefully designed DTMs will retain their place in medical student education after the COVID-19 pandemic. Beyond that, patients may benefit from easy-to-follow digital medical education tools provided by their doctors during the pandemic and thereafter [28].

The use of digital LMSs, such as ILIAS for medical student education, has been described by various authors and even more so since the emergence of COVID-19 (https://pubmed.ncbi.nlm.nih.gov/?term=digital+learning+management+system) (accessed on 27 June 2021) [29]. There is a wealth of ideas to promote the transition to digital teaching, including coverage of feedback mechanisms that are directed towards the students in settings similar to the situation at our department [30–34]. However, only little light has been shed upon the options digital medical student education provides for feedback that is directed towards the academic staff [31,33–35].

In our hands, the exploitation of the digital LMS feedback option with the lowest possible threshold, namely the retrospective analysis of students' overall evaluation of

DTMs with scores from 0 to 5, yielded novel, significant insights (Figures 1 and 2; Table 3): first, the average evaluation of a DTM was significantly correlated with the number of figures provided in the DTM, obviously following a saturation curve (Figure 1). Second, the number of evaluations of a DTM was significantly correlated with the number of figures provided in the DTM in a more or less linear manner (Figure 2).

The number of responses to our extra advertised, prominently placed online survey was disappointing. We assume that this low response rate is primarily owed to the high threshold that came with the survey, namely the considerable amount of time needed to answer all the questions. This part of our experience is similar to what Vielsmeier et al. [34] encountered at the ear, nose, and throat (ENT) department of a German university hospital: despite repetitive requests, there was a low willingness among students to give feedback through an online survey on the quality of digital education during the COVID-19 pandemic.

Such observations may explain why there is little literature on feedback towards the academic staff in digital medical education. The low overall response rate, the retrospective character of our analysis, and the fact that we report on a single-center experience are certainly the main limitations of our study. Nonetheless, we think that the response to the closed questions in our online survey contains a clear mandate to develop more DTMs in the future (Supplementary Table S1).

Although certainly lowest in number and, due to an approach that was qualitative in nature, the single response to the open question in our survey and the e-mail notifications as obtained from individual students brought some additional design advice: these respondents found interactive figures and clinical cases in the DTMs very helpful (Table 3).

Table 3. Characteristics of feedback as received through different feedback channels.

Feedback Channel	Threshold	Feedback Quantity	Feedback Quality
Scoring bar	(+)	(+++)	(+++)
Survey, closed questions	(+++)	(++)	(+)
Survey, open questions	(++)	(+)	(++)
Individual response by e-mail	(++)	(+)	(++)

(+) low, (++) medium, (+++) high.

5. Conclusions

Based on our pandemic-driven experience, we devised the following recommendations for the design of DTMs in medical student education:

- (Interactive) figures and illustrative cases apparently foster students' engagement with the content of the DTM; and
- To obtain valuable feedback from students, it is advised to offer low-threshold communication channels. These include a scoring option for each DTM, open survey questions, and provision of the e-mail address of a correspondent academic staff member.

Supplementary Materials: The following are available online at https://www.mdpi.com/article/10.3390/healthcare9091141/s1, Table S1: Students' answers to the closed questions in an online survey assessing 9 digital teaching modules.

Author Contributions: Conceptualization, R.R. and B.V.; methodology, R.R. and B.V.; validation, B.V. and R.R.; formal analysis, B.V. and R.R.; investigation, B.V. and R.R.; data curation, B.V. and R.R; writing—original draft preparation, B.V. and R.R.; writing—review and editing, C.N. and M.P.; visualization, B.V. and R.R.; supervision, C.N.; project administration, B.V. All authors have read and agreed to the published version of the manuscript.

Funding: This research received no external funding.

Institutional Review Board Statement: Ethical review and approval were waived for this study, due to its retrospective, anonymized design.

Informed Consent Statement: Obtaining informed consent was waived due to the retrospective, anonymized study design.

Data Availability Statement: All data can be obtained from the corresponding author upon reasonable request.

Conflicts of Interest: The authors declare no conflict of interest.

References

1. Hu, B.; Guao, H.; Zhou, P.; Shi, Z.L. Characteristics of SARS-CoV-2 and COVID-19. *Nat. Rev. Microbiol.* **2021**, *19*, 141–154. [CrossRef]
2. Sorci, G.; Faivre, B.; Morand, S. Explaining among-country variation in COVID-19 case fatality rate. *Sci. Rep.* **2020**, *10*, 18909. [CrossRef]
3. Meyerowitz-Katz, G.; Merone, L. A systematic review and meta-analysis of published research data on COVID-19 infection fatality rates. *Int. J. Infect. Dis.* **2020**, *101*, 138–148. [CrossRef]
4. Haug, N.; Geyrhofer, L.; Londei, A.; Dervic, E.; Desvars-Larrive, A.; Loreto, V.; Pinior, B.; Thurner, S.; Klimek, P. Ranking the effectiveness of worldwide COVID-19 government interventions. *Nat. Hum. Behav.* **2020**, *4*, 1303–1312. [CrossRef] [PubMed]
5. Pozo, J.I.; Pérez Echeverria, M.P.; Cabellos, B.; Sánchez, D.L. Teaching and Learning in Times of COVID-19: Uses of Digital Technologies During School Lockdown. *Front. Psychol.* **2021**, *12*, 656776. [CrossRef]
6. Motte-Signoret, E.; Labbé, A.; Benoist, G.; Linglart, A.; Gajdos, V.; Lapillonne, A. Perception of medical education by learners and teachers during the COVID-19 pandemic: A cross-sectional survey of online-teaching. *Med. Educ. Online* **2021**, *26*, 1919042. [CrossRef]
7. Asgari, S.; Trajkovic, J.; Rahmani, M.; Zhang, W.; Lo, R.C.; Sciortino, A. An observational study of engineering online education during the COVID-19 pandemic. *PLoS ONE* **2021**, *16*, e0250041. [CrossRef] [PubMed]
8. ILIAS. Available online: https://www.ilias.de (accessed on 27 June 2021).
9. k-MED. Available online: https://kmed.uni-giessen.de (accessed on 27 June 2021).
10. Besprechung der Bundeskanzlerin mit den Regierungschefinnen und Regierungschefs der Länder am 12. März 2020. Available online: https://www.bundesregierung.de/breg-de/themen/coronavirus/beschluss-zu-corona-1730292 (accessed on 27 June 2021).
11. Alsoufi, A.; Alsuyihili, A.; Msherghi, A.; Elhadi, A.; Atiyah, H.; Ashini, A.; Ashwieb, A.; Ghula, M.; Ben Hasan, H.; Abudabuos, S.; et al. Impact of the COVID-19 pandemic on medical education: Medical students' knowledge, attitudes, and practices regarding electronic learning. *PLoS ONE* **2020**, *15*, e0242905. [CrossRef]
12. Atreya, A.; Acharya, J. Distant virtual medical education during COVID-19: Half a loaf of bread. *Clin. Teach.* **2020**, *17*, 418–419. [CrossRef]
13. Jones, N.; Sanchez Tapia, I.; Baird, S.; Guglielmi, S.; Oakley, E.; Yadete, W.A.; Sultan, M.; Pincock, K. Intersecting barriers to adolescents' educational access during COVID-19: Exploring the role of gender, disability and poverty. *Int. J. Educ. Dev.* **2021**, *85*, 102428. [CrossRef]
14. Maity, S.; Sahu, T.N.; Sen, N. Panoramic view of digital education in COVID-19: A new explored avenue. *Rev. Educ.* **2021**, *9*, 405–423. [CrossRef]
15. Chen, T.; Peng, L.; Yin, X.; Rong, J.; Yang, J.; Cong, G. Analysis of user satisfaction with online education platforms in China during the COVID-19 pandemic. *Healthcare* **2020**, *8*, 200. [CrossRef] [PubMed]
16. Ramos, J.L.; Cattaneo, A.A.P.; de Jong, F.P.C.M.; Espadeiro, R.G. Pedagogical models for the facilitation of teacher professional development via video-supported collaborative learning. A review of the state of the art. *J. Res. Technol. Educ.* **2021**, [CrossRef]
17. Katz, N.; Nandi, N. Social media and medical education in the context of the COVID-19 pandemic: Scoping review. *JMIR Med. Educ.* **2021**, *7*, e25892. [CrossRef]
18. Corell-Almuzara, A.; Lopez-Belmonte, J.; Marin-Marin, J.-A.; Moreno-Guerrero, A.-J. COVID-19 in the field of education: State of the art. *Sustainability* **2021**, *13*, 5452. [CrossRef]
19. The R Project. Available online: https://www.r-project.org (accessed on 30 June 2021).
20. Keifenheim, K.E.; Teufel, M.; Ip, J.; Speiser, N.; Leehr, E.J.; Zipfel, S.; Herrmann-Werner, A. Teaching history taking to medical students: A systematic review. *BMC Med. Educ.* **2015**, *15*, 159. [CrossRef] [PubMed]
21. Lerchenfeldt, S.; Mi, M.; Eng, M. The utilization of peer feedback during collaborative learning in undergraduate medical education: A systematic review. *BMC Med. Educ.* **2019**, *19*, 321. [CrossRef]
22. O'Doherty, D.; Dromey, M.; Lougheed, J.; Hannigan, A.; Last, J.; McGrath, D. Barriers and solutions to online learning in medical education—An integrative review. *BMC Med. Educ.* **2018**, *18*, 130. [CrossRef]
23. Singal, A.; Bansal, A.; Chaudhary, P.; Singh, H.; Patra, A. Anatomy education of medical and dental students during COVID-19 pandemic: A reality check. *Surg. Radiol. Anat.* **2021**, *43*, 515–521. [CrossRef]
24. Lau, E.J.S.; Aslam, A.; Arshad, Z. How have digital resources been utilised in times of COVID-19? Opinions of medical students based in the United Kingdom. *Can. Med. Educ. J.* **2021**, *12*, e115–e117. [CrossRef]
25. Capsule. Available online: https://www.capsule.ac.uk (accessed on 27 June 2021).
26. Eurorad. Available online: https://www.eurorad.org (accessed on 27 June 2021).

27. Kyaw, B.M.; Posadzki, P.; Paddock, S.; Car, J.; Campbell, J.; Car, L.T. Effectiveness of Digital Education on Communication Skills Among Medical Students: Systematic Review and Meta-Analysis by the Digital Health Education Collaboration. *J. Med. Internet Res.* **2019**, *21*, e12967. [CrossRef] [PubMed]
28. Turkdogan, S.; Schnitman, G.; Wang, T.; Gotlieb, R.; How, J.; Gotlieb, W.H. Development of a Digital Patient Education Tool for Patients with Cancer During the COVID-19 Pandemic. *JMIR Cancer* **2021**, *7*, e23637. [CrossRef] [PubMed]
29. Pubmed Search for the Term "Digital Learning Management System". Available online: https://pubmed.ncbi.nlm.nih.gov/?term=digital+learning+management+system (accessed on 27 June 2021).
30. Darras, K.E.; Spouge, R.J.; de Bruin, A.B.H.; Sedlic, A.; Hague, C.; Forster, B.B. Undergraduate Radiology Education During the COVID-19 Pandemic: A Review of Teaching and Learning Strategies. *Can. Assoc. Radiol. J.* **2021**, *72*, 194–200. [CrossRef]
31. Heinzmann, A.; Bode, S.; Forster, J.; Berger, J. Interactive, case-based seminars in the digitized pediatrics block internship from the students' perspective. *GMS J. Med. Educ.* **2021**, *38*, Doc24. [CrossRef]
32. Langewitz, W.; Pleines Dantas Seixas, U.; Hunziker, S.; Becker, C.; Fischer, M.R.; Benz, A.; Otto, B. Doctor-patient communication during the Corona crisis—Web-based interactions and structured feedback from standardized patients at the university of Basel and the LMU Munich. *GMS J. Med. Educ.* **2021**, *38*, Doc81. [CrossRef] [PubMed]
33. Smith, E.; Boscak, A. A virtual emergency: Learning lessons from remote medical student education during the COVID-19 pandemic. *Emerg. Radiol.* **2021**, *28*, 445–452. [CrossRef]
34. Vielsmeier, V.; Auerswald, S.; Marienhagen, J.; Keil, S.; Müller, N. Digital teaching with interactive case presentations of ENT diseases—Discussion of utilization and motivation of students. *GMS J. Med. Educ.* **2020**, *37*, Doc100. [CrossRef]
35. He, M.; Tang, X.-Q.; Zhang, H.-N.; Luo, Y.-Y.; Tang, Z.-C.; Gao, S.-G. Remote clinical training practice in the neurology internship during the COVID-19 pandemic. *Med. Educ. Online* **2021**, *26*, 1899642. [CrossRef]

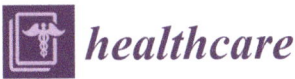

Article

An Interprofessional E-Learning Resource to Prepare Students for Clinical Practice in the Operating Room—A Mixed Method Study from the Students' Perspective

Ann-Mari Fagerdahl [1,2,*], Eva Torbjörnsson [1,3] and Anders Sondén [1,3]

1. Department of Clinical Science and Education, Karolinska Institutet, 118 83 Stockholm, Sweden; eva.torbjornsson@ki.se (E.T.); anders.sonden@ki.se (A.S.)
2. Wound Centre, Södersjukhuset, 118 83 Stockholm, Sweden
3. Department of Surgery, Södersjukhuset, Sjukhusbacken 10, 118 83 Stockholm, Sweden
* Correspondence: ann-mari.fagerdahl@ki.se

Abstract: The operating room is a challenging learning environment for many students. Preparedness for practice is important as perceived stress and the fear of making mistakes are known to hamper learning. The aim was to evaluate students' perspectives of an e-learning resource for achieving preparedness. A mixed methods design was used. Students ($n = 52$) from three educational nursing and medical programs were included. A questionnaire was used to explore demographics, student use of the e-learning resource, and how the learning activities had helped them prepare for their clinical placement. Five focus group interviews were conducted as a complement. Most students (79%) stated that the resource prepared them for their clinical placement and helped them to feel more relaxed when attending to the operating room. In total, 93% of the students recommended other students to use the e-learning resource prior to a clinical placement in the operating room. Activities containing films focusing on practical procedures were rated as the most useful. We conclude that an e-learning resource seems to increase students' perceived preparedness for their clinical practice in the operating room. The development of e-learning resources has its challenges, and we recommend student involvement to evaluate the content.

Keywords: clinical learning environment; e-learning; operating room; student preparedness

1. Introduction

The operating room (OR) environment is challenging for students in relation to achieving their learning objectives. Feelings of anxiety, humiliation, and other emotional obstacles for effective learning have been described by both medical and nursing students [1,2]. Some of these emotional barriers can be reduced if the students are well-prepared before their clinical practice [3,4]. Preparedness can be divided into a general part and a specific part. The general part should consist of information about the OR setting, etiquette, and the professional roles of the staff, in combination with workshops on practical skills. The specific part is the information needed on day-to-day basis, i.e., which supervisor the OR student should follow [1,2].

Methods for delivering general introductory sessions to students have been described by several authors, but there is weak evidence as to which arrangement is the most effective [2,5]. It has been concluded, however, that the introductory sessions should have an interprofessional perspective, as interprofessional teamwork is essential for creating a safe surgical environment for patients [6]. However, interprofessional learning (IPL) activities pose logistical and scheduling challenges [7]. One way to overcome these timetabling and geographic barriers is e-learning [8]. Another advantage of e-learning is that it is well-suited for learning practical skills within the perioperative setting, due to the possibility to incorporate multimedia [8,9].

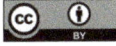

For many years, the medical students and the OR nurses in our OR department at Södersjukhuset, Karolinska Institutet have attended a pre-theatre workshop on surgical hand preparation and sterile gloving technique before entering the OR. The workshop contains a lecture, followed by practical training. The general nurses and anesthetic nurses have only a 15 min lecture about guidelines for clothes and aseptic techniques. A survey aimed at the medical students in 2016 showed that the students perceived that the general introduction was too sparse; moreover, the practical workshop was too short, and it lacked an interprofessional approach. Therefore, an interprofessional faculty at our institution created a complementary e-learning resource, defined as a software-based resource distributed online with the aim to enhance knowledge and performance [9] for all students attending the OR [10].

The aim of the e-learning resource was to better prepare the different student categories (nurses, OR nurses, anesthetic nurses, and medical students) and to reduce emotional barriers, hence creating a better foundation for learning. The focus of the learning outcomes in the e-learning resource was set on skills and interprofessional collaboration.

In 2018, we performed a pilot study evaluating the e-learning resource. It was concluded that it was valuable to the students, but it was difficult to draw conclusions on why and how it was valuable due to lack of qualitative data. Moreover, only medical students participated in the evaluation, so no conclusions could be drawn for the other student categories. There was also a lack of knowledge regarding ideas for improvement of the e-learning resource.

The aim of this study was thus to explore the perspectives of all student categories using the new e-learning resource, with a focus on preparedness for practice.

2. Materials and Methods

2.1. Design

An explanatory sequential mixed methods design was used, i.e., data was collected in two consecutive phases: first the quantitative data and then the qualitative data. Thereafter, the data was merged to achieve methodological integration [11,12]. Questionnaires were used to gather qualitative data. Focus group (FG) interviews were used to deepen the knowledge from the questionnaires and to obtain suggestions and ideas for improvement of the e-learning resource. This specific qualitative data collection method was chosen for its ability to help participants to explore and explain their perceptions further in interaction with others [13].

2.2. The E-Learning Resource

The e-learning resource used in this project was a package of online learning materials using Articulate Storyline® (Articulate Global, New York, NY, USA) and consisted of pre-recorded lectures and video demonstrations of skills which could be accessed on different digital devices such as computers or mobile phones. The software used to produce the learning material were PowerPoint® (Microsoft Corporation, Redmond, WA, USA) and Screencast-omatic ® (UserVoice, San Francisco, CA, USA), while the films were recorded using a regular camcorder with a microphone.

The resource was based on seven interprofessional learning outcomes, each one forming the base for a learning activity in the online program. The majority of the learning outcomes were considered generic, except "surgical hand preparation" and "gowning procedure" that were directed to the OR nurses and medical students exclusively (Table 1).

Four of the learning activities were followed by a formative assessment in order to give immediate feedback to students.

Table 1. Learning outcome and learning activities of the e-learning resource (Torbjornsson et al., 2018).

Learning Outcome	Learning Activity	Format	Running Time (min)
The student shall understand the structure of an operation ward	OR design	Recorded audio lecture	5.04
The student shall understand the different professions working at the OR and their responsibilities	Professions	Recorded audio lecture	4.24
The student shall have knowledge regarding the hygiene routine at the OR	Hygiene Routine	Recorded audio lecture	0.45
The student shall be able to describe the radiation safety at OR	Radiation Safety	Recorded audio lecture	2.34
The student shall be able to perform a sterile gloving technique	Gloving technique	Recorded audio movie	1.40
The student shall be able to perform a perioperative surgical hand preparation	Surgical hand preparation	Recorded audio movie	4.01

2.3. Participants

Students from three educational programs were included in the study: 4th year medical students ($n = 24$), 3rd year nursing students ($n = 12$), and 1st year perioperative specialist nursing students, specializing in either OR nursing or Anesthesiology nursing ($n = 16$). The medical and nursing students all had their clinical placement at the OR ward in the same hospital, while the perioperative nursing students did their clinical placement in two different hospitals in Stockholm connected to the university. The students received written information regarding the study in their ordinary online learning management system (Ping-Pong AB, Stockholm, Sweden) and verbal information in their course introduction at campus. An email to all eligible students was sent with information on the e-learning resource and the study, together with a link to the e-learning resource on their study platform. All nursing students had a link to the evaluation questionnaire on their study platform. The medical students were given the questionnaire on paper during their examination week at the end of the semester. All students received information regarding the focus groups (FG), and the students who were willing to participate were invited to contact the researcher by mail. In total, 52 students (33 women and 19 men) out of 117 enrolled in the studied programs answered the questionnaires, giving a response rate of 44%. Out of them, 65% had used the e-learning resource prior to their clinical placement (Table 2).

Table 2. Demographics of the study population.

	All Students $n = 52$	4th Year Medical Students $n = 24$	1st Year Perioperative Nursing Students $n = 16$	3rd Year Nursing Students $n = 12$
Age mean (range)	34.0 (21–55)	29.5 (22–47)	38.4 (26–55)	34.9 (21–52)
Gender (%)				
Male	33 (63)	13 (54)	4 (25)	2 (17)
Female	19 (37)	11 (46)	12 (75)	10 (83)
Previous experience of OR (%)				
Yes	31 (60)	12 (50)	13	6 (50)
No	19 (37)	10 (42)	3	6 (50)
Missing	2 (3)	2 (8)		0
Had used the e-resource (%)				
Yes	34 (65)	13 (54)	12 (75)	9 (75)
No	18 (36)	11 (46)	4 (25)	3 (25)
Missing	0	0	0	0

2.4. Data Collection

2.4.1. Questionnaire

The questionnaire was developed by the research group and was based on the questionnaire used in the pilot study by Torbjornsson et al. [10]. To address face and content validity, the questionnaire was discussed within the expert group and modified by adding further questions and using another scale for the answers (a 5-level Likert scale instead of a 4-level) [14]. None of the students asked questions about the questionnaire that suggested that they had difficulties to understand it.

The questionnaire consisted of 16 questions: 4 were demographic, 3 contained information regarding the use of the e-learning resource, and 9 were questions where the students rated how well the different learning activities had helped them prepare for their clinical placement in the OR (on a 5-level Likert scale: very little; little; some; large; very large). There was also one open-ended question where the students could give improvement suggestions on the resource (suppl Document S1).

2.4.2. Focus Group Interviews

The FG interviews focused on evaluating the e-learning resource and the students' perceptions regarding if and how it helped them to prepare for their clinical practice. The students were divided into groups based on their profession. The aim was to create homogeneity in the groups and avoid any form of hierarchy that may inhibit an open atmosphere enabling everyone to feel confident to speak out [13].

The FG were attended by a moderator and conducted by the first and second author. The FG interviews lasted 22–45 min and were documented by note-taking from the moderator. A semi-structured interview guide was used, and probing questions were used to further enable the participants to elaborate. Five FG interviews were conducted with a total of 17 students (2–5 students/FG): medical students ($n = 9$), nursing students ($n = 2$), and perioperative specialist nursing students ($n = 6$). All of the focus groups contained participants of the same educational program.

2.5. Data Analysis

2.5.1. Questionnaire—Quantitative Data

The quantitative data analysis was performed on the questionnaires from the students with descriptive statistics [15]. Continuous variables are presented with mean and standard deviation (SD) and categorical variables as n (percent). No comparative analyses between the different student categories were made. The quantitative analyses were performed with IBM SPSS statistics version 23.0 (IBM Inc., Chicago, IL, USA).

2.5.2. Focus Group Interviews—Qualitative Data

The notes from the FG were read and reread to identify patterns and tendencies. The text units were condensed into meaning units, labelled with a code, and sorted into different categories based on the focus areas of the questionnaire. The focus of the qualitative analysis was to extend and to deepen the knowledge from the questionnaires.

The analysis was performed by two members (AMF and ET) of the research group, and the result was discussed until consensus was reached. Directed content analysis using a deductive approach, based on the different areas of the questionnaire, was used [16].

2.6. Ethical Considerations

The study was performed in accordance with good clinical practice and research as per the Helsinki Declaration [17]. Before any data collection began, the students were informed that the participation in this study was voluntary with the purpose of a scientific analysis and publication. They were also informed that their participation in no way would affect their grades, that they could cease participation at any time, and that the collected data would be completely discarded if they were to withdraw from the study. Completing and returning the questionnaire implied their consent to participate. To ensure confidentiality, one of the three authors did the initial analysis of the questionnaires and FG interviews and matched the participants' data using numeric codes.

3. Results

The demographics of the study population is shown in Table 1. The majority of the students (79%) stated that the e-learning resource had prepared them for their clinical placement in the OR, and the medical students rated the e-learning resource as the least useful. However, three quarters of the medical students still rated the e-learning resource as useful to some extent and none rated it as not useful at all (Figure 1).

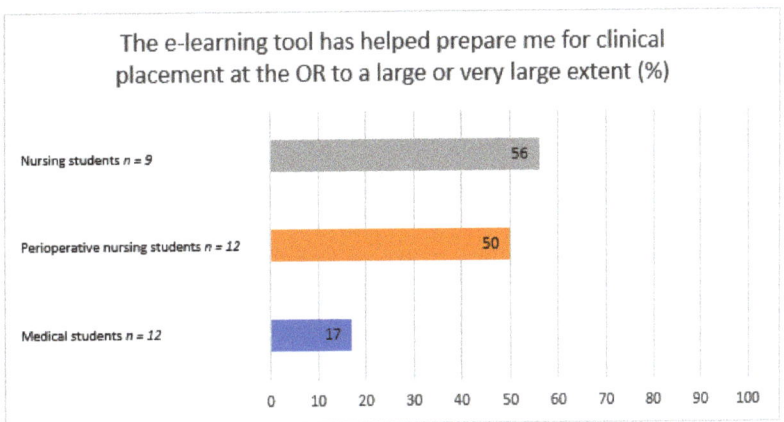

Figure 1. Feelings of preparedness for clinical placement at the OR.

In total, 93% of the students recommended other students to use the e-learning resource prior to a clinical placement at the OR ward. The differences between student groups are shown in Figure 2.

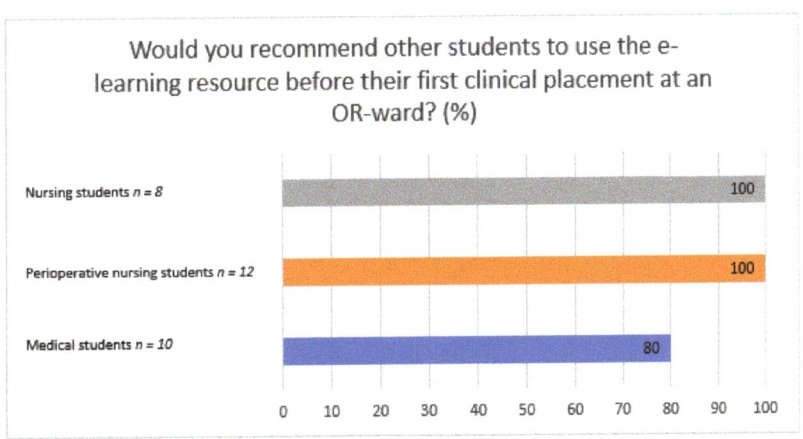

Figure 2. Students' recommendation of the resource to other students.

3.1. The E-Learning Resource in Preparation for Clinical Placement at the OR

The students were asked to what extent the different learning activities of the e-learning resource had helped them prepare for their placement at the OR. Eighty percent of the students perceived that all the different learning activities, at least to some extent, had helped them prepare for their clinical placement (Figure 3).

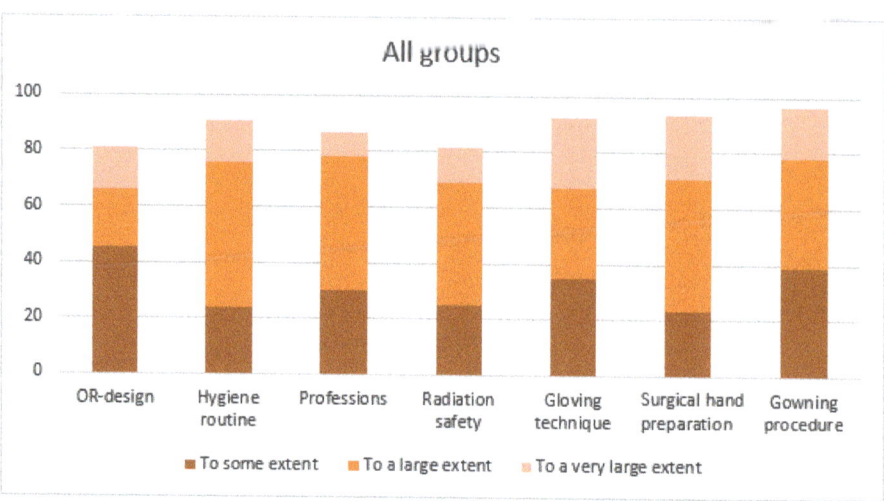

Figure 3. Preparedness for the clinical placement at the OR regarding the different learning activities.

The FG interviews revealed that many of the students felt different levels of anxiety prior to their clinical placement at the OR. The students explained that the main cause of this anxiety was the feeling of being in an unfamiliar environment and a sense of being out of place. These feelings gave rise to insecurity and stress and made them more sensitive and vulnerable to what people said or to events that occurred. Students from all programs thought that the e-learning resource was a way to reduce the perceived stress and had prepared them for the OR placement:

> "You want to be as well prepared as possible when you arrive. Although you may not be able to practice so much practically wearing gloves and such things, you want to be able to see ... because then it is good because then you can see it over and over again ... and you become a little more confident when you come out if you have seen it ... "
>
> (Perioperative nurse)

In the FG interviews, all three student categories commented that the e-learning resource should be a mandatory learning activity for all student groups prior to clinical placement at the OR.

The nursing students stated that the e-learning resource saved time for them: by being better prepared, they could use their time in the OR more efficiently. Medical students, having a two-hour OR preparation workshop prior to attending their clinical placement, thought the workshop per se prepared them well, but that the e-learning resource was a good complement.

3.2. The Students' Perception of the Content in the Learning Resource

In total, 52% of the students perceived, to a large or very large extent, that the e-learning resource contained all the elements needed to prepare them for their clinical placement. The perioperative nursing students rated the content highest (67%) while the medical students expressed a need for additional information.

The three learning activities containing films and focusing on practical procedures ('gloving technique', 'surgical hand preparation', and 'gowning procedure') were rated most useful (Figure 3). All of the medical students and a majority of the other student categories perceived that the latter two activities, to a very large extent, had prepared them for the OR.

The least valuable activities according to the students were 'OR-design' and 'radiation safety'. 'Radiation safety' got the lowest ratings of all activities, particularly by the medical and perioperative nursing students (Figure 4).

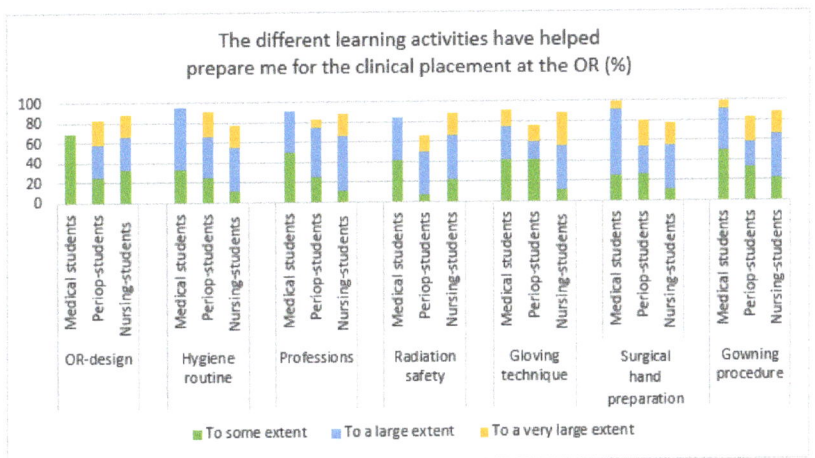

Figure 4. Preparedness for clinical placement at the OR regarding the different learning activities from an all-professions perspective.

The FG interviews revealed that the medical students and perioperative nursing students wanted more information directed to their special needs in their specific profession. The medical students expressed a wish for films that could give them a general overview of the workflow and patient process in the OR, together with instructions on what happens when something goes wrong—for example, what to do if they are unsterile during surgery. They thought this would ease the stress and fear of doing something wrong.

> "Another suggestion is to also inform about what happens when something goes wrong, for example when we get unsterile or similar. So that when and if it happens it will not be so huge but you know what to do if it happens and how to handle this. Takes a little bit of the stress boost ... "

(Medical student)

The medical students also requested films containing specific surgical specialties depending on what kind of surgery they were doing in their clinical placement. The perioperative nurses mentioned elements like positioning on the OR bed and instrument knowledge. The nursing students proposed that the e-learning resource should be divided into two parts: part 1 with basic interprofessional content, which would be mandatory for all students, and part 2 with optional, more profession-oriented content.

3.3. Design and Layout of the E-Learning Resource

The majority of the students stated that they had used the e-learning resource on their computer and not on their cell phone. The reason was that the resource was not adequately adapted to the cell phone format. The students thought that they would have used the e-learning resource more often if it was better adapted to the cell phone. This was particularly important for the activities containing films.

The perioperative nursing students and the nursing students experienced the resource as being too messy and lacking a well-defined flow. This was a major obstacle when conducting the activity.

"It is confusing the whole arrangement I think... you do not know which (learning activity) one is inside and so you click back, and you end up somewhere else... it is difficult to remember..."

(Perioperative nursing student)

The medical students agreed that there could be a more structured arrangement; however, they did not consider this to be a major issue.

All student groups commented that the technical form of the learning activity had some drawbacks. The most important part identified by all the focus groups was that the students wanted to be able to see which activities they had performed, which they had left, and finally when they had succeeded with the entire learning activity. Moreover, they wanted to see how long the films were, how much time had passed, and how much was left. One suggestion from the medical students was that the activities could change color when they had been performed. Students from all categories also wished for the possibility to pause and to rewind if they needed to repeat something, without the need to restart a module in the e-leaning resource.

The students all agreed that the maximum amount of time for this kind of learning resource should not be more than 30 min and that the films should not exceed five minutes each.

3.4. Interprofessional Perspective

The learning activity 'Professions' was rated differently by the student groups. Common for all student groups was that they considered the interprofessional knowledge in the e-learning resource an important feature, that it was important to learn about each other's responsibilities at the OR, and that this was essential for a successful interprofessional collaboration in the future. However, the FG interviews identified several requests for improvement regarding the interprofessional approach. Students wanted deeper knowledge regarding the task of the different professions working at the OR ward and not only, as earlier described, a film focusing on the patient process or journey throughout the surgical procedure at the OR. They also proposed an additional film following the different professions in their daily work.

"We are lacking an overall picture of what is happening at the operating room, a description of the flow. To be able to prepare even better. A kind of "patient journey" through the flow to the surgery department and also a "staff journey" to gain an increased understanding of other professions in the surgery. That is generally lacking in teaching in general."

(Medical student)

4. Discussion

Every semester, the OR receives students from different education healthcare programs. Many of them, regardless of student category, perceive the learning environment at the OR as extremely stressful [1,2]—something that is known to hamper their learning [18]. This study shows that an e-learning resource based on seven interprofessional learning outcomes enhanced the different student categories' perceived preparedness for their clinical placement. It did so by making the environment less unfamiliar by explaining the expected role of the student as well as the role of the other professions at the OR and how they interact. The e-learning resource also gave students the possibility to learn specific skills that are known to induce stress when performed in the real environment [19]. These learning activities could be seen "over and over again" and be repeated just before practice.

The students rated the activities that contained film and focused on practical skills as most valuable. This is consistent with previous findings that skills training such as sterility and operating room etiquettes have been seen as particularly important [2]. Radiation safety got the lowest rating. The rationale for that part could be discussed. It might have been better to name the activity 'safety in the OR' and include, for example, laser safety and how to manage surgical smoke. The lack of student involvement is probably one of the reasons that we missed that in the design. One can also argue that knowledge regarding radiation may be quite abstract for the students and that it does not seem as important as the practical skills [18]. Overall, the findings from the FG interviews conclude that it is important to have student involvement in the design phase of an e-learning resource. For example, there was a request from both the medical students and the perioperative nurses to have more films that contained information regarding specific skills, such as instrument knowledge and surgical skills.

The format is of importance when developing online learning material. The students in this study demanded easy access, preferably in cell phones, with short films and an easy way to find the different contents of the learning activities. Since digital use in society has exploded in recent years and the generation of today's students have been using digital devices their entire life, they would be a useful resource when creating different online activities. Haraldseid, Friberg, and Aase [20] concluded that active student involvement in the development of technological learning material for clinical skills training could enhance the knowledge of the most important learning needs of the students. It could also make the learning activities more effective and attractive [20].

Interprofessional collaboration is known as a major stressor for students attending the OR. Students fear to be despised by the surgeon or nurse when doing something wrong or for simply being in the room [2]. The students expressed the need for knowledge regarding actions when doing something wrong, to be better prepared for such situations. In the FG interviews, the students expressed that they had identified the importance of interprofessional collaboration by using the e-learning resource, and they requested a deeper knowledge of the functions of the different professions, despite the resource not being an IPL resource by definition [21]. The students expressed the IPL ground of learning with and particularly about each other as an area that should be expanded, since they experienced this as important for their psychological preparation for clinical placement at the OR.

Just in-time teaching (JiTT) is a learning model shown in research to enhance student motivation and to give the students a sense of control. JiTT is defined as a method where the students prepare just before the lesson and lesson time, focusing on specific questions that they experience as difficult and demanding [22]. This e-learning resource may be seen as a way of using the JiTT method, since the students can go through the activities just prior to the clinical task and be better prepared. The main advantage is to be able to repeat the specific element as many times as needed for the student in an easy-access way (on their cell phone, for instance). This creates the possibility for students to tailor their learning to meet their own specific individual learning needs [9,23], which is particularly important given that we address such a broad spectrum of different students. Furthermore, in a stressful environment like the OR, the stress and anxiety of students may inhibit learning and prolong the learning curve [2]. To prepare students by using e-learning in the practical procedures, they may feel less stress when arriving at the OR, and the threshold for learning can be lowered.

The development of an e-learning resource, such as the one that we have described, could be a useful learning method for student groups in other contexts where practical skills and interprofessional collaboration is important.

Limitations

It may be argued that a limitation of this study is that we did not have a control group and did not perform a comparative study to assess the effectiveness of the e-learning resource. The aim of the study was, however, not to measure student preparedness or specific knowledge or skills, but to evaluate and describe the students´ perceptions and to explore the value of the resource from the students´ perspective.

It is recommended that the ideal size of a focus group is six to ten people [24]. In our study, we had a convenience sample which was based on the voluntariness and interest of the students, and we unfortunately did not manage to receive further participants.

However, Cote-Arsenault and Morrison-Beedy [25] emphasize that the aim of the study together with developmental levels of the participants is more important than a set number. Since we included students with several years of university studies and we chose to have the FGs separated for the different categories, we believe that the low number of participants in the groups did not inhibit the creativity and data received, nor did we feel that the participants felt pressured to speak, which is described as being a risk in low-numbered FGs [25].

To only rely on notetaking during the FG interviews and not audiotapes is a limitation. However, as the moderators had high knowledge regarding the setting and the appearance of the e-learning resource, it was not perceived as a problem. The low response rate in the quantitative part of the study can seem to be a problem for the validity (44%). There is a risk of nonresponse bias; however, it is tempting to believe that it does not have the same impact on the result as it may have when it comes to sensitive data such as aspects on quality of life [26].

It also needs to be mentioned that the questionnaire was not evaluated with a psychometric test. However, we believe the fact that the questionnaire was evaluated in the expert group, as well as in the pilot study, increases the validity. Further, the use of FG gave a deeper knowledge regarding the e-learning resource.

5. Conclusions

We conclude that an e-learning resource seems to increase students' perceived preparedness for their clinical practice at the OR. The students stated that they felt more relaxed when attending the OR, which may, according to the literature, lead to a better learning environment and improved learning. The development of e-learning resources has its challenges, and we recommend student involvement to evaluate the content of the learning activities as well as to prevent technical issues.

Supplementary Materials: The following are available online at https://www.mdpi.com/article/10.3390/healthcare9081028/s1, Document S1: translated version of the questionnaire.

Author Contributions: Conceptualization, methodology, formal analysis, investigation, resources, data curation, writing—original draft preparation, and writing—review and editing, A.-M.F., E.T. and A.S. All authors have read and agreed to the published version of the manuscript.

Funding: The authors have received an unrestricted pedagogical grant from Karolinska Institutet, Department of Clinical Science and Education, Södersjukhuset.

Institutional Review Board Statement: The study was conducted according to the guidelines of the Declaration of Helsinki.

Informed Consent Statement: Informed consent was obtained from all subjects involved in the study.

Data Availability Statement: The data presented in this study are available on request from the corresponding author.

Conflicts of Interest: The authors declare no conflict of interest.

References

1. Meyer, R.; Van Schalkwyk, S.C.; Prakaschandra, R. The operating room as a clinical learning environment: An exploratory study. *Nurse Educ. Pract.* **2016**, *18*, 60–72. [CrossRef]
2. Croghan, S.M.; Phillips, C.; Howson, W. The operating theatre as a classroom: A literature review of medical student learning in the theatre environment. *Int. J. Med. Educ.* **2019**, *10*, 75–87. [CrossRef] [PubMed]
3. Zundel, S.; Wolf, I.; Christen, H.-J.; Huwendiek, S. What supports students' education in the operating room? A focus group study including students' and surgeons' views. *Am. J. Surg.* **2015**, *210*, 951–959. [CrossRef]
4. Chapman, S.; Hakeem, A.R.; Marangoni, G.; Prasad, K.R. How can we Enhance Undergraduate Medical Training in the Operating Room? A Survey of Student Attitudes and Opinions. *J. Surg. Educ.* **2013**, *70*, 326–333. [CrossRef] [PubMed]
5. Aliabad, H.B.; Bakhshi, M.; Hassanshahi, G. Students' perceptions of the academic learning environment in seven medical sciences courses based on DREEM. *Adv. Med. Educ. Pract.* **2015**, *6*, 195–203. [CrossRef]

6. Gillespie, B.M.; Gwinner, K.; Chaboyer, W.; Fairweather, N. Team communications in surgery—Creating a culture of safety. *J. Interprof. Care* **2013**, *27*, 387–393. [CrossRef] [PubMed]
7. West, C.; Graham, L.; Palmer, R.T.; Miller, M.F.; Thayer, E.K.; Stuber, M.L.; Awdishu, L.; Umoren, R.; Wamsley, M.A.; Nelson, E.A.; et al. Implementation of interprofessional education (IPE) in 16 U.S. medical schools: Common practices, barriers and facilitators. *J. Interprof. Educ. Pract.* **2016**, *4*, 41–49. [CrossRef] [PubMed]
8. Maertens, H.; Madani, A.; Landry, T.; Vermassen, F.; Van Herzeele, I.; Aggarwal, R. Systematic review of e-learning for surgical training. *J. Br. Surg.* **2016**, *103*, 1428–1437. [CrossRef]
9. Ruiz, J.G.; Mintzer, M.J.; Leipzig, R.M. The Impact of E-Learning in Medical Education. *Acad. Med.* **2006**, *81*, 207–212. [CrossRef]
10. Torbjörnsson, E.; Olivecrona, C.; Sonden, A. An interprofessional initiative aimed at creating a common learning resource for the operating room ward. *J. Interprof. Care* **2018**, *32*, 501–504. [CrossRef] [PubMed]
11. Schoonenboom, J.; Johnson, R.B. How to Construct a Mixed Methods Research Design. *KZfSS Kölner Zeitschrift für Soziologie und Sozialpsychologie* **2017**, *69*, 107–131. [CrossRef]
12. Warfa, A.-R.M. Mixed-Methods Design in Biology Education Research: Approach and Uses. *CBE-Life Sci. Educ.* **2016**, *15*, rm5. [CrossRef]
13. Kitzinger, J. Qualitative Research: Introducing focus groups. *BMJ* **1995**, *311*, 299–302. [CrossRef]
14. Holden, R.R. Face Validity. *Corsini Encycl. Psychol.* **2010**, 1–2. [CrossRef]
15. Halfens, R.; Meijers, J. Back to basics: An introduction to statistics. *J. Wound Care* **2013**, *22*, 248–251. [CrossRef] [PubMed]
16. Hsieh, H.-F.; Shannon, S.E. Three approaches to qualitative content analysis. *Qual. Health Res.* **2005**, *15*, 1277–1288. [CrossRef] [PubMed]
17. World Medical Association. World Medical Association Declaration of Helsinki: Ethical Principles for Medical Research Involving Human Subjects. *JAMA* **2013**, *310*, 2191–2194. [CrossRef]
18. McNamara, N. Preparing students for clinical placements: The student's perspective. *Nurse Educ. Pract.* **2015**, *15*, 196–202. [CrossRef]
19. Chu, L.F.; Ngai, L.K.; Young, C.A.; Pearl, R.G.; Macario, A.; Harrison, T.K. Preparing Interns for Anesthesiology Residency Training: Development and Assessment of the Successful Transition to Anesthesia Residency Training (START) E-Learning Curriculum. *J. Grad. Med. Educ.* **2013**, *5*, 125–129. [CrossRef]
20. Haraldseid, C.; Friberg, F.; Aase, K. How can students contribute? A qualitative study of active student involvement in development of technological learning material for clinical skills training. *BMC Nurs.* **2016**, *15*, 2. [CrossRef]
21. Parsell, G.; Bligh, J. Interprofessional learning. *Postgrad. Med. J.* **1998**, *74*, 89–95. [CrossRef] [PubMed]
22. Schuller, M.C.; DaRosa, D.A.; Crandall, M.L. Using Just-in-Time Teaching and Peer Instruction in a Residency Program's Core Curriculum. *Acad. Med.* **2015**, *90*, 384–391. [CrossRef] [PubMed]
23. Leong, C.; Louizos, C.; Currie, C.; Glassford, L.; Davies, N.M.; Brothwell, D.; Renaud, R. Student perspectives of an online module for teaching physical assessment skills for dentistry, dental hygiene, and pharmacy students. *J. Interprof. Care* **2014**, *29*, 1–3. [CrossRef]
24. Stalmeijer, R.E.; McNaughton, N.; Van Mook, W.N.K.A. Using focus groups in medical education research: AMEE Guide No. 91. *Med. Teach.* **2014**, *36*, 923–939. [CrossRef]
25. Côté-Arsenault, D.; Morrison-Beedy, D. Maintaining your focus in focus groups: Avoiding common mistakes. *Res. Nurs. Health* **2005**, *28*, 172–179. [CrossRef]
26. Groves, R.M. Nonresponse Rates and Nonresponse Bias in Household Surveys. *Public Opin. Q.* **2006**, *70*, 646–675. [CrossRef]

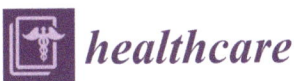

Article

Perception of the Online Learning Environment of Nursing Students in Slovenia: Validation of the DREEM Questionnaire

Lucija Gosak [1,*], Nino Fijačko [1], Carolina Chabrera [2], Esther Cabrera [2] and Gregor Štiglic [1,3,4]

1 Faculty of Health Sciences, University of Maribor, 2000 Maribor, Slovenia; nino.fijacko@um.si (N.F.); gregor.stiglic@um.si (G.Š.)
2 Research Group in Attention to Chronicity and Innovation in Health (GRACIS), TecnoCampus, Universitat Pompeu Fabra, 08002 Barcelona, Spain; cchabrera@tecnocampus.cat (C.C.); ecabrera@tecnocampus.cat (E.C.)
3 Faculty of Electrical Engineering and Computer Science, University of Maribor, 2000 Maribor, Slovenia
4 Usher Institute, University of Edinburgh, Edinburgh EH8 9YL, UK
* Correspondence: lucija.gosak2@um.si; Tel.: +386-2-300-47-35

Abstract: At the time of the outbreak of the coronavirus pandemic, several measures were in place to limit the spread of the virus, such as lockdown and restriction of social contacts. Many colleges thus had to shift their education from personal to online form overnight. The educational environment itself has a significant influence on students' learning outcomes, knowledge, and satisfaction. This study aims to validate the tool for assessing the educational environment in the Slovenian nursing student population. To assess the educational environment, we used the DREEM tool distributed among nursing students using an online platform. First, we translated the survey questionnaire from English into Slovenian using the reverse translation technique. We also validated the DREEM survey questionnaire. We performed psychometric testing and content validation. I-CVI and S-CVI are at an acceptable level. A high degree of internal consistency was present, as Cronbach's alpha was 0.951. The questionnaire was completed by 174 participants, of whom 30 were men and 143 were women. One person did not define gender. The mean age of students was 21.1 years (SD = 3.96). The mean DREEM score was 122.2. The mean grade of student perception of learning was 58.54%, student perception of teachers was 65.68%, student academic self-perception was 61.88%, student perception of the atmosphere was 60.63%, and social self-perception of students was 58.93%. Although coronavirus has affected the educational process, students still perceive the educational environment as positive. Nevertheless, there is still room for improvement in all assessed areas.

Keywords: education; learning environment; nursing student; transcultural adaptation; psychometric properties; health care

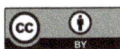

1. Introduction

Due to the coronavirus pandemic (COVID-19), which was reported in Wuhan, China [1–4] and soon after, the first major outbreak in Europe spread rapidly to Slovenia [5,6]. Governments issued directives on social isolation and living at home, so colleges and universities around the world were closed [7]. COVID-19 has forced education systems around the world to find alternatives to personal teaching [8]. Online distance learning platforms are the only available way of learning and teaching during unprecedented events such as the outbreak of COVID-19 [9–11]. However, it is important to distinguish between online distance education and distance learning in an emergency as a temporary solution. Online education provides students with flexibility and choice [12]. This involves implementing education using information and communication technology [13] and represents an easily accessible teaching method [14].

Online learning promotes student-centered learning, in which case courses are easy to manage [15], resulting in better knowledge and self-efficacy for some students [16]. It increases performance, encourages critical thinking, and improves writing skills for most students [17]. Through the accelerated use of online learning, educators and carers need to consider the pedagogical and practical challenges posed by the integration of online learning [18]. Negative aspects highlighted are a lack of appropriate infrastructure for some students, less effective communication and interaction, inability to implement practical applications, lack of socialization, lack of motivation, less objective exams, and the possibility of deteriorating health [19].

Despite growing evidence that online learning is just as effective as traditional learning tools, there is very little evidence of what works, when, and how online learning improves teaching and learning [20]. Therefore, in this study, we decided to evaluate the online learning environment of students using the Dundee Ready Education Environment Measure (DREEM) tool [21–23]. Any learning environment that meets students' internal and external needs is likely to lead to better and more promising learning outcomes [24]. Achieving an optimal educational environment must meet the expectations of students regarding the school atmosphere, teaching, teachers, students, school staff, educational equipment, and the physical environment [25]. A good learning environment for students in clinical practice depends on the structure of student admission, the pedagogical atmosphere, and the participation of those involved [26]. The educational environment has an impact on students' learning outcomes, preparation for practice, and student satisfaction [27]. Also, the perception of the learning environment is related to well-being and stress in students [28].

The main goal of the research is a validation of the questionnaire focusing on the assessment and perception of nursing students about the online learning environment. The goal is also to test psychometrically the DREEM tool [22,23]. The validation of the DREEM tool is performed within the Erasmus+ project Digital Toolbox for Innovation and Nursing Education (I-BOX), which aims to develop material for teaching nursing students and nurses. Based on the obtained results, we will also assess where the greatest deviations occur in the assessment of the learning environment and thus encourage the improvement of the learning environment for students.

2. Materials and Methods

2.1. Study Design

We used quantitative research methodology [29–31]. Data for assessing the educational environment by undergraduate and postgraduate nursing students were collected using an online questionnaire between November 2020 and January 2021. The survey questionnaire was previously translated into Slovenian language and validated in the Slovenian environment for the first time.

2.2. Assessment Tool

To assess the online educational environment, we used the DREEM tool [22,23]. DREEM is a validated tool for assessing the educational environment in health care professions worldwide [32]. In addition to being used to diagnose deficiencies in the current educational environment, DREEM is also used to compare different groups, monitor the same group over time, and assess factors influencing the educational environment [33,34]. The DREEM tool includes five subscales: students' perception of learning (SPL); students' perception of teachers (SPT); students' academic self-perception (SAP); students' perception of the atmosphere (SPA) and students' social self-perception (SSP). The maximum score is 200 [35]. The use of the questionnaire was previously authorized by the authors [22,23]. The survey questionnaire was translated from English into Slovenian and then back to the original language [36]: Independently by two researchers, the survey questionnaire was translated from English into Slovenian. Both researchers had the necessary knowledge of English, andragogy, and nursing. Thus, we obtained two versions of the translation, which we merged into one in the next step, based on consultation between experts. If disagreement was present, a third researcher was involved. In the last step, two experts with the necessary knowledge of English translated a joint version of the Slovenian questionnaire into English. Thus, we obtained two forms of reverse translation and subsequently merged them into a common form [29,30].

Questionnaires were distributed using an online survey platform ENKA from which the results were then downloaded and analysed using IBM SPSS Statistics 27.

2.2.1. Validation of Assessment Tool

We assessed the validity of the content and the validity of the construct in the survey questionnaire and performed confirmatory factor analysis [37,38]. To determine the content validity, we included experts who have the necessary knowledge in the field [29,30,37,39]. Based on the recommendations where six to ten experts are required [40], we included six experts who work as nursing teachers. The questions in the questionnaire were rated on a four-point scale from 1 to 4, where 1 represents statements that are not relevant; 2, deficient/poorly understood statements; 3, partially understandable/partially relevant statements; and 4, entirely understandable/completely relevant claims [41]. To assess the content validity of the questionnaire, we calculated the content validity of individual claims (I-CVI) and content validity of the whole questionnaire (S-CVI) [41–46]. For the internal reliability analysis, we calculated Cronbach's α, which presents us with a measure of internal reliability between several items [47]. Cronbach's alpha coefficients and interpreted the values as follows: ≥ 0.90, excellent; 0.80–0.89, good; 0.70–0.79, acceptable; 0.60–0.69, questionable; 0.50–0.59, poor; and <0.50, unacceptable [48]. Correlations between items are an essential element in the analysis of the items representing a specific concept. Correlations between items examine the extent to which ratings of one item are related to ratings of all other scale items [49–51].

I-CVI represents the quotient between the number of experts who rated each question with a grade of 3 or 4 and between the number of all experts, which in our case was six [42,44–46,52]. The probability of agreement was calculated using the formula $Pc = [N!/A! (N-A)!] \, 0{,}5N$ where N represents the number of evaluators, and A represents the number of consents [42,44–46,52,53]. We used the following formula to calculate the kappa determination of the compliance agreement: $k = (\text{I-CVI} - Pc)/(1 - Pc)$. I-CVI represents item content validity index, and Pc represents the probability of chance agreement [42,44–46,52]. The S-CVI represents the proportion of questions rated by two experts with a score of 3 or 4 [39,42,52].

2.2.2. Perception of the Learning Environment

The DREEM tool includes 50 items, 41 positive and nine negatives, related to learning perception (12 items), teacher perception (11 items), academic self-perception (eight items), atmospheric perception (12 items), and social self-perception (seven items). Each item is rated on a five-point Likert scale (from 1—strongly disagree to 5—strongly agree), where reverse-coding is used for nine statements [22,32]. Questions 4, 8, 9, 17, 25, 35, 39, 48, and 50 are reverse-coded [22,32,54]. The highest score indicates an ideal educational environment [22,32]. The categorization of the sub-scale for all items is as follows: lower than 50 represents a very poor level, range 51–75 is defined as a "plenty of problems" category, range 76–150 represents more positive than negative category, and higher than 150 represents an excellent score [35]. When analysing an individual item, it is necessary to pay attention to those with a mean score lower than 2. There are also possible improvements in the measured assumptions with a mean score between 2 and 3 [55–57].

2.3. Ethics of Research

Before the research, we obtained ethical permission from the institutional ethical commission (No. 038/2020/2176-02/504). The authors of the questionnaire were asked for permission to use and translate it. Individuals who submitted responses to the online questionnaire also agreed to participate in the survey [22,23]. As part of the research, we sent students an invitation to participate in the research by e-mail. The online questionnaire also informed the participants about the purpose and goals of the research. Participants had the opportunity to refuse to participate in the anonymous survey. The survey was conducted from November 2020 until January 2021. We also informed them that we would use the results exclusively for research. In doing so, we will not disclose information from which the individuals involved could be identified. The risks and burdens of research are minimal.

3. Results

Of the 298 invited participants, 174 participants completed the questionnaire (response rate: 58.4%). Of these, 17% ($n = 30$) were men and 83% ($n = 143$) were women (one person did not specify their gender). The average age of the participants was 21.1 years (SD = 3.96). The youngest person was 18 years old, and the oldest was 46 years old. Other basic characteristics of the students involved are shown in Table 1.

Table 1. Sample characteristics.

Gender	N (%)
Men	30 (17.2%)
Female	143 (82.2%)
Missing	1 (0.6%)
Age	**M (SD)**
	21.1 (3.96)
Study program	**N (%)**
Undergraduate 1st degree study programme Nursing Care	167 (96%)
Postgraduate 2nd degree study programme Nursing Care	3 (1.7%)
Postgraduate 3rd degree study programme Nursing Care	2 (1.1%)
Missing	2 (1.1%)
Study year	**N (%)**
1st year	86 (49.4%)
2nd year	59 (33.9%)
3rd year	23 (13.2%)
Senior	5 (2.9%)
Missing	1 (0.6%)

N = sample size; % = percent.

3.1. DREEM Tool Validation Results

The DREEM questionnaire was backtranslated from English into Slovenian by two experts. The content validity and reliability of the DREEM tool questionnaire in the Slovenian environment to assess the perception of the learning space in nursing students are presented below.

3.1.1. Content Validity of the Questionnaire

Table 2 presents the I-CVI, Pc, and k coefficient calculations for all questions in the DREEM tool. I-CVI for all questions in the Slovenian version of the questionnaire is acceptable. The I-CVI for all questions except question 20 was 1.000. The I-CVI for question twenty, "The teaching is well focused," was 0.833. The probability of agreement on all questions is 0.016, and on the twentieth question, 0.094. Kappa on the determination of the agreement on adequacy for all questions is 1. For the twentieth question, it is 0.816.

Table 2. Content validity of the DREEM tool.

No.	Question(s)	N	A	I-CVI	Pc	k	Interpretation
1	I am encouraged to participate in class.	6	6	1.000	0.016	1.000	Appropriate
2	The teachers are knowledgeable.	6	6	1.000	0.016	1.000	Appropriate
3	There is a good support system for students who get stressed.	6	6	1.000	0.016	1.000	Appropriate
4	I am too tired to enjoy this course.	6	6	1.000	0.016	1.000	Appropriate
5	Learning strategies which worked for me before continue to work for me now.	6	6	1.000	0.016	1.000	Appropriate
6	The teachers are patient with patients.	6	6	1.000	0.016	1.000	Appropriate
7	The teaching is often stimulating.	6	6	1.000	0.016	1.000	Appropriate
8	The teachers ridicule the students.	6	6	1.000	0.016	1.000	Appropriate
9	The teachers are authoritarian.	6	6	1.000	0.016	1.000	Appropriate
10	I am confident about my passing this year.	6	6	1.000	0.016	1.000	Appropriate
11	The atmosphere is relaxed during the ward teaching.	6	6	1.000	0.016	1.000	Appropriate
12	This school is well timetabled.	6	6	1.000	0.016	1.000	Appropriate
13	The teaching is student-centred.	6	6	1.000	0.016	1.000	Appropriate
14	I am rarely bored on this course.	6	6	1.000	0.016	1.000	Appropriate
15	I have good friends in this school.	6	6	1.000	0.016	1.000	Appropriate
16	The teaching is sufficiently concerned to develop my competence.	6	6	1.000	0.016	1.000	Appropriate
17	Cheating is a problem in this school.	6	6	1.000	0.016	1.000	Appropriate
18	The teachers have good communications skills with patients.	6	6	1.000	0.016	1.000	Appropriate
19	My social life is good.	6	6	1.000	0.016	1.000	Appropriate
20	The teaching is well focused.	6	5	0.833	0.094	0.816	Appropriate
21	I am feel am being well prepared for my profession.	6	6	1.000	0.016	1.000	Appropriate
22	The teaching is sufficiently concerned to develop my confidence.	6	6	1.000	0.016	1.000	Appropriate
23	The atmosphere is relaxed during lectures.	6	6	1.000	0.016	1.000	Appropriate
24	The teaching time is put to good use.	6	6	1.000	0.016	1.000	Appropriate
25	The teaching over-emphasizes factual learning.	6	6	1.000	0.016	1.000	Appropriate
26	Last year work has been a good preparation for this year's work.	6	6	1.000	0.016	1.000	Appropriate
27	I am able to memorize all I need.	6	6	1.000	0.016	1.000	Appropriate
28	I seldom feel lonely.	6	6	1.000	0.016	1.000	Appropriate
29	The teachers are good at providing feedback to students.	6	6	1.000	0.016	1.000	Appropriate
30	There are opportunities for me to develop interpersonal skills.	6	6	1.000	0.016	1.000	Appropriate
31	I have learned a lot about empathy in my profession.	6	6	1.000	0.016	1.000	Appropriate
32	The teachers provide constructive criticism here.	6	6	1.000	0.016	1.000	Appropriate
33	I feel comfortable in class socially.	6	6	1.000	0.016	1.000	Appropriate
34	The atmosphere is relaxed during seminars/tutorials.	6	6	1.000	0.016	1.000	Appropriate
35	I find the experience disappointing.	6	6	1.000	0.016	1.000	Appropriate
36	I am able to concentrate well.	6	6	1.000	0.016	1.000	Appropriate
37	The teachers give clear examples.	6	6	1.000	0.016	1.000	Appropriate
38	I am clear about the learning objectives of the course.	6	6	1.000	0.016	1.000	Appropriate
39	The teachers get angry in class.	6	6	1.000	0.016	1.000	Appropriate
40	The teachers are well prepared for their class.	6	6	1.000	0.016	1.000	Appropriate

Table 2. Cont.

No.	Question(s)	N	A	I-CVI	Pc	k	Interpretation
41	My problem-solving skills are being well developed here.	6	6	1.000	0.016	1.000	Appropriate
42	The enjoyment outweighs the stress of studying medicine.	6	6	1.000	0.016	1.000	Appropriate
43	The atmosphere motivates me as a learner.	6	6	1.000	0.016	1.000	Appropriate
44	The teaching encourages me to be an active learner.	6	6	1.000	0.016	1.000	Appropriate
45	Much of what I have to learn seems relevant to a career in medicine.	6	6	1.000	0.016	1.000	Appropriate
46	My accommodation is pleasant.	6	6	1.000	0.016	1.000	Appropriate
47	Long-term learning is emphasized over short-term.	6	6	1.000	0.016	1.000	Appropriate
48	The teaching is too teacher-centred.	6	6	1.000	0.016	1.000	Appropriate
49	I feel able to ask the questions I want.	6	6	1.000	0.016	1.000	Appropriate
50	The students irritate the teachers.	6	6	1.000	0.016	1.000	Appropriate

No. = Number of question; N = sample size; A = number of agreements; I-CVI = item content validity index; Pc = probability of chance agreement; k = kappa designating agreement on relevance.

The evaluation of two experts was included in the S-CVI assessment. None of them rated the question with a score of 1 or a score of 2 with a final S-CVI of 1.000 and is acceptable for the Slovenian environment (Table 3).

Table 3. Scale content validity of the DREEM tool.

	Expert Ratter No. 1	Expert Ratter No. 2	Total
Items rated 1 or 2	0	0	0
Items rated 3 or 4	50	50	100
Items rated 3	11	2	13
Items rated 4	39	48	87
S-CVI	50/50 = 1.000		

S-CVI = scale content validity.

3.1.2. Reliability of the Questionnaire

Supplementary Materials presents the correlations between the items in each scale in the DREEM tool questionnaire. Item correlations ranged between −0.038 and 0.620.

Cronbach's alpha was 0.951, which indicates a high level of internal consistency. Table 4 represents the values of Cronbach's alpha with specific items deleted. Removing any question other than question 17, "Cheating is a problem in this school," and question 25, "The teaching over-emphasizes factual learning," would reduce the value of Cronbach's alpha. Corrected item-total correlation for question 17 was 0.186, and 0.192 for question 25.

Table 4. Item-total statistics.

No.	Scale Mean if Item Deleted	Scale Variance if Item Deleted	Corrected Item-Total Correlation	Cronbach's Alpha if Item Deleted
1	127.8932	555.567	0.501	0.950
2	126.6893	555.765	0.507	0.950
3	127.9029	541.912	0.652	0.949
4	127.9223	552.896	0.468	0.951
5	127.0194	560.882	0.384	0.951
6	126.7864	557.052	0.443	0.951
7	127.2039	545.399	0.689	0.949

Table 4. *Cont.*

No.	Scale Mean if Item Deleted	Scale Variance if Item Deleted	Corrected Item-Total Correlation	Cronbach's Alpha if Item Deleted
8	126.5049	552.743	0.571	0.950
9	127.6019	554.673	0.435	0.951
10	126.7087	561.875	0.340	0.951
11	127.1456	550.283	0.557	0.950
12	128.0777	545.072	0.581	0.950
13	127.2136	549.189	0.596	0.950
14	127.5728	553.678	0.478	0.951
15	126.5340	563.898	0.339	0.951
16	126.7961	554.791	0.597	0.950
17	126.9806	567.862	0.186	0.952
18	126.6893	558.785	0.552	0.950
19	126.8738	557.053	0.423	0.951
20	126.9223	553.386	0.688	0.950
21	126.9709	558.715	0.419	0.951
22	127.1262	547.111	0.664	0.949
23	126.8932	553.430	0.683	0.950
24	126.7767	556.352	0.678	0.950
25	128.3204	567.573	0.192	0.952
26	126.8932	562.018	0.364	0.951
27	127.4660	549.800	0.557	0.950
28	127.1553	556.780	0.397	0.951
29	126.8835	550.006	0.668	0.950
30	126.8611	556.060	0.614	0.950
31	126.5631	562.621	0.450	0.951
32	126.9515	556.341	0.570	0.950
33	126.5728	558.208	0.549	0.950
34	126.6699	556.164	0.607	0.950
35	127.0583	545.820	0.715	0.949
36	127.1748	561.714	0.376	0.951
37	126.8932	549.077	0.700	0.949
38	126.9806	553.078	0.510	0.950
39	126.8252	555.655	0.513	0.950
40	126.8058	549.609	0.693	0.949
41	126.9612	548.979	0.780	0.949
42	127.4757	544.075	0.651	0.949
43	127.2718	545.769	0.663	0.949
44	127.2621	546.215	0.682	0.949
45	126.9806	560.706	0.361	0.951
46	126.3786	569.198	0.232	0.951
47	127.0000	544.843	0.672	0.949
48	127.1748	564.479	0.299	0.951
49	126.7184	556.322	0.520	0.950
50	126.7670	561.024	0.385	0.951

Figure 1 presents a graph for screen analysis. The graph shows the eigenvalue scree plot for 50 instrument elements and points at one factor.

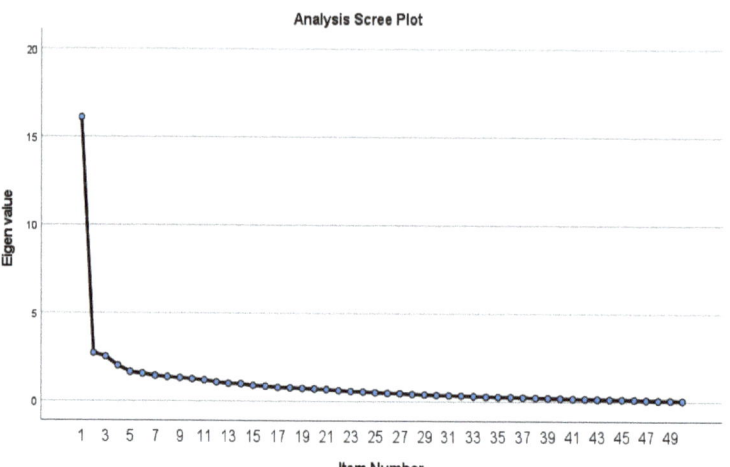

Figure 1. Analysis Scree Plot.

3.2. Results of Perception of the Learning Environment

Online teaching was perceived more positively than negatively. The mean assessment of student perception of learning is 28.1/48, student perception of teachers is 28.9/44, student academic self-perception is 19.8/32, student perception of the atmosphere is 29.1/48, and social self-perception of students is 16.5/28 (Table 5). All individual subscales are statistically related ($p < 0.001$).

Table 5. Mean score of DREEM tool.

Subscale	Items	Total Score	Mean Score (SD)	Maximum Score	Minimum Score	Interpretation
SPL	12	48	28.1 (7.92)	47	3	A more positive approach (25–36)
SPT	11	44	28.9 (7.31)	44	5	Moving in the right direction (23–33)
SAP	8	32	19.8 (5.26)	32	4	Feeling more on the positive side (17–24)
SPA	12	48	29.1 (8.35)	48	3	A more positive atmosphere (25–36)
SSP	7	28	16.5 (3.93)	28	2	Not too bad (15–21)
Total	50	200	122.2 (30.66)	196	20	More positive than negative (101–150)

SPL = Students perception of learning; SPT = Students perception of teachers; SAP = Students academic self-perception; SPA = Students perceptions of atmosphere; SSP = Students social self-perceptions; SD = standard deviation.

Based on the Shapiro–Wilk test for women and the Kolmogorov–Smirnov test for men, we found that the individual values of the scales in students were unevenly distributed according to gender. Based on the Mann–Whitney U test, we identified a statistically significant relationship between the assessment of student perception of learning by gender (U = 1346,500; $p = 0.024$). The mean SPL score for men was 24.9/48 (SD = 8.82). For women, this mean score was 28.9/48 (SD = 7.27). There is no statistically significant difference by gender between the other subscales. Nevertheless, in all subscales, the scores were higher for women than for men: subscale SPT (29.3 vs. 28.1), subscale SAP (20.0 vs. 19.0), subscale SPA (29.4 vs. 28.6), and subscale SSP (16.4 vs. 16.6) (Figure 2).

To show the relationship between age and individual subscales, we performed a Pearson correlation test. The age of students is statistically significantly related to the SAP subscale score ($r = 0.212$; $p = 0.007$) and the SPA subscale score ($r = 9.213$; 0.007).

Based on the Kruskal–Wallis test, we found that the study program attended by students affects the SAP score. The mean grade of SAP students attending the undergraduate first degree study program nursing care is 19.7/32 (SD = 5.05), the score of students attending the postgraduate second degree study program nursing care is 25.67/32 (1.53), and the score of students who attend a postgraduate third degree study program nursing care is 26/32 (SD = 8.49).

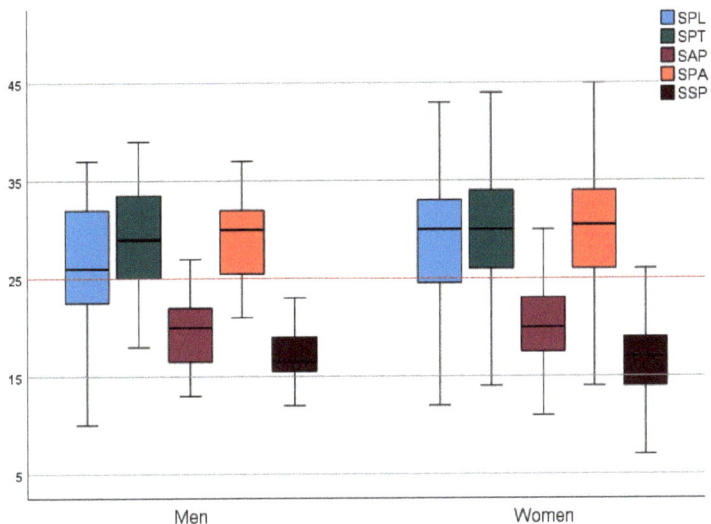

Figure 2. Gender comparison in subscales.

The mean assessment of student perception of learning is 28.1/48, which means a more positive perception. Problematic assumptions with a mean grade of ≤2 in the SPL subscale are "I am encouraged to participate in class," which has an average grade of 1.8 (SD = 0.83), and "The teaching over-emphasizes factual learning," which has a mean grade of 1.3 (SD = 0.68) (Table 6); 69.2% of men (n = 18) and 64% of women (n = 80) agree that teachers being encouraging to participate. Table S1 in Supplementary Materials present the links between SPL items.

Table 6. Subscale SPL.

No.	Question(s)	N	M (SD)
1	I am encouraged to participate in class.	160	1.8 (0.83)
7	The teaching is often stimulating.	160	2.5 (0.88)
13	The teaching is student-centred.	158	2.5 (0.94)
16	The teaching is sufficiently concerned to develop my competence.	160	2.8 (0.78)
20	The teaching is well focused.	159	2.7 (0.70)
22	The teaching is sufficiently concerned to develop my confidence.	150	2.6 (0.89)
24	The teaching time is put to good use.	152	2.9 (0.61)
25	The teaching over-emphasizes factual learning.	151	1.3 (0.68)
38	I am clear about the learning objectives of the course.	150	2.7 (0.86)
44	The teaching encourages me to be an active learner.	147	2.4 (0.91)
47	Long-term learning is emphasized over short-term.	147	2.7 (0.95)
48	The teaching is too teacher-centred.	148	2.5 (0.79)

No. = Number of question; N = sample size; M = mean; SD = standard deviation.

The mean score of student perception of teachers is 28.9/44, which means that it is moving in the right direction. The item "The teachers are authoritarian" received the lowest mean value of 1.9 (SD = 0.98) (Table 7); 39.4% of respondents (n = 62) do not agree with this statement, and 25.5% (n = 48) neither agree nor disagree with this statement. Table S2 in Supplementary Materials present the links between SPT items.

Table 7. Subscale SPT.

No.	Question(s)	N	M (SD)
2	The teachers are knowledgeable.	160	3.1 (0.84)
6	The teachers are patient with patients.	148	2.9 (0.88)
8	The teachers ridicule the students.	159	3.1 (0.83)
9	The teachers are authoritarian.	174	1.9 (0.98)
18	The teachers have good communications skills with patients.	144	3.0 (0.69)
29	The teachers are good at providing feedback to students.	150	2.8 (0.78)
32	The teachers provide constructive criticism here.	143	2.7 (0.72)
37	The teachers give clear examples.	151	2.8 (0.78)
39	The teachers get angry in class.	151	2.8 (0.84)
40	The teachers are well prepared for their class.	151	2.9 (0.79)
50	The students irritate the teachers.	147	2.9 (0.83)

No. = Number of question; N = sample size; M = mean; SD = standard deviation.

The mean score of students' academic self-perception is 19.8/32, representing that feelings are more on the positive side. None of the items in the SAP subscale received a lower mean score than 2 (Table 8). With the highest mean score, the item "I have learned a lot about empathy in my profession" stands out, with a mean score of 3.1 (SD = 0.65). A total of 89.9% of respondents (n = 134) agree that they learned a lot about empathy in the profession during their studies in the current year. Table S3 in Supplementary Materials present the links between SAP items.

Table 8. Subscale SAP.

No.	Question(s)	N	M (SD)
5	Learning strategies which worked for me before continue to work for me now.	157	2.6 (0.81)
10	I am confident about my passing this year.	161	2.9 (0.84)
21	I am feel am being well prepared for my profession.	149	2.7 (0.83)
26	Last year work has been a good preparation for this year's work.	113	2.7 (0.81)
27	I am able to memorize all I need.	152	2.2 (0.95)
31	I have learned a lot about empathy in my profession.	174	3.1 (0.65)
41	My problem-solving skills are being well developed here.	146	2.7 (0.74)
45	Much of what I have to learn seems relevant to a career in medicine.	147	2.7 (0.83)

No. = Number of question; N = sample size; M = mean; SD = standard deviation.

A score of students' perceptions of the atmosphere is 29.1/48, meaning that the atmosphere is more positive than negative. The lowest score was given to the statement "This school is well timetabled" and was 1.5 (SD = 1.10) (Table 9); 51.3% of respondents (n = 81) disagree that the schedule is well planned, 25.9% (n = 41) neither agree nor disagree with the statement. Table S4 in Supplementary Materials present the links between SPA items.

Table 9. Subscale SPA.

No.	Question(s)	N	M (SD)
11	The atmosphere is relaxed during the ward teaching.	144	2.5 (0.95)
12	This school is well timetabled.	159	1.5 (1.10)
17	Cheating is a problem in this school.	160	2.7 (0.87)
23	The atmosphere is relaxed during lectures.	151	2.8 (0.69)
30	There are opportunities for me to develop interpersonal skills.	152	2.7 (0.74)
33	I feel comfortable in class socially.	151	3.0 (0.69)
34	The atmosphere is relaxed during seminars/tutorials.	150	3.0 (0.66)
35	I find the experience disappointing.	151	2.7 (0.86)
36	I am able to concentrate well.	151	2.5 (0.79)
42	The enjoyment outweighs the stress of studying medicine.	147	2.1 (0.98)
43	The atmosphere motivates me as a learner.	147	2.4 (0.96)
49	I feel able to ask the questions I want.	147	3.0 (0.79)

No. = Number of question; N = sample size; M = mean; SD = standard deviation.

The mean score of students' social self-perception is 16.5/28, meaning that social perception is not too bad (Table 10). The item "There is a good support system for students who get stressed" and the item "I am too tired to enjoy this course" get a lower score of 2, more specifically 1.8 (SD = 1.06) and 1.7 (SD = 0.97). 43.1% of the surveyed (n = 69) students are too tired to participate in the lectures. Table S4 in Supplementary Materials present the links between SPL items.

Table 10. Subscale SSP.

No.	Question(s)	N	M (SD)
3	There is a good support system for students who get stressed.	161	1.8 (1.06)
4	I am too tired to enjoy this course.	161	1.7 (0.97)
14	I am rarely bored on this course.	159	2.1 (0.95)
15	I have good friends in this school.	159	3.0 (0.81)
19	My social life is good.	158	2.8 (0.96)
28	I seldom feel lonely.	151	2.5 (0.97)
46	My accommodation is pleasant.	146	3.2 (0.67)

No. = Number of question; N = sample size; M = mean; SD = standard deviation.

Supplementary Materials represents the inter-item correlations of the subscale.

4. Discussion

To the best of the authors 'knowledge, this is the first study to assess students' perceptions of the educational environment in Slovenia. We wanted to obtain information to assess the learning environment of nursing students. Our study was conducted during the COVID-19 pandemic, when colleges were forced to move their education online. Thus, despite the challenges of social distancing, isolation, and quarantine measures [58], they continued to provide education for nurses [59].

The assessment of the learning environment in the nursing student participants of this study is more positive than negative, as in many studies where this tool was used [15,35,54,60–68]. So far, only one study has been conducted that provides researchers with insight into the differences between personal and online teaching. In the United Kingdom, researchers conducted a national cross-sectional study to assess the learning environment during online teaching. They found that the assessment of the learning environment was lower than in live teaching [21].

We wanted to assess if there are differences between individual scales according to gender. In our study, differences were detected only in the assessment of learning perception (SPL), where women had a higher score than men (28.9 for women vs. 24.9 for men, $p = 0.024$). No statistically significant differences were detected in other subscales. The overall score is also higher for women (124.3; SD = 29.04) compared with men (116.1; SD = 32.1). Similar results were also obtained in another study where researchers found higher scores in women than in men [62]. This means that women have a better perception of the educational environment. Studies detect gender differences in study habits, which in turn affect student outcomes [69]. Also, female students are more willing to participate and work in a team than male students [70]. There are also differences in the acceptance of e-learning between men and women [71]. In contrast to our study, however, Fooladi found that perceptions of the learning environment are lower in women among vulnerable groups [72].

There is no statistically significant difference between years of enrolment in our study. The highest DREEM score is detected in the first year of study, where the mean grade is 124.15 (SD = 31.89). Other research finds that perception of the learning environment differs according to student performance, and also a difference between individual years of study [73]. Shrestha, et al., also note that the learning environment assessment is highest among students in the first year of study [74].

Of particular concern is that most students disagree with the claim that the schedule is well planned. Only 20.7% of respondents ($n = 36$) rate schedules as well-planned. This can also be related to the observation that 40.2% of students ($n = 70$) are often too tired to participate in lectures. Students are primarily concerned with time management in distance learning [75,76]. It is important to reduce the academic burden on students and help students develop time management skills, which significantly contributes to their success [77,78]. Stress and overload in nursing students can lead to burnout, anxiety, and depression [79].

Nebhinani, et al. point out that there is a great need to plan and implement various stress management programs [80]. Only 23.5% of respondents ($n = 41$) in our study agree that a good support system is in place in the presence of stress. Like our study, students in eastern Nepal perceived that they do not have a good support system during times of stress [74]. Numerous studies have found increased stress in students due to an outbreak of coronavirus disease [10,81–83], so support in this area is particularly important at this time. Stress connected with distance learning for students mainly leads to a lack of concentration, motivation, and technical difficulties [84].

56.3% of students ($n = 98$) believe that teachers focus too much on teaching based on data memorization, and 36.2% of students ($n = 63$) believe that teachers are too authoritative in their work. Nevertheless, most students ($n = 117$; 67.2%) believe that teaching is sufficiently focused on developing competencies related to their profession.

Health science students will receive such a good education, but its effectiveness must be rigorously and regularly evaluated [85]. Therefore, it is of the utmost importance that such research is continued, and the rate of improvement is assessed. Only in this way can we achieve the best possible learning environment for students.

Limitations

There is a possibility of bias due to low response to the survey questionnaire. The reason for this might be in the fact that questionnaires were sent to the students in an online form, which usually results in low response rates. The study also took place within one faculty and cannot be generalized on a wider scale. Also, the limitation is that the assessment of the educational environment was carried out only during online teaching and cannot be compared with the evaluation of the learning environment during the traditional implementation of the learning process. Another limitation is that the online survey was conducted only from November 2020 to January 2021 and not in other study periods.

5. Conclusions

Nursing students generally rate their learning environment more positively than negatively, but there is still room for improvement in all categories. Greater emphasis is needed on the organization and timing of lessons to achieve better concentration of students in classes and reduce their level of stress. Educational organizations are also recommended to set up a good support system for students. The need to change the approach by teachers and their role was also perceived. With an authoritative approach and too much emphasis on factual learning, we negatively affect the student's motivation and willingness to work. Teachers can improve this through appropriate pedagogical and andragogic education.

It is important that learning organizations and teachers also focus on providing a suitable and appropriate learning environment for students during distance learning. This is the only way they can contribute to positive learning outcomes and gain student experience. However, this presents a unique challenge, as the teacher has no contact with students when teaching online.

In the future, we plan to conduct a longitudinal study to observe the impact and variation of different factors in assessment of the learning environment over time.

Supplementary Materials: The following are available online at https://www.mdpi.com/article/10.3390/healthcare9080998/s1, Inter-item correlations of the subscale.

Author Contributions: Conceptualization, L.G., C.C., E.C., and G.Š.; Data curation, L.G., N.F., C.C., E.C., and G.Š.; Formal analysis, L.G. and G.Š.; Methodology, L.G., N.F., and G.Š.; Supervision, L.G. and G.Š.; Validation, L.G., N.F., and G.Š.; Visualization, L.G. and G.Š.; Writing—original draft, L.G. and G.Š.; Writing—review & editing, L.G., N.F., C.C., E.C., and G.Š. All authors have read and agreed to the published version of the manuscript.

Funding: The project "Digital Toolbox for Innovation in Nursing Education (I-BOX)" has been funded with support from the European Commission (2019-1-ES01-KA203-065836) under the Erasmus+ program. This publication reflects the views only of the authors, and the Commission cannot be held responsible for any use which may be made of the information contained therein. This study was also supported by the "knowledge through creative pathways 2016–2020" scheme cofunded by the European Union from the European Social Fund and the Republic of Slovenia and the Slovenian Research Agency (grant numbers N2-0101 and P2-0057).

Institutional Review Board Statement: The study was conducted according to the guidelines of the Declaration of Helsinki, and approved by the Ethics Committee of Faculty of Health Sciences, University of Maribor (038/2020/2176-02/504, 10.06.2020).

Informed Consent Statement: Participants agreed to participate in the research by completing and submitting a questionnaire.

Data Availability Statement: Data is currently not available for sharing, due to the further data collection process. Contact the first author for more information.

Conflicts of Interest: The authors declare no conflict of interest.

References

1. Pollard, C.A.; Morran, M.P.; Nestor-Kalinoski, A.L. The COVID-19 pandemic: A global health crisis. *Physiol. Genom.* **2020**, *52*, 549–557. [CrossRef] [PubMed]
2. Akande, O.W.; Akande, T.M. COVID-19 pandemic: A global health burden. *Niger. Postgrad. Med. J.* **2020**, *27*, 147. [CrossRef] [PubMed]
3. Alhajjaj, H.A. The effects of the covid-19 pandemic on students in Jordanian schools: A qualitative study. *PalArchs J. Archaeol. Egypt/Egyptol.* **2020**, *17*, 13787–13800.
4. Hiscott, J.; Alexandridi, M.; Muscolini, M.; Tassone, E.; Palermo, E.; Soultsioti, M.; Zevini, A. The global impact of the coronavirus pandemic. *Cytokine Growth Factor Rev.* **2020**, *53*, 1–9. [CrossRef] [PubMed]
5. Velikonja, N.K.; Erjavec, K.; Verdenik, I.; Hussein, M.; Velikonja, V.G. Association between preventive behaviour and anxiety at the start of the COVID-19 pandemic in Slovenia. *Slov. J. Public Health* **2020**, *60*, 17–24. [CrossRef]
6. Zadnik, V.; Mihor, A.; Tomsic, S.; Zagar, T.; Bric, N.; Lokar, K.; Oblak, I. Impact of COVID-19 on cancer diagnosis and management in Slovenia–preliminary results. *Radiol. Oncol.* **2020**, *54*, 329–334. [CrossRef]

7. Rajab, M.H.; Gazal, A.M.; Alkattan, K. Challenges to online medical education during the COVID-19 pandemic. *Cureus* **2020**, *12*, e8966. [CrossRef]
8. OECD Policy Responses to Coronavirus. Strengthening Online Learning When Schools Are Closed: The Role of Families and Teachers in Supporting Students during the COVID-19 Crisis. Available online: http://www.oecd.org/coronavirus/policy-responses/strengthening-online-learning-when-schools-are-closed-the-role-of-families-and-teachers-in-supporting-students-during-the-covid-19-crisis-c4ecba6c/ (accessed on 1 March 2021).
9. Mahdy, M.A.A. The impact of COVID-19 pandemic on the academic performance of veterinary medical students. *Front. Vet. Sci.* **2020**, *7*, 594261. [CrossRef] [PubMed]
10. Son, C.; Hegde, S.; Smith, A.; Wang, X.; Sasangohar, F. Effects of COVID-19 on college students' mental health in the United States: Interview survey study. *J. Med. Internet Res.* **2020**, *22*, e21279. [CrossRef] [PubMed]
11. Shawaqfeh, M.S.; Al Bekairy, A.M.; Al-Azayzih, A.; A Alkatheri, A.; Qandil, A.M.; A Obaidat, A.; Al Harbi, S.; Muflih, S.M. Pharmacy Students Perceptions of Their Distance Online Learning Experience During the COVID-19 Pandemic: A Cross-Sectional Survey Study. *J. Med. Educ. Curric. Dev.* **2020**, *7*, 2382120520963039. [CrossRef]
12. Bozkurt, A.; Sharma, R.C. Emergency remote teaching in a time of global crisis due to CoronaVirus pandemic. *Asian J. Distance Educ.* **2020**, *15*, i–vi.
13. Lawn, S.; Zhi, X.; Morello, A. An integrative review of e-learning in the delivery of self-management support training for health professionals. *BMC Med. Educ.* **2017**, *17*, 1–16. [CrossRef]
14. Dhawan, S. Online learning: A panacea in the time of COVID-19 crisis. *J. Educ. Technol. Syst.* **2020**, *49*, 5–22. [CrossRef]
15. Mukhtar, K.; Javed, K.; Arooj, M.; Sethi, A. Advantages, Limitations and Recommendations for online learning during COVID-19 pandemic era. *Pak. J. Med. Sci.* **2020**, *36*, S27. [CrossRef]
16. Tannenbaum, C.; Van Hoof, K. Effectiveness of online learning on health researcher capacity to appropriately integrate sex, gender, or both in grant proposals. *Biol. Sex Differ.* **2018**, *9*, 1–8. [CrossRef]
17. Gernsbacher, M.A. Why internet-based education? *Front. Psychol.* **2015**, *5*, 1530. [CrossRef] [PubMed]
18. Ellman, M.S.; Schwartz, M.L. Article Commentary: Online Learning Tools as Supplements for Basic and Clinical Science Education. *J. Med. Educ. Curric. Dev.* **2016**, *3*, JMECD–S1893. [CrossRef] [PubMed]
19. Radu, M.C.; Schnakovszky, C.; Herghelegiu, E.; Ciubotariu, V.A.; Cristea, I. The Impact of the COVID-19 Pandemic on the Quality of Educational Process: A Student Survey. *Int. J. Environ. Res. Public Health* **2020**, *17*, 7770. [CrossRef]
20. Regmi, K.; Jones, L. A systematic review of the factors–enablers and barriers–affecting e-learning in health sciences education. *BMC Med. Educ.* **2020**, *20*, 1–18. [CrossRef]
21. Dost, S.; Hossain, A.; Shehab, M.; Abdelwahed, A.; Al-Nusair, L. Perceptions of medical students towards online teaching during the COVID-19 pandemic: A national cross-sectional survey of 2721 UK medical students. *BMJ Open* **2020**, *10*, e042378. [CrossRef]
22. Roff, S. The Dundee Ready Educational Environment Measure (DREEM)—A generic instrument for measuring students' perceptions of undergraduate health professions curricula. *Med. Teach.* **2005**, *27*, 322–325. [CrossRef] [PubMed]
23. Roff, S.; McAleer, S.; Harden, R.M.; Al-Qahtani, M.; Ahmed, A.U.; Deza, H.; Groenen, G.; Primparyon, P. Development and validation of the Dundee ready education environment measure (DREEM). *Med. Teach.* **1997**, *19*, 295–299. [CrossRef]
24. Irfan, F.; Al Faris, E.; Al Maflehi, N.; Karim, S.I.; Ponnamperuma, G.; Saad, H.; Ahmed, A.M. The learning environment of four undergraduate health professional schools: Lessons learned. *Pak. J. Med. Sci.* **2019**, *35*, 598. [CrossRef] [PubMed]
25. Aghamolaei, T.; Shirazi, M.; Dadgaran, I.; Shahsavari, H.; Ghanbarnejad, A. Health students' expectations of the ideal educational environment: A qualitative research. *J. Adv. Med. Educ. Prof.* **2014**, *2*, 151.
26. Ekstedt, M.; Lindblad, M.; Löfmark, A. Nursing students' perception of the clinical learning environment and supervision in relation to two different supervision models—A comparative cross-sectional study. *BMC Nurs.* **2019**, *18*, 1–12. [CrossRef]
27. Flott, E.A.; Linden, L. The clinical learning environment in nursing education: A concept analysis. *J. Adv. Nurs.* **2016**, *72*, 501–513. [CrossRef] [PubMed]
28. Helou, M.A.; Keiser, V.; Feldman, M.; Santen, S.; Cyrus, J.W.; Ryan, M.S. Student well-being and the learning environment. *Clin. Teach.* **2019**, *16*, 362–366. [CrossRef]
29. Polit, D.F.; Beck, C.T. *Nursing Research: Principles and Methods*; Lippincott Williams and Wilkins: Philadelphia, PA, USA, 2004.
30. Polit, D.F.; Beck, C.T. *Nursing Research: Generating and Assessing Evidence for Nursing Practice*; Lippincott Williams and Wilkins: Philadelphia, PA, USA, 2008.
31. Creswell, J.W. *Educational Research: Planning, Conducting, and Evaluating Quantitative and Qualitative Research*; Pearson: London, UK, 2004.
32. Riga, V.; Kossioni, A.; Lyrakos, G. Can DREEM Instrument (Dundee Ready Education Environment Measure) measure the learning environment in a School of Education? *Educ. J. Univ. Patras UNESCO Chair* **2015**, *2*, 59–69.
33. Whittle, S.R.; Whelan, B.; Murdoch-Eaton, D.G. DREEM and beyond; studies of the educational environment as a means for its enhancement. *Educ. Health* **2007**, *20*, 7.
34. Jeyashree, K.; Shewade, H.D.; Kathirvel, S. Development and psychometric testing of an abridged version of Dundee Ready Educational Environment Measure (DREEM). *Environ. Health Prev. Med.* **2018**, *23*, 1–6. [CrossRef]
35. Bhosale, U. Medical students' perception about the educational environment in western Maharashtra in medical college using DREEM scale. *J. Clin. Diagn. Res. JCDR* **2015**, *9*, JC01. [CrossRef]

36. Colina, S.; Marrone, N.; Ingram, M.; Sánchez, D. Translation quality assessment in health research: A functionalist alternative to back-translation. *Eval. Health Prof.* **2017**, *40*, 267–293. [CrossRef]
37. Artino, A.R., Jr.; La Rochelle, J.S.; Dezee, K.J.; Gehlbach, H. Developing questionnaires for educational research: AMEE Guide No. 87. *Med. Teach.* **2014**, *36*, 463–474. [CrossRef] [PubMed]
38. Tsang, S.; Royse, C.F.; Terkawi, A.S. Guidelines for developing, translating, and validating a questionnaire in perioperative and pain medicine. *Saudi J. Anaesth.* **2017**, *11*, S80. [CrossRef]
39. Waltz, C.F.; Strickland, O.L.; Lenz, E.R. (Eds.) *Measurement in Nursing and Health Research*; Springer Publishing Company: New York, NY, USA, 2010.
40. Rubio, D.M.; Berg-Weger, M.; Tebb, S.S.; Lee, E.S.; Rauch, S. Objectifying content validity: Conducting a content validity study in social work research. *Soc. Work Res.* **2003**, *27*, 94–104. [CrossRef]
41. Yusoff, M.S.B. ABC of content validation and content validity index calculation. *Resource* **2019**, *11*, 49–54. [CrossRef]
42. Cilar, L.; Pajnkihar, M.; Štiglic, G. Validation of the Warwick-Edinburgh Mental Well-being Scale among nursing students in Slovenia. *J. Nurs. Manag.* **2020**, *28*, 1335–1346. [CrossRef]
43. Fijačko, N.; Fekonja, Z.; Denny, M.; Sharvin, B.; Pajnkihar, M.; Štiglic, G. Using content validity for the development of objective structured clinical examination checklists in a Slovenian Undergraduate Nursing program. In *Teaching and Learning in Nursing*; IntechOpen: London, UK, 2017.
44. Polit, D.F.; Beck, C.T. The content validity index: Are you sure you know what's being reported? Critique and recommendations. *Res. Nurs. Health* **2006**, *29*, 489–497. [CrossRef] [PubMed]
45. Polit, D.F.; Beck, T.; Owen, S.V. Focus on research methods is the CVI an acceptable indicator of content validity. *Res. Nurs. Health* **2007**, *30*, 459–467. [CrossRef]
46. Boateng, G.O.; Neilands, T.B.; Frongillo, E.A.; Melgar-Quiñonez, H.R.; Young, S.L. Best practices for developing and validating scales for health, social, and behavioral research: A primer. *Front. Public Health* **2018**, *6*, 149. [CrossRef] [PubMed]
47. Bujang, M.A.; Omar, E.D.; Baharum, N.A. A review on sample size determination for Cronbach's alpha test: A simple guide for researchers. *Malays. J. Med. Sci. MJMS* **2018**, *25*, 85. [CrossRef]
48. Balk, E.M.; Gazula, A.; Markozannes, G.; Kimmel, H.J.; Saldanha, I.J.; Resnik, L.J.; Trikalinos, T.A. *Lower Limb Prostheses: Measurement Instruments, Comparison of Component Effects by Subgroups, and Long-Term Outcomes*; Agency for Healthcare Research and Quality: Rockville, MD, USA, 2018.
49. Cohen, R.J.; Swerdlik, M.E.; Phillips, S.M. *Psychological Testing and Assessment: An Introduction to Tests and Measurement*; Mayfield Publishing Co.: California City, CA, USA, 1996.
50. Piedmont, R.L. Encyclopedia of quality of life and well-being research. In *Inter-Item Correlations*; Springer: Berlin/Heidelberg, Germany, 2014; pp. 3303–3304.
51. Piedmont, R.L.; Hyland, M.E. Inter-item correlation frequency distribution analysis: A method for evaluating scale dimensionality. *Educ. Psychol. Meas.* **1993**, *53*, 369–378. [CrossRef]
52. Vrbnjak, D.; Pahor, D.; Nelson, J.W.; Pajnkihar, M. Content validity, face validity and internal consistency of the Slovene version of Caring Factor Survey for care providers, caring for co-workers and caring of managers. *Scand. J. Caring Sci.* **2017**, *31*, 395–404. [CrossRef] [PubMed]
53. Larsson, H.; Tegern, M.; Monnier, A.; Skoglund, J.; Helander, C.; Persson, E.; Malm, C.; Broman, L.; Aasa, U. Content validity index and intra-and inter-rater reliability of a new muscle strength/endurance test battery for Swedish soldiers. *PLoS ONE* **2015**, *10*, e0132185. [CrossRef] [PubMed]
54. Al-Natour, S.H. Medical Students' Perceptions of their Educational Environment at a Saudi University. *Saudi J. Med. Med. Sci.* **2019**, *7*, 163. [CrossRef] [PubMed]
55. McAleer, S.; Roff, S. A practical guide to using the Dundee Ready Education Environment Measure (DREEM). *AMEE Med. Educ. Guide* **2001**, *23*, 29–33.
56. Miles, S.; Swift, L.; Leinster, S.J. The Dundee Ready Education Environment Measure (DREEM): A review of its adoption and use. *Med. Teach.* **2012**, *34*, e620–e634. [CrossRef] [PubMed]
57. Vaughan, B.; Carter, A.; Macfarlane, C.; Morrison, T. The DREEM, part 1: Measurement of the educational environment in an osteopathy teaching program. *BMC Med. Educ.* **2014**, *14*, 1–11. [CrossRef]
58. Dewart, G.; Corcoran, L.; Thirsk, L.; Petrovic, K. Nursing education in a pandemic: Academic challenges in response to COVID-19. *Nurse Educ. Today* **2020**, *92*, 104471. [CrossRef] [PubMed]
59. Morin, K.H. Nursing education after COVID-19: Same or different? *J. Clin. Nurs.* **2020**, *29*, 3117–3119. [CrossRef] [PubMed]
60. Al-Mohaimeed, A. Perceptions of the educational environment of a new medical school, Saudi Arabia. *Int. J. Health Sci.* **2013**, *7*, 150. [CrossRef] [PubMed]
61. Badiee Aval, S.; Morovatdar, N. Perceptions of Students toward the Educational Environment Based on the DREEM Tool in a New Nursing Scholl in Iran. *J. Patient Saf. Qual. Improv.* **2018**, *6*, 1–6.
62. Bakhshialiabad, H.; Bakhshi, G.; Hashemi, Z.; Bakhshi, A.; Abazari, F. Improving students' learning environment by DREEM: An educational experiment in an Iranian medical sciences university (2011–2016). *BMC Med. Educ.* **2019**, *19*, 1–10. [CrossRef] [PubMed]
63. Edgren, G.; Haffling, A.C.; Jakobsson, U.L.F.; Mcaleer, S.; Danielsen, N. Comparing the educational environment (as measured by DREEM) at two different stages of curriculum reform. *Med. Teach.* **2010**, *32*, e233–e238. [CrossRef] [PubMed]

64. Farooq, S.; Rehman, R.; Hussain, M.; Dias, J.M. Comparison of undergraduate educational environment in medical and nursing program using the DREEM tool. *Nurse Educ. Today* **2018**, *69*, 74–80. [CrossRef]
65. Hamid, B.; Faroukh, A.; Mohammadhosein, B. Nursing students' perceptions of their educational environment based on DREEM model in an Iranian university. *Malays. J. Med. Sci. MJMS* **2013**, *20*, 56.
66. Hongkan, W.; Arora, R.; Muenpa, R.; Chamnan, P. Perception of educational environment among medical students in Thailand. *Int. J. Med. Educ.* **2018**, *9*, 18. [CrossRef]
67. Keskinis, C.; Bafitis, V.; Karailidou, P.; Pagonidou, C.; Pantelidis, P.; Rampotas, A.; Sideris, M.; Tsoulfas, G.; Stalkos, D. The use of theatre in medical education in the emergency cases school: An appealing and widely accessible way of learning. *Perspect. Med. Educ.* **2017**, *6*, 199–204. [CrossRef]
68. Ogun, O.A.; Nottidge, T.E.; Roff, S. Students' perceptions of the learning environment in two Nigerian medical schools offering different curricula. *Ghana Med. J.* **2018**, *52*, 116–121. [CrossRef]
69. Alzahrani, S.S.; Soo Park, Y.; Tekian, A. Study habits and academic achievement among medical students: A comparison between male and female subjects. *Med. Teach.* **2018**, *40*, S1–S9. [CrossRef]
70. Wilhelmsson, M.; Ponzer, S.; Dahlgren, L.O.; Timpka, T.; Faresjö, T. Are female students in general and nursing students more ready for teamwork and interprofessional collaboration in healthcare? *BMC Med. Educ.* **2011**, *11*, 1–10. [CrossRef] [PubMed]
71. Ramírez-Correa, P.E.; Arenas-Gaitán, J.; Rondán-Cataluña, F.J. Gender and acceptance of e-learning: A multi-group analysis based on a structural equation model among college students in Chile and Spain. *PLoS ONE* **2015**, *10*, e0140460.
72. Fooladi, M.M. Gender influence on nursing education and practice at Aga Khan university school of nursing in Karachi, Pakistan. *Nurse Educ. Pract.* **2008**, *8*, 231–238. [CrossRef] [PubMed]
73. Ahmed, Y.; Taha, M.H.; Al-Neel, S.; Gaffar, A.M. Students' perception of the learning environment and its relation to their study year and performance in Sudan. *Int. J. Med. Educ.* **2018**, *9*, 145. [CrossRef]
74. Shrestha, E.; Mehta, R.S.; Mandal, G.; Chaudhary, K.; Pradhan, N. Perception of the learning environment among the students in a nursing college in Eastern Nepal. *BMC Med. Educ.* **2019**, *19*, 1–7. [CrossRef] [PubMed]
75. Fidalgo, P.; Thormann, J.; Kulyk, O.; Lencastre, J.A. Students' perceptions on distance education: A multinational study. *Int. J. Educ. Technol. High. Educ.* **2020**, *17*, 1–18. [CrossRef]
76. Parker, E.B.; Howland, L.C. Strategies to manage the time demands of online teaching. *Nurse Educ.* **2006**, *31*, 270–274. [CrossRef]
77. Ghiasvand, A.M.; Naderi, M.; Tafreshi, M.Z.; Ahmadi, F.; Hosseini, M. Relationship between time management skills and anxiety and academic motivation of nursing students in Tehran. *Electron. Physician* **2017**, *9*, 3678. [CrossRef]
78. Quina Galdino, M.J.; Preslis Brando Matos de Almeida, L.; Ferreira Rigonatti da Silva, L.; Cremer, E.; Rolim Scholze, A.; Trevisan Martins, J.; Haddad, F.L.; do Carmo, M. Burnout among nursing students: A mixed method study. *Investig. Educ. Enferm.* **2020**, *38*, e07. [CrossRef] [PubMed]
79. Chaabane, S.; Chaabna, K.; Bhagat, S.; Abraham, A.; Doraiswamy, S.; Mamtani, R.; Cheema, S. Perceived stress, stressors, and coping strategies among nursing students in the Middle East and North Africa: An overview of systematic reviews. *Syst. Rev.* **2021**, *10*, 1–17. [CrossRef]
80. Nebhinani, M.; Kumar, A.; Parihar, A.; Rani, R. Stress and coping strategies among undergraduate nursing students: A descriptive assessment from Western Rajasthan. *Indian J. Community Med. Off. Publ. Indian Assoc. Prev. Soc. Med.* **2020**, *45*, 172. [CrossRef] [PubMed]
81. Aiyer, A.; Surani, S.; Gill, Y.; Ratnani, I.; Sunesara, S. COVID-19 anxiety and stress survey (cass) in high school and college students due to coronavirus disease 2019. *Chest* **2020**, *158*, A314. [CrossRef]
82. Lai, A.Y.K.; Lee, L.; Wang, M.P.; Feng, Y.; Lai, T.T.K.; Ho, L.M.; Lam, V.S.F.; Ip, M.S.M.; Lam, T.H. Mental health impacts of the COVID-19 pandemic on international university students, related stressors, and coping strategies. *Front. Psychiatry* **2020**, *11*, 584240. [CrossRef]
83. Rodríguez-Hidalgo, A.J.; Pantaleón, Y.; Dios, I.; Falla, D. Fear of COVID-19, Stress, and Anxiety in University Undergraduate Students: A Predictive Model for Depression. *Front. Psychol.* **2020**, *11*, 3041. [CrossRef] [PubMed]
84. Lischer, S.; Safi, N.; Dickson, C. Remote learning and students' mental health during the Covid-19 pandemic: A mixed-method enquiry. *Prospects* **2021**, 1–11. [CrossRef]
85. Khalil, R.; Mansour, A.E.; Fadda, W.A.; Almisnid, K.; Aldamegh, M.; Al-Nafeesah, A.; Alkhalifah, A.; Al-Wutayd, O. The sudden transition to synchronized online learning during the COVID-19 pandemic in Saudi Arabia: A qualitative study exploring medical students' perspectives. *BMC Med. Educ.* **2020**, *20*, 1–10. [CrossRef]

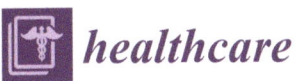

Article

Medical Faculty's and Students' Perceptions toward Pediatric Electronic OSCE during the COVID-19 Pandemic in Saudi Arabia

Lana A. Shaiba [1,2,†], Mahdi A. Alnamnakani [1,3,†], Mohamad-Hani Temsah [1,4,5,*], Nurah Alamro [1,6], Fahad Alsohime [1,4], Abdulkarim Alrabiaah [1,7], Shahad N. Alanazi [1], Khalid Alhasan [1,8], Adi Alherbish [1,8], Khalid F. Mobaireek [1,9], Fahad A. Bashiri [1,10] and Yazed AlRuthia [11]

1. College of Medicine, King Saud University, Riyadh 11362, Saudi Arabia; lshaiba@ksu.edu.sa (L.A.S.); malnamnakani@ksu.edu.sa (M.A.A.); nmalamro@ksu.edu.sa (N.A.); fAlsohime@ksu.edu.sa (F.A.) Alrabiaah@ksu.edu.sa (A.A.); Shahad.n.f.a@gmail.com (S.N.A.); kalhasan@ksu.edu.sa (K.A.); aalherbish@KSU.EDU.SA (A.A.); KHALIDFM1@yahoo.com (K.F.M.); fbashiri@ksu.edu.sa (F.A.B.)
2. Neonatal Intensive Care Unit, Department of Pediatrics, College of Medicine, King Saud University Medical City, King Saud University, Riyadh 11362, Saudi Arabia
3. General Pediatric Unit, Department of Pediatrics, College of Medicine, King Saud University Medical City, King Saud University, Riyadh 11362, Saudi Arabia
4. Pediatric Intensive Care Unit, Pediatric Department, College of Medicine, King Saud University Medical City, King Saud University, Riyadh 11362, Saudi Arabia
5. Undergraduate Committee, Pediatric Department, King Saud University, Riyadh 11362, Saudi Arabia
6. Department of Family and Community Medicine, College of Medicine, King Saud University Medical City, King Saud University, Riyadh 11362, Saudi Arabia
7. Pediatric Infectious Diseases Unit, Pediatric Department, College of Medicine, King Saud University Medical City, King Saud University, Riyadh 11362, Saudi Arabia
8. Pediatric Nephrology Unit, Pediatric Department, King Saud University Medical City, King Saud University, Riyadh 11362, Saudi Arabia
9. Pulmonary Medicine Unit, Pediatric Department, King Saud University Medical City, King Saud University, Riyadh 11362, Saudi Arabia
10. Pediatric Neurology Unit, Pediatric Department, College of Medicine, King Saud University Medical City, King Saud University, Riyadh 11362, Saudi Arabia
11. Department of Clinical Pharmacy, College of Pharmacy, King Saud University, Riyadh 11451, Saudi Arabia; yazeed@ksu.edu.sa
* Correspondence: mtemsah@ksu.edu.sa; Tel.: +966-114-692-132; Fax: +966-114-672-439
† First two authors contributed equally to this work.

Abstract: Background: The educational process in different medical schools has been negatively affected by the COVID-19 pandemic worldwide. As a part of the Saudi government's attempts to contain the spread of the virus, schools' and universities' educational activities and face-to-face lectures have been modified to virtual classrooms. The purpose of this study was to explore the perceptions of the faculty and the students of an electronic objective structured clinical examination (E-OSCE) activity that took place during the COVID-19 pandemic in the oldest medical school in Saudi Arabia. Methods: An e-OSCE style examination was designed for the final-year medical students by the pediatrics department, College of Medicine at King Saud University in Riyadh, Saudi Arabia. The examination was administered by Zoom™ video conferencing where both students and faculty participated through their laptop or desktop computers. In order to explore the students' and the faculty's perceptions about this experience, a newly designed 13-item online questionnaire was administered at the end of the e-OSCE. Results: Out of 136 participants (23 faculty and 112 students), 73 respondents (e.g., 54% response rate) filled out the questionnaire. Most of the respondents (69.8%) were very comfortable with this new virtual experience. Most participants (53.4%) preferred the e-OSCE compared to the classic face-to-face clinical OSCE during the pandemic. Regarding the e-OSCE assessment student tool, 46.6% reported that it is similar to the classic face-to-face OSCE; however, 38.4% felt it was worse. Conclusions: The e-OSCE can be a very effective alternative to the classic face-to-face OSCE due to the current circumstances that still pose a significant risk of infection transmission. Future studies should examine different virtual strategies to ensure effective OSCE delivery from the perspective of both faculty and students.

Citation: Shaiba, L.A.; Alnamnakani, M.A.; Temsah, M.-H.; Alamro, N.; Alsohime, F.; Alrabiaah, A.; Alanazi, S.N.; Alhasan, K.; Alherbish, A.; Mobaireek, K.F.; et al. Medical Faculty's and Students' Perceptions toward Pediatric Electronic OSCE during the COVID-19 Pandemic in Saudi Arabia. *Healthcare* **2021**, *9*, 950. https://doi.org/10.3390/healthcare9080950

Academic Editors: Luís Proença, José João Mendes, João Botelho and Vanessa Machado

Received: 6 June 2021
Accepted: 24 July 2021
Published: 28 July 2021

Publisher's Note: MDPI stays neutral with regard to jurisdictional claims in published maps and institutional affiliations.

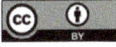

Copyright: © 2021 by the authors. Licensee MDPI, Basel, Switzerland. This article is an open access article distributed under the terms and conditions of the Creative Commons Attribution (CC BY) license (https://creativecommons.org/licenses/by/4.0/).

Keywords: final year medical students; COVID-19; pandemic; distance learning; assessment; educational; pediatric; OSCE

1. Introduction

The educational process throughout the different undergraduate and graduate medical institutes has been immensely disrupted due to the concern of COVID-19 infection transmission as well as the precautionary lockdown and other preventive actions that have been taken to contain the pandemic worldwide [1]. Therefore, many medical schools across the world have adopted and implemented the electronic Objective Structured Clinical Examination (e-OSCE) as a tool to evaluate their medical students with great success [1–4]. In Saudi Arabia, as part of the government's attempts to contain the spread of the virus, the face-to-face activities of all educational institutions were converted to the virtual classroom to promote social distancing. Many studies suggested that 90% of the teachers were motivated to implement social education despite having diverse students with different cultural backgrounds [5,6].

The school of medicine at King Saud University offers a 6-year Bachelor of Medicine and Bachelor of Surgery (MBBS) program where the first year includes basic sciences followed by three years of basic clinical courses (e.g., anatomy, physiology, pharmacology, biochemistry), and the last two years are mainly applied clinical courses (e.g., surgery, internal medicine, otorhinolaryngology, ophthalmology, family medicine, and pediatrics). The pediatrics course consists of two major parts (theoretical and clinical). This course is divided into three parts and is delivered throughout the academic year. However, the course delivery has been disrupted by the COVID-19 pandemic, especially for students in their last two years. Therefore, the different online assessment tools, such as the e-OSCE, have been commonly utilized during this pandemic to ensure the continuity of education for medical students and to assess the quality of the educational outcomes [4]. In this study, our objective was to examine the perceptions of students and faculty on the implementation of e-OSCE during COVID-19 lockdown in King Saud University in Riyadh, Saudi Arabia. The perceptions of the fifth-year medical students as well as their faculty members who participated in assessing their performance in the pediatric e-OSCE delivered through Zoom™ teleconferencing platform (Zoom Video Communication, Inc., San Jose, CA, USA) at King Saud University in Riyadh, Saudi Arabia, were explored using a newly developed online-based questionnaire. Furthermore, the steps taken to prepare and conduct this new virtual experiment in the oldest medical school in Saudi Arabia are described.

2. Methods

2.1. Study Design

This was an online questionnaire-based cross-sectional study that followed a pediatric e-OSCE for the fifth-year medical students to explore the students' and faculty perceptions toward this new experience during this unprecedented pandemic time at King Saud University in Riyadh, Saudi Arabia. The students underwent an intensive overview and teaching of common pediatrics case presentations two months prior to the e-OSCE over a two-week period. Students were divided into small groups for case discussion, and each group was assigned two faculty members to facilitate the case discussion and observe the performance of each group using a standardized assessment scale. The students were given 120 min (2 h) to discuss the cases, and discussions were held on Zoom™ breakout rooms, given the students' familiarity with this application. This e-OSCE was conducted as a part of the clinical evaluation for the last course in the fifth-year of medical school. The clinical cases were carefully chosen and included different parts to assess the history and physical examination skills as well as the skills in interpreting radiological and laboratory results. These cases were predesigned and prepared by the undergraduate committee in the department of pediatrics, but did not include real patients. The students were informed about the exam through an email that was sent by the director of the exam committee and included a clear description of the examination process as well as the date/time of the exam and the registration process.

2.2. Electronic-OSCE Procedures

The following were steps taken to ensure smooth conduct of the examination:
- Zoom™ breakout rooms were created by the examination committee.
- Students arrived 15 min before the start of the exam and were admitted to waiting virtual breakout rooms.
- The students and the examiners were asked to keep their cameras on throughout the exam.
- The students were admitted to their assigned virtual breakout rooms where their examiners were waiting for them there (e.g., two examiners in each breakout room).
- The examiners then presented students with three different clinical scenarios, which included patient history taking, an emergency case, and a chronic pediatric problem.
- The students were then given eight minutes to answer all post-encounter prompts.
- While one of the examiners was observing and grading the students, the other examiner acted as a standardized patient as needed based on the case scenario.
- At the end of the encounter (24 min in total), a five-minute break was given to allow timely admission of the next group of students.
- A 15-min break between each student and the next was taken to complete the checklist and mark the students by each examiner separately for the three stations.
- The case scenarios were changed for each group with a total of 18 scenarios.

There were 18 different grading subcommittees with two pediatric consultants (e.g., examiners) in each, which brought the total number of pediatric consultants to 36. The e-OSCE lasted about 2 h per day and was completed in two days.

The objectives of the OSCE stations were to test the student's ability to take a comprehensive history; including the different unique components in common pediatric cases. The e-OSCE stations were similar in themes and structure to the traditional OSCE that were conducted face-to-face before the COVID-19 crisis.

The general themes of the stations included: taking developmental history and estimating the child's developmental age, the asthma station with questions in acute management and long-term management, the bronchiolitis station. Also included was a febrile seizure station, and the questions included history taking, differential diagnosis, and distinguishing between febrile seizures and other types of seizures. In addition, a station included interpretation of different patterns of the growth chart. A station was targeted at identifying different equipment in pediatrics and the ability to describe the indications, contradictions, and adverse events.

Furthermore, case stations including abdominal pain and abdominal mass, as well as neonatology or critical care station, were also encompassed. Each station's allocated time was 8 min per station. Each student had five stations to go through. Each station of the OSCE had 3–4 questions with 2 min of time allocated to answer each question.

2.3. Faculty's and Students' Perceptions of e-OSCE

In order to evaluate the faculty's and students' perceptions of the pediatric e-OSCE during the COVID-19 pandemic, a-13 item online questionnaire was developed by the undergraduate programs committee at the department of pediatrics. This questionnaire consisted of two parts. The first part consists of four questions about demographic characteristics (e.g., age, gender, title) and previous exposure to a teleconferencing experience (e.g., Zoom™, Microsoft teams, webinars); and the second part consists of nine questions about the likelihood to recommend this experience to other students and faculty members, how comfortable this experience was, personal preference to face-to-face or virtual OSCE, how the virtual OSCE affected the quality of student's assessment, the personal rating of this experience, whether this experience resulted in lower stress and anxiety in comparison to the classic face-to-face experience, and whether it should be incorporated in the future assessment of medical students especially after the end of this pandemic, the different positive aspects of this experience, and the obstacles faced during this experience (Appendix A). The face and content validity of the questionnaire were checked by five faculty members, and the reliability was checked using the Cronbach's alpha method. All students (103 students) and faculty members (36 faculty) who participated in this e-OSCE were invited to participate in this survey directly after the end of the assessment. Those who accepted the invitation were asked to consent to participate before filling out the questionnaire. No personal identifiers were collected, and the study adhered to the ethical principles of the Helsinki declaration.

2.4. Statistical Analysis

The mean and standard deviation were used to describe continuous variables and frequencies and percentages for the categorical variables. The median values were quoted for the bivariate comparisons with the non-parametric comparison methods. The multiple response dichotomy analysis was used to describe the questions measured with multiple option selections. The chi-squared test of association was used to assess the correlations between categorically measured variables. The non-parametric Mann–Whitney U test was used to compare people's perceptions of the e-OSCE across binary categorical variable levels. Alpha significance level was considered at 0.050 level. All statistical analyses were performed using SPSS 21 (IBM Corp., Armonk, NY, USA).

3. Results

Out of 136 participants in the pediatric e-OSCE who were invited to participate in the questionnaire upon the completion of the examination, 73 individuals (23 faculty and 50 students) filled out the questionnaire (54% response rate). The majority of the participants were female (86%) and aged 30 years and younger (68.5%). Almost all participants (98.6%) had previous experience with the Zoom™ videoconferencing platform (Table 1). The questionnaire showed good internal consistency (e.g., Cronbach's alpha = 0.955).

Table 1. The e-OSCE survey participating subjects characteristics ($n = 73$).

Characteristic	Frequency	Percentage
Sex		
Female	63	86.3
Male	10	13.7
Age		
≤30 years	50	68.5
>30 years	23	31.5
Role		
Academic teacher	23	31.5
Medical student	50	68.5
Previously used teleconference methods		
Face time	26	35.6
Zoom	72	98.6
Webinar	40	54.8
Work-related online meetings	26	35.6
Online learning interfaces	35	47.9
Telephonic conference	15	20.5
Other methods/tools	1	1.4

Most of the participants (69.8%) felt very comfortable or extremely comfortable during their participation in the pediatric e-OSCE. Moreover, most participants preferred the e-OSCE over the classic face-to-face OSCE (53.4%) or did not prefer classic face-to-face (15.1%). In addition, most of the participants (74%) reported that the participation in e-OSCE had either reduced their level of stress or anxiety or did not have any effect in comparison to the classic face-to-face OSCE. However, less than 40% of the participants recommended incorporating e-OSCE in the curriculum after the end of the COVID-19 pandemic, and 74% did not recommend the use of remote students' assessment in the future (Table 2). When asked on a 1–10 Likert scale about how likely is it that they would recommend such virtual assessment (e-OSCE) to a colleague, their mean (SD) 7.75 (1.63) indicated that most of them would recommend it.

Table 2. Characteristics of the e-OSCE experience by the faculty and students (n = 73).

Question	Frequency	Percentage (%)
How comfortable did you feel participating in this remote clinical exam (via Zoom or any other similar application)?		
Not at all comfortable	1	1.4
Not so comfortable	7	9.6
Somewhat comfortable	14	19.2
Very comfortable	35	47.9
Extremely comfortable	16	21.9
In regard to your previous experience with "classic face-to-face" clinical OSCE, what is the preferred OSCE style for you during the COVID-19 Pandemic?		
Virtual OSCE (e-OSCE) is preferred	39	53.4
Classic face-to-face is preferred	23	31.5
Both are equally preferred for me	11	15.1
How do you think these remote clinical exams (e-OSCE) affected the quality of the student's assessment?		
Similar assessment to the face-to-face OSCE	34	46.6
Better assessment than face-to-face OSCE	11	15.1
Worse assessment than face-to-face OSCE	28	38.4
Doing remote video assessment during the COVID-19 pandemic decreased my anxiety-mean (SD) 1–5 Likert agreement.		
Strongly disagree	6	8.2
Disagree	13	17.8
Neither agree or disagree	18	24.7
Agree	26	35.6
Strongly agree	10	13.7
Video conferencing as an assessment tool for the pediatric course should be incorporated in next year's courses.		
Strongly disagree	5	6.8
Disagree	20	27.4
Neither agree or disagree	19	26
Agree	24	32.9
Strongly agree	5	6.8
Do you suggest continuing on remote student assessments (via Zoom or similar platforms) after the COVID crisis?		
Yes	19	26
No	54	74

Abbreviations: OSCE: objective structured clinical examination, e-OSCE: electronic objective structured clinical examination.

The participants perceived the following as the top three positive contributors to e-OSCE: clear instructions provided, the organizers' prompt communications, and the free use of the zoom application (Figure 1). Conversely, the slow internet connectivity and the vague instructions, as well as other negative aspects that were not clearly specified, were the most commonly reported negative aspects of the e-OSCE, as shown in Table 3.

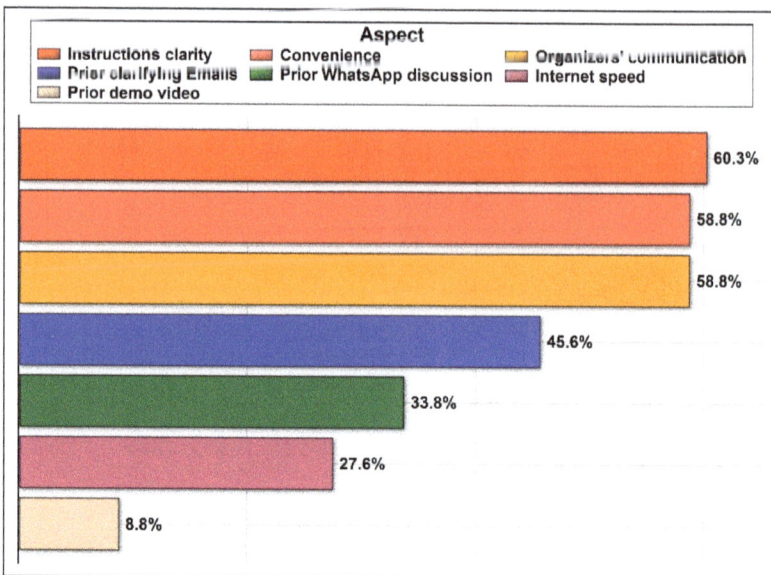

Figure 1. Different aspects of the OSCE experience that were viewed positively by the participants.

Table 3. The e-OSCE teleconference participants perceived "Positive" versus "Negative" aspects about the experience.

Characteristic	Frequency	Percentage (%)
The participants perceived Positive aspects of the Online OSCE experience		
The clear instructions provided	41	60.3
Organizers' prompt communications	40	58.8
The free use of the zoom application	40	58.8
Clarifying emails received from the organizers	31	45.6
The WhatsApp group discussion that related specifically to this event	23	33.8
The fast internet speed	19	27.9
The demo of videoconference before connecting	5	7.4
Other	6	8.8
The participants perceived negative aspects of the Online OSCE experience		
Slow internet speed	30	44.1
Unclear demo video	18	26.4
Unclear instructions	10	14.7
Unfamiliarity with the application	6	8.8
Not receiving clarification emails	2	2.9
Other	23	33.8

To better understand why participants had perceived different quality of e-OSCE assessment, a bivariate analysis was conducted (Table 4). The resulted findings showed that the student's sex did not correlate significantly on their perception of the quality of e-OSCE assessment, but ages older than thirty years perceived the quality of e-OSCE assessment significantly worse ($p = 0.030$). Also, medical students perceived the quality of e-OSCE assessment significantly worse than teachers ($p = 0.030$) according to the chi-squared test of independence. The non-parametric Mann–Whitney U test showed that physicians who perceived worse e-OSCE quality were significantly less willing to recommend this virtual assessment (Median = 6) as compared to those who perceived it as better or similar to the face-face assessment (Median = 8) on average (U = 350.5, df = 73, p = 0.003).

Table 4. Bivariate analysis of participants' e-OSCE quality of assessment.

Variable	How Do You Think These Remote Clinical Exams (e-OSCE) Affected the Quality of the Student's Assessment?		Test Statistic	p-Value
	Similar/Better	Worse		
Sex				
Female	40 (88.9)	23 (82.1)	$\chi^2(1) = 0.22$	0.642
Male	5 (11.1)	5 (17.9)		
Age				
≤30 years	35 (77.8)	15 (53.6)	$\chi^2(1) = 4.70$	0.030
>30 years	10 (22.2)	13 (46.4)		
Role				
Academic teacher/coordinator	10 (22.2)	13 (46.4)	$\chi^2(1) = 4.670$	0.030
Medical student	35 (77.8)	15 (53.6)		
How likely is it that you would recommend virtual assessment (e-OSCE) to a friend or colleague?-median Likert rating	8	6	U(73) = 380.5	0.003
How comfortable did you feel participating in this remote clinical exam (via Zoom or any other similar application)?—median Likert rating	4	3.4	U(73) = 418	0.010
In regard to your previous experience with "classic face-to-face" clinical OSCE, what is the preferred OSCE style for you during the COVID Pandemic?				
virtual OSCE (e-OSCE) is preferred	29 (64.4)	10 (35.7)	$\chi^2(2) = 7.60$	0.022
classic face-to-face is preferred	9 (20)	14 (50)		
Both are equally preferred for me	7 (15.6)	4 (14.3)		
Doing remote video assessment during the COVID-19 pandemic decreased my anxiety-median Likert agreement	4	3	U(73) = 487	0.093
Video conferencing as an assessment tool for the pediatric course should be incorporated in next year's courses-median value	4	2	U(73) = 223.5	<0.001

Another non-parametric Mann–Whitney U test showed that the students who perceived worse e-OSCE quality had perceived significantly lower comfort (Median = 3.4) than those who had perceived the e-OSCE equivalent or better with respect to the quality of assessment compared to the face-face methods (U = 418, df = 73, p = 0.010). Even so, participants who preferred the face-face OSCE assessment were found to be significantly more predictable of perceiving the e-OSCE as being significantly worse than face-face methods (p = 0.022). People's perception of anxiety during the e-OSCE did not correlate significantly with their perceived quality of the virtual assessment (p = 0.093). However, those who perceived the e-OSCE as worse had measured significantly lower willingness to incorporate virtual assessments in future courses (median = 2) compared to people who were satisfied with the quality of the e-OSCE method (median = 4) according to a Mann–Whitney U test ($p < 0.001$).

4. Discussion

The current COVID-19 pandemic has emerged as the greatest threat to global educational and healthcare systems and imposed an enormous challenge. Over the last year, virtual education played a vital role in mitigating the impact of this pandemic on the educational process by providing an interactive communication platform. These platforms, such as Microsoft teams®, Zoom™, Skype®, and Cisco Web™, have been increasingly adopted by all the medical schools across the country to overcome the raised challenges during the COVID-19 pandemic and try to maintain/rescue the educational process through distance learning [7,8]. As the pandemic persisted, another challenge was raised by the end of the academic year of how to safely but reliably assess the performance of the medical students. To ensure the safety of staff and students during this period and maintain physical distancing, the pediatric department implemented an online exam using an interactive communication platform and applied a final online multimodal exam for the fifth-year medical students. This multimodal exam approach used predesigned clinical scenarios that assessed various competencies, including history taking, clinical examination findings, communication skills, laboratory, and diagnostic image interpretation. However, despite adopting this novel approach, it was essential to study the effect of this newly implemented virtual assessment method on both students and faculty. Therefore, we explored the perceptions of the students and faculty toward this newly implemented online multimodal exam, the challenges, limitations, and the overall satisfaction of the participants.

In this study, around 90% of the participants stated that they were familiar and had previous experience with different virtual interactive communication platforms and apps, such as the Zoom™ platform. Over the previous few months, different virtual education platforms had been adopted and implemented by the faculty of medicine and ensured that all students and faculty had unrestricted access to these platforms. This project was adopted by the pediatric department to empower, support, and facilitate distance learning among its staff and students. This went along with the worldwide transition as most academic institutions converted to use online learning platforms as an alternative during this period of pandemic and lockdown to ensure the safety of staff and students [9].

This study demonstrated that a comprehensive multi-format, the high-stakes exam, could be run online uneventfully with an acceptable level of satisfaction by all stakeholders as nearly 84% of participants in the study felt comfortable. Although we expected that students would be anxious about how they would perform in this online exam due to their unfamiliarity with this type of exam, many of them reported that taking the OSCE online reduced their anxiety levels. One possible explanation is that their anxiety toward acquiring COVID-19 during a face-to-face OSCE surpassed their anxiety of being examined online for the first time. This explanation could be supported by the preference of most participants not to continue the remote assessment after the COVID-19 pandemic [10].

However, during an infectious disease outbreak, the literature reported that medical students expressed anxiety during coronavirus disease, with an increased level of social avoidance during the outbreaks [11–13]. Previous reports in an academic teaching hospital setting with MERS-CoV experience showed increased knowledge and adherence to protective hygienic practices, and reduced anxiety towards COVID-19 [14].

Our results showed no gender correlations with the perceptions about the e-OSCE experience. Yet, it is important to consider gender-specific should be evaluated in future vitual OSCE, considering the previously reported differences between female and male students [15]. Also, the older age group who perceived lower quality of e-OSCE in our study suggest that more emphasis on their virtual assessment experience may be warranted in the future. Our medical students also perceived the quality of e-OSCE assessment to be significantly worse than the teachers. Kim et al., found that while students were generally prepared for e-learning, there was a significant improvement in their OSCE performance after e-learning interventions [16]. Still, there were gender differences but no age associations; with their readiness being higher for males than females ($p < 0.05$), without differences across ages ($p = 0.24$) [16].

Although participants were overall satisfied with the e-OSCE, they rated some aspects of this new experience more favorably than others. The highly-rated positive aspects of this experience were clear instructions provided prior to the e-OSCE exam and the presence of a team of coordinators, and their prompt responses. Similar findings were observed by Khalaf et al. [17]. Of note, we observed that the participants preferred communication through emails compared to the WhatsApp® group. However, as there were no previous studies with similar findings; this new finding might be due to the perception among the surveyed participants that emails are still being viewed as a more official way of communication in comparison to WhatsApp® [18]. Moreover, some studies have shown that students who had prior exposure to online education were more satisfied with the e-OSCE than those who had not undergone such an experience before. This is understandable and expected as the former are more adept at using online communication platforms than the latter [17,19].

In this study, participants who perceived worse e-OSCE quality were significantly less willing to recommend this virtual assessment in the future. Therefore, more efforts are needed to improve such virtual assessments and mitigate any negative aspects of the experience, for both the students and faculty. Some participants reported minor technical problems as a negative aspect of e-OSCE, such as a slow-speed internet. Similarly, findings were observed by Pal D et al. with the use of Microsoft® teams as an online learning platform during the current COVID-19 pandemic [20]. However, these problems can be overcome with a high-speed internet, better exam coordination, and IT support to provide the required help and support to students who may encounter any technical issues during the exam, as well as clear instructions and guidance given to them prior to the exam.

Although the pediatric e-OSCE was perceived favorably by most students and faculty, it has several limitations. As the COVID-19 pandemic evolved rapidly, the decision to implement the e-OSCE project was taken urgently. Consequently, the sample size was small from a single institution which limits the generalizability of the findings. Information bias is another limitation that cannot be ruled out as well. In addition, this survey was administered to students and faculty in the pediatrics rotation, and their perceptions may differ from students in other clinical rotations. The survey also used closed-ended questions, which may limit the examination of beliefs and attitudes. Despite these limitations, this is the first study that has explored the perceptions of both the students and faculty members about pediatric e-OSCE in Saudi Arabia. Additionally, the positive and negative aspects of this new experience were revealed from both the medical faculty's and students' perceptions.

5. Conclusions

In this study, a novel way of e-OSCE was implemented to ensure medical education continuity and quality during the COVID-19 crisis. This virtual method of assessment was generally well-perceived by both students and faculty, but older ages were less satisfied with the quality of this virtual assessment. While e-OSCE provides a valuable alternative to the classic face-to-face OSCE during infectious disease outbreaks, more research on improving this virtual assessment tool is warranted. Sharing innovative educational experiences, such as the e-OSCE, in these circumstances is beneficial as the pandemic continues to pose a global threat that could continue to affect medical education and evaluation for a long time. The findings of this study should guide the future direction and decisions toward the optimization of this innovative virtual experiment as well as inform any upcoming studies that are aimed to explore and assess the educational outcomes of different virtual strategies during this unconventional time.

Author Contributions: Conceptualization, L.A.S., M.A.A., M.-H.T., K.A. and K.F.M.; Data curation, L.A.S., F.A., S.N.A. and K.A.; Formal analysis, M.A.A. and N.A.; Methodology, N.A.; Project administration, M.-H.T.; Resources, M.-H.T.; Supervision, A.A. (Abdulkarim Alrabiaah) and K.A.; Validation, Y.A.; Writing—original draft, L.A.S., M.A.A., N.A., F.A., A.A. (Abdulkarim Alrabiaah) and S.N.A.; Writing—review & editing, L.A.S., M.A.A., M.-H.T., A.A. (Adi Alherbish), F.A.B. and Y.A. All authors have read and agreed to the published version of the manuscript.

Funding: This research was funded by the Researchers Supporting Project (grant number RSP-2021/16), King Saud University, Riyadh, Saudi Arabia.

Institutional Review Board Statement: The study was approved by the institutional review board of the College of Medicine at King Saud University, Riyadh, Saudi Arabia (approval number KSUMC/8702998-287).

Informed Consent Statement: Informed consent was acquired from candidates participating in the project.

Data Availability Statement: The data are available upon reasonable request from the corresponding author.

Conflicts of Interest: The authors declare no conflict of interest.

Appendix A

Table A1. Questionnaire on faculty's and students' perceptions of the pediatric e-OSCE.

1. **What is your gender?**

   ☐ Male.

   ☐ Female.

2. **Your title:**

   ☐ Faculty (Dr., Professor).

   ☐ Student.

3. **What is your age?**

   ☐ 18–30 years.

   ☐ 31–40 years.

   ☐ 41–50 years.

   ☐ 51–60 years.

   ☐ 61–70 years.

   ☐ 71 years or older.

4. **How likely is it that you would recommend virtual assessment (e-OSCE) to a friend or colleague?**

   NOT AT ALL LIKELY   EXTREMELY LIKELY

   0   1   2   3   4   5   6   7   8   9   10

Table A1. *Cont.*

5. **Previous teleconferencing experience (please check all that apply).**

   ☐ Facetime.

   ☐ Zoom.

   ☐ Webinars.

   ☐ Work-related online meetings.

   ☐ Online learning.

   ☐ Telephone conferencing.

   ☐ Other (please specify).

6. **How comfortable did you feel participating in this remote clinical exam (via Zoom or any other similar application)?**

   ☐ Extremely comfortable.

   ☐ Very comfortable.

   ☐ Somewhat comfortable.

   ☐ Not so comfortable.

   ☐ Not at all comfortable.

7. **In regards to your previous experience with "classic face-to-face" clinical OSCE, what is the preferred OSCE style for you during the COVID Pandemic?**

   ☐ Virtual OSCE (e-OSCE) is preferred.

   ☐ Classic face-to-face is preferred.

   ☐ Both are equally preferred for me.

8. **How do you think these remote clinical exams (e-OSCE) affected the quality of the student's assessment?**

   ☐ Similar assessment to the face-to-face OSCE.

   ☐ Better assessment than face-to-face OSCE.

   ☐ Worse assessment than face-to-face OSCE.

Table A1. *Cont.*

9. How much do you rate this Zoom clinical assessment experience?

   Worst   Best

10. How much do you agree with the following statements regarding this video interview?

a. Doing remote video assessments during the COVID-19 pandemic decreased my anxiety.

☐ Strongly disagree.

☐ Disagree.

☐ Neither agree nor disagree.

☐ Agree.

☐ Strongly agree.

b. Video conferencing as an assessment tool for the pediatric course should be incorporated in next year's courses.

☐ Strongly disagree.

☐ Disagree.

☐ Neither agree nor disagree.

☐ Agree.

☐ Strongly agree.

11. Do you suggest to continue on remote student's assessment (via Zoom or similar platforms) after the COVID-19 crisis?

☐ Yes.

☐ No.

Table A1. *Cont.*

12. **What are the positive aspects of your e-OSCE experience in our previous Pediatric course? (Please choose all that apply)**

    ☐ Organizers' communication.

    ☐ WhatsApp group discussion that related specifically to this event.

    ☐ Emails from the organizers.

    ☐ Demo of the video conferencing App before the event.

    ☐ Clear instructions.

    ☐ Free application (Zoom).

    ☐ Fast internet speed.

    ☐ Other (please specify):_____

13. **What are the obstacles you faced during your remote clinical exam (via Zoom)? (please choose all that apply)**

    ☐ Not receiving the emails that were sent from the organizers.

    ☐ Not having a Demo of the video conferencing App before the event.

    ☐ The unclear instructions.

    ☐ Application related (for example: unfamiliar with Zoom).

    ☐ Slow or interrupted internet speed.

    ☐ Other (please specify):_____

References

1. Major, S.; Sawan, L.; Vognsen, J.; Jabre, M. COVID-19 pandemic prompts the development of a Web-OSCE using Zoom teleconferencing to resume medical students' clinical skills training at Weill Cornell Medicine-Qatar. *BMJ Simul. Technol. Enhanc. Learn.* **2020**, bmjstel-2020-000629. [CrossRef]
2. Lara, S.; Foster, C.W.; Hawks, M.; Montgomery, M. Remote Assessment of Clinical Skills During COVID-19: A Virtual, High-Stakes, Summative Pediatric Objective Structured Clinical Examination. *Acad. Pediatr.* **2020**, *20*, 760–761. [CrossRef] [PubMed]
3. Pitt, M.B.; Li, S.T.; Klein, M. Novel Educational Responses to COVID-19: What is Here to Stay? *Acad. Pediatr.* **2020**, *20*, 733–734. [CrossRef] [PubMed]
4. Elham, A. Implementing eOSCE During COVID-19 Lockdown. *J. Adv. Pharm. Educ. Res.* **2020**, *10*, 174–180.
5. Alsoufi, A.; Alsuyihili, A.; Msherghi, A.; Elhadi, A.; Atiyah, H.; Ashini, A.; Ashwieb, A.; Ghula, M.; Ben Hasan, H.; Abudabuos, S.; et al. Impact of the COVID-19 pandemic on medical education: Medical students' knowledge, attitudes, and practices regarding electronic learning. *PLoS ONE* **2020**, *15*, e0242589. [CrossRef] [PubMed]
6. Alea, L.A.; Fabrea, M.F.; Roldan, R.D.A.; Farooqi, A.Z. Teachers' Covid-19 awareness, distance learning education experiences and perceptions towards institutional readiness and challenges. *Int. J. Learn. Teach. Educ. Res.* **2020**, *19*, 127–144.
7. Walsh, K. Online assessment in medical education-current trends and future directions. *Malawi Med. J.* **2015**, *27*, 71–72. [CrossRef] [PubMed]

8. Palmer, R.T.; Biagioli, F.E.; Mujcic, J.; Schneider, B.N.; Spires, L.; Dodson, L.G. The feasibility and acceptability of administering a telemedicine objective structured clinical exam as a solution for providing equivalent education to remote and rural learners. *Rural. Remote Health* **2015**, *15*, 3399. [PubMed]
9. School, H.M. Coronavirus Communications. Available online: https://hms.harvard.edu/coronavirus/coronavirus-communications (accessed on 18 October 2020).
10. Stowell, J.R.; Bennett, D. Effects of online testing on student exam performance and test anxiety. *J. Educ. Comput. Res.* **2010**, *42*, 161–171. [CrossRef]
11. Batais, M.A.; Temsah, M.H.; AlGhofili, H.; AlRuwayshid, N.; Alsohime, F.; Almigbal, T.H.; Al-Rabiaah, A.; Al-Eyadhy, A.A.; Mujammami, M.H.; Halwani, R.; et al. The coronavirus disease of 2019 pandemic-associated stress among medical students in middle east respiratory syndrome-CoV endemic area: An observational study. *Med. (Baltim.)* **2021**, *100*, e23690. [CrossRef] [PubMed]
12. Al-Rabiaah, A.; Temsah, M.H.; Al-Eyadhy, A.A.; Hasan, G.M.; Al-Zamil, F.; Al-Subaie, S.; Alsohime, F.; Jamal, A.; Alhaboob, A.; Al-Saadi, B.; et al. Middle East Respiratory Syndrome-Corona Virus (MERS-CoV) associated stress among medical students at a university teaching hospital in Saudi Arabia. *J. Infect. Public Health* **2020**. [CrossRef] [PubMed]
13. Saddik, B.; Hussein, A.; Sharif-Askari, F.S.; Kheder, W.; Temsah, M.H.; Koutaich, R.A.; Haddad, E.S.; Al-Roub, N.M.; Marhoon, F.A.; Hamid, Q.; et al. Increased Levels of Anxiety Among Medical and Non-Medical University Students During the COVID-19 Pandemic in the United Arab Emirates. *Risk Manag. Healthc Policy* **2020**, *13*, 2395–2406. [CrossRef] [PubMed]
14. Temsah, M.H.; Alhuzaimi, A.N.; Alrabiaah, A.; Al-Sohime, F.; Alhasan, K.; Kari, J.A.; Almaghlouth, I.; Aljamaan, F.; Al-Eyadhy, A.; et al. Knowledge, attitudes and practices of healthcare workers during the early COVID-19 pandemic in a main, academic tertiary care centre in Saudi Arabia. *Epidemiol. Infect.* **2020**, *148*, e203. [CrossRef] [PubMed]
15. Graf, J.; Smolka, R.; Simoes, E.; Zipfel, S.; Junne, F.; Holderried, F.; Wosnik, A.; Doherty, A.M.; Menzel, K.; Herrmann-Werner, A. Communication skills of medical students during the OSCE: Gender-specific differences in a longitudinal trend study. *BMC Med. Educ.* **2017**, *17*, 75. [CrossRef] [PubMed]
16. Kim, K.-J.; Lee, Y.J.; Lee, M.J.; Kim, Y.H. E-Learning for Enhancement of Medical Student Performance at the Objective Structured Clinical Examination (OSCE) in the COVID-19 Era. 2020. Available online: https://assets.researchsquare.com/files/rs-126355/v1/6f83ee43-4189-432e-a706-48b6a3bf9376.pdf?c=1609139666 (accessed on 18 October 2020).
17. Khalaf, K.; El-Kishawi, M.; Moufti, M.A.; Al Kawas, S. Introducing a comprehensive high-stake online exam to final-year dental students during the COVID-19 pandemic and evaluation of its effectiveness. *Med. Educ. Online* **2020**, *25*, 1826861. [CrossRef] [PubMed]
18. Elledge, R.; Williams, R.; Fowell, C.; Green, J. Maxillofacial education in the time of COVID-19: The West Midlands experience. *Br. J. Oral Maxillofac. Surg.* **2020**. [CrossRef] [PubMed]
19. Petrisor, M.; Marusteri, M.; Simpalean, D.; Carasca, E.; Ghiga, D. Medical students' acceptance of online assessment systems. *Acta Med. Marisiensis* **2016**, *62*, 30–32. [CrossRef]
20. Pal, D.; Vanijja, V. Perceived usability evaluation of Microsoft Teams as an online learning platform during COVID-19 using system usability scale and technology acceptance model in India. *Child. Youth Serv. Rev.* **2020**, *119*, 105535. [CrossRef] [PubMed]

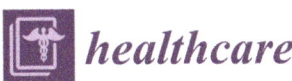

Article

Lapnurse—A Blended Learning Course for Nursing Education in Minimally Invasive Surgery: Design and Experts' Preliminary Validation of Its Online Theoretical Module

Juan Francisco Ortega-Morán [1,*], Blas Pagador [1], Juan Maestre-Antequera [1], Javier Sánchez-Fernández [1], Antonio Arco [2], Francisco Monteiro [2] and Francisco M. Sánchez-Margallo [1]

[1] Jesús Usón Minimally Invasive Surgery Centre, Ctra. N-521, Km. 41.8, 10071 Cáceres, Spain; jbpagador@ccmijesususon.com (B.P.); jmaestre@ccmijesususon.com (J.M.-A.); jsanchez@ccmijesususon.com (J.S.-F.); msanchez@ccmijesususon.com (F.M.S.-M.)

[2] Polytechnic Institute of Portalegre, Praça do Município, 11, 7300-110 Portalegre, Portugal; a.arco@ipportalegre.pt (A.A.); franciscomonteiro@ipportalegre.pt (F.M.)

* Correspondence: jfortega@ccmijesususon.com; Tel.: +34-927181032

Abstract: Background: The implantation of Minimally Invasive Surgery (MIS) leads to the specialization of nurses in this surgical field. However, there is no standard curriculum of MIS Nursing in Europe. Spanish and Portuguese nurses are inexperienced and have poor training in MIS. For that, a blended learning course for nursing education in MIS (Lapnurse) has been developed. This work aims to detail the course design and to preliminary validate by experts its online theoretical module. Methods: Lapnurse consists of an online module with nine theoretical lessons and a face-to-face module with three practical lessons. The e-learning environment created to provide the online module, with didactic contents based on surgical videos and innovative 3D designs, has been validated by two technicians (functionality) and four nurses with teaching experience in MIS (usability and content). Results: The E-learning platform meets all technical requirements, provides whole and updated multimedia contents correctly applied for educational purposes, incorporates interactivity with 3D designs, and has an attractive, easy-to-use and intuitive design. Conclusions: The lack of knowledge in MIS of Spanish and Portuguese nurses could be addressed by the blended learning course created, Lapnurse, where the e-learning environment that provides theoretical training has obtained a positive validation.

Keywords: blended learning; design; education; e-learning; laparoscopy; minimally invasive surgery; nursing; training course; validation

1. Introduction

Health professionals' mobility between countries has been a common practice for many years. As an example of this, the migration of nurses between Spain and Portugal is easier because of their geographical contiguity and cultural affinity, and it has always existed in both directions [1]. That cross-border migration of nurses is enriching for both destination and origin countries, as long as these health professionals are adequately trained to practice in the destination country. Minimally Invasive Surgery (MIS) techniques have been implanted in recent years as a routine surgical practice, making it necessary to meet the training needs of professionals in this surgical field [2], including nurses. However, as far as we know, there is no standard curriculum of MIS Nursing in Europe. Thus, appropriate means should be available for nurses to acquire the knowledge that allows them to develop new attitudes and skills in the workplace [3], as required in MIS.

E-learning may be a good tool to improve the quality of education [4], allowing students flexibility in time, place, and access to content. Furthermore, it improves their learning ability by allowing them to progress at the most appropriate speed [5]. However, those education programs carried out entirely online can raise inequalities for users with computer illiteracy [6]. Moreover, e-learning has a series of interrelation drawbacks between teachers and students, such as the inability of students to receive immediate feedback from the teacher [5]. For that, blended learning, which combines both online and face-to-face learning, is a method that allows overcoming these barriers of e-learning, combining the flexibility of timing and the convenience of online delivery with the spontaneity and interpersonal interaction of face-to-face learning [7].

Although the benefits of e-learning and blended learning have been demonstrated in several studies, not enough is known about what nurses think about continuing education through e-learning [8,9] or blended learning [10]. For that, a study has been performed to firstly identify and compare training needs and level of experience in MIS of Spanish and Portuguese nurses, in order to check if they are qualified to work in this field, and to also check whether e-learning technologies would be useful for a successful MIS training. A total of 81 nurses from Extremadura (Spain) and 113 nurses from Alentejo (Portugal) participated by filling in a questionnaire that showed a lack of experience and training of nurses in MIS. In order to meet their training needs, they consider essential the implementation of e-learning environments that offer courses with useful contents for their work and a focus on clinical practice, to incorporate interactivity into these environments, and to use surgical videos in online training processes. Such study indicated that nurses are technologically competent to be trained by e-learning, and the blended learning is their preferred method to learn MIS.

Therefore, we have designed and developed a laparoscopic training course for nursing, named Lapnurse, through blended learning method with interactive didactic contents. The main objectives of this study were to:

- Detail how the course has been designed and developed based on the training needs demanded by nurses; and
- Preliminary assess by experts in a pilot study the functionality, content, and usability of the e-learning environment that provides the theoretical module of Lapnurse.

2. Materials and Methods

2.1. Course Design

Blended learning method, as preferred by nurses, has been selected to implement the Lapnurse course. This course consists of (1) a theoretical module with nine lessons, to be taught through an e-learning web environment, and (2) a practical module with three lessons, to be carried out in person in a specialized reference centre (Figure 1).

The contents of the course have been designed based on the role of nurses in MIS. The tasks of circulating nurses are mainly focused on maintaining a safe and comfortable environment in the surgical room during the surgery. They do not participate in intervention and work outside of the sterile field, and have been responsible for the inspection of surgical equipment and instruments, and also the preparation of the documentation related to the surgery and the patient. However, the scrub nurses are directly involved in the surgical intervention working within the sterile field. They prepare the operating room for the patient and the instruments. They assist the surgical team by donning sterile masks, gloves, and gowns, as well as by passing the instruments during surgery. For this, surgical nurses need to acquire the necessary knowledge about instruments, equipment, and techniques related to laparoscopic interventions in order to perform their work in a safe way. Different sections of the developed course have been designed to meet all these training needs in MIS.

As the e-learning environment used to provide the theoretical module of Lapnurse, the Moodle web application [11] has been selected (Figure 2). This free distribution course management system is very useful in the educational field, since it allows for incremental performance and satisfaction when compared to traditional didactic lectures [12].

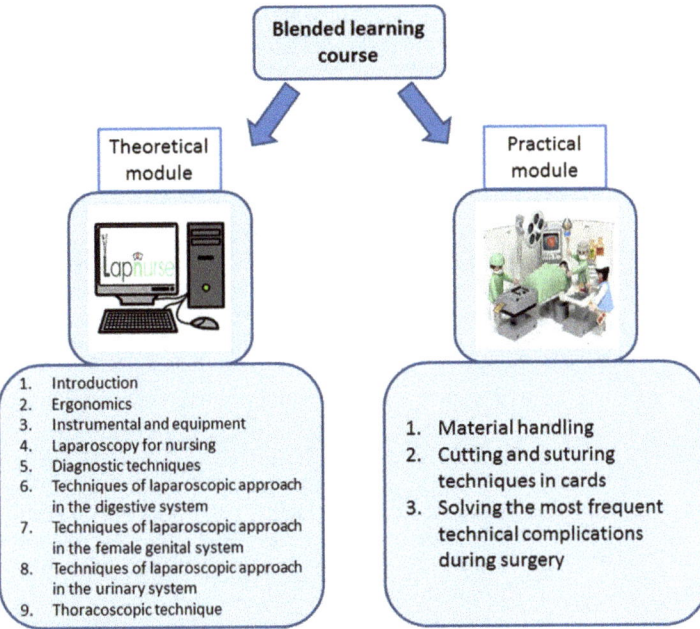

Figure 1. Blended learning course.

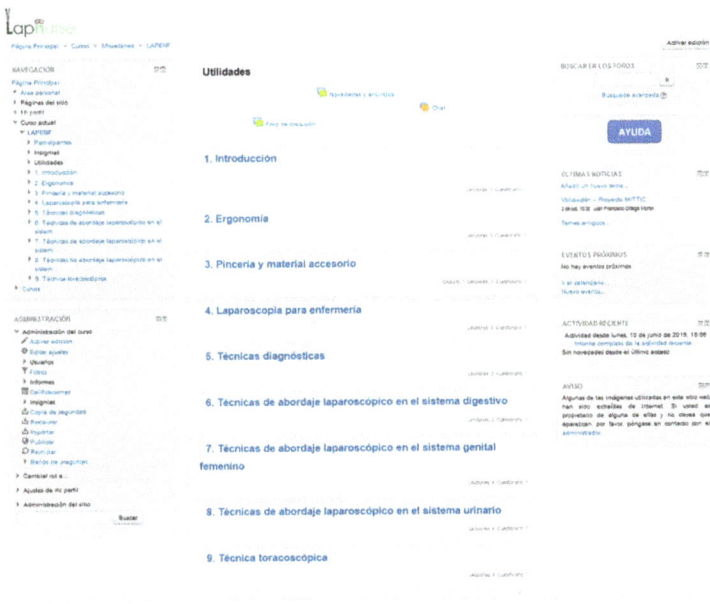

Figure 2. The Spanish version of the e-learning environment used to provide the theoretical module of Lapnurse.

Lessons consist of sequential pages providing all resources of the course (text, images, videos, and 3D designs), in Spanish and Portuguese languages. On the left side of the environment, the menu of each lesson is displayed, so that the user can view the tabs that the lesson contains and can navigate through them. At the end of each lesson, a questionnaire evaluates the knowledge acquired by the students through multiple choice and true/false questions, with two attempts to answer them within a limited time. Each attempt is automatically scored and the results are saved in the gradebook, although they are displayed to the user, with feedback comments and correct answers.

To encourage collaborative learning, synchronous and asynchronous means for communication between users have been included (chat and two forums, respectively). The chat allows participants to have a discussion in text format in a synchronous way in real time. Chats are especially useful when a group does not have the possibility to meet physically to talk face-to-face. The forum allows participants to have asynchronous discussions that take place over an extended period of time. The automatically created forum "News and announcement" indicates what is happening in the course, and it is only posted by teachers and an administrator. Additionally, the "Discussion forum" has been created, in which all users can add or reply to posts.

The main roles interacting with the system are the following:

- Student: They will be the main receiver of didactic contents in an active knowledge search. For aspects of formal and non-formal learning, the student acts as a consumer of content, e.g., accessing didactic content and courses, but without permission to create new content or edit existing ones. For aspects of informal learning, the student is considered an active participant within the professional network of the environment. They will participate in forums and discussions, and will interact with other users in the community.
- Teacher: A MIS surgeon with broad experience in teaching. As such, the main role of the teacher will be as a content provider for formal learning, creating and editing didactic contents, and loading them into the environment. For informal learning, they will be considered an active participant within the professional network of the environment. They will be able to upload multimedia content, participate as a tutor solving doubts in forums and debates, and interact with other users in the community.
- Administrator: The administrator will normally be an expert in computer systems, responsible for all management and technical aspects of the environment. Among their tasks are user management, system monitoring, and technical assistance.

2.2. Didactic Surgical Videos

Surgical videos are the basis of the didactic contents offered by Lapnurse, since they are very important and useful for nurses in online training processes and have increasingly been used for continuing medical education in e-learning technologies [13,14].

These are endoscopic videos corresponding to digestive, gynaecological, thoracic, and urologic surgical interventions. Video sections of interest to users have been selected from raw videos, avoiding long duration because the time away from work is the main drawback of health professionals who want training [15] and short contents are ideal for them [16]. A wide sample of up-to-date videos of each surgical specialty has been included to provide innovative information on advances in applied technology in line with the current surgical trend.

2.3. Interactive 3D Designs

New interactive 3D designs of laparoscopic instrumental and equipment have been developed to incorporate the interactivity demanded by nurses. They are PDF files with the 3D model (Figure 3), which allow the user to perform some interactive actions over the objects, such as rotate and move the model, zoom in or out, generate defined views, add comments, make 3D measurements, make section views, and select visualization of each component of the design, among others.

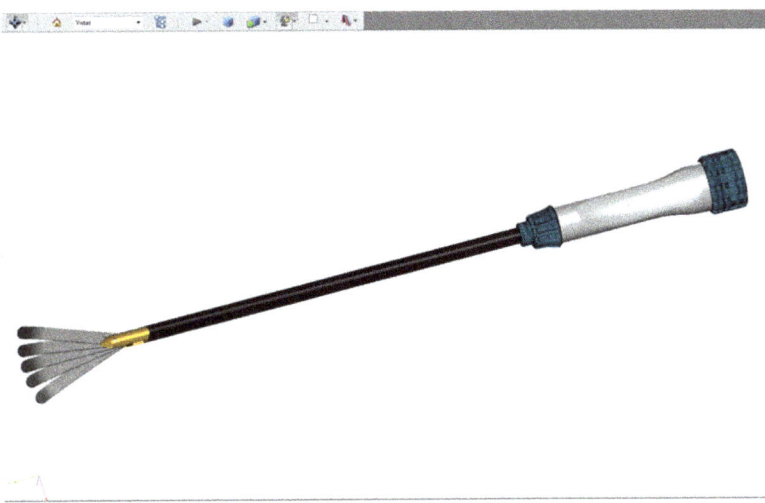

Figure 3. Interactive 3D design.

All interactive 3D designs have been included in a Glossary within lesson 3. When any term of the glossary appears in the text of the course, that word is highlighted so that users can click it to visualize and interact with interactive 3D designs without having to visit the glossary.

2.4. Preliminary Validation by Experts of the Online Theoretical Module

A pilot study for a preliminary validation by experts of the online theoretical module of Lapnurse has been performed according to the scheme shown in Figure 4.

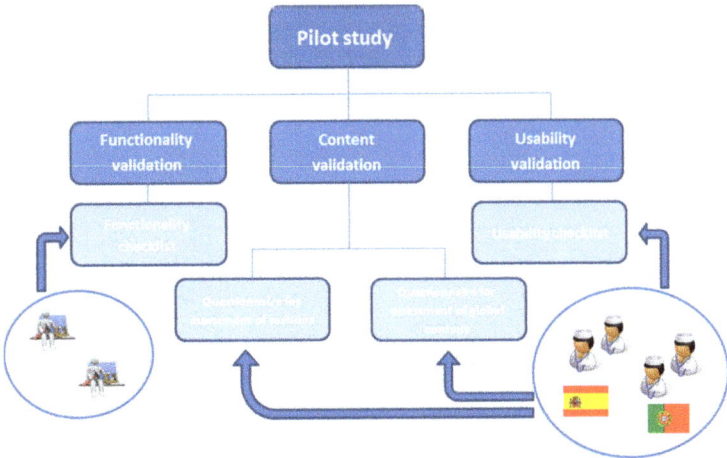

Figure 4. Scheme of the validation methodology.

Functionality, contents, and usability tests have been performed in order to get an e-learning platform of high quality [17]. Functionality validation checks the correct functioning of the system, as well as compliance with the functional requirements, through a checklist (see Appendix A). Content validation evaluates the suitability of the lessons and contents offered to meet the learning requirements. For that, a five-point Likert scale survey (1—completely disagree, to 5—completely agree) has been used to subjectively evaluate the specific content of each lesson and the global content of the course (see Appendix B). The minimum threshold for considering a validation as positive has been set to 3.5 out of 5 points in the Likert scale, according to 70% of agreement [18]. A "yes/no" checklist with a list of requirements regarding the usability of the e-learning platform has been used to assess the design and layout of the web environment (see Appendix C).

Two technicians with extensive experience in the development of distance training tools (functionality validation) and four nurses (two from Spain and two from Portugal) with teaching experience and advanced knowledge in MIS (content and usability validation) carried out such tests. Participants had no relationship with the course or its creators, and the non-probability convenience sampling technique has been used to conduct sampling of participants once the course was developed, where emails were sent to contacts whose data are stored in databases of partners involved in the study. Four to five participants are enough for detecting usability problems in a preliminary validation of a web environment [19], and a questionnaire is the most usual method [20–22]. Results were not statistically analysed looking for significant differences between Spanish and Portuguese participants because it is not appropriate in groups of two users each. The analysis of the data was carried out using mean values, standard deviations, and percentages with the software SPSS 15.0 for Windows (IBM, Armonk, NY, USA).

3. Results

The two technical evaluators verified that the e-learning platform meets all technical requirements related to access management, user profile and interactions, environment maintenance, and formal and informal learning.

Averaged results from the validation of specific contents of each lesson are shown in Tables 1 and 2, and of the global contents in Figure 5. In both cases, all issues far exceed the validation threshold, most of them reaching almost the highest score.

Table 1. Results from the validation of specific contents of lessons 1–5 (Mean values ± Standard deviation).

Question	Lesson 1	Lesson 2	Lesson 3	Lesson 4	Lesson 5
	Mean ± SD	Mean ± SD	Mean ± SD	Mean ± SD	Mean ± SD
Q1	4.75 ± 0.50	4.75 ± 0.50	5.00 ± 0.00	5.00 ± 0.00	5.00 ± 0.00
Q2	5.00 ± 0.00	5.00 ± 0.00	5.00 ± 0.00	4.75 ± 0.50	4.75 ± 0.50
Q3	5.00 ± 0.00	4.75 ± 0.50	4.50 ± 0.58	5.00 ± 0.00	4.50 ± 0.58
Q4	4.75 ± 0.50	5.00 ± 0.00	5.00 ± 0.00	5.00 ± 0.00	5.00 ± 0.00
Q5	4.25 ± 0.50	4.75 ± 0.50	4.00 ± 1.41	4.75 ± 0.50	4.75 ± 0.50

Table 2. Results from the validation of specific contents of lessons 6–9 (Mean values ± Standard deviation).

Question	Lesson 6	Lesson 7	Lesson 8	Lesson 9
	Mean ± SD	Mean ± SD	Mean ± SD	Mean ± SD
Q1	4.75 ± 0.50	5.00 ± 0.00	5.00 ± 0.00	5.00 ± 0.00
Q2	4.75 ± 0.50	4.75 ± 0.50	4.50 ± 0.58	5.00 ± 0.00
Q3	4.25 ± 0.50	5.00 ± 0.00	5.00 ± 0.00	4.75 ± 0.50
Q4	5.00 ± 0.00	5.00 ± 0.00	5.00 ± 0.00	5.00 ± 0.00
Q5	4.75 ± 0.50	4.75 ± 0.50	4.75 ± 0.50	4.75 ± 0.50

Lessons most important for experts are instrumental and equipment, ergonomics, and laparoscopy for nursing, and the least interesting are those related to diagnostic and approach techniques. Resources most important are lessons and didactic contents, while the least interesting are the means of communications between users (chat and forum).

Subjective usability results related to the design of the e-learning environment show a positive answer from all experts to all questions, as shown in Figure 6.

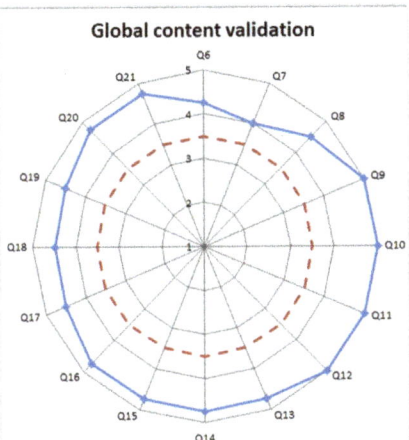

Figure 5. The blue continuous line represents the results of the validation of the global content of the course (1—Completely disagree, to 5—completely agree). The red dashed line indicates the minimum threshold necessary for positive validation.

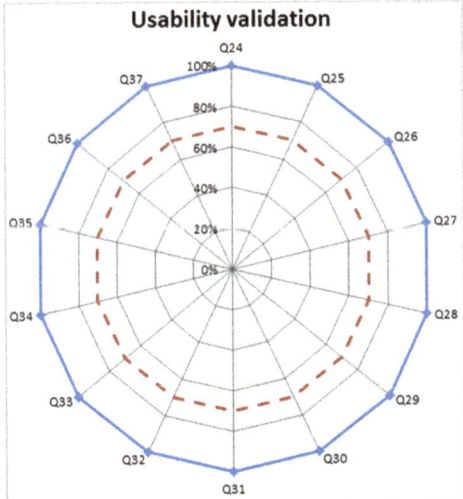

Figure 6. The blue continuous line represents the results of usability validation (% surgeons agree). The red dashed line indicates the minimum threshold necessary for positive validation.

4. Discussion

The traditional used method for MIS training consisting of the attendance of nurses to in-person courses requires incorporating the technological multimedia innovation according to the growth and evolution of this emerging surgical technique. For that, the laparoscopic training course for nursing Lapnurse through the blended learning method has been developed, with a face-to-face practical module and an online theoretical module. Findings obtained in this study regarding the successful design and preliminary validation by experts of the online module of the course suggest that Lapnurse could contribute to meet the training needs in MIS of Spanish and Portuguese nurses. In this way, they could be better able to work in the MIS field in their country or in another. Since the 1990s, changes in education policy, international relations, and the labor market facilitated the migration of nurses to work in other European countries. The recognition of qualifications under the OECD has facilitated such mobility of health workers [23]. In 2016, 145,487 nurses lived in a member state other than their country of citizenship [24]. Despite this high mobility rate, as far as we know, a standard curriculum of MIS nursing in Europe is still missing. Therefore, a new EU framework for nurses in MIS techniques should be developed. The content of courses such as Lapnurse should be applicable to European regulations so that such nurses trained in MIS could increase their employability in Europe and also contribute to the implantation of MIS at the European level.

Most studies about the validation of e-learning platforms are oriented to be performed by end users [17,25], but only few studies have been focused on instructors' satisfaction [26,27]. The instructor's point of view is often omitted but is also important [28], since the instructor is one of the main players of the learning process [29]. For that, in our work the validation tests have been performed by nurses with teaching experience in MIS.

One rather neglected issue in the validation tests is the reliability assessment of the e-learning environment. Due to its flexibility and ease of use, Moodle has been selected as the e-learning platform to provide the theoretical module of Lapnurse. It offers sufficient guarantees because it has been validated in several fields [30–33]. In this sense, system quality of an e-learning environment, in terms of navigability, accessibility, and stability [34,35], is critical for a good user experience of e-learning [36] and has a positive impact on use and satisfaction [37]. Therefore, we have successfully performed a functionality evaluation from a technical point of view, which takes into account the possible interaction between user, content, and technology.

The positive validation of contents highlights that they are whole and complete, updated, and correctly applied for educational purposes. This agrees with Back [38], who indicates that medical e-learning environments should be designed with availability of all relevant contents, always up-to-date, and with relevance for practical clinical work. Participants value contents as unique and innovative, but without reaching a score as high as the other questions. This feature should be improved in future editions of the course because one of the key webpage factors to obtain good SERP (Search Engine Ranking Positions) rating score from a search engine is the quality of contents, in the sense of being original and unique [39].

Some e-learning scenarios only provide unidirectional information for online use or downloads [38]. However, the learning outcomes and the engagement of users in their learning process can be favorably influenced by integrating interactivity [40], thus avoiding user dropouts in the e-learning environment. In Lapnurse, interactivity has been included through 3D designs of the glossary, which have been valued by participants as useful and complete, with interactive, realistic, and good quality 3D objects. The innovative 3D tools offered by this course provide originality and suppose a novelty compared with other e-learning scenarios. They would allow nurses to better know the instruments and equipment they have to manage during surgical interventions, since they could interact with them and not only see them in a simple picture or video as before in other online platforms.

Surgical videos and multimedia contents are important resources for the experts, agreeing thus with Bloomfield and Jones [41], which promotes video clips with clinical demonstrations as the most useful feature of e-learning due to being visual aids that can help students develop mental representations in their learning process. However, the incorporation of interactive components in surgical videos would be welcome, since interactive videos are being increasingly applied to skills-based training to overtake traditional passive watching of video-based training material [42].

User engagement with the e-learning platform can be achieved with usability features such as user-friendliness and ease of use [43]. Positive results from our usability validation show that the developed e-learning environment is attractive, organized, easy to use, and has a consistent design and layout with intuitive navigation. Despite this, ease of use has no influence on instructor satisfaction, but perceived usefulness and services quality on using the e-learning environment [29]. Participants have indicated that contents have good quality, provide added value and useful information, and are correctly applied for educational purposes. Moreover, they consider that the e-learning platform includes useful tools for users, such as the glossary of 3D designs, chat, and forums.

The Lapnurse course could be used as a basis for creating similar courses for training other surgical staff involved in laparoscopic interventions, such as surgeons or anesthetists. There are contents and sections related to laparoscopy in general that are common to any staff, such as ergonomics, instruments and equipment (including the glossary of interactive 3D designs), and diagnostic and approach techniques. It would only be necessary to adapt to the target staff some specific sections, such as laparoscopy for nursing. Moreover, this course could be generalized to other surgical disciplines for which the surgical staff need training, such as endoscopy, microsurgery, cardiovascular, etc. For that, taking into account the successful validation of usability and functionality of the e-learning platform, the structure and layout could be the same, and only the content of the course should be adapted to the surgical discipline. However, nowadays mobile internet and smartphones are increasingly popular in nursing education and practice [44], so structure and layout of the course can change from a PC to a mobile phone. According to Back [38], medical e-learning environments should have compatibility for all operating systems and unrestricted mobile access via tablet or smartphone.

There is a growing trend in the use of Massive Open Online Courses (MOOCs) in traditionally taught courses through this blended method [45]. But nevertheless, according to the definition of MOOC [46], maybe we cannot categorize our course as blended MOOC. First, a MOOC is massive, allowing the registration of thousands of participants. However, if we allow the registration of such a large number of participants in the online theoretical module of the course, it would be practically unfeasible to manage the practical module of the course, since this part is usually performed in specialized centres with capacity of 10–15 people each time. And second, a MOOC is open, in which any type of participants could register without any kind of restriction in prerequisite terms. However, Lapnurse is a specialization course of surgical staff, for which a minimum requirement of being a nurse is needed.

4.1. Study Limitations

More studies are needed to provide additional evidence from students at a national and international level performing a user-level validation, since only technicians and expert teachers have been involved in this preliminary validation.

4.2. Comparison with Prior Work

As far as we know, there are no similar blended learning laparoscopic courses specially addressed to nurses, so this original course with innovative 3D designs could improve their training in MIS as members of surgical teams involved in the interventions.

5. Conclusions

Although surgery is commonly present in training programs for nursing, Portuguese and Spanish nurses are inexperienced in MIS. Therefore, a laparoscopic training course for nursing has been developed through the blended learning method. The e-learning environment developed for the online theoretical module facilitates the accessibility to high quality didactic material to nurses in a remote and asynchronous way, allowing a greater implementation of the new MIS techniques in health systems.

Positive preliminary validation of Lapnurse could motivate developers to design similar courses. First, this kind of e-learning platform should preliminarily be validated to guarantee instructors' satisfaction so that contents offered to final users can meet learning requirements. Second, contents should be complete, updated, and relevant for clinical practice and educational purposes, but also unique and innovative to attract users and thus stand out from the contents of similar e-learning platforms. Additionally, interactivity should be included in the platform, and even in surgical videos, to favor learning outcomes and to get users' engagement. And, finally, reliability and quality of the system should be assessed for a good user experience. Such e-learning environments should be easy to use, attractive, and with intuitive navigation to favor users' engagement, but with useful and quality services to meet the instructors' satisfaction. Moreover, this kind of course should be developed for PC and mobile devices so that users can perform them anywhere, anytime, and on any device.

Successful preliminary validation of functionality, contents, and usability suggests that Lapnurse can solve the gap of training needs in MIS of both Spanish and Portuguese nurses. So, they could be properly qualified to work in this field in their own country, but also in the neighboring one. Since the obtained results were largely positive for valuing the e-learning environment and the blended learning method, it is a good starting point for considering in future studies the created course as a tool that could improve learning outcomes.

Author Contributions: Conceptualization, J.F.O.-M. and B.P.; methodology, J.F.O.-M., B.P., J.M.-A., J.S.-F., A.A. and F.M.; software, J.F.O.-M., B.P., J.M.-A., J.S.-F., A.A. and F.M.; validation, J.F.O.-M. and A.A.; formal analysis, J.F.O.-M. and A.A.; investigation, J.F.O.-M., B.P., A.A. and F.M.; writing—original draft preparation, J.F.O.-M.; writing—review and editing, J.F.O.-M., B.P., J.M.-A., J.S.-F., A.A., F.M. and F.M.S.-M.; supervision, F.M.S.-M.; project administration, J.F.O.-M. and A.A.; funding acquisition, J.F.O.-M., B.P., A.A. and F.M.S.-M. All authors have read and agreed to the published version of the manuscript.

Funding: This study was carried out under the MITTIC Project (0606_MITTIC_4_E), Technological Modernisation and Innovation based on ICT in strategic and traditional sectors, financed jointly by the European Regional Development Fund (ERDF), through the Operational Program of Cross-border Cooperation Spain—Portugal (POCTEP) 2007–2013. The APC was funded by "Consejería de Economía, Ciencia y Agenda Digital, Junta de Extremadura" and co-funded by European Union (ERDF "A way to make Europe"). Grant number GR18199.

Institutional Review Board Statement: Ethical review and approval were waived for this study by the Ethical Committee of the Jesús Usón Minimally Invasive Surgery Centre because it was not within the scope of Law 14/2007 of 3rd July on Biomedical Research. This national regulation indicates that human health-related research involving invasive procedures needs approval by the ethical committee, but in this study the participants were not involved in invasive procedures.

Informed Consent Statement: Patient consent was waived for this study because it was not within the scope of Law 14/2007 of 3rd July on Biomedical Research. This national regulation indicates that human health-related research involving invasive procedures needs patient consent, but in this study the participants were not involved in invasive procedures. For this reason, it was not considered necessary for participants to sign a written informed consent. Only verbal informed consent was considered sufficient. All participants were informed about the objectives, length, and procedure of the study, the institutions responsible for the research, the contact people, the confidentiality and anonymity of the research data, and that their participation was voluntary, and they could withdraw from the study at any time if they wished to.

Data Availability Statement: The data presented in this study are available on request from the corresponding author.

Acknowledgments: The authors would like to gratefully acknowledge all technical and nursing experts from Spain and Portugal who willingly participated in the study.

Conflicts of Interest: The authors declare no conflict of interest. The funders had no role in the design of the study; in the collection, analyses, or interpretation of data; in the writing of the manuscript, or in the decision to publish the results.

Appendix A

This appendix includes the functional requirements evaluated:

- Access management requirements: user registration, login, logout, password recovery, and password change.

- Requirements of user profile and interactions: consultation and editing of personal data, user search, and language selection.
- Environmental maintenance requirements: user administration, monitoring, maintenance and updating of the environment, detection and notification of errors, and contingency response.
- Requirements for formal learning: creation, editing, and elimination of new courses, search for courses, request for subscription to courses, consultation of courses enrolled, accept/reject the subscription to a course, evaluation of skills acquired and progress evaluation.
- Requirements for informal learning: comment or raise questions in the forum, create new topics in the forum, and establish communication between users in the chat.

Appendix B

This appendix includes the questionnaire for content validation.

Note: This questionnaire has been translated into English for the readers of this article. The original one that was used during the validation process was in Spanish and Portuguese.

Questionnaire for Content Validation

Please read the different statements listed below concerning the specific content of each lesson of the theoretical module of the course and select the answer that best indicates the extent to which you agree with each of them, where 1 stands for "completely disagree" and 5 for "completely agree".

- Q1: Contents have good technical quality
- Q2: The amount of content is appropriate
- Q3: The content distribution is appropriate
- Q4: Multimedia contents (images, videos, and 3D designs) are of quality, provide added value and useful information
- Q5: The questionnaire is adequate in terms of number of questions and difficulty

Please read the different statements listed below concerning the global content of the theoretical module of the course and select the answer that best indicates the extent to which you agree with each of them, where 1 stands for "completely disagree" and 5 for "completely agree".

- Q6: The contents are unique, that is, the different types of content are not offered by similar e-learning environments
- Q7: The e-learning environment provides innovative content
- Q8: The e-learning environment uses professional language and appropriate content for users
- Q9: The content is whole and complete
- Q10: The e-learning environment uses multimedia content correctly applied for educational purposes
- Q11: Contents are updated
- Q12: Contents are easily understood
- Q13: 3D designs are interactive
- Q14: 3D designs are realistic and have good quality
- Q15: Contents are realistic and relevant to professional practice
- Q16: Surgical videos have good image quality
- Q17: The e-learning environment provides adequate means (questionnaires) to assess users' knowledge on the learned topics
- Q18: The discussion forum of the e-learning environment is suitable and useful for users
- Q19: The e-learning environment provides a useful chat for communication between users

- Q20: Contents satisfactorily cover the theoretical aspects of a nursing laparoscopy course
- Q21: The glossary of 3D designs is useful and complete

Please answer the next two open questions:

- Q22: Indicate which lessons you consider more and less important
- Q23: Indicate which resources (glossary, chat, discussion forum, multimedia didactic content, lessons, questionnaires) you consider more and less important

Appendix C

This appendix includes the questionnaire for usability validation.

Note: This questionnaire has been translated into English for the readers of this article. The original one that was used during the validation process was in Spanish and Portuguese.

Questionnaire for Usability Validation

Please read the different statements concerning the usability of the e-learning environment listed below and indicate whether or not you agree with each of them

- Q24: The text-background color contrast is appropriate
- Q25: The font type and size facilitates reading
- Q26: Navigation labels are clear and concise
- Q27: The e-learning environment is attractive
- Q28: Appropriate number of buttons/links
- Q29: The e-learning environment uses colors properly
- Q30: The e-learning environment is organized
- Q31: The overall design of the e-learning environment is consistent (consistency and uniformity in style, structures and colors on all pages)
- Q32: Web pages within the e-learning environment are not long
- Q33: Navigation through the e-learning environment is intuitive
- Q34: Correct use is made of the visual space of the e-learning environment
- Q35: Information overload is avoided
- Q36: I like the graphic aspect and the general layout of the e-learning environment
- Q37: The e-learning environment is easy to use

References

1. Leone, C.; Conceição, C.; Dussault, G. Trends of cross-border mobility of physicians and nurses between Portugal and Spain. *Hum. Resour. Health* **2013**, *11*, 36. [CrossRef]
2. Sánchez-Peralta, L.F.; Sánchez-Fernández, J.; Pagador, J.B.; Sánchez-Margallo, F.M. New technologies in minimally invasive surgery training: What do surgeons demand? *Cir. Cir.* **2013**, *81*, 412–419.
3. Graue, M.; Bjarkøy, R.Ø.; Iversen, M.M.; Haugstvedt, A.; Harris, J. Integrating evidence-based practice into the diabetes nurse curriculum in Bergen. *Eur. Diabetes Nurs.* **2010**, *7*, 10–15. [CrossRef]
4. Kim, K.K. Development of a web-based education program for nurses working in nursing homes on human rights of older adults. *J. Korean Acad. Nurs.* **2010**, *40*, 463–472. [CrossRef] [PubMed]
5. Öztürk, D.; Dinç, L. Effect of web-based education on nursing students' urinary catheterization knowledge and skills. *Nurse Educ. Today* **2014**, *34*, 802–808. [CrossRef]
6. McVeigh, H. Factors influencing the utilisation of e-learning in post-registration nursing students. *Nurse Educ. Today* **2009**, *29*, 91–99. [CrossRef]
7. Ward, J.A.; Beaton, R.D.; Bruck, A.M.; de Castro, A.B. Promoting occupational health nursing training: An educational outreach with a blended model of distance and traditional learning approaches. *AAOHN J.* **2011**, *59*, 401–406. [CrossRef] [PubMed]
8. Sowan, A.K.; Jenkins, L.S. Designing, delivering and evaluating a distance learning nursing course responsive to students needs. *Int. J. Med. Inf.* **2013**, *82*, 553–564. [CrossRef]
9. Lahti, M.; Kontio, R.; Pitkänen, A.; Välimäki, M. Knowledge transfer from an e-learning course to clinical practice. *Nurse Educ. Today* **2014**, *34*, 842–847. [CrossRef]
10. Smyth, S.; Houghton, C.; Cooney, A.; Casey, D. Students' experiences of blended learning across a range of postgraduate programmes. *Nurse Educ. Today* **2012**, *32*, 464–468. [CrossRef] [PubMed]
11. MOODLE. Available online: https://moodle.org/ (accessed on 15 June 2021).

12. Fernández-Alemán, J.L.; López-González, L.; González-Sequeros, O.; Jayne, C.; López-Jiménez, J.J.; Toval, A. The evaluation of i-SIDRA–a tool for intelligent feedback–in a course on the anatomy of the locomotor system. *Int. J. Med. Inf.* **2016**, *94*, 172–181. [CrossRef] [PubMed]
13. Rapp, A.K.; Healy, M.G.; Charlton, M.E.; Keith, J.N.; Rosenbaum, M.E.; Kapadia, M.R. YouTube is the most frequently used educational video source for surgical preparation. *J. Surg. Educ.* **2016**, *73*, 1072–1076. [CrossRef]
14. Sowan, A.K.; Idhail, J.A. Evaluation of an interactive web-based nursing course with streaming videos for medication administration skills. *Int. J. Med. Inf.* **2014**, *83*, 592–600. [CrossRef]
15. Wallace, T.; Birch, D.W. A needs-assessment study for continuing professional development in advances minimally invasive surgery. *Am. J. Surg.* **2007**, *193*, 593–596. [CrossRef]
16. Callisen, L. Why Micro Learning Is the Future of Training in the Workplace. eLearning Industry. Available online: http://elearningindustry.com/micro-learning-future-of-training-workplace (accessed on 15 June 2021).
17. Ortega-Morán, J.F.; Pagador, J.B.; Sánchez-Peralta, L.F.; Sánchez-González, P.; Noguera, J.; Burgos, D.; Gómez, E.J.; Sánchez-Margallo, F.M. Validation of the three web quality dimensions of a minimally invasive surgery e-learning platform. *Int. J. Med. Inf.* **2017**, *107*, 1–10. [CrossRef] [PubMed]
18. De Góes Fdos, S.; Fonseca, L.M.; de Camargo, R.A.; de Oliveira, G.F.; Felipe, H.R. Educational technology "Anatomy and Vital Signs": Evaluation study of content, appearance and usability. *Int. J. Med. Inf.* **2015**, *84*, 982–987. [CrossRef] [PubMed]
19. Davids, M.R.; Chikte, U.; Grimmer-Somers, K.; Halperin, M.L. Usability testing of a multimedia e-learning resource for electrolyte and acid-base disorders. *Br. J. Educ. Technol.* **2014**, *45*, 367–381. [CrossRef]
20. Guerrero-Martínez, I.M.; Portero-Prados, F.J.; Romero-González, R.C.; Romero-Castillo, R.; Pabón-Carrasco, M.; Ponce-Blandón, J.A. Nursing Students' Perception on the Effectiveness of Emergency Competence Learning through Simulation. *Healthcare* **2020**, *8*, 397. [CrossRef]
21. Wu, X.V.; Chi, Y.; Selvam, U.P.; Devi, M.K.; Wang, W.; Chan, Y.S.; Wee, F.C.; Zhao, S.; Sehgal, V.; Ang, N.K.E. A Clinical Teaching Blended Learning Program to Enhance Registered Nurse Preceptors' Teaching Competencies: Pretest and Posttest Study. *J. Med. Internet Res.* **2020**, *22*, e18604. [CrossRef]
22. Musharyanti, L.; Haryanti, F.; Claramita, M. Improving Nursing Students' Medication Safety Knowledge and Skills on Using the 4C/ID Learning Model. *J. Multidiscip. Healthc.* **2021**, *14*, 287. [CrossRef]
23. Galbany-Estragués, P.; Nelson, S. Factors in the drop in the migration of Spanish-trained nurses: 1999–2007. *J. Nurs. Manag.* **2018**, *26*, 477–484. [CrossRef]
24. Fries-Tersch, E.; Tugran, T.; Bradley, H. 2017 Annual Report on Intra-EU Labour Mobility. European Commission. 2018. Available online: https://ec.europa.eu/futurium/en/system/files/ged/2017_report_on_intra-eu_labour_mobility.pdf (accessed on 15 June 2021).
25. Ali, M.; Han, S.C.; Bilal, H.S.M.; Lee, S.; Kang, M.J.Y.; Kang, B.H.; Razzaq, M.A.; Amin, M.B. iCBLS: An interactive case-based learning system for medical education. *Int. J. Med. Inf.* **2018**, *109*, 55–69. [CrossRef] [PubMed]
26. Swartz, L.B.; Cole, M.T.; Shelley, D.J. Instructor satisfaction with teaching business law: Online vs. onground. *Int. J. Inf. Commun. Technol. Educ. (IJICTE)* **2010**, *6*, 1–16. [CrossRef]
27. Margalina, V.M.; De-Pablos-Heredero, C.; Botella, J.L.M. Achieving Job Satisfaction for Instructors in E-Learning: The Relational Coordination Role. In *Social Issues in the Workplace: Breakthroughs in Research and Practice*; IGI Global: Hershey, PA, USA, 2018; pp. 521–537. [CrossRef]
28. Yengin, I.; Karahoca, A.; Karahoca, D. E-learning success model for instructors' satisfactions in perspective of interaction and usability outcomes. *Procedia Comput. Sci.* **2011**, *3*, 1396–1403. [CrossRef]
29. Almarashdeh, I. Sharing instructors experience of learning management system: A technology perspective of user satisfaction in distance learning course. *Comput. Hum. Behav.* **2016**, *63*, 249–255. [CrossRef]
30. Costa, C.; Alvelos, H.; Teixeira, L. The Use of Moodle e-learning Platform: A Study in a Portuguese University. *Procedia Technol.* **2012**, *5*, 334–343. [CrossRef]
31. Amandu, G.M.; Muliira, J.K.; Fronda, D.C. Using Moodle E-learning Platform to Foster Student Self-directed Learning: Experiences with Utilization of the Software in Undergraduate Nursing Courses in a Middle Eastern University. *Procedia Soc. Behav. Sci.* **2013**, *93*, 677–683. [CrossRef]
32. Paragina, F.; Paragina, S.; Jipa, A.; Savu, T.; Dumitrescu, A. The benefits of using MOODLE in teacher training in Romania. *Procedia Soc. Behav. Sci.* **2011**, *15*, 1135–1139. [CrossRef]
33. Escobar-Rodriguez, T.; Monge-Lozano, P. The acceptance of Moodle technology by business administration students. *Comput. Educ.* **2012**, *58*, 1085–1093. [CrossRef]
34. Butzke, M.A.; Alberton, A. Estilos de aprendizagem e jogos de empresa: A percepção discente sobre estratégia de ensino e ambiente de aprendizagem. *REGE-Rev. Gestão* **2017**, *24*, 72–84. [CrossRef]
35. Tarhini, A.; Hone, K.; Liu, X.; Tarhini, T. Examining the moderating effect of individual-level cultural values on users' acceptance of e-learning in developing countries: A structural equation modeling of an extended technology acceptance model. *Interact. Learn. Environ.* **2017**, *25*, 306–328. [CrossRef]
36. Cidral, W.A.; Oliveira, T.; Di Felice, M.; Aparicio, M. E-learning success determinants: Brazilian empirical study. *Comput. Educ.* **2018**, *122*, 273–290. [CrossRef]
37. Aparicio, M.; Bacao, F.; Oliveira, T. Grit in the path to e-learning success. *Comput. Hum. Behav.* **2017**, *66*, 388–399. [CrossRef]

38. Back, D.A.; Behringer, F.; Haberstroh, N.; Ehlers, J.P.; Sostmann, K.; Peters, H. Learning management system and e-learning tools: An experience of medical students' usage and expectations. *Int. J. Med. Educ.* **2016**, *7*, 267–273. [CrossRef]
39. Rasheed, K.; Noman, M.; Imran, M.; Iqbal, M.; Khan, Z.M.; Abid, M.M. Performance comparison among local and foreign universities websites using seo tools. *ICTACT J. Soft Comput.* **2018**, *8*. Available online: http://ictactjournals.in/paper/IJSC_Vol_8_Iss_2_Paper_3_1597_1610.pdf (accessed on 15 June 2021).
40. Liaw, S.Y.; Wong, L.F.; Chan, S.W.; Ho, J.T.; Mordiffi, S.Z.; Ang, S.B.; Goh, P.S.; Ang, E.N. Designing and evaluating an interactive multimedia Web-based simulation for developing nurses' competencies in acute nursing care: Randomized controlled trial. *J. Med. Internet Res.* **2015**, *17*, e5. [CrossRef] [PubMed]
41. Bloomfield, J.G.; Jones, A. Using e-learning to support clinical skills acquisition: Exploring the experiences and perceptions of graduate first-year pre-registration nursing students—A mixed method study. *Nurse Educ. Today* **2013**, *33*, 1605–1611. [CrossRef] [PubMed]
42. Hammond, J.; Cherrett, T.; Waterson, B. Making in-class skills training more effective: The scope for interactive videos to complement the delivery of practical pedestrian training. *Br. J. Educ. Technol.* **2015**, *46*, 1344–1353. [CrossRef]
43. Mai, N.; Heykyung, P.; Min-Jae, L.; Jian-Yuan, S.; Ji-Young, O. Technology Acceptance of Healthcare E-Learning Modules: A Study of Korean and Malaysian Students' Perceptions. *TOJET Turk. Online J. Educ. Technol.* **2015**, *14*, 181–194.
44. Pimmer, C.; Brysiewicz, P.; Linxen, S.; Walters, F.; Chipps, J.; Gröhbiel, U. Informal mobile learning in nurse education and practice in remote areas—A case study from rural South Africa. *Nurse Educ. Today* **2014**, *34*, 1398–1404. [CrossRef]
45. Bralić, A.; Divjak, B. Integrating MOOCs in traditionally taught courses: Achieving learning outcomes with blended learning. *Int. J. Educ. Technol. High. Educ.* **2018**, *15*, 2. [CrossRef]
46. Gonçalves, B.; Osório, A. Massive Open Online Courses (MOOC) to improve teachers' professional development. *D-Rev. Educ. Distância Elearning* **2018**, *1*, 52–63.

Analysis of the Content and Comprehensiveness of Dermatology Residency Training Websites in Taiwan

Po-Yu Chen [1,2], Ying-Xiu Dai [2,3], Ya-Chuan Hsu [4] and Tzeng-Ji Chen [1,2,*]

1. Department of Family Medicine, Taipei Veterans General Hospital, Taipei 112, Taiwan; barry50710@gmail.com
2. School of Medicine, National Yang Ming Chiao Tung University, Taipei 112, Taiwan; daiinxiu@gmail.com
3. Department of Dermatology, Taipei Veterans General Hospital, Taipei 112, Taiwan
4. Department of Family Medicine, Kinmen Hospital, Ministry of Health and Welfare, Kinmen 891, Taiwan; ych97160@gmail.com
* Correspondence: tjchen@vghtpe.gov.tw; Tel.: +886-2-2875-7458; Fax: +886-2-2873-7901

Abstract: With a growing trend in the popularity of web-based resources, it is important to evaluate residency program websites for providing accurate information for dermatology residency applicants. Little is known about the quality of dermatology residency websites in Taiwan. The aim of the study is to assesses the quality of official websites of dermatology training programs in Taiwan. A literature search for all related studies from inception to 31 July 2020 was performed using PubMed without restriction on language. We used criteria that had 6 domains and 25 items to evaluate 23 official websites of the dermatology training programs in Taiwan from August to September 2020. Of the 23 training programs, only 6 (26%) of the websites met more than half of the criteria. Notably, the items "features of the department" and "comprehensive faculty listing" were included in all websites. The criteria for interview process, board pass rates, social activities and information on the surrounding area were not met by all websites. Evidently, there is much room for improvement for the dermatology training program websites in Taiwan.

Keywords: dermatology; residency website; residency training

1. Introduction

1.1. Health Information on the Internet

In modern society, the Internet has gradually become more and more important for humans. According to statistics from the International Telecommunication Union, the percentage of Internet users worldwide increased from 16% in 2005 to 53.6% in 2019 [1]. In Taiwan in 2019, 92.78% of people used the Internet. It has become a convenient and generalized tool for acquiring information in Taiwan. A previous study reported that 80% of Internet users use the Internet to acquire healthcare information [2], and medical staff search it for information they need. Online resources for medical knowledge have become available to medical students and patients through computers and smart phones [3]. For physicians, clinicians and students, online resources represent an extensive source of continuing education in different specializations [4–6]. Patients can find several educational materials on the Internet, especially professional websites. In fact, a previous study showed that online patient education materials from the websites of major dermatology associations, such as the American Academy of Dermatology, was written well and appropriate for the general population [7]. Indeed, Internet has become a rather significant tool for physicians, medical students and patients.

1.2. Taiwanese Residency Training Programs: Dermatology

Since 2019, in Taiwan, medical students have been required to obtain a medical license after graduation and to finish postgraduate year training (PGY) within 2 years if they decide to receive advanced residency training [8]. Thereafter, they need to choose a specialization and complete residency training; for this purpose, they apply to several programs all over Taiwan, but many young doctors in the PGY-2 level are unfamiliar with the processes. Of all 23 specializations, dermatology is one of the most popular in Taiwan. The training period for dermatology residency is 4 years. Due to the advance of aesthetic medicine and the national health insurance system, there is tough competition to be accepted into a dermatology training program. Approximately 1400 medical students are able to obtain their medical license every year, but only about 28 positions per year are available for dermatology residency training. Even though this capacity can be adjusted by an agreement between the Taiwanese Dermatological Association and the Ministry of Health and Welfare, it is still much less than other specializations [9].

In the past, information on the training programs was difficult to obtain. Applicants often have to ask their senior residents or teachers for information or search the public information on the program websites. Applicants are less competitive without knowing people in dermatology departments. With widespread use, the Internet has become a common source of information for medical students applying for residency. Previous studies have indicated that the website content influenced an applicant's decision-making, especially for those who had never been engaged in the department [10]. Prospective applicants rely heavily on the websites of residency training programs to obtain significant information regarding the application process, as well as the unique aspects of the different programs [11]. Therefore, the importance of maintaining an informative and accessible website continues to grow. Many studies abroad have evaluated the website content of different specialties, including dermatology [12–18]. However, there had been no research that studied the contents of websites on residency training programs in Taiwan. In this study, standardized criteria were used to evaluate the websites of dermatology training programs in Taiwan. It is expected to provide dermatology programs information about how to enrich the content and display the strengths of their program to applicants. By enhancing their websites, the training programs also can attract more excellent applicants.

2. Materials and Methods

2.1. Establishing the Criteria

We searched for previous research that evaluated the websites of different residency or fellowship programs through the online literature database PubMed, using the keywords "Internet standards," "internship and residency," "fellowship and scholarship," and "information dissemination" from April to May 2020. We found 6 studies that performed questionnaire surveys to understand what content is important for applicants. After reevaluation, we developed a set of evaluation criteria with 25 content items categorized into 6 domains: recruitment information, department information, education and research, clinical work, incentives and frequently asked questions and answers (Table 1) [10,11,19–23]. The process of establishing the criteria is shown in Figure 1. The evaluation criteria were published previously in the *Taiwan Journal of Family Medicine* [23]. This is the first study to use these criteria to evaluate residency program websites in Taiwan.

2.2. Internet Search for Taiwanese Dermatology Training Program Websites

Thereafter, using the keywords "dermatology" and "training capacity," we performed Google search for the online official website of the Taiwanese Dermatological Association to check for the list of qualified dermatology training hospitals. We linked our search to the website of the Taiwan Ministry of Health and Welfare to review the publication list of qualified dermatology training hospitals and the training capacity after revision in July 2020 [9]. The number of items that met the criteria was calculated for each website. We conducted the evaluations twice with different reviewers. The first review was conducted by the first author around August 2020. A second review was conducted by the second author around September 2020, blinded to the results of the first review. Since this study did not involve human subjects, it did not need institutional review board approval.

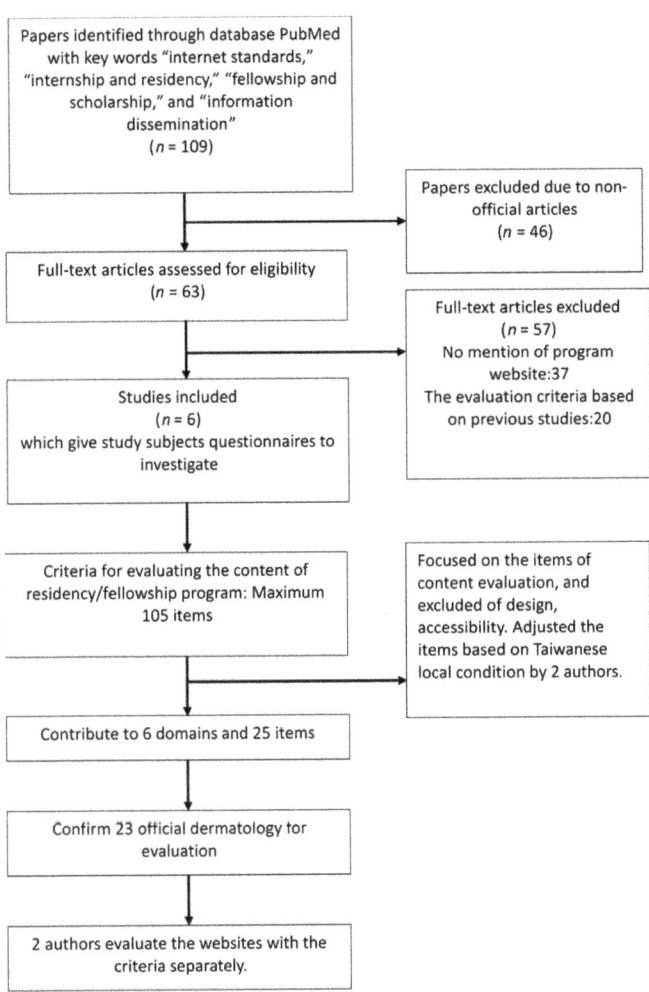

Figure 1. Flowchart of establishing the criteria and evaluating the websites.

Table 1. Criteria for evaluating the websites of residency and fellowship programs.

Domains (6)	Items (25)
Recruitment information	Recruitment criteria Interview process * Contact information
Department information	History of the department Features of the department Comprehensive faculty listing Message from the chairman/program director List of current residents/fellows Board pass rates Alumni information and outcomes Description of environment and equipment Social activities Information on the surrounding area [†]

Table 1. Cont.

Domains (6)	Items (25)
Education and research	Program goals Research activities and accomplishments Educational resources available to residents Conference schedule Elective opportunities
Clinical work	Work hours Rotation schedule Expected case load [§] On-call expectation
Incentive	Salary Ancillary benefit [‖]
Frequently asked questions and answers	Frequently asked questions and answers

[*] How to proceed with the recruitment (e.g., written tests, face to face interview, etc.). [†] The location of the department/hospital. [§] The number of inpatient cases or weekly outpatient cases per resident. [‖] Independent office, independent rest room when on-call, etc.

3. Results

Website Evaluation

Overall, 23 dermatology residency training programs were approved by the Taiwan Ministry of Health and Welfare, and their official websites were evaluated in this study. The name of the training programs/departments and their website links are listed in Supplement Table S1. Based on the common administrative regional classification in Taiwan, the distribution of the training programs among the 23 hospitals was as follows: 56.6% (13 programs) in the northern area, 17.4% (4 programs) in the central area, 21.7% (5 programs) in the southern area and 4.3% (1 program) in the eastern area. Of the 23 hospitals, 39.1% (9 programs) were public and 60.9% (14 programs) were private.

In comparison with the results of 2 surveys, there was no difference. The final results are listed in Table 2. The websites met a mean and median of 13 of 25 items (52%) of the criteria, with a maximum of 18 items (72%) and a minimum of 4 items (16%). Over half of the criteria were met by 26% (6 of 23 programs) of the dermatology departments, of which 3 were at public hospitals and 3 were at private hospitals. However, the dermatology websites of Cathay General Hospital, Taipei City Hospital, Renai Branch and Heping Fuyou Branch met only four items (16%) of the criteria.

The distribution of the items on the websites is listed in Table 3 and Figure 2. Most of the websites (over 85%, 20 of 23 programs) contained information on the following 4 items: features of the department (100%, 23 programs); comprehensive faculty listing (100%, 23 programs); description of the environment and equipment (91.3%, 21 programs); and history of the department (87%, 20 programs). Notably, the items on interview process, board pass rates, social activities and information on the surrounding area were not posted on any dermatology website.

We further analyzed and compared the proportion of public and private programs/departments that contained each item in our criteria. Public and private programs had the tendency to show similar information on most items ($p > 0.05$) in the 6 domains. These results are listed in detail in Table 3.

Table 2. Conditions of training program websites.

Name of Hospital	Public/Private	Criteria Matched (Percentage, %)
Northern Area (13) *		
Keelung Chang Gung Memorial Hospital and Lovers Lake Branch	Private	5 (20%)
Taipei Veterans General Hospital	Public	16 (64%)
National Taiwan University Hospital	Public	10 (40%)
Tri-service General Hospital	Public	18 (72%)
Mackay Memorial Hospital	Private	13 (52%)
Taipei Municipal Wangfang Hospital †	Public	8 (32%)
Taipei Medical University Hospital	Private	8 (32%)
Shin Kong Wu Ho Su Memorial Hospital	Private	12 (48%)
Cathay General Hospital	Private	4 (16%)
Taipei City Hospital, Renai Branch and Heping Fuyou Branch	Public	4 (16%)
Taipei and Linkou Chang Gung Memorial Hospital	Private	12 (48%)
Far Eastern Memorial Hospital	Private	13 (52%)
Shuang Ho Hospital, Ministry of Health and Welfare †	Public	5 (20%)
Central Area (4) *		
Taichung Veterans General Hospital	Public	12 (48%)
China Medical University Hospital	Private	5 (20%)
Chung Shan Medical University Hospital	Private	6 (24%)
Changhua Christian Hospital	Private	5 (20%)
Southern Area (5) *		
National Cheng Kung University Hospital	Public	16 (64%)
Chi Mei Medical Center	Private	16 (64%)
Kaohsiung Medical University Chung-Ho Memorial Hospital	Private	7 (28%)
Kaohsiung Veterans General Hospital	Public	10 (40%)
Kaohsiung Chang Gung Memorial Hospital	Private	8 (32%)
Eastern Area (1) *		
Hualien Tzu Chi Hospital	Private	6 (24%)

* The hospitals were divided into four areas (i.e., northern, central, southern and eastern), according to location, Council for Economic Planning and Development, Executive Yuan. † The Taipei Municipal Wangfang Hospital; Shuang Ho Hospital, Ministry of Health and Welfare were regarded as public hospitals even if these were managed by the Taipei Medical University.

Table 3. Percentage of dermatology residency websites that contain publicly accessible information on the 25 list items.

Criteria	Total ($n = 23$) (%)	Public ($n = 9$) (%)	Private ($n = 14$) (%)	p Value
Recruitment information				0.31
Recruitment criteria	1 (4.3%)	0 (0)	1 (7.1%)	
Interview process	0 (0)	0 (0)	0 (0)	
Contact information	18 (78.3%)	8 (88.9%)	10 (71.4%)	
Department information				0.42
History of the department	20 (87.0%)	7 (77.8%)	13 (92.9%)	
Features of the department	23 (100%)	9 (100%)	14 (100%)	
Comprehensive faculty listing	23 (100%)	9 (100%)	14 (100%)	
Message from the chairman/program director	1 (4.3%)	0 (0)	1 (7.1%)	
List of current residents/fellows	13 (56.5%)	7 (77.8%)	6 (42.9%)	
Board pass rates	0 (0)	0 (0)	0 (0)	
Alumni information and outcomes	5 (21.7%)	3 (33.3%)	2 (14.3%)	
Description of environment and equipment	21 (91.3%)	8 (88.9%)	13 (92.9%)	
Social activities	0 (0)	0 (0)	0 (0)	
Information on the surrounding area	0 (0)	0 (0)	0 (0)	

Table 3. Cont.

Criteria	Total (n = 23) (%)	Public (n = 9) (%)	Private (n = 14) (%)	p Value
Education and research				0.48
Program goals	13 (56.5%)	6 (66.7%)	7 (50.0%)	
Research activities and accomplishments	13 (56.5%)	6 (66.7%)	7 (50.0%)	
Educational resources available to residents	18 (78.3%)	8 (88.9%)	10 (71.4%)	
Conference schedule	13 (56.5%)	7 (77.8%)	6 (42.9%)	
Elective opportunities	9 (39.1%)	4 (44.4%)	5 (35.7%)	
Clinical work				0.27
Work hours	4 (17.4%)	3 (33.3%)	1 (7.1%)	
Rotation schedule	9 (39.1%)	4 (44.4%)	5 (35.7%)	
Expected case load	4 (17.4%)	3 (33.3%)	1 (7.1%)	
On-call expectation	4 (17.4%)	3 (33.3%)	1 (7.1%)	
Incentive				0.70
Salary	1 (4.3%)	0 (0)	1 (7.1%)	
Ancillary benefit	4 (17.4%)	2 (22.2%)	2 (14.3%)	
Frequently asked questions and answers				0.42
Frequently asked questions and answers	2 (8.7%)	2 (22.2%)	0 (0)	

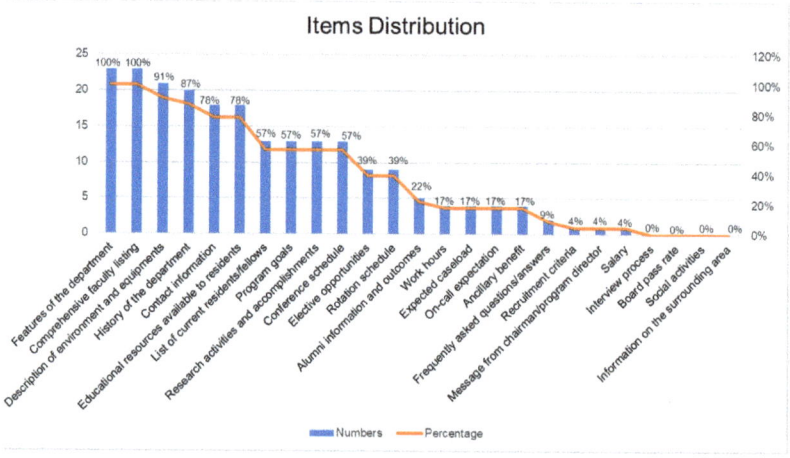

Figure 2. Item distribution over all programs.

4. Discussion

4.1. Analysis of Website Contents

Previous related studies, most of which were from the United States of America (USA) and Canada, have been conducted to evaluate the websites of residency and fellowship specializations [14–20]. To our best knowledge, this study was the first to evaluate the content of dermatology residency program websites in Taiwan. Our study found highly variable content and quality among these websites. Most programs need improvements in the functioning of their webpages.

Among the criteria items, the most common information addressed were "features of the department" and "comprehensive faculty listing." Through this, people can learn more about the development of the department and choose which doctor they prefer. Applicants can also learn of senior role models for their medical careers. Over half of the websites included "list of current residents/fellows," but only 21.7% mentioned "alumni information and outcomes." This information could show close relationships between the department and its staff, but it was not valued by most programs. The items of "program goals," "research activities and accomplishments" and "educational resources available to residents" were included in more than half of websites. Information on the research achievements and education resources allow applicants to compare different activities and resources. Patients and the general public can also improve their medical knowledge.

Among the least common and poorly represented information were program-related specifics, such as "recruitment criteria," "message from the chairman/program director," "salary," "interview process," "board pass rates," "social activities," and "information on the surrounding area." In most websites, announcements on the "recruitment criteria" and "interview process" appeared only during the period of application; at other times, we could not find the relevant information. Simple statements on recruitment would encourage more excellent applicants to apply and provide them with an understanding of the process. Notably, "message from the chairman/program director" was often neglected among the websites evaluated in this study but had been more frequent in foreign websites [13,18].

Salary is an item that most people and organizations do not disclose to the public in Taiwan. Most applicants might presume that the directors would think that these issues are not directly related with clinical training: "if you ask about these, it means you are only interested in the money and benefits, and do not have a passion for the medical training." This observation had been reported in the USA and Taiwan [16].

Information about clinical work for residents was less clear on the internet. Information on "work hours," "expected caseload," and "on-call expectation" was provided in fewer than 10% of websites. Recently, the case loading and work hours of residency have been hot topics due to cases of death from overwork. Since residency doctors were included in the regulations of the 2019 Taiwanese Labor Standards Act, programs have been required to follow the Guideline of Residents Labor Rights Protection and Working Hours. Disclosure of this information is important for applicants [24].

4.2. Comparison with Research from the USA

Prior research includes one 2016 study about dermatology residency program websites in the USA [15]. We compared this with our study to understand the differences and found the following similarities and differences. Similarities with the USA study: program contact information, 83.5%; program description, 95.7%; research opportunities, 86.1%; current resident listing and 64.3%; current faculty listing, 89.6%. Our results were also all >50%. Other percentages >50% in the USA study were rotations and electives, 87.8%; applicant information, 88.7%; interview process, 64.3% (all >50%). In our study, these items were <40%. Most dermatology residency websites in the USA and Taiwan included content that described programs and listed faculty, residents and research accomplishments. However, Taiwanese websites rarely had information about recruitment, interviews and rotation. The disparity suggested much room for improvement in the website content in Taiwan.

4.3. Limitations

There were several limitations in our study. First, the criteria were according to foreign studies and may not be applicable to programs in Taiwan. In addition, the reliability and validity need to be verified further in the future. Second, our results represented a single snapshot in time. Owing to differences in navigability among the websites based on individual subjectivity, some information may have been overlooked during data collection. However, the likelihood that the differences in collection would change the nature of the presented data was low, even is this study was primarily descriptive in nature. Finally, our study focused only on the content of the websites and did not assess website design and quality. Each website has a unique design; therefore, quality can be difficult to compare. This aspect may be further analyzed in future.

5. Conclusions

Most of the dermatology websites from Taiwan did not contain sufficient information, especially recruitment, board pass rate, alumni, social activities, surrounding area, clinical work, salary, ancillary benefits and frequently asked questions and answers were especially neglected.

Supplementary Materials: The following are available online at https://www.mdpi.com/article/10.3390/healthcare9060773/s1, Table S1: Dermatology residency websites included in this study.

Author Contributions: Conceptualization, T.-J.C.; methodology, P.-Y.C. and Y.-C.H.; formal analysis, P.-Y.C. and Y.-X.D.; investigation, P.-Y.C. and Y.-X.D.; writing—original draft preparation, P.-Y.C. and Y.-X.D.; writing—review and editing, Y.-C.H. and T.-J.C.; supervision, T.-J.C. All authors have read and agreed to the published version of the manuscript.

Funding: The study was supported by a grant (V109E-002-1) from Taipei Veterans General Hospital.

Institutional Review Board Statement: Not applicable.

Informed Consent Statement: Not applicable.

Data Availability Statement: Data is contained within the article.

Conflicts of Interest: The authors declare no conflict of interest.

References

1. International Telecommunication Union. Available online: https://www.itu.int/en/ITU-D/Statistics/Pages/stat/default.aspx (accessed on 12 November 2020).
2. Cline, R.J.; Haynes, K.M. Consumer health information seeking on the internet: The state of the art. *Health Educ. Res.* **2001**, *16*, 671–692. [CrossRef]
3. Laughter, M.; Zangara, T.; Maymone, M.; Rundle, C.; Dunnick, C.; Hugh, J.; Sadeghpour, M.; Dellavalle, R. Social media use in dermatology. *Dermatol. Sin.* **2020**, *38*, 28–34.
4. Hanson, A.H.; Krause, L.K.; Simmons, R.N.; Ellis, J.I.; Gamble, R.G.; Jensen, J.D.; Noble, M.N.; Orser, M.L.; Suarez, A.L.; Dellavalle, R.P. Dermatology education and the internet: Traditional and cutting-edge resources. *J. Am. Acad. Dermatol.* **2011**, *65*, 836–842. [CrossRef] [PubMed]
5. Craddock, M.F.; Blondin, H.M.; Youssef, M.J.; Tollefson, M.M.; Hill, L.F.; Hanson, J.L.; Bruckner, A.L. Online education improves pediatric residents' understanding of atopic dermatitis. *Pediatr Dermatol.* **2018**, *35*, 64–69. [CrossRef] [PubMed]
6. Jayakumar, N.; Brunckhorst, O.; Dasgupta, P.; Khan, M.S.; Ahmed, K. E-learning in surgical education: A systematic review. *J. Surg. Educ.* **2015**, *72*, 1145–1157. [CrossRef]
7. John, A.M.; John, E.S.; Hansberry, D.R.; Lambert, W.C. Assessment of online patient education materials from major dermatologic associations. *J. Clin. Aesthet. Dermatol.* **2016**, *9*, 23–28.
8. Lo, W.L.; Lin, Y.G.; Pan, Y.J.; Wu, Y.J.; Hsieh, M.C. Faculty development program for general medicine in Taiwan: Past, present, and future. *Ci Ji Yi Xue Za Zhi* **2014**, *26*, 64–67. [CrossRef]
9. Taiwanese Dermatological Association. Annual Training Capacity. Available online: http://www.dermateach.org.tw/hospital/HospitalSheet.asp? (accessed on 23 June 2020).
10. Mahler, S.A.; Wagner, M.J.; Church, A.; Sokolosky, M.; Cline, D.M. Importance of residency program web sites to emergency medicine applicants. *J. Emerg. Med.* **2009**, *36*, 83–88. [CrossRef]
11. Gaeta, T.J.; Birkhahn, R.H.; Lamont, D.; Banga, N.; Bove, J.J. Aspects of residency programs' web sites important to student applicants. *Acad. Emerg. Med.* **2005**, *12*, 89–92. [CrossRef]
12. Miller, V.M.; Padilla, L.A.; Schuh, A.; Mauchley, D.; Cleveland, D.; Aburjania, Z.; Dabal, R. Evaluation of cardiothoracic surgery residency and fellowship program websites. *J. Surg. Res.* **2020**, *246*, 200–206. [CrossRef] [PubMed]
13. Stoeger, S.M.; Freeman, H.; Bitter, B.; Helmer, S.D.; Reyes, J.; Vincent, K.B. Evaluation of general surgery residency program websites. *Am. J. Surg.* **2019**, *217*, 794–799. [CrossRef]
14. Ruddell, J.H.; Eltorai, A.E.M.; Tang, O.Y.; Suskin, J.A.; Dibble, E.H.; Oates, M.E.; Yoo, D.C. The current state of nuclear medicine and nuclear radiology: Workforce trends, training pathways, and training program websites. *Acad. Radiol.* **2020**, *27*, 1751–1759. [CrossRef] [PubMed]
15. Ashack, K.A.; Burton, K.A.; Soh, J.M.; Lanoue, J.; Boyd, A.H.; Milford, E.E.; Dunnick, C.; Dellavalle, R.P. Evaluating dermatology residency program websites. *Dermatol. Online. J.* **2016**, *22*, 8.
16. Svider, P.F.; Gupta, A.; Johnson, A.P.; Zuliani, G.; Shkoukani, M.A.; Eloy, J.A.; Folbe, A.J. Evaluation of otolaryngology residency program websites. *JAMA Otolaryngol. Head Neck Surg.* **2014**, *140*, 956–960. [CrossRef] [PubMed]
17. Sugrue, G.; Hamid, S.; Vijayasarathi, A.; Niu, B.; Nicolaou, S.; Khosa, F. An evaluation of the content of Canadian radiology fellowship websites. *Curr. Probl. Diagn. Radiol.* **2019**, *49*, 243–247. [CrossRef] [PubMed]

18. Goerlitz-Jessen, M.; Behunin, N.; Montijo, M.; Wilkinson, M. Recruiting the digital-age applicant: The impact of ophthalmology residency program web presence on residency recruitment. *J. Acad. Ophthalmol.* **2018**, *10*, e32–e37. [CrossRef]
19. Chu, L.F.; Young, C.A.; Zamora, A.K.; Lowe, D.; Hoang, D.B.; Pearl, R.G.; Macario, A. Self-reported information needs of anesthesia residency applicants and analysis of applicant-related web sites resources at 131 United States training programs. *Anesth. Analg.* **2011**, *112*, 430–439. [CrossRef]
20. Reilly, E.F.; Leibrandt, T.J.; Zonno, A.J.; Simpson, M.C.; Morris, J.B. General surgery residency program websites: Usefulness and usability for resident applicants. *Curr. Surg.* **2004**, *61*, 236–240. [CrossRef] [PubMed]
21. Embi, P.J.; Desai, S.; Cooney, T.G. Use and utility of web-based residency program information: A survey of residency applicants. *J. Med. Internet Res.* **2003**, *5*, 85–95. [CrossRef]
22. Winters, R.C.; Hendey, G.W. Do web sites catch residency applicants? *Acad. Emerg. Med.* **1999**, *6*, 968–972. [CrossRef]
23. Chen, P.Y.; Hsu, Y.C.; Chen, T.J. Criteria for evaluating the websites of residency and fellowship programs. *Taiwan J. Fam. Med.* **2020**, *30*, 196–203.
24. Ministry of Health and Welfare. Guideline of Residents Labor Rights Protection and Working Hours. Available online: https://dep.mohw.gov.tw/doma/cp-2713-7808-106.html (accessed on 22 May 2020).

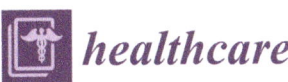

Article

Facilitating Interprofessional Education in an Online Environment during the COVID-19 Pandemic: A Mixed Method Study

Jitendra Singh * and Barbara Matthees

School of Nursing & Healthcare Leadership, College of Science, Health, & the Environment, Minnesota State University Moorhead, Moorhead, MN 56563, USA; matthees@mnstate.edu
* Correspondence: jitendra.singh@mnstate.edu

Abstract: With the COVID-19 crisis and rapid increase in cases, the need for interprofessional education (IPE) and collaborative practice is more important than ever. Instructors and health professionals are exploring innovative methods to deliver IPE programs in online education This paper presents a mixed methods study where an interprofessional education program was delivered/taught using online instruction. Using a survey/questionnaire adapted from the Readiness for Interprofessional Learning Scale (RIPLS) and qualitative discussions, students' readiness towards online IPE program and the importance of such preparation was examined. Out of two hundred fifteen students who completed the IPE program, one hundred eighty five students from clinical and non-clinical health disciplines responded to the questionnaire (86.04% response rate). Additional qualitative content analysis was conducted on a total of seven hundred and thirty six online discussions. Data analysis across all the four subscales of RIPLS suggests that students felt positively about teamwork and collaboration, and valued opportunities for shared learning with other healthcare students. Qualitative data analysis demonstrated that IPE increases awareness of team members' roles, enhances communication and collaboration and can lead to better care for COVID-19 patients.

Keywords: interprofessional education (IPE); COVID-19; pandemic; nursing; healthcare; health care; online education; communication; collaboration; mixed methods study

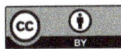

1. Introduction

Interprofessional Education (IPE) is defined as "occasions when two or more professions learn with, from and about each other to improve collaboration and the quality of care" [1]. Errors in processes, failure to work as part of a team and lack of a coordinated effort result in medical complications or even patient deaths in healthcare settings. These events not only lead to patient safety issues, but also result in increased costs to the healthcare system [2]. Understanding team members' roles in patient care processes and a team-based approach that involves collaboration among the different units and departments of an organization can be used to make the system safer for consumers of healthcare services [3]. Interprofessional education and the ability to work in collaboration with other health professionals can lead to reductions in difficulties faced by health organizations in different countries [4]. Teamwork, collaboration, and involvement of employees from different disciplines (who may have been operating in silos) promotes interaction among colleagues, which, in turn, could lead to a fresh look at existing issues/problems and identification of potential solutions to those problems [3,5].

With the global health crisis and rapid increase in COVID cases, there is an increased need for interprofessional education and collaborative programs. As interprofessional practice continues to evolve, instructors and health professionals are exploring innovative methods to deliver IPE programs in online medium of practice. While using online platform/medium for interprofessional learning is a laudable goal for academic institutions [6], there is extremely limited evidence on online IPE programs where clinical and non-clinical health students learn together in a team-based setting. This preparation will help students in undergraduate programs who wish to serve in clinical and/or non-clinical environments in healthcare settings. While clinical disciplines include nursing, athletic training, and other field of study, non-clinical disciplines include (but are not limited to) programs such as health administration, gerontology, social work, and public health. Inclusion of IPE programs during the first year of education will allow students to learn from each other and appreciate what team members can accomplish as a team in a complex healthcare environment.

Background

As problems posed by the COVID-19 pandemic continue to grow, it is imperative that clinical providers work in close coordination with professionals from different disciplines, departments and sectors of healthcare. Evidence suggests that patients and families experience fragmented care, especially when health professionals are unable to work as one team within healthcare settings. The consequences of failing to work effectively in a team-based setting results in increased costs, inefficiency, lower quality of care and decreased patient satisfaction. Further, failure to work as part of a team and lack of a coordinated effort may result in medical complications or even patient deaths in healthcare settings [7]. Wakely et al. (2013) conducted a study where students from several health disciplines participated in a program that incorporated interprofessional learning modules [8]. It was found that learning about various health disciplines led to improvement in student attitudes (indicated by scores on readiness for interprofessional learning scale). Sani et al. (2011) assessed changes in students' attitudes after they completed interprofessional learning module. This study reported noteworthy improvements in scores on collaboration and team work [9].

A case study conducted by Evans et al. (2012) examined the effect of inclusion of interprofessional learning modules on students who were studying dentistry and dental technology at the Griffith University. Closer analysis of results suggested that inclusion of interprofessional practices led to positive professional identity and better communication between students [10]. In a quantitative study (Evans et al., 2013), perceptions regarding roles, responsibilities, communication, and team work were compared across two student groups enrolled in dental technology programs. While one group was exposed to a program with content in interprofessional education, other group was a part of traditional program. Results indicated that exposure to interprofessional learning led to changes in attitudes and resulted in improved collaboration among students [11]. Research suggests that interprofessional education and knowledge-sharing among the different disciplines can lead to highly-coordinated, effective patient care in health care settings [12]. This, in turn, can lead to better patient outcomes, increased satisfaction for the provider, and better usage of existing resources. While there are several studies that show importance of interprofessional education programs, it is important to note that health care disciplines still operate in silos and there is a very little opportunity for students in different disciplines to learn together [13].

Research on IPE has focused on clinical programs and traditional on-campus/university based programs. Given that the COVID-19 crisis will continue, academic institutions need to explore new methods to offer IPE and prepare a next generation of leaders who are not afraid to utilize methods that could transform healthcare delivery. There is a scarcity of literature that examines how interprofessional education can be delivered using online medium of instruction [6]. With growth in online education, especially in the field of healthcare, it is important to explore opportunities where professionals from different disciplines can learn together. Using a mixed methods approach, this study aimed to examine students' readiness and attitudes towards online interprofessional education and importance of such preparation during COVID-19, a public health crisis that has resulted in more than 70 million cases and approximately 1.6 million deaths worldwide.

2. Materials and Methods

2.1. Participants and Study Design

A total of 215 students, enrolled in an undergraduate healthcare program focused on interprofessional education and learning, were invited to participate in the study. It is important to focus on undergraduate healthcare students because education/training of the majority of these students takes place in silos with a very little chance to collaborate with professionals from different disciplines. An email describing the purpose of the study was sent to all the students. In order to assess impact of IPE training, a pre and post-test methodology was used. All the students were required to complete a survey/questionnaire adapted from Readiness for Interprofessional Learning Scale (RIPLS) prior to beginning of the IPE curriculum and once they finished the IPE curriculum. Qualitative content analysis was completed to analyze students' responses recorded during IPE program. This provided direct insights into students' thoughts about collaboration and team-work as they worked in interprofessional teams. The study commenced once approval to conduct the study was obtained from the Institutional Review Board at the university.

2.2. Description of IPE Program

The entire IPE educational program was divided into five online modules. These modules were based on the core competencies outlined by Interprofessional Collaborative Practice [14]. The first module focused on introduction of participants and discussion of key concepts in the field of IPE. Student introductions were recorded and used later to form interprofessional teams needed to work on case studies.

In the second module, quality and safety concepts were discussed such as problems related to COVID-19 pandemic, medical complications, and shortage of medical staff. Instructor engaged students in conversations/topics focused on the importance of IPE and need for interprofessional team work required to treat serious COVID patients who suffer from complex medical conditions or conditions that require health care professionals from different disciples to work together.

The third module focused on roles and responsibilities of team members in clinical and administrative processes in healthcare settings. More specifically, content included readings and videos on trainings of providers, importance of engaging family and care givers in the plan of care, and scope of knowledge and abilities of team members as they work on providing safe, high quality and efficient care to patients.

The fourth module focused on the importance of communication between providers during the patient care processes especially in COVID-19 cases. The learning material allowed students to think critically about problems due to faulty communication, fragmented systems of care and adverse events that may lead to patient/resident deaths in facilities. Further, content on utilization of standardized format for communication, importance of respectful communication to patient, providers and families and several communication strategies were included.

The readings and material in the fifth module focused on the importance of team work between providers as they provide care to critical patients in healthcare facilities. Content related to the process of team development, ethical guidelines, shared decision making, problem solving and leadership practices was covered.

2.3. Interprofessional Case Studies and Assignments

The entire program included four quizzes, three discussion questions, and two case studies. While quizzes focused on basic understanding of the content, discussion questions and case studies required students to demonstrate in-depth understanding of the material. Case study and discussions focused on scenarios where providers from different disciplines worked as a team when severe cases of COVID-19 were admitted to healthcare facility, roles of providers, team-work, and collaboration. Students completed these cases and discussions via zoom meetings. Students also submitted written response to discussion question via online learning management system. Practitioners from different health disciplines, both clinical and non-clinical, were invited, electronically, to meet with students and present their point of view while dealing with COVID 19 cases.

2.4. Quantitative Study Instrument

The Readiness for Interprofessional Learning Scale (RIPLS) was used to collect data for this study. The RIPLS has gained wide acceptance amongst researchers who focus on interprofessional education and learning in healthcare. This scale consists of 19 items, divided into four different subscales. These subscales are as follows: (a) *team work and collaboration* (items 1–9), (b) *negative professional identity* (10–12), (c) *positive professional identity* (13–16), and (d) *roles and responsibilities* [15–17]. Researchers have demonstrated statistical validity of the research instrument [18]. Demographic items were added to the scale to collect information about the students.

2.5. Quantitative Data Analysis

The data analysis program, IBM SPSS 23.0 was utilized for storing data and analysis. Descriptive statistics were used to examine demographic information. For all the RIPLS subscale, items were summed and scores were calculated. T-tests (independent) were conducted to compare pre-test and post test scores.

3. Results

3.1. Results of Survey

A total of 185 students responded to the RIPLS (86.04% response rate). Approximately 73% of the participants were females. The median age of the participants was 21 years (IQR = 15) and ranged from 23 to 67 years. The median amount of time spent in their academic program was 10 months and ranged between 1 and 28 months. The participants were mainly white and non-Hispanic or Latino. The majority of the participants worked in healthcare organizations and were from health administration and nursing program (see Table 1).

Table 1. Characteristic of Sample (N = 185).

Subscale Scores	Mdn.	IQR	f(n)	%
Age (Years)	21	15		
Time in education program (Months)	10	12		
Sex				
Male			50	27
Female			135	73
Race				
White/Caucasian			142	76
Black/African American			26	14
Asian			6	3
Native Hawaiian or Pacific Islander			0	0
American Indian or Native America			3	1.6
Other			8	4.3
Ethnicity				
Hispanic or Latino			16	8.64
Non-Hispanic or Latino			169	91.35
Education Program				
Health Services Administration (HSAD)			108	58
Nursing			20	10.8
Social Work			17	9.1
Health & Medical Sciences			12	6.48
Psychology			14	7.56
Athletic Training			5	2.7
Gerontology			9	4.8
Work place				
Health care			125	67.56
Education			18	9.7
Other			42	22.7

3.2. Comparison of RIPLS Scores

Results of the RIPLS scores demonstrated that there was no significant difference between disciplines/fields of study. More specifically, scores on pre-test (Mean = 69.25 ± 10.06) were not very different from scores on post-test (Mean = 72.12 ± 9.01) across different disciplines'. The RIPLS pre-test score ranged between 67.42 ± 9.32 and 71.54 ± 7.28 with psychology scoring the lowest among the disciplines and athletic training scoring the highest. RIPLS pre-test score for Health Administration was lower than athletic training and health and medical science students. The pre-test score of social work students was lower than health administration students.

The RIPLS post test scores ranged between 68.42 ± 9.34 and 71.94 ± 8.62. There were improvements in groups of students who were from health administration, psychology, and nursing programs. Further, students in gerontology, health and medical sciences and social work demonstrated increase in their post-test scores (see Table 2).

Table 2. Comparison of Scores.

Education Program	Pre-Test Scores (Mean ± SD)	Post-Test Scores (Mean ± SD)	p Value
Health Administration	69.25 ± 8.42	70.24 ± 9.64	0.73
Nursing	67.42 ± 9.32	70.68 ± 9.21	0.68
Social Work	68.21 ± 8.63	68.42 ± 9.34	0.83
Health and Medical Sciences	70.21 ± 8.34	70.12 ± 8.68	0.50
Psychology	66.54 ± 9.45	69.32 ± 9.67	0.64
Athletic Training	71.54 ±7.28	71.94 ± 8.62	0.76
Gerontology	69.41 ± 9.48	70.42 ± 8.54	0.89

3.3. Online Discussions and Qualitative Data Analysis

Online open-ended discussion questions were included as one of the data sources for the study. These open-ended questions allowed students to express their own thoughts. Response time and the amount of text was not restricted and these questions enabled students to explain themselves freely [19] and describe how they felt about teamwork, communication, and shared learning especially during the public health crisis. This can be extremely hard to achieve when questionnaires or surveys are used. Researchers made every effort to reduce bias and did not influence participants' responses. The students were asked to describe (1) how interprofessional education and team work can be used to enhance patient safety and care for patients suffering with COVID-19, (2) their perceptions regarding how members of interprofessional teams strive to work on clinically complex cases and (3) the importance of awareness of team members' roles and communication between members while caring for COVID-19 cases.

An inductive approach using content analysis was utilized to conduct the analysis of participants' discussion posts. A total of seven hundred and thirty six posts were analyzed. Content analysis allows researchers to examine participants' responses by carefully coding and finding themes in the collected data. It is noteworthy that content analysis has been widely utilized on written texts irrespective of the data collection approach. The principal investigator of the study hired two research assistants to perform data analysis of the study. Both the assistants were trained in research methods and had prior experience in working on qualitative research projects. Upon completion of open coding, researchers independently created codes, subcategories, generic categories, and main categories. Once individual data analysis was completed, the team met to discuss data analysis and reach to final consensus on categories and results [19,20]. The summary of findings are reported here.

3.4. Result of Qualitative Content Analysis

The final analysis resulted in generation of 38 codes, 15 sub categories, six generic categories and three main categories. The main categories were (1) IPE increases awareness of team members' roles and enhances collaboration (2) Increased communication and cohesion among members of teams is critical during the pandemic (3) IPE can lead to better care for COVID-19 patients (See Table 3)

Table 3. Categories.

Category 1	Category 2	Category 3
Awareness of roles and collaboration	Communication and cohesion	Better care for patients

3.4.1. IPE Increases Awareness of Team Members' Roles and Enhances Collaboration

Interprofessional education and experience as part of a diverse healthcare team allows team members to learn about roles and responsibilities of different practitioners. This allows team members to break past professional barriers and build more collaborative infrastructure.

One of the students noted:

"Increased communication and training on how to collaborate with other departments/specialties, outside facilities, and better communication between provider and patients would be the most significant methods and approaches to increased patient safety and satisfaction."

Using complex COVID cases as example, another student noted, "IPE leads to better communication between different departments in a facility, its affiliated clinics, and between providers and patients. It also makes it easier to forward information to outside facilities or other hospital companies (with appropriate patient authorization). This allows for more of a "whole person" treatment plan vs. segmented treatment plans from each department. Everyone can see what has been done, is currently being done, and what hasn't been tried yet."

Furthermore, another participant indicated:

"One unique feature of the interprofessional education is that the professionals working together are expected to not only be an expert in their own field, but to understand the basics of the disciplines they work with. By understanding the basics of disciplines beyond their own, they can better understand a patient's condition, and this contributes information to paint a better picture of how to help a patient, leading to better results and better quality."

Participants indicated that knowing both one's role and place amidst the team is an important attribute, as well. By understanding their responsibilities to the team, a professional can fulfill their role effectively and take responsibility for their actions. The shared identity of a team is another key component for success. Being able to trust and work with one another is essential for providing patient care in an efficient manner.

Another student clearly stated "the balance between the two is perhaps the most important; knowing when one's role overlaps another, and what matters they should or should not get involved with. Further, making sure the information they are relaying to the team is relevant and will assist other professionals in their jobs."

Adding to this claim, a student who works as nurse mentioned "in midst of pandemic, I have seen that team members are so rushed and may not demonstrate knowledge of how team works as a cohesive unit. Although each discipline is knowledgeable about their individual role, they are not knowledgeable of other roles and there is a lack of coordination and collaboration. This gap could lead to a delay in the length of stay, errors in communication, and even in safety for the patient."

As students completed the IPE program, they clearly indicated that when there is an interprofessional team approach, each discipline works in parallel to the other and crosses over with collaboration and coordination to meet the needs of the patient. This might look like bedside huddles, situational awareness of the whole person and environment, and a well-coordinated series of tasks that feel very safe and flowing to the patient. The patient and caregivers will feel confident in the care of the team and this will increase satisfaction.

3.4.2. Increased Communication and Cohesion among Members of Teams Is Critical during the Pandemic

Students described that IPE leads to an increase in communication and cohesion among team members. This results in improved care for patients and families dealing with COVID-19 crisis.

For example, a student who worked as a nursing home administrator indicated that "communication between healthcare teams is super important when it comes to safety and collaboration. In health care the goal is to care for patients which includes keeping them safe. With interprofessional education/practice we can increase the safety of the patients by all of the nurses, doctors, surgeons, etc. involved with them updating each other on the patient. Some patients have a long journey of medical problems when they are admitted to the facility and having all the care providers working together will ensure them that they know what they are doing."

Another student reemphasized how a patient suffering with a COVID-19 problem will need to interact with doctors, nurses, long term care workers, pharmacists, physical therapists, and a whole host of other team members throughout the process. The student further added *"if this team of care providers have effective communication and collaboration between them the patient will receive better, more effective quality care. Training health care professionals with different backgrounds and areas of focus to work together and collaborate is where interprofessional learning and education can play a major role. Interprofessional education is when students from different care professions learn from and with each other to improve patient care."*

Students used various examples to explain their points. One example that is worth noting is the infection control nurse's role which includes the responsibility for policies/procedures that keep staff, visitors, and patients safe. This student added *"one staff member cannot do it all. These committees arise to complete a task or tasks that one individual could not do on their own. An example of working together is implementation of a policy for patient safety during the current pandemic. Upon arrival to the clinic, masks are passed out to patients who are symptomatic, and they are brought back to be treated quickly to help stop the spread of the virus. Team members have to develop a process through collaboration. They then have to implement it to other staff members through education. Not one person alone can develop a policy that doesn't affect others around them; interprofessional communication/teamwork is necessary in any healthcare setting."*

3.4.3. IPE Can Lead to Better Care for COVID-19 Patients

Students recognized the effect of the COVID-19 crisis on healthcare system including personal lives of patients, care providers, and professionals who work in public health and data collection. Students called for collaboration and better training to improve the response to emergency situations such as the current pandemic. To avoid adverse events which could lead to deaths, students felt the need for IPE programs where professionals from multiple disciplines can collaborate and work as a part of team.

For instance, a public health nurse indicated:

"Interprofessional education can help in dealing with challenges related to the pandemic especially when researchers and data analysts work with providers of clinical services. This would allow us to better plan, prioritize who needs urgent care, coordinate care, identify and deal with gaps and avoid duplication of services. We can use data to identify population with chronic diseases and others who are more vulnerable to the problem"

Students mentioned how IPE can help in building trust and establishing clear lines of communication between members of the patient care team and families. Supporting this claim, a student in Social Work mentioned *"IPE can help in providing foundation for our response. Important relationships between acute care providers, public health professionals, data collection people, and skilled nursing facilities needs to be built. We should make efforts to understand the needs of the community and then focus our attention on the section of community that needs urgent attention."*

Students expressed themselves freely and used personal examples to demonstrate that they have seen applications of IPE when their relatives were admitted to the hospital. For example, one of the students indicated that *"interprofessional team not only provided assistance to the patient but they worked collaboratively together to come up with a care plan which best fit our needs. They would meet regularly to compare notes and come up with a schedule of care that would benefit the patient. They were so clear about what they were doing and acted quickly when our patient was admitted."*

Corroborating previous statements and participants response, another student who works in a frontline position at an acute care hospital mentioned that *"you'd much rather have a team of professionals working together than to just have one doctor try to do all the work and fail. A patient is more likely to feel assured when they see a group of health care professionals collaborating to find a solution. That patient will be satisfied and content with the care they are receiving due to the collaboration."*

4. Discussion

Interprofessional collaboration and communication in healthcare has been shown to improve patient outcomes [21]. It is expected that including experience and practice in interprofessional practice during the professionals' education leads to more successful interprofessional collaboration in practice. This interprofessional education lays the groundwork for effective practice.

Research has shown that the setting for learning is critical [21]. Ideally, these educational experiences happen in a face to face, live simulation experience with a mixture of professional practice students, guided by expert educators/practitioners. Research has shown that students' learning improves as carefully developed interdisciplinary simulations mimic reality closely [22]. However, in the current state of COVID-19 restrictions, live experiences in simulation or a clinical setting may not be easy to perform. At the same time, interprofessional collaboration has never been more important. An alternative educational format becomes necessary to accomplish the outcome of practice professionals entering the clinical arena with interprofessional communication and collaboration skills.

Online education provides access to programs for many working professionals, especially those distant from the educational setting or unable to attend 'class' due to work schedules or other constraints. Indeed, much of higher and professional education has moved to online settings, even prior to the advent of COVID. With the arrival of the pandemic, a great majority of coursework and clinical experiences pivoted rapidly into an online delivery methodology. Usage of e-learning tools has not been consistent across different health profession programs and countries [23]. Recent studies suggested that inclusion of mobile applications and virtual hospitals were well received by students [23–25]. It has also been suggested that if used correctly, e-learning can enhance teaching and learning methods in clinical programs [23]. The questions then become whether IPE can be done in an online setting, and whether it is effective in practitioner development.

This study provides important insight into the opportunities that online asynchronous education offers for healthcare students' understanding of their interprofessional roles. Both quantitative and qualitative methodologies were utilized. Use of a mixed-methods approach may address the 'what' and 'how' of an IPE intervention and its outcomes [21].

This online IPE program focused on four areas: key concepts in the field of IPE, quality and safety, roles and responsibilities of the various providers, and the importance of communication and teamwork. Several different health-related majors were represented by the enrolled students, which is consistent with professional practice. A variety of educational tools including quizzes, discussion questions, and case studies, are reflected in this mixed methods study.

The quantitative Readiness for Interprofessional Learning Scale (RIPLS) found that students clearly reflected the positive outcomes of IPE, even in the online setting. Qualitatively, students responded to discussion questions and described that:

(1) IPE increases awareness of team members' roles and enhances collaboration

(2) Increased communication and cohesion among members of teams is critical during the pandemic and
(3) IPE can lead to better care for COVID-19 patients.

These RIPLS quantitative results and qualitative student perspectives provide optimism that IPE can be learned effectively in an online environment, which will be critical moving forward as healthcare aims to improve care through interprofessional collaboration, even in an online, asynchronous environment. This study is unique in that the students were entirely online during a pandemic and represented a variety of healthcare roles. More work needs to be done to expand the understanding of the most effective online teaching/learning tools. Follow up with program graduates will be significant as they move into their professional positions.

5. Limitations

Because many students were working in healthcare and other institutions, they did not check their university email regularly. As a result, faculty members struggled to reach out to students and communicate in a timely fashion. This program was offered at a single academic institution located in the Midwest US. While findings and methodology can be utilized at other institutions, these findings may not be generalizable across the US or the globe. COVID-19 pandemic academic management posed additional problems for the implementation of the program. It was hard to invite healthcare practitioners to the class as they were extremely busy in dealing with COVID cases in their roles. As online education in healthcare disciplines continue to grow, more research is needed that can explore students attitudes towards online IPE program across several university campuses.

6. Conclusions

The aim of this mixed method study was to examine attitudes and readiness towards interprofessional education and significance of this preparation during the pandemic. Findings suggest that students from both clinical and non-clinical programs valued opportunities for learning together and felt that IPE enhances awareness of team members' roles and responsibilities and improves collaboration. Participants further suggested that IPE increases communication and cohesion, and results in better care of patients' which is extremely important while working with COVID patients. Further studies across medical centers and academic settings are needed to explore attitudes of students towards IPE programs. Inclusion of different education settings and additional clinical and non-clinical programs not currently represented in the study sample will allow better understanding of IPE especially while working with patients during public health crisis.

Author Contributions: Conceptualization, J.S.; methodology, J.S.; software, J.S.; validation, J.S., B.M.; formal analysis, J.S.; investigation, J.S.; resources, J.S.; data curation, J.S.; visualization, J.S.; supervision, J.S.; project administration, J.S. All authors have read and agreed to the published version of the manuscript.

Funding: This research received no external funding.

Institutional Review Board Statement: The study was conducted according to the guidelines of the Declaration of Helsinki, and approved by the Institutional Review Board of Minnesota State University Moorhead.

Informed Consent Statement: Informed consent was obtained from all subjects involved in the study.

Data Availability Statement: Data available on request due to restrictions.

Conflicts of Interest: The authors declare no conflict of interest.

References

1. Center for the Advancement of Interprofessional Education. The Definition and Principles of Interprofessional Education. Available online: http://caipe.org.uk/about-us/the-definitionand-principles-of-interprofessional-education/ (accessed on 1 January 2021).
2. Farup, P.G. Are measurements of patient safety culture and adverse Events Valid and reliable? Results from a cross sectional study. *BMC Health Serv. Res.* **2015**, *15*, 186. [CrossRef] [PubMed]
3. Mitchell, P.; Wynia, M.; Golden, R.; McNellis, B.; Okun, S.; Webb, C.E.; Von Kohorn, I. Core Principles & Values of Effective Team-Based Health Care. Available online: https://www.nationalahec.org/pdfs/VSRT-Team-Based-Care-Principles-Values.pdf (accessed on 11 May 2021).
4. World Health Organization. Framework for Action on Interprofessional Education & Collaborative Practice. Geneva: World Health Organization. Available online: http://whqlibdoc.who.int/hq/2010/WHO_HRH_HPN_10.3_eng.pdf (accessed on 11 May 2021).
5. Young, H.M.; Siegel, E.O.; McCormick, W.C.; Fulmer, T.; Harootyan, L.K.; Dorr, D.A. Interdisciplinary collaboration in geriatrics: Advancing health for older adults. *Nurs. Outlook* **2011**, *59*, 243–250. [CrossRef] [PubMed]
6. Solomon, P.; Baptitste, S.; Hall, P.; Luke, R.; Orchard, C.; Rukholm, E.; Damiani-Taraba, G. Students' Perceptions of Interprofessional Learning through Facilitated Online Learning Modules. *Med. Teach.* **2010**, *32*, e391–e398. Available online: https://www.atsu.edu/pdf/student_perceptions_of_interprofessional_learning.pdf (accessed on 11 May 2021). [CrossRef] [PubMed]
7. Miller, R.; Scherpbier, N.; van Amsterdam, L.; Guedes, V.; Pype, P. Inter-professional education and primary care: EFPC position paper. *Prim. Health Care Res. Dev.* **2019**, *20*, e138. [CrossRef] [PubMed]
8. Wakely, L.; Brown, L.; Burrows, J. Evaluating interprofessional learning modules: Health students' attitudes to interprofessional practice. *J. Interprof. Care* **2013**, *27*, 424–425. [CrossRef] [PubMed]
9. Saini, B.; Shah, S.; Keary, P.; Bosnic-Anticevich, S.; Grootjans, J.; Armour, C. Instructional design and assessment: An interprofessional learning module on asthma health promotion. *Am. J. Pharm. Educ.* **2011**, *75*, 201–208. [CrossRef] [PubMed]
10. Evans, J.; Henderson, A.; Johnson, N.W. Interprofessional learning enhances knowledge of roles but is less able to shift attitudes: A case study from dental education. *Eur. J. Dent. Educ.* **2012**, *16*, 239–245. [CrossRef] [PubMed]
11. Evans, J.; Henderson, A.; Johnson, N.W. Traditional and Interprofessional Curricula for Dental Technology: Perceptions of Students in Two Programs in Australia. *J. Dent. Educ.* **2013**, *77*, 1225–1236. Available online: http://www.jdentaled.org/content/77/9/1225.full?sid=8a28bd98-1cc7-4c6e-8de1-5d91f1ffd90b (accessed on 11 May 2021). [CrossRef] [PubMed]
12. Doherty, R.B.; Crowley, R.A. Principles supporting dynamics of clinical care team: An American college of physicians position paper. *Ann. Intern. Med.* **2013**, *159*, 620–626. [CrossRef] [PubMed]
13. Chan, L.K.; Ganotice, F.; Wong, F.K.Y.; Lau, C.S.; Bridges, S.M.; Chan, C.H.Y.; Yum, T.P. Implementation of an interprofessional team-based learning program involving seven undergraduate health and social care programs from two universities, and students' evaluation of their readiness for interprofessional learning. *BMC Med. Educ.* **2017**, *17*, 221. [CrossRef] [PubMed]
14. IPEC. Core Competencies for Interprofessional Collaborative Practice. 2016. Available online: https://hsc.unm.edu/ipe/resources/index.html (accessed on 11 May 2021).
15. Hertweck, M.L.; Hawkins, S.R.; Bednarek, M.L.; Goreczny, A.J.; Schreiber, J.L.; Sterrett, S.E. Attitudes toward inter-professional education: Comparing physician assistant and other health care professions students. *J. Phys. Assist. Educ.* **2012**, *23*, 8–15. [CrossRef]
16. Wilhelmsson, M.; Ponzer, S.; Dahlgren, L.O.; Timpka, T.; Faresjö, T. Are female students in general and nursing students more ready for teamwork and interprofessional collaboration in healthcare? *BMC Med. Educ.* **2011**, *11*, 15. [CrossRef] [PubMed]
17. Singh, J.; Salisbury, H. Attitudes and Perceptions of Non- Clinical Health Care Students Towards Interprofessional Learning. *Health Interprof. Pract. Educ.* **2019**, *3*, eP1179. [CrossRef]
18. Reid, R.; Bruce, D.; Allstaff, K.; McLernon, D. Validating the Readiness for Interprofessional Learning Scale (RIPLS) in the postgraduate context: Are health care professionals ready for IPL? *Med. Educ.* **2006**, *40*, 415–422. [CrossRef]
19. Lovric, R.; Farcic, N.; Miksic, S.; Vcev, A. Studying during the COVID-19 pandemic: A qualitative inductive content analysis of nursing students' perceptions and experiences. *Educ. Sci.* **2020**, *10*, 188. [CrossRef]
20. Bengtsson, M. How to plan and perform a qualitative study using content analysis. *Nurs. Plus. Open* **2016**, *2*, 8–14. [CrossRef]
21. Measuring the Impact of Interprofessional Education on Collaborative Practice and Patient Outcomes. Available online: https://www.ncbi.nlm.nih.gov/books/NBK338360/ (accessed on 11 May 2021).
22. Bryant, K.; Aebersold, M.L.; Jeffries, P.R.; Kardong-Edgren, S. Innovations in simulation: Nursing leaders' exchange of best practices. *Clin. Simul. Nurs.* **2020**, *41*, 33–40. [CrossRef]
23. Varvara, G.; Bernardi, S.; Bianchi, S.; Sinjari, B.; Piattelli, M. Dental Education Challenges during the COVID-19 Pandemic Period in Italy: Undergraduate Student Feedback, Future Perspectives, and the Needs of Teaching Strategies for Professional Development. *Healthcare* **2021**, *9*, 454. [CrossRef] [PubMed]
24. Mladenovic, R.; Bukumiric, Z.; Mladenovic, K. Influence of a dedicated mobile application on studying traumatic dental injuries during student isolation. *J. Dent. Educ.* **2020**, 1–3. [CrossRef] [PubMed]
25. Stoopler, E.T.; Tanaka, T.I.; Sollecito, T.P. Hospital-based dental externship during COVID-19 pandemic: Think virtual! *Spec. Care Dent.* **2020**, *40*, 393–394. [CrossRef] [PubMed]

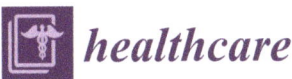

Article

Experiences of Pathology Course among Hospital Management Graduates

Jung Hee Park [1], Woo Sok Han [2], Jinkyung Kim [2] and Hyunjung Lee [3,*]

[1] Department of Emergency Medical Service, Konyang University, Daejeon 35365, Korea; jhpug@konyang.ac.kr
[2] Department of Hospital Management, Konyang University, Daejeon 35365, Korea; wshan@konyang.ac.kr (W.S.H.); jkim@konyang.ac.kr (J.K.)
[3] College of Nursing, Konyang University, Daejeon 35365, Korea
* Correspondence: leehj18@konyang.ac.kr; Tel.:+82-42-600-8584

Abstract: The purpose of this study was to explore hospital management graduates' experience in pathology courses. Data were gathered through four focus group interviews by 16 hospital management graduates who attended pathology courses. Data were collected from June to August, 2020. Conventional content analysis was used for data analysis. Six categories were extracted that described hospital management graduates' experience in pathology courses, as follows: "Suggestions for the curriculum," "Students' preference for pathology professor," "Demands for various teaching methods," "Broad and difficult class content," "Recognition of pathology courses during college years," and "The importance of studying the pathology course realized after graduation." The findings suggest that it is important to identify hospital management graduates' perspectives to improve pathology curriculum in the educational process. Additionally, it is necessary to continuously connect educational and practical environments for the effective management of pathology courses.

Keywords: hospital management; pathology; qualitative study

1. Introduction

The department of hospital management encourages and trains professionals in the field of health administration by teaching theories and practices that are essential for the effective management of different health care organizations, with an emphasis on basic medical education [1]. Students majoring in hospital management build their careers in the health and medical industry, and most of the graduates are employed in medical institutions. Different departments associated with health administration, such as the department of public health, department of health care management, department of health administration, department of health policy, and department of hospital management, follow a similar curriculum. In South Korea, since the 1980s, health administration departments have distributed their curriculum over four-year bachelor courses at colleges, demonstrating how four-year-course college departments are gradually subdividing and specializing in accordance with the current trends and the social demand [2].

Currently, with the advancement of information technology, life science, and genetics, the medical industry is rapidly changing [3]. Thus, practitioners in the field of health administration are expected to show multiple competencies such as basic medical knowledge, knowledge about the systems used in the medical field, operation, and management skills [1]. The primary duties assigned to health administration majors in medical institutions include medical records and insurance reviews alongside computerized data management, hospital administration, planning and public relations, human resources, supplies, and the general administration of the hospital. As such, it is necessary to cultivate professionalism that can be used in overall work related to hospital management. Previous study findings revealed that the level of satisfaction among college students majoring in health administration had a positive correlation with career preparation and decisions [2,4,5], and the level of satisfaction with the curriculum of their major had a significant effect on becoming qualified and employed in the respective fields [6]. Therefore, colleges with four-year-courses offering majors in hospital management include classes on basic medical fields such as anatomy, pathology, and physiology in their curriculum; this aids in strengthening the competencies of students majoring in hospital management [7,8]. Additionally, the department of health administration belongs to the colleges of health or medical science, with the department of hospital management. Furthermore, it was found that basic medical education, including pathology, was chiefly taught by professors majoring in basic medicine or nursing [1,4]. Previous studies on basic medicine have largely focused on students majoring in nursing or medical engineering [9]; however, there have been very few studies on the effectiveness of basic medicine as a subject for departments related to health administration. This gap may have occurred due to the lack of importance given to basic medicine compared to other subjects. However, this subject is central because students from the department of hospital management are often employed in fields relevant to medicine; therefore, they need to have knowledge about diseases to enable seamless communication with other medical workers and to understand patients. In addition, hospital management graduates can be put into overall hospital management-related tasks. Since medical knowledge is required to support the work of healthcare workers, the awareness of the importance of pathology is increasing in clinical practice [1,3]. However, the hospital management department belongs to the college of health sciences or medical sciences, which focus on hospital management, health insurance claims, administration, and statistics rather than professional knowledge in medicine. To that end, both professors and students have difficulties in teaching and studying pre-clinical medical classes such as pathology and anatomy [6]. The results of overall course evaluations, which are customarily done at the university level, have only shown a formal quantitative score and have limitations in understanding students' needs. Thus, more in-depth exploration was required. Moreover, it is important to understand the students' educational needs and implement effective instructional strategies to promote competencies among learners [6,9]. Therefore, with the rapid development in the multidisciplinary field of medicine, it is essential to examine the pathology course curriculum from the perspective of students majoring in hospital management.

The ADDIE (Analysis, Design, Development, Implementation, and Evaluation) model, which structures the teaching–learning planning in different stages (analysis, design, development, implementation, and evaluation) [10], enables educators to create programs using a systematic approach designed to meet learner's needs. Thus, this study aimed to thoroughly understand the experience of students attending pathology courses who are majoring in hospital management; this study conducted focus group interviews and analyzed the results to serve as basic data for the effective management of pathology courses by reflecting on the perspectives of the graduates.

2. Materials and Methods

2.1. Study Design

This phenomenological qualitative study aimed to obtain insights into the essence of hospital management graduates' experiences by vividly describing the experiences of a pathology course in at Konyang University.

2.2. Participants

Participants were recruited in this study by posting a recruitment notice on an online portal with an active audience of hospital administration graduates. Graduates who agreed to participate in the research further introduced the researchers to their colleagues. The inclusion criteria for the participants of this study were: (1) those who had majored in hospital administration, (2) those who had attended pathology courses when enrolled in hospital administration, (3) those who had graduated in the last five years, and (4) those who were employed in fields relevant to their major. A total of 16 individuals met all the inclusion criteria and provided informed consent to participate in the study. It is recommended to conduct three or more focus groups with four to six participants in each to extract and obtain reliable data [11,12]. Therefore, participants were divided into four groups as per their workplace (medical records office group, hospital administration group, hospital office group of the same university hospital, and insurance company group) to ensure the homogeneity of participants and free flowing discussions in each group (Table 1).

Table 1. General characteristics of study participants (N = 16).

	Participant	Age (Years)	Sex	Degree	Working Experience
	1	25	F	Bachelor	3 years
L	2	25	F	Master	3 years
	3	26	M	Bachelor	2 years
	4	26	F	Bachelor	4 years
	1	27	F	Bachelor	4 years
P	2	26	M	Bachelor	1 years
	3	26	F	Bachelor	2 years
	4	27	F	Bachelor	1 years
	1	26	F	Master	3 years
K	2	24	F	Bachelor	1 years
	3	24	F	Bachelor	1 years
	4	23	F	Bachelor	1 years
	1	23	F	Bachelor	1 years
H	2	23	F	Bachelor	1 years
	3	27	M	Bachelor	2 years
	4	24	F	Bachelor	1 years

L: medical records office team; P: Insurance company team; K: hospital administration team; H: hospital office team.

2.3. Interviews

The questions were formed in accordance with the format recommendations of Krueger and Casey; our interview questionnaire comprised an opening question, introductory questions, transitional questions, main questions, and a closing question in an open-ended question format [11,12]. The questions were reviewed by a qualitative research expert before the final completion to ensure that their content did not deviate from the research investigation. The overall purpose of the interview was to obtain an answer to "How was your experience of taking pathology courses while in school?" Other questions are shown in Table 2.

2.4. Data Collection

Qualitative research uses the principle of "appropriacy" for sampling; therefore, it is important to select participants who can provide the most relevant information about the research topic and objective [13]. Focus group interviews, in particular, enable a broader understanding of the research topic since intensive conversations among participants with common characteristics generate detailed research material [11,12]. Thus, four interviewees were assigned to each group to facilitate effective conversation management and enable participants to freely express their feelings.

Table 2. Questions for this study.

Opening Question	Please Share Your Experience of the Pathology Courses You Attended While You Were in College.
Introductory questions	Please share the satisfying experiences you had during the course.
	Please share the unsatisfying experiences you had during the course.
	Please share about any difficulties you had during the course.
Transitional questions	Do you think taking pathology classes helped you with your current job?
	Please share your overall experience at your professor's lectures.
	Please share your overall experience at your pathology courses curriculum
Closing question	Please share anything you may want to mention.

Focus groups were led by skilled moderators experienced in qualitative research and familiar with the scope of this research. The first author attended most of the focus groups. If this was not possible for logistic reasons, another co-author familiar with the interview protocol took over. The data collection period was from 25 July to 15 August 2020, and the interviews were conducted in a quiet and comfortable location as per the participants' convenience and availability. There were two times of interview at each group, approximately 1 h and 1 h and 20 min long for each session, and participants were notified of the topic and questions of the study prior to the interview. Data collection was finished after second interview when no new information was generated from the interviews; therefore, data from 4 previously selected groups with 16 participants were finally included.

2.5. Data Analysis

The data transcribed by two assistant researchers were analyzed based on the consensual qualitative research (CQR) developed by Hill et al. [14]. The analysis followed an in-depth process. First, the researchers repeatedly listened to the recorded interviews, accurately transcribed the interviews, and then reviewed the participant protocols several times to identify and understand the underlying emotions throughout the interviews. Second, the researchers recorded the initial feelings experienced by the participants, the first thoughts that occurred to them, and the initial analysis of the data, and then they generated codes for their statements. Third, the researchers conducted a detailed discussion to record sub-themes for core factors of the responses; additionally, the extracted sub-themes were combined to form clusters of themes with similar contents, and these theme clusters were grouped into domains. Throughout the entire data analysis process, the researchers met several times and continuously contacted each other to compare, discuss, and agree on the data analyzed by each of them. In addition, to evaluate the appropriateness of the extracted codes, sub-themes, and theme clusters, the process was repeated to reconfirm and revise the original statements. Researchers proceeded with the analysis immediately after the data were collected, and repeatedly interviewed the participants until there was no new content in the following interviews. Once the statements, concepts, and themes started to appear repeatedly in the data analysis, the process was deemed to have reached theoretical saturation. The first and co-authors separately coded and analyzed the data, and the corresponding author supervised this process.

Data were sent to the participants via e-mail after analysis and reporting to identify their accuracy with the participants' experiences and to improve the credibility of the study; furthermore, participant feedback was obtained for this purpose. In order to maintain neutrality, the researchers conducted an extensive literature review on the research subject, and all judgments were reserved throughout the process to avoid researchers' prejudice or bias as much as possible.

2.6. Pre-Understanding

The researchers of this study were professors who have experience in teaching pathology courses, in addition to clinical and hospital administration experience at university hospitals. They have continuously participated in seminars to conduct qualitative studies, explored and discussed qualitative research methods, and developed their capabilities for qualitative research. Moreover, a mentor professor provided general guidance on qualitative research performance over the course of this study. In addition, the corresponding author of this study studied qualitative research in graduate school, conducted qualitative research for the last five years, and published it in academic journals.

2.7. Ethical Considerations

This study was approved by the Institutional Review Board of Konyang University, which the authors were affiliated prior to data collection (IRB No 2020-096-01). Participants were informed about withdrawing their participation at any time during the study with no disadvantages, and their consent was obtained to record the interview. The audio files and transcripts of the recordings were coded to prevent the identification of the participants' identities, and separate unique numbers were assigned. Documents were stored in a document storage box with a lock, and they were discarded using a shredder after the completion of the study.

3. Results

A total of 232 meaningful statements were extracted from the original data provided by the 16 participants. We extracted two broad content areas: (1) regarding course management and (2) regarding the learners. These areas were further classified into six theme clusters and 12 themes (Table 3).

Table 3. Area, theme clusters, and themes of hospital management graduates' pathology course experiences.

Area	Theme Clusters	Themes
Course management	Suggestions for the curriculum	The need to assign relevant courses The necessity to understand the educational level and needs of students
	Students' preference for pathology professor	Desire to learn before or after the clinical practice Professor with extensive hospital clinical experience Professor who interacts with students and teaches in a way that students can easily learn
	Demands for various teaching methods	Memorable case-based, role-play classes Boring lecture-style classes
	Broad and difficult class content	Excessive amount of learning content Difficulties in concentrating on basic medical content
The learners	Recognition of pathology courses during college years	Lack of motivation to learn The memorization subject participants wanted to give up
	The importance of studying the pathology course realized after graduation	Coming to know that pathology is an important course that is helpful in clinical practice Helpful in obtaining a major-related qualification

3.1. Area: Course Management

The course management area included four theme clusters: "Suggestions for the curriculum," "Students' preference for pathology professor," "Demands for various teaching methods," and "Broad and difficult content." Participants provided their opinions based on their personal experience of the pathology course.

3.1.1. Theme Cluster: Suggestions for the Curriculum

This theme cluster was composed of three themes: "the need to assign relevant courses," "the necessity to understand the educational level and needs of students," and "the desire to learn before or after the hospital placement." The participants shared their subjective experiences and existing difficulties with the curriculum.

Theme: The Need to Assign Relevant Courses

Participants frequently experienced the need to study the relevant material prior to attending these classes due to the use of technical terminology and unfamiliar diseases in the pathology course. It was also considered necessary to learn by sequentially assigning the pathology course and subjects relevant to pathology courses to help with education in pathology, which was considered difficult to learn.

"I think it would be better to study (pathology) together with a field or part such as pharmacology or anatomical physiology, and ... such subjects will be more beneficial, so I think it will be more beneficial if pathology was studied together during the semester that pharmacology or anatomical physiology is studied." (H3)

Theme: The Necessity to Understand the Educational Level and Needs of Students

Pathology is an unfamiliar area of study for these students and provides basic medical knowledge. Therefore, participants hoped to learn smoothly without difficulties by being taught at an eye-level; they wanted the professors to consider the students' educational level while teaching. In addition, participants suggested that understanding the educational needs of the students will help in establishing an in-depth course for students who wish to learn in-depth contents in accordance with the diverse interests and concerns of the pathology course.

"Because the professor teaches from a completely different background of knowledge from us, when we are trying to accept the content, um ... I thought it would have been good if the professor could explain it more easily and extensively." (P4)

"For students who want to learn pathology even during their undergraduate years because they find it fun, this would be an opportunity for them to choose... so, if there is an opportunity to receive the education then I think the students who want to study further could do so and use it in their future somehow." (L1)

Theme: Desire to Learn before or after the Clinical Practice

The participants' opinions about the study period of the pathology course varied. Several participants had hoped to learn pathology during the second or third year in order to ensure practical application during their clinical practice in hospitals. Participants generally agreed that pathology courses had a positive influence on clinical practice at hospitals.

"I think the semester students can usually focus is around the second year. I don't think there will be a lot to do for employment or to attain other qualifications, so I think it would be good to learn intensively before the clinical practice." (H3)

"Now that I have completed the clinical practice, I think learning in the first semester of the third year and then immediately following it with clinical practice would be a good idea." (P1)

3.1.2. Theme Cluster: The Pathology Professor the Students Want

This theme cluster consisted of two themes: "the professor with extensive hospital clinical experience" and "the professor who interacts with students and teaches in a way that students can easily learn." Participants presented their opinions about the characteristics they desired in their professors based on their experiences and impressions formed during classes.

Theme: Professor with Extensive Hospital Clinical Experience

In accordance with the unfamiliarity and difficulty of the pathology course, students desired a professor who could help them easily understand the topic. Professors, who taught using their real-life clinical experiences and case studies, engaged the students' interest in a fun and memorable way during the pathology course.

> "The vivid experiences of the clinical field encountered through the professors enriched the pathology course memories." (K4)

> "We are now graduating and moving forward because the professor gave lectures to us while working in the hospital field and ... professors are normally employed in hospitals or insurance companies, which enables us to hear a lot about the direct experiences that they had while working, so ... that helped a lot." (P4)

Theme: Professor Who Interacts with Students and Teaches in a Way That Students Can Easily Learn

Since pathology was a difficult subject, learners reflected their positive experience with professors based on the highest learning effect. Participants positively evaluated those professors who usually attempted to interact with students, and their efforts subsequently led to high learning outcomes.

> "The professor asked the students if anyone had ever suffered a disease, and how and where they were sick. The professor asked a lot of questions like this, so I think that helped a lot learn intensively before the pathology was conducted pleasant classes, which ... was a good method." (H1)

3.1.3. Theme Cluster: Demands for Various Teaching Methods

This theme cluster consisted of two themes: "memorable case-based role-play classes" and "boring lecture-style classes." The participants desired learner-centered teaching methods based on their previous learning experience.

Theme: Memorable Case-Based Role-Play Classes

In terms of learning methods, participants wanted learner-centered class plans conducted through various mediums that were easy to approach and participate in.

> "It is good when they give case scenarios and give some time to think about the examinations or diagnosis ... ". (L2)

> "It wasn't just lectures, but we were grouped together we were given a disease each and did something like a role play. So, I think it was good that I was able to learn and understand more specifically about the disease while directly participating in the role play, in addition to the theoretical part of the disease ... ". (P1)

> "We did something like a role-play in the last class of pathology. Each group was assigned the name of a disease and played the roles of a doctor, a patient, and a nurse for such situation. It was followed by an evaluation, and I wondered why we were doing such a thing back then. Looking back now, I think that was what helped me." (L4)

Theme: Boring Lecture-Style Classes

In general, there were many negative evaluations for lecture-style classes (professor-centered).

> "When I listened to the lecture, had to wrote it down without thinking, so I became much less attentive and ... just listening to lectures was not suitable for me". (L2)

> "I wasn't able to concentrate due to um ... incomprehensive terminology and boring lecture ... ". (K2)

3.1.4. Theme Cluster: Broad and Difficult Class Content

This theme cluster consisted of two themes. "excessive amount of learning content" and "difficulties in concentrating on basic medical content." The participants had various content requirements based on their current employment, and they wanted practical contents that could be applied to their job duties.

Theme: Excessive amount of Learning Content

Participants' primary memory of the pathology classes was the difficulty faced due to the unfamiliarity and large proportion of the curriculum. The excessiveness of the content was especially higher for liberal arts students who were completely unaware of basic medicine.

> "There were too many disease to learn and memorize." (H1)

> "It was difficult because the amount of study was too much compared to other subjects." (K4)

Theme: Difficulties in Concentrating on Basic Medical Content

Participants complained about difficulties in concentrating during the classes due to the use of unfamiliar and technical pathological terminology of pathology, which is starkly different from those used in other hospital administration courses, and the rapid progression into specialized medical content.

> "Due to the nature of the pathology, there is a lot of medical knowledge and a lot of information to be delivered ... Personally, it was difficult to understand because there was a lot of information being given at once." (P4)

> "Incomprehensible terminology gave me hard time ... ". (P1)

3.2. Area: The Learners

This area consisted of two theme clusters: "recognition of pathology courses during college years" and "the importance of pathology courses participants learned after graduation." Study participants suggested ideas to help the future students gain a positive experience, based on their personal experiences. This was classified as the learners' area.

3.2.1. Theme Cluster: Recognition of Pathology Courses during College Years

This theme cluster consisted of two themes: "lack of motivation to learn" and "subjects requiring memorization that participants wanted to give up." Participants emphasized the necessity and importance of learning pathology and the role of learners who are the focal point of education in accordance with their real-life experiences.

Theme: Lack of Motivation to Learn

The participants believed that there was a lack of awareness about the effect of pathology courses on their future practice.

> "Since we do not do practical work but rather do administrative work, I think I attended the pathology classes with an underlying opinion that pathology is not important." (K4)

Theme: The Memorization Subjects That Participants Wanted to Give Up

Participants revealed that a lack of motivation for learning pathology, the excessive amount of studying, and the realization that pathology requires memorization negatively affected the learning outcomes.

> "Students give up because there is so much to learn ... hard to understand and probably because they do not want to memorize." (L3)

> "All I can recall is the memorization techniques." (P2)

3.2.2. Theme Cluster: The Importance of Studying the Pathology Course Realized after Graduation

This theme cluster consisted of two themes: "coming to know that pathology is an important course that is helpful in clinical practice" and "helpful in obtaining a major-related qualification."

Theme: Coming to Know That Pathology Is an Important Course That Is Helpful in Clinical Practice

The participants emphasized the importance and usefulness of the pathology course based on their positive experiences during their employment practice; although they did not recognize this importance while attending the classes.

> "It helped me greatly to understand which areas are diseases with high severity and to understand whether patients have high severity when reading the list." (H3)

> "I think once you go to work after understanding the subject called pathology, you can communicate more comfortably with people in the medical department, nurses, or even with the patients you directly encounter." (K4)

> "It is content you need to know after you get a job and results will change according to how you study so I hope students study hard and learn a lot." (L2)

Theme: Helpful in Obtaining a Major-Related Qualification

The participants in this study vividly remembered their experiences while preparing for employment after graduation. Participants conveyed the pre-requisite role of the pathology course in obtaining further certification related to their major, such as that of a health information manager. Additionally, they acknowledged that studying the course provided practical guidance for obtaining the certification.

> "There are a lot of places that require a certificate than you would expect...They prefer people with a certificate...and it's a very good certificate to have...I think studying pathology will be absolutely indispensable to get a certificate such as health information manager certificate in the future." (K1)

> "I think it was helpful when I was taking the medical recorder's license exam. It really helped my studies when I looked through the materials I had studied before." (L3)

4. Discussion

This paper presents a qualitative study that aimed to understand the underlying experience of studying in a pathology course among hospital management graduates, and six theme clusters were subsequently extracted. An unexpected question from the participants during the interview was when they asked for an explanation of what a pathology course entails. This was surprising because all the participants had opted into this course and had only graduated within the last five years. Therefore, this indicates the relatively low importance attached to basic courses in hospital management majors, as administration and management courses are considered more essential. However, a general understanding of disease is becoming necessary with the increased engagement in medicine-related duties. Fortunately, the participants began to comprehensively reminisce about the overall experience of the course management and learning throughout the rest of the interview.

Pathology involves the in-depth study of disease mechanisms; H3 of the hospital office team expressed the desire to sequentially study relevant courses such as medical terminology, anatomy, physiology, and clinical practice. H3 also suggested the need for conducted pathology courses, before or after hospital placements, at the medical institutions in consideration with the educational level and needs of the students. Previous studies with students of health and medical department-related subjects have revealed that satisfaction with the major subject was high if high satisfaction was experienced with the curriculum and field placement [4–6,15]. This demonstrates that a systematically designed curriculum has a significant influence on overall course satisfaction. Similarly, other participants of the current study also wanted the pathology course to be taught before or after hospital placements. Therefore, it is necessary to conduct detailed discussions about the completion period of the course while designing the curriculum in order to increase student satisfaction with basic courses among hospital management graduates. These changes in curriculum design will aid the clinical placement of students, which can be an important turning point for those studying subjects relevant to health and medical departments; moreover, it will help in satisfying their intellectual curiosity related to their major and in fostering their potential [15]. Furthermore, due to the adaptive and dynamic nature of the curriculum, the pathology content may be added or reduced according to the educational needs of learners [4–6,15]; therefore, it is necessary to assess student satisfaction with the pathology course for those who are currently enrolled.

The second theme cluster in course management was concerned with student preferences for the professor of the course. Students preferred pathology professors who had clinical experience in hospitals and taught students in an interactive way that facilitated easy learning. Since professors enjoy a high degree of autonomy in class planning and evaluation, their competency acts as a crucial factor in determining the quality of their classes [16]. Students preferred professors with practical clinical experience who facilitate easy learning for students using real-life clinical cases during the pathology lectures. The results of a previous study reported that highly prioritized competencies in college professors are "systematic compositions" and "the explanation capacity" [17]. The current study findings were consistent with the results of this previous study. Thus, professors must seek techniques to systematically organize the contents of the pathology curriculum to easily explain the contents for students studying hospital administration while emphasizing important core contents.

Participants also expressed difficulty to motivate themselves to learn pathology during their college years, as the subject dealt with the mechanism of diseases. Therefore, professors with specialized knowledge and experience should use clinical case studies to make pathology classes less technical and more practical.

These requests were categorized into the third theme cluster of course management concerning the demands for various teaching methods, which included classes using audio–visual materials and case-based, role-playing techniques as the preferred lesson methods in order to tackle the difficulties expressed by the participants to engage in learning with lecture-based lessons due to boredom. The characteristics of excellent instructors are well-organized class content, clear delivery, and harmonious interactions with students [18]. Rote learning with professor-centered education to deliver extensive amounts of knowledge was the method preferred in the past when knowledge itself was the resource. However, modern day students require learner-centered classes (e.g., problem-based and team-based learning) to acquire and apply knowledge by participating in various learning activities based on student–professor interactions [9]. Due to the gap in previous research on the management of basic courses such as pathology for hospital management students, this study reviewed the available literature on the educational needs of nursing students, which is another health-related department. The reviewed literature revealed that nursing students also preferred performance-oriented education that enabled learning through direct participation and experiential learning, which was similar to those studying hospital administration [19]. Role-playing education, which participants positively recalled, involves the process of autonomously constructing specific scenarios, planning roles, and promoting the understanding of diseases; it can be an effective learning method that improves problem-solving and self-directed learning skills A previous study identified "media and technology utilization " as a component of an appealing class [20]; therefore, professors must seek methods to appropriately use relevant audio–visual materials to promote the interests and understanding in learners regarding unfamiliar disease mechanisms and terminology.

In the fourth theme cluster about the broad and difficult class content, the participants' complaints regarding the excessive amount of learning material and the basic medical contents that were difficult to concentrate on were recorded. Participants expressed the following concerns: (1) difficulty due to technical terminologies, (2) unfamiliarity with the content, (3) limitations due to the excessive amount of study material, (4) treating the course as a memorization subject, and (5) giving up learning altogether.

This is connected with the recognition of pathology courses during college years, which was the first theme cluster in the learner's area. Participants suggested that they were indifferent to the pathology course during their school years due to a lack of motivation to learn and because it was a subject that they wanted to give up studying due to the extensive amount of memorization involved. However, participants independently confirmed the importance of basic knowledge about diseases during their employment after graduation; they eventually realized the importance of the pathology course. Such factors are important for motivating students studying hospital management to learn pathology. As the learning and academic achievement increases, the purpose of taking a class becomes clearer for a learner [21]. These experiences of graduates can have a positive effect on inducing learning motivation for students who are currently enrolled.

A lack of effort or awareness in a learner who is the focus of education can prevent correct learning and lead to the abandonment of an course altogether [21]. In other words, a learner's proactive learning attitude is a determining factor in achieving learning outcomes.

Participants suggested that their experience of taking a pathology course as a student was crucial for reviewing and determining medical records at work in the medical institutions and insurance companies where they currently work. However, they expressed regret over not recognizing this importance during college. These findings demonstrate highly meaningful statements for professors teaching pathology in the field of education. Since the career paths of students studying hospital management are associated with medical institutions, it is imperative to improve their ability to seamlessly communicate with other health care workers and to understand their patients. Therefore, specific goals need to be determined for students studying hospital management to achieve the learning outcomes of the pathology course. Furthermore, there is also an urgency to seek solutions that consider the educational needs and the academic achievement of students while planning pathology classes to implement education at the eye-level for students who are studying hospital management.

5. Conclusions

This study divided the experience of the pathology course among graduates of hospital management into the areas of: (1) course management and (2) learners. The graduates commonly and consensually expressed a lack of motivation to study pathology and difficulties in concentrating on the course content due to the excessive amount of study material. However, graduates appeared to have recognized the importance of the pathology course after graduation during their employment in fields relevant to their major.

There are limitations in generalizing these results because this study conducted focus group interviews with the graduates of hospital management from the same local university. However, this study is significant because it has provided a deeper understanding of the experience of studying the pathology course in hospital management students amidst an insufficiency of relevant literature.

Based on the results of this study, the following recommendations are proposed: (1) the current management of basic courses, including pathology, in the department of hospital management must be evaluated and recognized; (2) pathology course curriculum should facilitate practical learning for effective the study management of pathological courses, which could be facilitated through collaborations with the employment centers where students can work after their graduation; and (3) learning contents should be constructed based on major diseases to enhance learning motivation. The findings of this study will be helpful for developing pathology course for hospital management students.

Author Contributions: Conceptualization, H.L.; methodology, J.H.P., and H.L.; software, J.H.P. and J.K.; validation, J.H.P., W.S.H., J.K., and J.H.P.; formal analysis, J.H.P., W.S.H., J.H.P. and H.L.; investigation, W.S.H., J.K., and H.L.; resources, W.S.H., J.K.; data curation, J.H.P., and H.L.; writing—original draft preparation, J.H.P.; writing—review and editing, J.H.P., W.S.H., J.K., and H.L.; supervision, H.L.; project administration, J.H.P. All authors have read and agreed to the published version of the manuscript.

Funding: This research was funded by Konyang University Research Fund in 2020.

Institutional Review Board Statement: The study was conducted according to the guidelines of the Declaration of Helsinki, and approved by the Institutional Review Board of Konyang University (IRB No 2020-096-01).

Informed Consent Statement: Informed consent was obtained from all subjects involved in the study.

Data Availability Statement: The data presented in this study are available on request from the corresponding author. The data are not publicly available due to data restriction policies.

Acknowledgments: The authors deeply thank the graduates who participated in this research.

Conflicts of Interest: The authors declare no conflict of interest.

References

1. Terzic-Supic, Z.; Bjegovic-Mikanovic, V.; Vukovic, D.; Santric-Milicevic, M.; Marinkovic, J.; Vasic, V.; Laaser, U. Training hospital managers for strategic planning and management: A prospective study. *BMC Med. Educ.* **2015**, *15*, 25. [CrossRef] [PubMed]
2. Cheon, E.Y.; Nam, Y.H.; Kwon, H.J. The relationship between career decision-making, self-efficacy, social support, career education experience, career attitude maturity for college students with major in health administration. *Health Pol. Manag.* **2009**, *19*, 166–182. [CrossRef]
3. Reibling, N.; Ariaans, M.; Wendt, C. Worlds of Healthcare: A Healthcare System Typology of OECD Countries. *Health Policy* **2019**, *123*, 611–620. [CrossRef] [PubMed]
4. Lee, H.S. Impact of major satisfaction of university students majoring public health administration on the career decision level and career prepare behaviors: Career decision-making self-efficacy as mediating factors. *J. Digit. Converg.* **2019**, *17*, 359–368.
5. Kim, Y.H. An analysis of differences in the recognition of career choice, satisfaction, and major adjustment among university students-Focused on the comparison between Health-care majors and Social science majors. *Crisisonomy* **2013**, *9*, 165–182.
6. Seo, H.J.; Park, H.J. The impact of satisfaction with major curriculum on acquisition of certification and employment for college students with major in Healthcare. *Korean J. Hosp. Manag.* **2017**, *22*, 51–60.
7. Lee, Y. Curriculum analysis on health management schools in Republic of Korea: Focusing on relationship with license and certification. *Health Pol. Manag.* **2018**, *28*, 23–34.
8. Hwang, C.I.; Hwang, J. A comparison on major curriculum of 2-year, 3-year, and 4-year health administration colleges in Korea. *Health Pol. Manag.* **2013**, *23*, 224–232. [CrossRef]
9. Park, J.H.; Han, W.S.; Kim, J.; Lee, H. Strategies for flipped learning in the health professions education in South Korea and their effects: A systematic review. *Educ. Sci.* **2021**, *11*, 1–10.
10. Morrison, G.R.; Ross, S.M.; Kalman, H.K.; Kemp, J.E. *Designing Effective Instruction*, 6th ed.; John Wiley & Sons: Hoboken, NJ, USA, 2010.
11. Krueger, R.A.; Casey, M.A. *Focus Group: A Practical Guide for Applied Research*; SAGE Publication: Thousand Oaks, CA, USA, 2009.
12. Krueger, R.A.; Casey, M.A. *Focus Group*, 3rd ed.; SAGE Publication: Thousand Oaks, CA, USA, 2000.
13. Morse, J.; Field, P.A. *Qualitative Research Methods for Health Professionals*; SAGE Publication: Thousand Oaks, CA, USA, 1995.
14. Hill, C.E.; Thompson, B.J.; Williams, E.N. A guide to conducting consensual qualitative research. *Couns. Psychol.* **1997**, *25*, 517–572. [CrossRef]
15. Kim, J.H.; Park, J.Y.; Yang, B.S. A study on the curricular satisfactions and curriculum improvements of the students majoring in Clinical Pathology. *Korean J. Clin. Lab. Sci.* **2012**, *44*, 239–244.
16. Sunal, D.W.; Wright, E.L.; Bland, J. *Reform in Undergraduate Science Teaching for the 21st Century*; Information Age Publishing: Greenwich, CT, USA, 2006.
17. Ha, O.S. University professor's teaching competency factor derivation from the learner's perspective and analysis of difference in lecture. *J. Educ. Res.* **2017**, *15*, 1–26. [CrossRef]
18. Kim, M.S. Characteristics and types of caring professors perceived by college students. *Korean J. Educ. Psychol.* **2011**, *25*, 61–86.

19. Kim, N.H.; Park, J.Y.; Jun, S.E. The effects of case-based learning (CBL) on learning motivation and learning satisfaction of nursing students in a Human Physiology course. *J. Korean Biol. Nurs. Sci.* **2015**, *17*, 78–87. [CrossRef]
20. Pollock, W.; Rea, P.M. The use of social media in anatomical and health professional education: A systematic review. *Adv. Exp. Med. Biol.* **2019**, *1205*, 149–170. [CrossRef] [PubMed]
21. Han, M.Y.; Kim, M.S. Experience in Microbiology course of nursing students: Qualitative content analysis. *J. Korean Biol. Nurs. Sci.* **2018**, *20*, 244–251. [CrossRef]

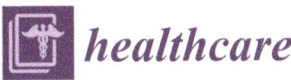 healthcare

Article

The Usefulness of the QR Code in Orthotic Applications after Orthopedic Surgery

Jaeho Cho [1,†], Gi-Won Seo [2,†], Jeong Seok Lee [2], Hyung Ki Cho [2], Eun Myeong Kang [2], Jahyung Kim [2], Dong-Il Chun [2], Young Yi [3] and Sung Hun Won [2,*]

1. Department of Orthopaedic Surgery, Chuncheon Sacred Heart Hospital, Hallym University, 77, Sakju-ro, Chuncheon-si 24253, Korea; hohotoy@nate.com
2. Department of Orthopaedic Surgery, Soonchunhyang University Seoul Hospital, 59, Daesagwan-ro, Yongsan-gu, Seoul 04401, Korea; 102980@schmc.ac.kr (G.-W.S.); 124856@schmc.ac.kr (J.S.L.); 125134@schmc.ac.kr (H.K.C.); 129741@schmc.ac.kr (E.M.K.); hpsyndrome@naver.com (J.K.); orthochun@gmail.com (D.-I.C.)
3. Department of Orthopaedic Surgery, Seoul Foot and Ankle Center, Inje University Seoul Paik Hospital, 85, 2-ga, Jeo-dong, Jung-gu, Seoul 04551, Korea; 20vvin@naver.com
* Correspondence: orthowon@gmail.com; Tel.: +82-10-709-9250; Fax: +82-2-710-3191
† Jaeho Cho and Gi-Won Seo contributed equally to this work.

Abstract: The purpose of this study is to evaluate the utility of QR (quick response) codes in explaining the proper method for orthotic use after orthopedic surgery. A questionnaire survey was adopted to evaluate patient satisfaction with education and training in orthotic applications after orthopedic surgery. The study periods were 1 April to 30 April 2017, and 1 October to 31 October 2017. The oral training involving the conventional orthoses was conducted in April, and the videos with the orthosis on the QR code were captured in October. The QR code containing the data was distributed and the education was conducted. A total of 68 patients (QR-code group: 33) participated in the questionnaire survey. After the QR code application, the number of retraining cases increased from 62.9 to 93.9% (p-value < 0.01). The mean scores of the four items measuring the comprehension increased from 10.97 to 14.39. The satisfaction level rose from 7.14 to 9.30, and the performance increased from 7.14 to 9.52 (p-value < 0.01). The QR code is expected to be a valuable method for explaining the orthotic application after orthopedic surgery, and especially when repeated explanations are needed for elderly patients.

Keywords: QR code; orthosis; orthopedic surgery; patient education

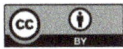

1. Introduction

Interest in the improvement of the quality of medical care and patient safety is growing. The obligation to explain all the procedures performed by the medical staff is greatly emphasized. The provision of accurate information to the patients enables understanding of the medical services, providing them with opportunities to actively participate in the treatment [1]. However, with the increasing number of elderly patients in recent years, patient's lack of understanding is expected, thereby increasing the necessity for repeated education, which is a burden not only for the patient but also for the healthcare personnel [2].

In orthopedic departments, nonsurgical treatments, intra-articular injections, splint fixation, and physical therapy are also used in addition to surgical treatment. The effort and patience required are especially high for patients wearing braces [3]. The medical personnel are required to provide the corresponding explanation to the patients and their caregivers.

With the recent advances in information technology (IT), it has become easier to access various audiovisual materials such as photographs and videos. In particular, this accessibility is facilitated by the smartphone popularization. The usefulness of online video tutorials is reported in medical fields, especially in the field of training of medical staff or students and in video descriptions for patients [4,5].

It has been reported that approximately 14% of the medical information provided orally is remembered correctly by the patients [6]. To address this challenge, it has been reported that the usage of pictography during medical explanations increased patient memory by 80% [7,8]. Sandberg et al. [9] reported that even if the information was not remembered at first, the patient recall ability increased to 67% when a clue was provided. Therefore, it is important to provide visual data and repeated interventions to ensure communication of medical information is memorized by the patient.

The QR (Quick Response) code is a matrix barcode (or two-dimensional barcode) that represents information in a black-and-white plaid pattern; these barcodes comprise vertical and horizontal information and contain up to 7089 numeric characters, or 4296 alphanumeric characters, or 2953 bytes (binary data). They can be used to encode specific URLs linking to sounds, pictures, and video information. Recently, the number of scanner applications capable of recognizing QR codes in smartphones has increased, and it is easier to obtain the desired information by simply recognizing the QR code with a smartphone rather than browsing the information online using a web-browser URL. Accordingly, this code technology is increasingly popular. A recent study reported the effectiveness of QR codes on a mobile phone in improving patient surveys [10].

Recently, the usage of QR codes in elderly patients with heart disease has led to increased medication compliance [11]. Likewise, they have the advantage of increasing medical accessibility to older age or chronic disease patients who require repetitive and continuous education.

This study evaluates the usefulness and patient satisfaction with orthopedic orthoses for which the QR code is used.

2. Materials and Methods

All research was performed in accordance with the relevant guidelines and regulations. The study periods were 1–30 April 2017 and 1–31 October 2017. The oral training involving conventional braces was conducted in April, and the videos with the braces on the QR code were captured in April. Therefore, we investigated two groups: the QR group as a case group and the oral training group as a control. The QR code containing the data was distributed before the education was provided. The QR code was distributed in the form of a business-card-size print and sticker, which was attached to the brace (Figure 1), while the length of each video varied from 1 to 2 min.

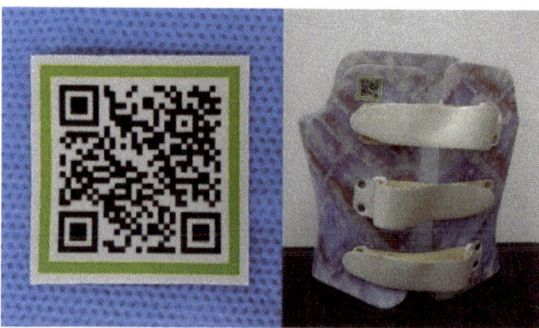

Figure 1. The QR code was distributed in the form of a business card-sized print and sticker and the sticker was attached to the brace.

To evaluate the satisfaction with the training in wearing the orthosis and the degree of satisfaction associated with the orthosis after the orthopedic surgery (orthoses included shoulder-abductor brace, thoracolumbosacral orthosis (TLSO), hip-abductor brace, corset,

Philadelphia cervical collar brace (P-brace)), a questionnaire was administered to patients who needed to wear it in October. The questionnaire included simple demographic data such as the patient's gender and age, and the frequency and timing of training in orthosis wearing, along with the training contents. In order to evaluate comprehension, the questionnaire included the following items: understanding the position of the orthosis, the duration of post-discharge orthosis wearing, the precautions for orthosis wearing, and the timing of the wearing and removal of the orthosis. To evaluate patient satisfaction, the patient was asked to provide subjective scores on a scale of 1 to 10. Finally, a performance score ranging from 1 to 10 was measured by the medical staff to determine if the patient was wearing the orthosis correctly, including the wear position, fixation strength and wearing order (Figure 2). A descriptive analysis of all the variables was performed, including the mean and the standard deviation or frequency. The data normality was tested using the Kolmogorov–Smirnov test. The Student's t-test was utilized to compare continuous variables, and the chi-square test was used to compare the categorical variables between the two groups.

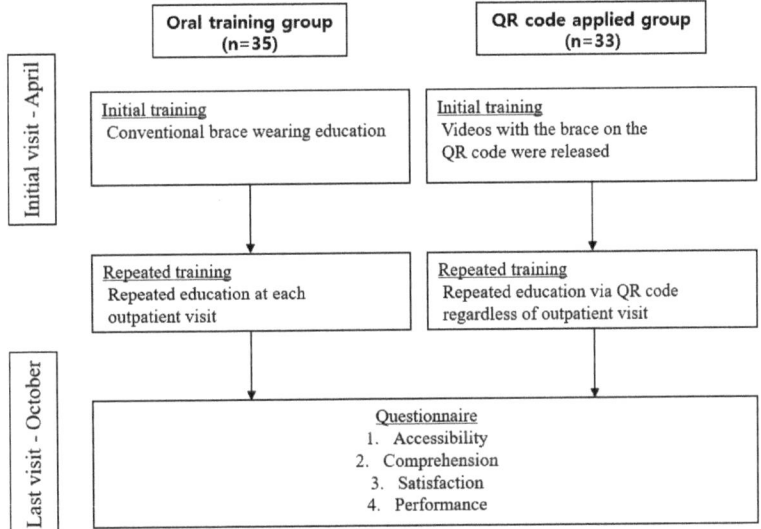

Figure 2. Flow chart of the study process.

3. Results

A total of 68 patients participated in the questionnaire survey. The mean age was 61.0 years (range: 10–88 years). The TLSO constitutes 33.8%, followed by the shoulder-abductor orthosis (32.4%), corset brace (14.7%), hip-abductor orthosis (13.2%), and P-brace (5.9%) (Table 1).

Table 1. Patient demographics.

		Group		Total (%)	p Value
		Oral Training Group	QR Code Applied Group		
Age	Mean ± SD	58.60 ± 16.20	63.55 ± 15.93	61.0 ± 16.14	0.209 *
	Range (Min–Max)	10–88	15–85	10–88	
Sex	Male	20	19	39 (57.4)	0.971 †
	Female	15	14	29 (42.6)	
Orthosis	Shoulder abduction brace	15	7	22 (32.4)	0.354 †
	TLSO	11	12	23 (33.8)	
	Hip abduction brace	4	5	9 (13.2)	
	Corset	4	6	10 (14.7)	
	P-brace	1	3	4 (5.9)	

p values calculated by * t-test or † Chi-square test. SD = standard deviation; Min = minimum; Max = maximum; TLSO = thoracolumbosacral orthosis.

At least two-thirds of the training time in both groups was spent wearing the orthosis. The orally trained group and the group supplied with QR code were exposed to repeated training three times in 11% and 29% of the cases, respectively. Meanwhile, with the application of the QR code, the frequency of retraining (accessibility) increased from 62.9 to 93.9% (p-value < 0.01) (Figure 3).

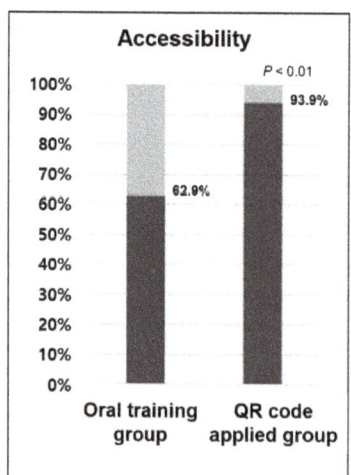

Figure 3. The difference in frequency of retraining (accessibility) between the oral training group and QR code applied group.

The mean scores of the four items that measured the comprehension increased from 10.97 to 14.39 (p-value < 0.01), and the satisfaction level increased from 7.14 to 9.30. The performance increased from 7.14 to 9.52 (p-value < 0.01) (Figure 4).

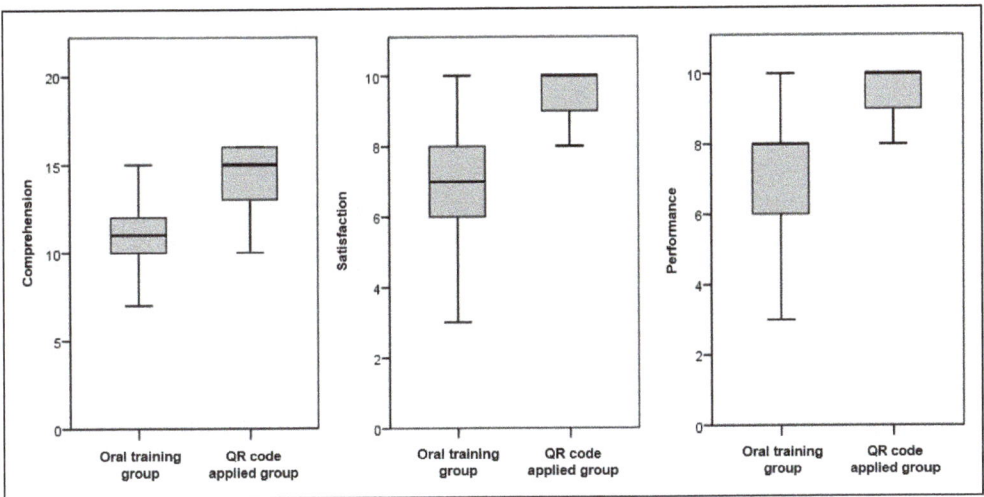

Figure 4. The mean scores of the four items measuring comprehension, satisfaction level, and performance score.

4. Discussion

In this first reported study using a QR code to explain orthosis wearing to patients after orthopedic surgery, the patients who used the QR code showed sound outcomes in terms of both the wearing competency and understanding of the orthosis compared with patients who received only an oral explanation.

Yuzer et al. [12] reported that patients with stroke most often declined to wear an orthosis because they felt it was unnecessary and inconvenient. It is important for the patient to wear a brace continuously and correctly. Improper wearing of the orthosis results in discomfort, which may reduce patient compliance. There are many types of orthosis that are worn differently for varying durations. Furthermore, it is necessary for the patient to be repeatedly educated about the orthosis.

It is difficult for the patient to fit into some of the orthotic types without the help of a caregiver; therefore, the caregiver needs to have precise information. It is also difficult, however, for all caregivers to accompany the medical staff at the time of explanation, suggesting the need for a handy educational tool. Consequently, it is expected that the caregiver education will increase the compliance of patients.

As the smartphone technology becomes widespread, the QR code will be used in various industries. Because the memorizing of the URL is unnecessary and the smartphone is portable, the QR code can be used to access information conveniently and repeatedly. Accordingly, the use of the QR code for accurate drug administration in the elderly population has been reported [13]. In the orthopedic field, it has been used in cast management and sound clinical outcomes have been reported [14].

As the Internet has become widespread, various types of information can be accessed quickly and easily, but it is also difficult to identify accurate information. In the case of a nonmedical person, it is difficult to understand the correct terminology, which complicates the search and often introduces inaccuracies in medical knowledge conveyed to the patient. The usage of the QR code prevents the dissemination of false orthosis information to the patients, because it provides audiovisual information in an easy way via a smart phone. This study shows that the QR code can be used more effectively by repeated patient education and accessibility than conventional oral training in an outpatient clinic. It is expected the patient compliance will be improved by minimizing the inconvenience due to wearing of the correct orthosis and enhancing the understanding of the importance of wearing the orthosis.

Spaulding et al. described three major variables in orthotis and prosthesis care; (1) the state of functioning, disability, and health (International Classification of Functioning, Disability and Health); (2) orthotic and prosthetic technical properties, procedures, and appropriateness; and (3) professional service as part of orthotic and prosthetic interventions [15]. The usage of a QR code may enhance the provision of professional service throughout the orthotic care of patients.

Although this study is the first study demonstrating the usefulness of the QR code for orthosis application after orthopedic surgery, limitations have been identified. First, the number of the observed patients is small and the follow-up period is short. However, it is significant that the QR code, which has the advantages of repeatability and convenience, was newly used in the orthotic field. Further, the QR code is widely available in various medical fields beyond orthopedics. Second, our study compared QR codes with oral explanations about the overall understanding of orthosis after orthopedic surgery. Because this is the first attempt at orthopedic surgery, we have investigated a number of orthoses, suggesting possible heterogeneity. In future studies, each orthosis application and training will be investigated comprehensively. Third, our study did not compare online educational tutorials containing educational videos with our QR code containing an educational video. This is considered a study limitation, and it will be necessary to compare the two videos in the future. However, the advantages of our study are two-fold. First, the educational and training videos included in this study are tailored to the patient and individual circumstances. Therefore, patients can obtain a better understanding of brace application. Second, it is easier for elderly patients to access information using the QR code than to search the Internet for every educational video. Lastly, although we did not compare QR code education with a conventional paper education brochure, because of its repeatability and better visualization, QR code education can be a better option for patients.

5. Conclusions

The QR code is a valuable method for training patients and caregivers regarding brace applications after orthopedic surgery. It has gained popularity among other medical fields. Even though it has the limitation that there are few studies showing superiority compared to conventional education modalities, the authors believe that the QR code will be used in several medical fields in the future because of its repeatability and accessibility.

Author Contributions: Conceptualization, S.H.W.; formal analysis, J.S.L.; investigation, H.K.C.; resources, E.M.K.; writing—original draft, J.C.; writing—review and editing, G.-W.S.; visualization, J.K.; supervision, D.-I.C., Y.Y.; project administration, S.H.W.; funding acquisition, S.H.W. All authors have read and agreed to the published version of the manuscript.

Funding: This work was supported by the Soonchunhyang University Research Fund.

Institutional Review Board Statement: The study was conducted according to the guidelines of The Declaration of Helsinki, and approved by the Ethical Committee of the Soonchunhyang university Seoul hospital.

Informed Consent Statement: Informed consent was obtained from all subjects involved in this study.

Data Availability Statement: The data presented in this study are available on request from the corresponding author. The data are not publicly available due to data restriction policies.

Acknowledgments: The authors are grateful for the collaboration of all nurses in the orthopedic surgery department of Soonchunhyang University Seoul Hospital.

Conflicts of Interest: The authors declare that they have no competing interests.

References

1. Daack-Hirsch, S.; Campbell, C.A. The role of patient engagement in personalized healthcare. *Pers. Med.* **2014**, *11*, 1–4. [CrossRef] [PubMed]
2. Lundby, C.; Graabaek, T.; Ryg, J.; Søndergaard, J.; Pottegård, A.; Nielsen, D.S. Health care professionals' attitudes towards deprescribing in older patients with limited life expectancy: A systematic review. *Br. J. Clin. Pharmacol.* **2019**, *85*, 868–892. [CrossRef] [PubMed]
3. Miller, D.J.; Franzone, J.M.; Matsumoto, H.; Gomez, J.A.; Avendaño, J.; Hyman, J.E.; Roye, D.P., Jr.; Vitale, M.G. Electronic monitoring improves brace-wearing compliance in patients with adolescent idiopathic scoliosis: A randomized clinical trial. *Spine* **2012**, *37*, 717–721. [CrossRef] [PubMed]
4. Judd, T.; Elliott, K. Selection and Use of Online Learning Resources by First-Year Medical Students: Cross-Sectional Study. *JMIR Med. Educ.* **2017**, *3*, e17. [CrossRef] [PubMed]
5. Srikesavan, C.; Williamson, E.; Cranston, T.; Hunter, J.; Adams, J.; Lamb, S.E. An Online Hand Exercise Intervention for Adults With Rheumatoid Arthritis (mySARAH): Design, Development, and Usability Testing. *J. Med. Internet Res.* **2018**, *20*, e10457. [CrossRef] [PubMed]
6. Kessels, R.P. Patients' memory for medical information. *J. R. Soc. Med.* **2003**, *96*, 219–222. [CrossRef] [PubMed]
7. Houts, P.S.; Bachrach, R.; Witmer, J.T.; Tringali, C.A.; Bucher, J.A.; Localio, R.A. Using pictographs to enhance recall of spoken medical instructions. *Patient Educ. Couns.* **1998**, *35*, 83–88. [CrossRef]
8. Houts, P.S.; Witmer, J.T.; Egeth, H.E.; Loscalzo, M.J.; Zabora, J.R. Using pictographs to enhance recall of spoken medical instructions II. *Patient Educ. Couns.* **2001**, *43*, 231–242. [CrossRef]
9. Sandberg, E.H.; Sharma, R.; Sandberg, W.S. Deficits in retention for verbally presented medical information. *Anesthesiology* **2012**, *117*, 772–779. [CrossRef] [PubMed]
10. Chien, T.W.; Lin, W.S. Improving Inpatient Surveys: Web-Based Computer Adaptive Testing Accessed via Mobile Phone QR Codes. *JMIR Med. Inform.* **2016**, *4*, e8. [CrossRef] [PubMed]
11. Capranzano, P.; Francaviglia, B.; Sardone, A.; Agnello, F.; Valenti, N.; Frazzetto, M.; Legnazzi, M.; Occhipinti, G.; Scalia, L.; Calvi, V.; et al. Suitability for elderly with heart disease of a QR code-based feedback of drug intake: Overcoming limitations of current medication adherence telemonitoring systems. *Int. J. Cardiol.* **2021**, *327*, 209–216. [CrossRef]
12. Nakipoğlu Yüzer, G.F.; Koyuncu, E.; Çam, P.; Özgirgin, N. The regularity of orthosis use and the reasons for disuse in stroke patients. *Int. J. Rehabil. Res.* **2018**, *41*, 270–275. [CrossRef] [PubMed]
13. Tseng, M.H.; Wu, H.C. A cloud medication safety support system using QR code and Web services for elderly outpatients. *Technol. Health Care Off. J. Eur. Soc. Eng. Med.* **2014**, *22*, 99–113. [CrossRef] [PubMed]
14. Gough, A.T.; Fieraru, G.; Gaffney, P.; Butler, M.; Kincaid, R.J.; Middleton, R.G. A novel use of QR code stickers after orthopaedic cast application. *Ann. R. Coll. Surg. Engl.* **2017**, *99*, 476–478. [CrossRef]
15. Spaulding, S.E.; Yamane, A.; McDonald, C.L.; Spaulding, S.A. A conceptual framework for orthotic and prosthetic education. *Prosthet. Orthot. Int.* **2019**, *43*, 369–381. [CrossRef] [PubMed]

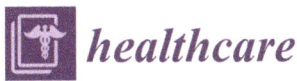

Article

The Impact of Teammates' Online Reputations on Physicians' Online Appointment Numbers: A Social Interdependency Perspective

Jingfang Liu, Xin Zhang *, Jun Kong and Liangyu Wu

School of Management, Shanghai University, Shanghai 200444, China; jingfangliu@shu.edu.cn (J.L.); charlottek@shu.edu.cn (J.K.); skyrim@shu.edu.cn (L.W.)
* Correspondence: 513651789@i.shu.edu.cn; Tel.: +86-1982-1834-368

Received: 15 September 2020; Accepted: 17 November 2020; Published: 23 November 2020

Abstract: Online medical team is an emerging online medical model in which patients can choose a doctor to register and consult. A doctor's reputation cannot be ignored. It is worth studying how that online reputation affects the focal doctor's appointment numbers on the online medical team. Based on the online reputation mechanism and social interdependence theory, this study empirically studied the impact of the focal doctor's own reputation and other teammates' reputation on his/her appointment numbers. Our data include 31,143 doctors from 6103 online expert teams of Guahao.com. The results indicate that for a leader doctor, his/her appointment numbers are not related to his/her own reputation, and there was an inverted U-shaped relationship with the ordinary doctors' reputations on the team. For an ordinary doctor, his/her appointment numbers were positively correlated with his/her own reputation and positively correlated with his/her leader's reputation and there was an inverted U-shaped relationship with the other ordinary doctors' reputations. The research showed that there is a positive spillover effect on the team leader's reputation. There are two relationships between team doctors: competition and cooperation. This study provides guidance for the leader to select team members and the ordinary doctor to select a team.

Keywords: online medical team; online reputation; appointment numbers; leader; teammates; inverted U-shaped relationship; competition; cooperation; social interdependence theory

1. Introduction

The coordination and delivery of safe, high-quality care require reliable teamwork and collaboration across organizational, disciplinary, technical, and cultural boundaries [1,2]. Offline medical teams are very common in Western countries. Effective team cooperation provides safe and effective care for all levels of the medical system [3,4]. In most developed countries, team medicine has become a standard of diagnosis and treatment. Both the leading family doctors and the famous Mayo Clinic work in doctor-collaboration teams [5]. The importance of teamwork is also evident in the response to COVID-19 [6]. Team medicine is helpful for both patients and doctors. For patients, team medical cooperative treatment can effectively improve the diagnosis and treatment ability and efficiency of complex diseases, provide comprehensive nursing and rehabilitation design for patients, and make each patient's treatment more personalized [7,8]. For the team's medical staff, it is necessary to change their focus from the concept of emergency to long-term disease prevention and health care. They can learn new technologies and make new breakthroughs in the diagnosis and treatment of each patient and require the medical staff to focus on their professional fields [9,10]. On the team, young doctors can also obtain better training and experience. With the development of the "Internet + healthcare", online medical teams have begun to appear on online medical service platforms in China. China's haodf.com and guahao.com have set up expert teams. The expert teams are led by brand doctors, joined by ordinary doctors and young doctors, and collaboration teams are established to jointly diagnose and treat patients. The emergence of online medical teams can alleviate the problem that senior experts have no time for branding, and young doctors and grassroots doctors have time but no brand, so that doctors can better allocate time, share experience, and share brands. This will make the distribution of valuable medical resources more reasonable. Online medical teams are a new type of virtual team, so it is necessary to study and analyze them.

As the basis for online transactions, the online reputation mechanism provides an important basis for consumers' purchase decisions [11,12]. Online reputation is a kind of public praise formed by the evaluation feedback of purchased goods or services after consumers consume online [13,14]. In the past, many scholars have studied online reputation based on online markets such as eBay, Taobao, Yelp, Uber, and Airbnb [15–17]. Medical and health services are a typical trust product [18]. Because of information asymmetry, it is difficult for patients to judge the medical service level of doctors. At this time, doctors know their own medical level, but patients do not know the real medical level of doctors before they receive the doctor's services. So, the patient can only judge the doctor's medical level through the information on the doctor's website. At this time, a doctor's online reputation is particularly important. As a signal of a doctor's medical service level, the doctor's online reputation provides a decision-making basis for patients to register online [19–21]. Many studies have confirmed the influence of brand on the sales volume of goods or the purchase intention of consumers [22]. In a medical team, the team leader is usually a doctor with high status, whose reputation is equivalent to the brand of the team. Therefore, the reputation of the leader of the team conveys the image of the team to the patients, provides an important basis for the patients to infer the medical level of the team, and reduces the perceived risk and information cost of the patients.

Interdependence and social classification are the foundation of team formation [23]. Koffka demonstrated that the team is a dynamic whole, with different forms and degrees of dependence among members [24]. Lewin proposed that the essence of a team is the interdependence among members of the team. The state change in any member or subteam in a team will affect the state of other members or subteams [25]. According to McGrath, a team is a social collection of existing mutual understanding and potential interactions between members [26]. When the results of individuals are influenced by their own and others' behaviors, social interdependence is produced [27]. Morton Deutsch put forward the theory of social interdependence in 1949. There are two types of social interdependence: positive (when the individual's behavior promotes the realization of common goals) and negative (when the individual's behavior hinders the realization of another's goals) [28]. When there is a positive-positive relationship between the goals and means of different individuals, there is a cooperative relationship between them, such as the relationship between football team players [29]. Under the condition of task interdependence and resource interdependence, students more easily achieve better results than students who study alone [30]. When there is a negative dependence on the target means of different individuals, there is a competitive relationship between them, such as boxing. When a person needs the resources of other team members but has no common goal (that is, he or she does not share resources with others, but only obtains resources from others), the result will affect another's productivity [28]. Colasante et al. found that intrateam competition can significantly reduce free-riding behavior [31].

In the field of health care, few people study the relationship between doctors working in the same organization. If an organization has a good reputation, all its members are considered to have a good reputation [32]. Wu et al. found that there are both cooperative relationships and competitive relationships between doctors and colleagues [33]. From the perspective of "cooperation", the reputations of a doctor and all his or her colleagues form the reputation of his or her team. When the reputation of the team is high, the team can attract more patients. At this time, the reputations of the doctor's colleagues has a positive impact on him or her. From the perspective of "competition", when patients register online, they will select the doctor of the expert team according to the doctor's online reputation and other signals. At this time, if the doctor's colleagues have a high online reputation, the doctor's colleagues are more likely to be selected. At this point, a colleague's online reputation has a negative impact on the doctor.

Therefore, it is meaningful to study the impact of teammates' online reputations in the online medical team on the focal doctor's appointment numbers.

Since there are two types of doctors in an online medical team, this study divided the doctors in an online medical team into two types, leader doctor and ordinary doctor, and conducted the study separately. The team is led by the leader doctor, and other doctors can join. The leader doctor is often a more senior doctor. Ordinary doctors are the team members other than the leader doctor. Most of them are young doctors and doctors with less seniority. This study mainly solves the following problems:

When the leader acts as the focal doctor:

Research question1: How does the focal doctor's reputation affect his/her own appointment numbers in the online medical team?

Research question12: How does the reputation of ordinary doctors of the online medical team affect the focal doctor's appointment numbers?

When the ordinary doctor acts as the focal doctor:

Research question11: How does the focal doctor's reputation affect his/her own appointment numbers in the online medical team?

Research question12: How does his/her leader' reputation affect the focal doctor's appointment numbers?

Research question13: How does the reputation of other ordinary doctors of the online medical team affect the focal doctor's appointment numbers?

In this study, we tested the research hypotheses using the data collected from Guahao.com. Guahao.com is one of the main online medical service platforms in China focusing on registration services. Guahao.com created a team medical model. A team consists of a well-known team leader doctor and several ordinary doctors. Patients can first select an expert team and then select a doctor from the expert team to register, consult, or purchase other services.

In August 2019, we collected data from 31,143 doctors from 6103 online expert teams of Guahao.com. Each dataset included the doctor's appointment numbers, title, department, hospital and city, review numbers, likes, scores, and team size. Then, we used an econometric method to verify our research hypothesis.

2. Materials and Methods

2.1. Research Model and Hypotheses Development

The purpose of this study was to investigate the impact of the focal doctor's own reputation and his/her teammates' reputations of an online medical team on the focal doctor's appointment numbers. In our research context, there were two types of doctors in an online medical team, leader and ordinary doctors. Therefore, we separated the leader and ordinary doctors to establish different research models.

2.1.1. Hypotheses of Leaders

The leader's conceptual model is shown in Figure 1.

Reputation is formed by patients' feedback on a doctor's service quality, so it is a kind of information including doctor service quality. Online health platforms are set with scoring, likes, comments, and other functions so that patients who have received online medical services can give feedback on the services they have received. This kind of feedback may include a doctor's medical level and service attitude. Online medical services are a kind of trust product. Patients have no accurate judgment on the service quality of doctors in advance. Users' online feedback can alleviate information asymmetry and increase patients' trust in doctors. Patients' satisfaction with mobile Internet services and willingness to continue using mobile Internet services have a significant positive impact on word of mouth [20]. A good reputation is usually obtained by a high level of diagnosis and treatment and a positive service attitude [34]. Therefore, a doctor's reputation is usually positively related to his or her service quality (diagnosis and treatment level and service attitude). So, having a high reputation can increase the chance of being selected by patients.

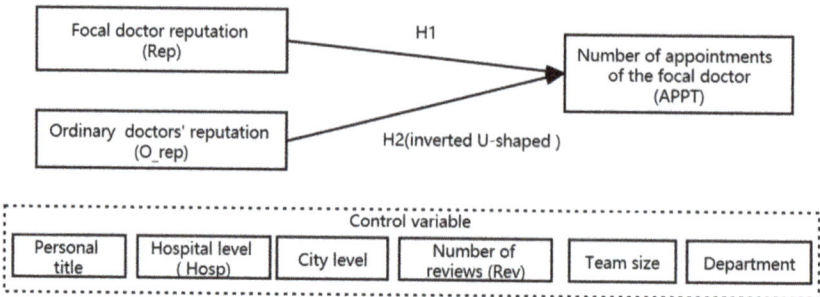

Figure 1. Conceptual model of leader.

Hypothesis 1. *There is a positive correlation between the focal doctor's reputation and appointment numbers.*

In a team, leaders and other team members have similar goals and means. They all compete for a patient's choice by displaying online information in the online medical service platform. Therefore, there is a dependency between the leader and the rest of the team. This dependence may be positive or negative. For the leader, the impact of the reputation of ordinary doctors in his or her team on his or her number of appointments may be positive or negative. On the one hand, ordinary doctors on the team belong to the same team as the leader. Their reputation together forms the reputation of the whole team. Improving the reputation of the team can also increase the chance that the leader is selected. At this time, he or she and ordinary doctors on the team form a cooperative relationship. On the other hand, when the reputations of ordinary doctors on the team are high enough, it shows that, in addition to the leader, there are many ordinary doctors with high service quality on the team for patients to choose from. At this point, there is a competitive relationship between the leader and the rest of the team. At this time, improving the reputation of ordinary doctors is detrimental to the number of appointments of the leader. Therefore, this paper believes that there is a theoretical basis for an inverted U-shaped relationship between ordinary doctors and leaders. Over time, we assume that the number of appointments for leaders will decrease as the reputation of ordinary doctors on the team increases to a certain value. Therefore, we assumed the following:

Hypothesis 2. *There is a nonlinear relationship (inverted U-shaped relationship) between the ordinary doctors' reputations on the team and the focal doctor's appointment numbers.*

2.1.2. Hypotheses of Ordinary Doctors

The ordinary doctor's conceptual model is shown in Figure 2.

The patient's feedback to the service of the ordinary doctor includes the service quality, service attitude, and other information in the online medical process of the ordinary doctor. During the appointment process, the patient can increase the understanding and trust of the ordinary doctor through his or her reputation. Therefore, we proposed the following assumptions:

Hypothesis 3. *There is a positive correlation between the focal doctor's reputation and appointment numbers.*

In our research, most of the leaders are well-known experts from high-level hospitals that have formed a brand effect. Leader reputation has a positive effect on team performance [35]. That is to say, the reputation of the team leader has a positive spillover effect on the number of appointments of the ordinary doctor. When patients make a choice among these doctors, the reputation of the leader can be transferred to the quality assessment of ordinary doctors. The reputation of the leader is equivalent to the brand of the team, which can attract patients to choose the team and then increase the chance of the ordinary doctor of the team to be selected. To this end, we proposed the following assumptions:

Hypothesis 4. *The reputation of the team's leader has a positive impact on the focal doctor's appointment numbers.*

In a medical team, doctors have similar goals and means, so they are dependent on each other. Therefore, the reputation of other ordinary doctors on the team will have a spillover effect on their own performance, which may be positive or negative. On the one hand, because they belong to the same team, their reputations add up to form the reputation of the whole team. At this time, the team doctors form a cooperative relationship. On the other hand, when the reputation of other ordinary doctors on the team is high enough, there is a competitive relationship between focal doctor and other ordinary doctors on the team. This paper argues that there is a theoretical basis for the inverted U-shaped relationship between other ordinary doctors on the team and the appointment quantity of the focal doctor. Therefore, we assumed the following:

Hypothesis 5: *There is a nonlinear relationship (inverted U-shaped relationship) between other ordinary doctors' reputations on the team and the focal doctor's appointment numbers.*

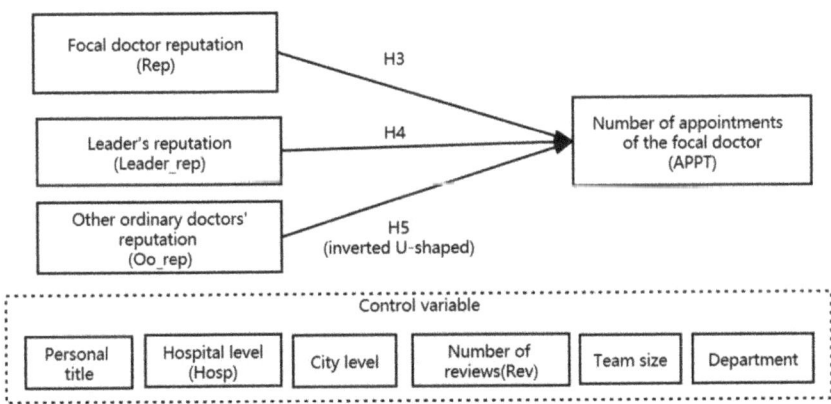

Figure 2. Conceptual model of ordinary doctor.

2.2. Research Methodology

2.2.1. Variables' Design

When the leader is the focal doctor, the dependent variable is his/her cumulative appointment numbers (APPT) and the independent variable is his/her own reputation (Rep) and ordinary doctors' average reputations on the team (O_rep). When the ordinary doctor is the focal doctor, the dependent variable is his/her cumulative appointment numbers (APPT) and the independent variable is his/her own reputation (Rep), leader's reputation (Leader_rep), and other ordinary doctors' average reputations on the team (Oo_rep).

Reputation was measured by two indicators: doctors' likes and scores. The patient can like and rate the doctor on the doctor's homepage after being served. Since these two variables may have different ranges, they are standardized and then averaged to create a composite variable.

Control variables at the individual level include the title, hospital level, city level, department, and review numbers and at the team level include team size. Tables 1 and 2 are variables' description of leaders and ordinary doctors.

Table 1. Variables' description of leaders.

Variables	Variables Symbol	Explanation
Dependent variable	APPT	The cumulative number of patients who have made a appointment with the focal doctor.
Independent variables	Rep	Reputation of the focal doctor was obtained by averaging the number of likes and score of the focal doctor after standardization.
	O_rep	The average reputation of other doctors in the team except the focal doctor, that is, the average reputation of all ordinary doctors. It is calculated as follows. For each team, we first sum up the reputation of all members of the team, then subtract the reputation of the focal doctor, and divide the value obtained by the number of team members minus 1.
	O_rep2	The square of the average reputation of all ordinary doctors on the team.
Control variables	Title	1 to 5, with 1 being the lowest and 5 being the highest.
	City	1 to 7, with 1 being the lowest and 7 the highest.
	Hosp	1 to 4, with 1 being the lowest and 4 the highest.
	Rev	The number of reviews received by the focal doctor.
	TeamSize	The number of people of the team.

Notes: APPT = number of appointments; Rep = online reputation; O_rep = the average reputation of all ordinary doctors in the team; O_rep2 = The square of the average reputation of all ordinary doctors on the team; City = city level; Hosp = hospital level; Rev = review number; TeamSize = team size.

Table 2. Variables' description of ordinary doctors.

Variables	Variables Symbol	Explanation
Dependent variable	APPT	The cumulative number of patients who have made an appointment with the focal doctor.
Independent variables	Rep	Reputation of the focal doctor was obtained by averaging the number of likes and score of the focal doctor after standardization.
	Leader_rep	The reputation of the leader physician on the team.
	Oo_rep	The average reputation of other doctors in the team except the focal doctor and the leader doctor, that is, the average reputation of other ordinary doctors except the focal doctor. For each team, we first sum up the reputation of all members of the team, then subtract the reputation of the focal doctor and the reputation of the leader doctor, and divide the value obtained by the number of people in the team minus the value after 2.
	Oo_rep2	The square of the average reputation of other ordinary doctors on the team.
Control variables	Title	1 to 5, with 1 being the lowest and 5 being the highest.
	City	1 to 7, with 1 being the lowest and 7 the highest.
	Hosp	1 to 4, with 1 being the lowest and 4 the highest.
	Rev	The number of reviews received by the focal doctor.
	TeamSize	The number of people of the team.

Notes: APPT = number of appointments; Rep = online reputation; Oo_rep = the average reputation of other ordinary doctors in the team; Oo_rep2 = The square of the average reputation of other ordinary doctors on the team; City = city level; Hosp = hospital level; Rev = review number; TeamSize = team size.

2.2.2. Empirical Model and Test Method

For the leader:

$$APPT = \beta_0 + \beta_1 Title + \beta_2 HospitalLevel + \beta_3 CityLevel + \beta_4 ReviewNumber + \beta_5 TeamSize \\ + \beta_6 Reputation + \beta_7 O\_rep + \beta_8 Reputation * O\_rep + Department\ dummies + \varepsilon, \quad (1)$$

For the ordinary doctor:

$$APPT = \beta_0 + \beta_1 Title + \beta_2 HospitalLevel + \beta_3 CityLevel + \beta_4 ReviewNumber + \beta_5 TeamSize \\ + \beta_6 Reputation + \beta_7 Leader\_Rep + \beta_8 Oo\_rep + \beta_9 Reputation * Leader\_rep + \beta_{10} Reputation \\ * Oo\_rep + \beta_{11} Leader\_Rep * Oo\_rep + Department\ dummies + \varepsilon, \quad (2)$$

In most empirical identification of U-shaped relationships, researchers will include a nonlinear (usually quadratic) term in a standard linear regression model [36–38]. If this term is significant, and the estimated extreme point is within the data range, it is considered that there is a U-shaped relationship. Therefore, we add the quadratic term to the empirical model to perform a standard regression analysis to test whether the quadratic term is significant to test whether the extreme points are within the data range.

However, Lind and Mehlum demonstrated that this standard is too weak [39]. When the true relationship is convex and monotonous, the model estimate will erroneously produce an extreme point and a U-shaped relationship. Lind and Mehlum used the general framework developed by Sasabuschi to test whether there is a U-shaped and inverted U-shaped relationship between two variables, and used this test principle to write the utest test command [39]. Utest provides an "exact test" for the existence of a U-shaped (or inverted U-shaped) relationship in an interval. Therefore, we continued to use the utest command to perform an inverted U test of our empirical model.

3. Results

3.1. Results for Leaders

3.1.1. Descriptive Statistic and Correlation for Leaders

The descriptive statistics and correlations for the key variables used in leader's research model are presented in Tables 3 and 4.

Table 3. Description statistics of leaders.

Variable	Obs	Mean	Std. Dev.	Min	Max
APPT	6103	543.64	2538.225	0.00	63,812
Rep	6103	0.196	1.072	−0.353	25.498
O_rep	6103	−0.094	0.831	−0.489	20.558
O_rep2	6103	0.699	6.849	0.00	422.621
Rev	6103	54.337	267.715	0.00	11,328
TeamSize	6103	5.107	3.025	1	88
Title	6103	4.774	0.433	1	5
Hosp	6103	2.978	0.164	1	3
City	6103	5.397	1.244	1	7

Note: APPT = number of appointments; Rep = online reputation; O_rep = the average reputation of all ordinary doctors in the team; O_rep2 = The square of the average reputation of all ordinary doctors on the team; City = city level; Hosp = hospital level; Rev = review number; TeamSize = team size, Obs = observation, Std. Dev. = Standard Deviation, Min = minimum, Max= maximum.

3.1.2. Regression Results of Leader's Research Model

Linear regression and hierarchical multiple regressions were used to estimate empirical results, while statistical significance was established at a p-value less than 0.05. All data were analyzed using STATA.

Table 4. Matrix of correlations of leaders.

Variables	(1)	(2)	(3)	(4)	(5)	(6)	(7)	(8)	(9)
(1) APPT	1.000								
(2) Rep	0.515	1.000							
(3) O_rep	0.377	0.374	1.000						
(4) O_rep2	0.114	0.073	0.672	1.000					
(5) Rev	0.810	0.543	0.346	0.120	1.000				
(6) TeamSize	0.082	0.159	0.047	−0.014	0.103	1.000			
(7) Title	0.048	0.073	0.052	0.010	0.025	0.112	1.000		
(8) Hosp	0.022	0.023	0.028	0.009	0.015	0.002	0.053	1.000	
(9) City	0.197	0.270	0.227	0.026	0.177	0.022	0.026	−0.038	1.000

Note: APPT = number of appointments; Rep = online reputation; O_rep = the average reputation of all ordinary doctors in the team; O_rep2 = The square of the average reputation of all ordinary doctors on the team; City = city level; Hosp = hospital level; Rev = review number; TeamSize = team size.

The regression results for the team leader are shown in Table 5. At this time, ordinary doctors on the team refer to doctors other than the leader on the team. From Model 2, it is noted that Rep ($\beta = 0.0495$, $p > 0.1$) has no effect on APPT. This may be because most leaders have busy offline tasks and limited online appointment opportunities. Therefore, their appointment numbers will not increase with his/her reputation's improvement. H1 is not supported (**H1:** *There is a positive correlation between the focal doctor's reputation and appointment numbers.*).

Table 5. Results of regression analyses of leaders.

	(1)	(2)
	model1	model2
Title	0.233 ***	0.218 ***
	(0.0591)	(0.0589)
City	0.328 ***	0.306 ***
	(0.0199)	(0.0198)
Hosp	0.212	0.178
	(0.146)	(0.142)
lnRev	0.992 ***	0.898 ***
	(0.0178)	(0.0304)
lnTeamSize	0.167 **	0.164 **
	(0.0804)	(0.0802)
Rep		0.0455
		(0.0527)
O_rep		0.472 ***
		(0.0689)
O_rep2		−0.0364 ***
		(0.0115)
_cons	−3.326 ***	−2.825 ***
	(0.529)	(0.521)
N	6103	6103
R2	0.552	0.559

Note: The numbers in the tables are mostly beta-values. The numbers in brackets are the standard errors. Department virtual variables are included in the model but are not shown in the table.; ** $p < 0.01$, *** $p < 0.001$; APPT = number of appointments; Rep = online reputation; O_rep = the average reputation of all ordinary doctors in the team; O_rep2 = The square of the average reputation of all ordinary doctors on the team; City = city level; Hosp = hospital level; Rev = review number; TeamSize = team size.

The coefficient of O_rep 's quadratic term ($\beta = -0.0363$ ***, $p < 0.01$) is negative and significant. This implies that the relationship between O_rep and APPT is nonlinear. Ordinary doctors' reputations have an inverted U relationship with the focal doctor's appointment numbers on the team, indicating that H2 is confirmed and in line with the social Interdependence theory (**H2:** *There is a nonlinear* relationship (inverted U-shaped relationship) between the ordinary doctors' reputations on the team and the focal doctor's appointment numbers.).

We used the utest command to test the inverted U-shaped curves in the empirical models.

For the leader's model, we tested the inverted U-shaped relationship between O_rep and APPT, and we saw that the extreme point was 6.477 and the range of O_rep was [−0.489, 20.557]. It can be seen that the extreme point is within the data range. $p > |t| = 0.00802$, the result is significant at a statistical level of 5%, which proves that there is an inverted U-shaped relationship between O_rep and APPT. The utest results for leader doctors are shown in Table 6.

Table 6. U–test results of leader.

Dependent Variable: APPT		
Test: H1: Inverse U Shape vs. H0: Monotone or U Shape		
Specification: $f(x) = x^2$ Extreme Point: 6.477339		
	Lower bound	Upper bound
Interval	−0.4888113	20.55774
Slope	0.507623	−1.026038
t-value	6.543666	−2.408667
$p > |t|$	3.25×10^{-11}	0.0080203
Overall test of presence of a Inverse U shape: t-value = 2.4 $p > |t| = 0.00802$		
95% Fieller interval for extreme point: [4.5529598; 13.757446]		

3.2. Results for Ordinary Doctors

3.2.1. Descriptive Statistic and Correlation for Ordinary Doctors

The descriptive statistics and correlations for the key variables used in ordinary doctors' research model are presented in Tables 7 and 8.

Table 7. Description statistics of ordinary doctors.

Variable	Obs	Mean	Std. Dev.	Min	Max
APPT	25,040	254.081	1,846.458	0	70,117
Rep	25,040	−0.048	0.713	−0.353	26.053
Leader rep	25,040	0.016	0.827	−0.479	13.106
Oo rep	25,040	0.027	0.815	−0.329	34.38
Oo rep2	25,040	0.666	12.253	0	1182.011
Rev	25,040	30.975	220.643	0	12,499
TeamSize	25,040	7.326	7.553	2	88
Title	25,040	3.678	0.915	1	5
Hosp	25,040	2.958	0.241	1	3
City	25,040	5.381	1.277	1	7

Notes: APPT = number of appointments; Rep = online reputation; Oo_rep = the average reputation of other ordinary doctors in the team; Oo_rep2 = The square of the average reputation of other ordinary doctors on the team; City = city level; Hosp = hospital level; Rev = review number; TeamSize = team size, Obs = observation, Std. Dev. = Standard Deviation, Min = minimum, Max= maximum.

Table 8. Matrix of correlations of ordinary doctors.

Variables	(1)	(2)	(3)	(4)	(5)	(6)	(7)	(8)	(9)	(10)
(1) APPT	1.000									
(2) Rep	0.497	1.000								
(3) Leader_rep	0.252	0.360	1.000							
(4) Oo_rep	0.301	0.358	0.318	1.000						
(5) Oo_rep2	0.058	0.040	0.026	0.658	1.000					
(6) Rev	0.716	0.530	0.217	0.244	0.048	1.000				
(7) TeamSize	0.015	0.031	0.296	0.004	−0.015	0.018	1.000			
(8) Title	0.110	0.184	−0.001	0.061	0.002	0.057	−0.062	1.000		
(9) Hosp	0.023	0.038	−0.115	0.002	0.003	0.004	−0.243	0.090	1.000	
(10) City	0.138	0.247	0.237	0.197	0.010	0.113	−0.088	0.070	−0.023	1.000

Notes: APPT = number of appointments; Rep = online reputation; Oo_rep = the average reputation of other ordinary doctors in the team; Oo_rep2 = The square of the average reputation of other ordinary doctors on the team; City = city level; Hosp = hospital level; Rev = review number; TeamSize = team size.

3.2.2. Regression Results of Ordinary Doctors' Research Model

The regression results for ordinary doctors are shown in Table 9. From Model 4, it is noted that Rep ($\beta = 0.329$, $p < 0.01$) and Leader_rep ($\beta = 0.318$, $p < 0.01$) have a positive effect on APPT. Therefore, H3 and H4 are supported (**H3:** *There is a positive correlation between the focal doctor's reputation and appointment numbers.* **H4:** *The reputation of the team's leader has a positive impact on the focal doctor's appointment numbers.*).

Table 9. Results of regression analyses of ordinary doctors.

	(3)	(4)
	Model3	Model4
Title	0.493 ***	0.512 ***
	(0.0118)	(0.0114)
City	0.234 ***	0.175 ***
	(0.00751)	(0.00727)
Hosp	0.216 ***	0.319 ***
	(0.0327)	(0.0325)
lnRev	0.810 ***	0.548 ***
	(0.0120)	(0.0324)
lnTeamSize	0.113 ***	−0.0153
	(0.0229)	(0.0230)
Rep		0.334 ***
		(0.0836)
Leader_rep		0.316 ***
		(0.0243)
Oo_rep		0.481 ***
		(0.0364)
Oo_rep2		−0.0194 ***
		(0.00396)
_cons	−3.560 ***	−3.116 ***
	(0.142)	(0.138)
N	25,040	25,002
R2	0.492	0.525

Note: The numbers in the tables are mostly beta values. The numbers in brackets are the standard errors. Department virtual variables are included in the model but are not shown in the table; *** $p < 0.001$.

Further, we note that the coefficient of Oo_rep's quadratic term ($\beta = -0.0198$, $p < 0.01$) is negative and significant. It means that the relationship between Oo_rep and APPT is nonlinear. Oo_rep has an inverted-U relationship with focal doctor's appointment numbers on the team, indicating that H5 is confirmed and in line with the social Interdependence theory (**H5:** *There is a nonlinear relationship (inverted U-shaped relationship) between other ordinary doctors' reputations on the team and the focal doctor's appointment numbers.*).

We used the utest command to test the inverted U-shaped curves in the empirical models.

For the ordinary doctor's model, we tested the inverted U-shaped relationship between Oo_rep and APPT, and we can see that the extreme point is 12.381 and the range of Oo_rep is [−11.467, 34.380]. It can be seen that the extreme point is within the data range. $p > |t| = 0.000262$, the result is significant at a statistical level of 5%, which proves that there is an inverted U-shaped relationship between Oo_rep and APPT. The utest results for leader doctors are shown in Table 10.

Table 10. Utest results of ordinary doctors.

Dependent Variable: APPT		
Test: H1: Inverse U shape vs. H0: Monotone or U Shape		
Specification: $f(x) = x^{\wedge}2$ Extreme Point: 12.38148		
	Lower bound	Upper bound
Interval	−11.46711	34.38039
Slope	0.92726	−0.8553423
t-value	7.7152	−3.468163
$p > |t|$	6.25×10^{-15}	0.0002625
Overall test of presence of a Inverse U shape: t-value = 3.47 $p > |t| = 0.000262$		
95% Fieller interval for extreme point: [9.6079864; 18.563818]		

4. Discussion

In this paper, the doctors in an online medical team were divided into the leaders and ordinary doctors. When the leader was the focal doctor, we studied the influence of the reputation of the focus doctor and the reputation of ordinary doctors on the team on the number of appointments of the focal doctor. The main findings were as follows.

The focal doctor's reputation has no impact on his or her own appointment numbers, which means that his or her appointment numbers will not change due to his or her reputation. The leader doctor who takes the lead in setting up the online medical team is ordinarily a senior expert with rich experience in diagnosis and treatment and high social status. When a patient makes an appointment, the reputation of the leader doctor is not the main consideration of the patient. Another possible explanation is that the leader doctor is usually a senior expert, with busy offline tasks and limited appointment opportunities on the Internet. Due to the ceiling effect, the number of online appointments of the leader doctor will not increase with the improvement of senior reputation.

The relationship between the reputation of ordinary doctors on the team and the focal doctor's appointment numbers is nonlinear, showing an inverted U-shaped relationship. This means that when the reputations of ordinary doctors on the team are at a low level, the reputations of ordinary doctors on the team have a positive spillover effect on the number of appointments of the focal doctor. At this time, these doctors cannot compete with the focal doctor. The higher the reputation of ordinary doctors on the team, the higher the focal doctor's appointment numbers, and the cooperative relationship between them; when the reputations of ordinary doctors on the team are high, the reputations of ordinary doctors on the team have a negative spillover effect on the focal doctor's appointment numbers. A high reputation represents a high quality of service. At this time, the service quality of ordinary doctors is also very high. They form a competitive relationship with the focal doctor.

When the ordinary doctor was the focal doctor, we studied the influence of his/her reputations, his/her leader's reputation, and other ordinary doctors' reputations on his/her number of appointments. The main findings are as follows.

The focal doctor's reputation has a positive impact on his/her own appointment numbers. This means that the number of appointments for ordinary doctors increases with their reputation. For ordinary doctors, online reputation reflects their service quality. The higher the online reputation is, the higher the service quality is and the chance of being selected by patients increases. As a result, the number of appointments for ordinary doctors will increase with their reputations.

The reputation of the leader doctor has a positive impact on the focal doctor's appointment numbers. This means that in an online health care team, the higher the reputation of the leader doctor, the higher the focal doctor's appointment numbers. As the brand of the team, the leader doctor has a greater visibility impact. The higher his or her reputation is, the more opportunities his/her team's doctors have to be selected.

There is a nonlinear relationship (inverted U-shaped relationship) between the reputation of other ordinary doctors on the team and the number of appointments of the focal doctor on the team. This means that when the reputations of other ordinary doctors on the team are at a low level, the reputations of other ordinary doctors on the team have a positive spillover effect on the number of appointments of the focal doctor. At this time, other ordinary doctors on the team are not enough to pose a competitive threat to the focal doctor; when the reputations of other ordinary doctors on the team are high, the reputations of other ordinary doctors on the team have a negative spillover effect on the number of appointments of the focal doctor. At this time, other ordinary doctors on the team compete with the focal doctor.

5. Conclusions

5.1. Key Findings

There were several major findings in this study. For a leader doctor, his/her appointment numbers are not related to his/her own reputation, and there was an inverted U-shaped relationship with the ordinary doctors' reputations on the team. For an ordinary doctor, his/her appointment numbers were positively correlated with his/her own reputation and positively correlated with his/her leader's reputation and there was an inverted U-shaped relationship with the other ordinary doctors' reputations. The research shows that there is a positive spillover effect on the team leaders' reputation. There are two relationships between team doctors: competition and cooperation. This study provides guidance for the leader to select team members and the ordinary doctor to select a team.

5.2. Implications for Research

Online medical team is a new model of online health care. It is important to help hierarchical treatment, balance medical resources, and improve medical efficiency. Existing research has focused on the overall performance of the team [1,27]. However, there are few studies on team member relationships in this field. This study examined the impact of teammates' online reputations on physicians' online appointment numbers. It is important not only for doctors but also for platform providers of electronic consultation websites to understand the factors that affect doctors' online reputations because it is a goal of platform providers to stimulate doctors to continue to participate and provide services.

Second, our research adds new insights to existing reputation theories. Previous research on online market reputation has focused on the analysis of individuals. Our research reveals the importance of member interaction. Our results provide evidence that teammates' online reputations affect the focal doctor's appointment numbers. This result suggests that when we study individuals in a team, we should bring the individual into the organizational environment and consider the influence of other team members.

This study expands and enriches the scope and meaning of the application of social interdependence theory. Social interdependence theory is mainly applied in the fields of psychology, education, and physical education. This study extends the social interdependence theory to the online health. This study explored the influence of the teammates' reputations on the focal doctor's appointment numbers. We found that there are two types of dependence between the leader doctor and the general doctor and between the general doctor and the general doctor, namely competition and cooperation.

5.3. Practical Significance

For the leader doctor, the results show that the leader doctor's own reputation has no effect on the number of appointments. This suggests that the leader doctor does not need to spend too much effort on reputation building. An increase in the reputation of an ordinary doctor whose reputation is in the lower range has a positive spillover effect on the leader doctor's appointment numbers. An increase in the reputation of an ordinary doctor whose reputation is in the higher range has a negative spillover effect on the leader doctor's appointment numbers. Therefore, the leader doctor may select the ordinary doctor with a medium reputation as his/her member.

For ordinary doctors, both their own reputations and the leader doctors' reputation have a positive impact on their appointment numbers. Therefore, ordinary doctors can concentrate on improving their service quality to help improve their reputation. They can also choose to join a team of the leader with a high reputation. There is a nonlinear relationship (inverted U-shaped relationship) between the reputation of other ordinary doctors on the team and the focal doctor's appointment numbers. It shows that when the reputations of other ordinary doctors on the team are at a low level, there is a cooperative relationship between them. When the reputations of other ordinary doctors on the team are at a high level, there is a competitive relationship. Therefore, a team with low reputations among other ordinary doctors on the team should be selected to join.

For designers and providers of online health platforms, this research helps them retain doctors and promote the prosperity of the platform. The results can help designers and providers of online health platforms understand how to improve the performance of doctors, especially how to help specific groups of doctors improve their performance. For example, a recommendation mechanism can be set up to recommend young doctors and general doctors with low reputations to the leader doctor as team members. It can also recommend online medical teams for young doctors and general doctors based on the reputation of the leader doctor and the overall reputations of the team's ordinary doctors.

6. Limitations and Future Work

(1) A multilevel approach was not possible due to a lack of data on the team level. Since the website currently does not have team-level data, we were unable to design team-level variables. We believe that the data will be enriched with the improvement of website. Once the team-level data are available, we will consider further adding the team-level variables to our study for multilevel analysis.

(2) This study examined the effect of teammates' reputations on the focal doctor's appointment numbers. Since other attributes of teammates may also have an effect on the focal doctor's appointment numbers, such as teammates' effort and status. In a future study, we intend to examine the effect of other attributes of teammates, such as teammates' effort and status, on the focal doctor's appointment numbers. This will further enrich the social interdependence theory.

(3) This study examined only Guahao.com's team of experts. Future research could be extended to medical teams or organizations on other online platforms. For example, China's haodf.com has established a similar online medical team. To test whether our findings are still valid in other circumstances, we considered collecting data from other online health care platforms for future studies.

(4) Due to data limitations, cross-sectional data were used in this study. It is possible that some of the independent variables relevant to our work may have been missed. The panel data can effectively

reduce or eliminate the impact of this problem. Therefore, the panel data will be considered for further research.

Author Contributions: Conceptualization, X.Z.; data curation, X.Z. and J.W.; formal analysis, Y.Z.; methodology, X.Z. and J.K.; writing–original draft, X.Z.; writing–review and editing, J.L. All authors have read and agreed to the published version of the manuscript.

Funding: This research was funded by the Natural Science Foundation of Shanghai, grant number 19ZR1419400.

Conflicts of Interest: The authors declare no conflict of interest.

References

1. Salas, E.; Zajac, S.; Marlow, S.L. Transforming Health Care One Team at a Time: Ten Observations and the Trail Ahead. *Group Organ. Manag.* **2018**, *43*, 357–381. [CrossRef]
2. Moyal, A. Team practice in multi-professional healthcare homes: A division of labour under medical control. *Rev. Fr. Aff. Soc.* **2020**, *1*, 103–123. [CrossRef]
3. Schmutz, J.B.; Meier, L.L.; Manser, T. How effective is teamwork really? The relationship between teamwork and performance in healthcare teams: A systematic review and meta-analysis. *BMJ Open* **2019**, *9*, e028280. [CrossRef]
4. Lacagnina, S.; Moore, M.; Mitchell, S. The Lifestyle Medicine Team: Health Care That Delivers Value. *Am. J. Lifestyle Med.* **2018**, *12*, 479–483. [CrossRef]
5. Berry, L.L.; Beckham, D. Team-Based Care at Mayo Clinic: A Model for ACOs. *J. Health Manag.* **2014**, *59*, 9–13. [CrossRef]
6. El-Awaisi, A.; O'Carroll, V.; Koraysh, S.; Koummich, S.; Huber, M. Perceptions of who is in the healthcare team? A content analysis of social media posts during COVID-19 pandemic. *J. Interprof. Care* **2020**, *34*, 622–632. [CrossRef] [PubMed]
7. Rosen, M.A.; DiazGranados, D.; Dietz, A.S.; Benishek, L.E.; Thompson, D.; Pronovost, P.J.; Weaver, S.J. Teamwork in healthcare: Key discoveries enabling safer, high-quality care. *Am. Psychol.* **2018**, *73*, 433–450. [CrossRef]
8. Johnson, A.; Nguyen, H.; Groth, M.; White, L. Reaping the Rewards of Functional Diversity in Healthcare Teams: Why Team Processes Improve Performance. *Group Organ. Manag.* **2018**, *43*, 440–474. [CrossRef]
9. Maynard, M.T.; Mathieu, J.E.; Rapp, T.L.; Gilson, L.L.; Kleiner, C. Team leader coaching intervention: An investigation of the impact on team processes and performance within a surgical context. *J. Appl. Psychol.* **2020**. [CrossRef]
10. Samuriwo, R.; Laws, E.; Webb, K.; Bullock, A.D. "I didn't realise they had such a key role." Impact of medical education curriculum change on medical student interactions with nurses: A qualitative exploratory study of student perceptions. *Adv. Health Sci. Educ.* **2019**, *25*, 75–93. [CrossRef]
11. Li, H.; Fang, Y.; Lim, K.H.; Wang, Y. Platform-Based Function Repertoire, Reputation, and Sales Performance of E-Marketplace Sellers. *MIS Q.* **2019**, *43*, 207–236. [CrossRef]
12. Anagnostopoulou, S.C.; Buhalis, D.; Kountouri, I.L.; Manousakis, E.G.; Tsekrekos, A.E. The impact of online reputation on hotel profitability. *Int. J. Contemp. Hosp. Manag.* **2020**, *32*, 20–39. [CrossRef]
13. Youness, C.; Valette-Florence, P.; Herrmann, J.-L. The Effects of Customer-Based Online Reputation on WOM and WPP: The Mediating Role of BRQ: An Abstract. In Proceedings of the 2008 Academy of Marketing Science (AMS) Annual Conference, Porto, Portugal, 26–29 June 2018; pp. 893–894.
14. Al-Yazidi, S.; Berri, J.; Al-Qurishi, M.; Al-Alrubaian, M. Measuring Reputation and Influence in Online Social Networks: A Systematic Literature Review. *IEEE Access* **2020**, *8*, 1. [CrossRef]
15. Tadelis, S. Reputation and Feedback Systems in Online Platform Markets. *Annu. Rev. Econ.* **2016**, *8*, 321–340. [CrossRef]
16. Gavilan, D.; Avello, M.; Martinez-Navarro, G. The influence of online ratings and reviews on hotel booking consideration. *Tour. Manag.* **2018**, *66*, 53–61. [CrossRef]
17. Luca, M. *Reviews, Reputation, and Revenue: The Case of Yelp.com*; Harvard Business School NOM Unit Working Paper: Boston, MA, USA, 2016.
18. Patel, S.; Cain, R.; Neailey, K.; Hooberman, L.; Alemi, F.; Lagu, T. Exploring Patients' Views Toward Giving Web-Based Feedback and Ratings to General Practitioners in England: A Qualitative Descriptive Study. *J. Med. Internet Res.* **2016**, *18*, e217. [CrossRef]

19. Burkle, C.M.; Keegan, M.T. Popularity of internet physician rating sites and their apparent influence on patients' choices of physicians. *BMC Health Serv. Res.* **2015**, *15*, 416. [CrossRef]
20. Gu, D.; Yang, X.; Li, X.; Jain, H.K.; Liang, C. Understanding the Role of Mobile Internet-Based Health Services on Patient Satisfaction and Word-of-Mouth. *Int. J. Environ. Res. Public Health* **2018**, *15*, 1972. [CrossRef]
21. Davydovich, A.R.; Shmeleva, T.V.; Syrkova, I.S. The medical organization of primary care: Competitiveness and reputation. *Probl. Soc. Hyg. Public Health Hist. Med.* **2020**, *28*, 729–735. [CrossRef]
22. Sattler, H.; Völckner, F.; Riediger, C.; Ringle, C.M. The impact of brand extension success drivers on brand extension price premiums. *Int. J. Res. Mark.* **2010**, *27*, 319–328. [CrossRef]
23. Platow, M.J.; Grace, D.M.; Smithson, M.J. Examining the Preconditions for Psychological Group Membership. *Soc. Psychol. Pers. Sci.* **2011**, *3*, 5–13. [CrossRef]
24. Koffka, K. *Principles of Gestalt Psychology. A Harbinger Book*; Harbinger: London, UK, 2005; Volume 20, pp. 623–628.
25. Kurt, L. A Dynamic Theory of Personality. *J. Nerv. Ment. Dis.* **1936**, *85*, 612–613.
26. Polley, R.B.; McGrath, J.E. Groups: Interaction and Performance. *Adm. Sci. Q.* **1984**, *29*, 469. [CrossRef]
27. Johnson, D.W.; Johnson, R.T. *Cooperation and Competition: Theory and Research*; Interaction Book Company: Edina, MN, USA, 1989; p. viii, 253.
28. Johnson, D.W.; Johnson, R.T. An Educational Psychology Success Story: Social Interdependence Theory and Cooperative Learning. *Educ. Res.* **2009**, *38*, 365–379. [CrossRef]
29. Bruner, M.W.; Eys, M.; Evans, M.B.; Wilson, K. Interdependence and Social Identity in Youth Sport Teams. *J. Appl. Sport Psychol.* **2015**, *27*, 351–358. [CrossRef]
30. Bertucci, A.; Johnson, D.W.; Johnson, R.T.; Conte, S. The Effects of Task and Resource Interdependence on Achievement and Social Support: An Exploratory Study of Italian Children. *J. Psychol.* **2011**, *145*, 343–360. [CrossRef]
31. Colasante, A.; García-Gallego, A.; Morone, A.; Temerario, T. The Utopia of Cooperation: Does Intra-Group Competition Drive out Free Riding? 2017. Available online: http://www.doctreballeco.uji.es/wpficheros/Colasante_et_al_08_2017.pdf (accessed on 23 November 2020).
32. Rogelberg, S.G. *The SAGE Encyclopedia of Industrial and Organizational Psychology*, 2nd ed.; SAGE Publication Inc.: Charlotte, NC, USA, 2017.
33. Wu, H.; Lu, N. How your colleagues' reputation impact your patients' odds of posting experiences: Evidence from an online health community. *Electron. Commer. Res. Appl.* **2016**, *16*, 7–17. [CrossRef]
34. Deng, Z.; Hong, Z.; Zhang, W.; Evans, R.M.; Chen, Y.; Hao, H.; Bidmon, S.; Li, L. The Effect of Online Effort and Reputation of Physicians on Patients' Choice: 3-Wave Data Analysis of China's Good Doctor Website. *J. Med. Internet Res.* **2019**, *21*, e10170. [CrossRef]
35. Liu, X.; Chen, M.; Li, J.; Ma, L. How to Manage Diversity and Enhance Team Performance: Evidence from Online Doctor Teams in China. *Int. J. Environ. Res. Public Health* **2019**, *17*, 48. [CrossRef]
36. Wu, H.; Lu, N. Service provision, pricing, and patient satisfaction in online health communities. *Int. J. Med. Inform.* **2018**, *110*, 77–89. [CrossRef]
37. Montani, F.; Vandenberghe, C.; Khedhaouria, A.; Courcy, F. Examining the inverted U-shaped relationship between workload and innovative work behavior: The role of work engagement and mindfulness. *Hum. Relat.* **2019**, *73*, 59–93. [CrossRef]
38. Rezvani, E.; Assaf, A.G.; Uysal, M.; Lee, M. Learning from own and others: The moderating role of performance aspiration. *Int. J. Hosp. Manag.* **2019**, *81*, 113–119. [CrossRef]
39. Lind, J.T.; Mehlum, H. With or Without U? The Appropriate Test for a U-Shaped Relationship. *Oxf. Bull. Econ. Stat.* **2010**, *72*, 109–118. [CrossRef]

Publisher's Note: MDPI stays neutral with regard to jurisdictional claims in published maps and institutional affiliations.

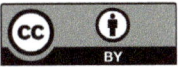

© 2020 by the authors. Licensee MDPI, Basel, Switzerland. This article is an open access article distributed under the terms and conditions of the Creative Commons Attribution (CC BY) license (http://creativecommons.org/licenses/by/4.0/).

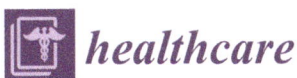

Article

Development of a Novel Interactive Multimedia E-Learning Model to Enhance Clinical Competency Training and Quality of Care among Medical Students

Yu-Ting Hsiao [1], Hsuan-Yin Liu [2] and Chih-Cheng Hsiao [3,4,*]

1. Department of Ophthalmology, Kaohsiung Chang Gung Memorial Hospital, Kaohsiung 83301, Taiwan; yuting1008@cgmh.org.tw
2. Department of Medical Education, Kaohsiung Chang Gung Memorial Hospital, Kaohsiung 83301, Taiwan; liu.hsuanyin@gmail.com
3. Division of Hematology/Oncology, Department of Pediatrics, Kaohsiung Chang Gung Memorial Hospital and Chang Gung University College of Medicine, Kaohsiung 83301, Taiwan
4. Chang Gung Memorial Hospital Research Centre for Medical Education, Taoyuan 333, Taiwan
* Correspondence: hsiaojc@cgmh.org.tw; Tel.: +886-7731-7123 (ext. 8701)

Received: 12 October 2020; Accepted: 18 November 2020; Published: 20 November 2020

Abstract: Clinical competencies consisting of skills, knowledge, and communication techniques should be acquired by all medical graduates to optimize healthcare quality. However, transitioning from observation to hands-on learning in clinical competencies poses a challenge to medical students. The aim of this study is to evaluate the impact of a novel interactive multimedia eBook curriculum in clinical competency training. Ninety-six medical students were recruited. Students in the control group ($n = 46$) were taught clinical competencies via conventional teaching, while students in the experimental group ($n = 50$) were taught with conventional teaching plus interactive multimedia eBooks. The outcomes of clinical competencies were evaluated using Objective Structured Clinical Examination (OSCE) scores, and feedback on their interactive eBook experiences was obtained. In the experimental group, the average National OSCE scores were not only higher than the control group (214.8 vs. 206.5, $p < 0.001$), but also showed a quicker improvement when comparing between three consecutive mock OSCEs ($p < 0.001$). In response to open-ended questions, participants emphasized the importance of eBooks in improving their abilities and self-confidence when dealing with 'difficult' patients. Implementing interactive multimedia eBooks could prompt a more rapid improvement in clinical skill performance to provide safer healthcare, indicating the potential of our innovative module in enhancing clinical competencies.

Keywords: eBooks; medical education; clinical competencies; interactive; e-learning

1. Introduction

The two essential bonds in health care and medical education—doctor–patient and teacher–learner relationships—have been at the core of medicine for decades. As patients rightfully trust the systems to adequately train doctors that are caring for them, the focus on establishing patient safety in medical education can provide confirmation of that trust, and therefore is of interest among medical educators. Furthermore, e-learning has become increasingly utilized in medical education globally, and educators must embrace the need for strategic improvement if knowledge for healthcare safety is to find its way to their students [1]. As many rapid advances in online medical educational systems have been made, there are several e-learning resources to provide different strategies for medical students to enhance their knowledge and performance [2–4]. Therefore, the question of its effectiveness and its integration into the medical education curriculum is a matter of importance [5–7].

Emphasis on patient safety and high-value care necessitates the acquisition of clinical skills, knowledge and attitudes as competencies in medical practice. During the final years of study, medical students are required to do rotations at hospitals and clinics, and play an active role in patient care. The concept of competencies is important as it implies a developmental transition from a medical student to, ultimately, a skilled and expert practitioner. To evaluate the complex notion of clinical competence, the Objective Structured Clinical Examination (OSCE) has developed into a mainstream assessment method in the education and licensing of physicians. OSCE testing has quickly become the standard process of certification, and is a part of the Medical Licensing Examination for medical graduates in various regions, including the U.S., Canada, the United Kingdom, and Taiwan. In 2011, the Taiwan Medical College Accreditation Council established 81 clinical competencies that should be acquired upon graduating. The clinical competencies included fields in physical examination skills, image interpretations, laboratory diagnosis techniques, procedure skills, treatment techniques and other activities [8,9]. Although the learning objectives are clearly defined, there is still a lack of well-organized curriculums to teach the clinical competencies, which in turn could result in inadequate clinical skills and poor doctor–patient relationships. A study has reported that 55.9% of students were confident that they had acquired the clinical skills required to become a resident, and 70.7% were satisfied with the quality of their medical education [10]. As such, in order to acquire sufficient knowledge and clinical skills, medical students have to spend more time self-studying clinical skills. Medical schools may also hold small sets of OSCE testing to help students in clinical competency training and to also pass the required assessment. However, the labor- and resource-intensive nature of OSCE testing makes it difficult for most medical schools to consistently invest this amount of time and money [11]. For example, Quebec Medical College reported spending USD 1080 for each student in a comprehensive OSCE [12]. Therefore, not only is it important to integrate clinical competencies into a new curriculum to help students, but also to provide students with suitable self-studying learning resources to optimize healthcare quality and patient safety.

Thanks to the advances in network technology, medical students are able to enhance their knowledge on patient care by e-learning nowadays. Ekenze et al. reported that most medical students are familiar with Internet tools and use them for learning, and they believe that the tools may be useful in integrating e-learning modality in the traditional mode of surgical education [13]. In fact, administrators and learners both find that e-learning enhances the teaching and learning experience [2]. E-learning is more efficient in allowing learners to gain knowledge and skills faster than traditional instructor-led methods [2,14]. In turn, this efficiency may be converted into improved motivation for learning. Evidence further suggests that e-learners have demonstrated increased retention rates and better utilization of content, resulting in better learning outcomes [14]. Furthermore, e-learners can select from a large variety of multimedia designs, including interactivity, feedback, and practice exercises to accommodate their different learning styles. This advantage in e-learning improves content accessibility, provides a personalized learning experience, further ensuring students are equipped with the knowledge, skills and attitudes necessary to function safely [15,16].

Despite the many benefits of e-learning, one problem is often faced: e-learning generally provides passive ways of learning, which lacks interactive instructional strategies and one-on-one guidance [3,17]. It is acknowledged that interactive learning offers a stronger learning reinforcement and helps to maintain the learner's interest [2]. For medical students to develop clinical competencies, they should learn by relating acquired knowledge to clinical experiences, and further applying these skills in daily practice [2,18]. Therefore, classes in empathy, medical knowledge, patient care, clinical skills, and communication are integrated into the curriculum in medical schools, and the use of simulated models or standardized patients places theory in a clinical scenario [19]. However, at present, there are no practical interactive, self-studying tools for strengthening clinical competencies.

In this study, an eBook editing software (SimMAGIC eBook, Hamastar technology company, Taiwan) with simple and highly customizable interface was employed to create 81 interactive multimedia eBooks for training and learning clinical competencies. This eBook software has a wide array of editing functions and enables editors to produce a simulative eBook by integrating various forms of multimedia into each eBook. Students are required to take simulated tests by interacting with the content in eBooks, and initial feedback could be given immediately to enhance the learning experience. A learning-management system was also designed to track the students' outcome assessments [20]. The aim of this study is to investigate the effect of interactive eBooks on the enhancement of clinical competencies, and their impact on the students' OSCE performance. The second objective of this study is to provide a further understanding of how the interactive eBooks are perceived by medical students in practical healthcare settings.

2. Materials and Methods

2.1. Study Design and Participants

The participants enrolled in this study were medical students who were in their final year of medical school and doing clinical rotations in Kaohsiung Chang Gung Memorial Hospital, Taiwan. The control group consisted of 46 students who were taught clinical skills via conventional teaching, which consisted of teaching through direct patient care by a group of clinical teachers and senior physicians. The experimental group consisted of 50 students, which were taught by conventional teaching plus interactive multimedia eBooks. The learning outcomes of clinical competencies were evaluated using mock OSCEs and OSCE scores in the Taiwan's National Medical Licensing Examination (National OSCE) to measure the clinical skill performance. Three mock OSCEs were held by Kaohsiung Chang Gung Memorial Hospital in August, November, and February. In the end, their final performance of clinical competencies was evaluated by the National OSCE. For an in-depth understanding of student experience with the eBooks, students in the experimental group were asked to perform a pre- and post-test included in each eBook session and anonymously answer a Likert-scale questionnaire. The experimental timeline is illustrated in Figure 1.

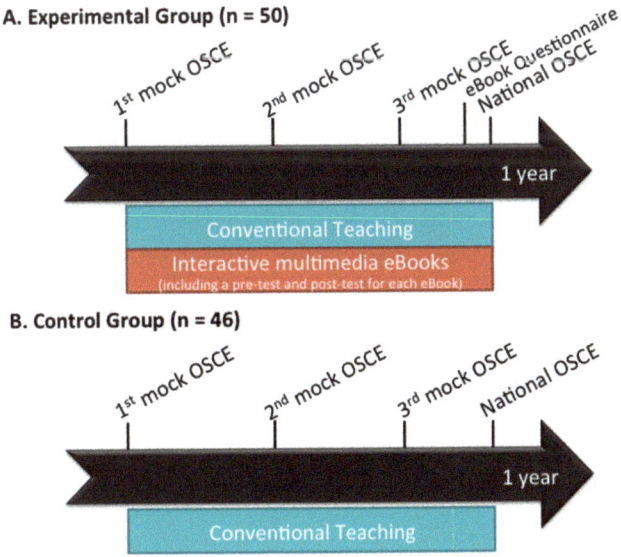

Figure 1. Schematic illustration of the experimental timeline.

In this study, we used SimMAGIC eBook software to create 81 interactive multimedia eBooks for learning clinical skills. SimMAGIC eBook editing software was introduced in a previous study [20], allowing editors to use various interactive functions such as drag and drop, filling in the blanks, matching and sorting exercises, pop-ups, animations, and clips of audio and videos to create eBooks (Figure 2). The saved eBook can be edited or updated anytime, and anyone can use the eBook software. In this program, at first, we collected the PowerPoint slides of clinical competencies from clinical teachers. The contents were classified into different fields including physical examination (31 topics), visual image interpretation (6 topics), laboratory examination (8 topics), procedure skills (16 topics), therapeutic skills (14 topics) and others (6 topics). The contents were reviewed by other clinical teachers, who made sure the contents followed and covered the learning objectives.

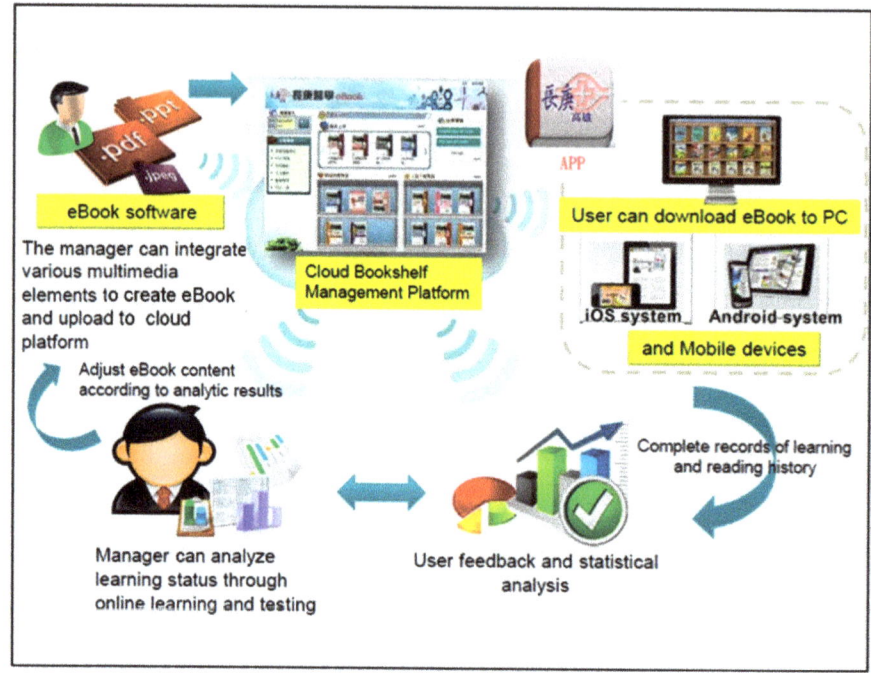

Figure 2. Establishment of the Bookshelf Management Cloud Platform.

Next, we integrated multimedia resources such as PowerPoint text, images, video, and audio into each interactive multimedia eBook, and emphasis was given to transitioning passive and instructor-led lectures into simulative and interactive educational materials (Figure 3). Afterwards, we uploaded the newly created eBooks to a Bookshelf Management Cloud Platform, which was compatible with eBook file formats. The eBooks can be downloaded to PC, tablets and mobile phones anytime and anywhere, permitting increased accessibility. A learning-management system is available on the platform, allowing medical educators to track the learners' accession of each module and their achievement of competencies. The Bookshelf Management Cloud Platform enables offline reading, and the offline user history is recorded and uploaded to the platform upon connection to the Internet.

In both groups, learning outcomes of clinical competencies were accessed by holding 3 mock OSCEs to measure the learners' clinical skill performance; the first mock OSCE was conducted on participants prior to commencement of the study, the second was arranged during the study period, and the third mock OSCE was held before the approaching National OSCE. National OSCE scores were also taken into account in both the control and experimental groups. In the experimental group, besides participants being asked to complete a pre-test and a post-test which were included in each eBook learning session, the students also took a feedback questionnaire on eBook satisfaction and its impact in healthcare practice near the end of the study period. Each student was given a different username and password for the eBook module in order to track their learning process individually.

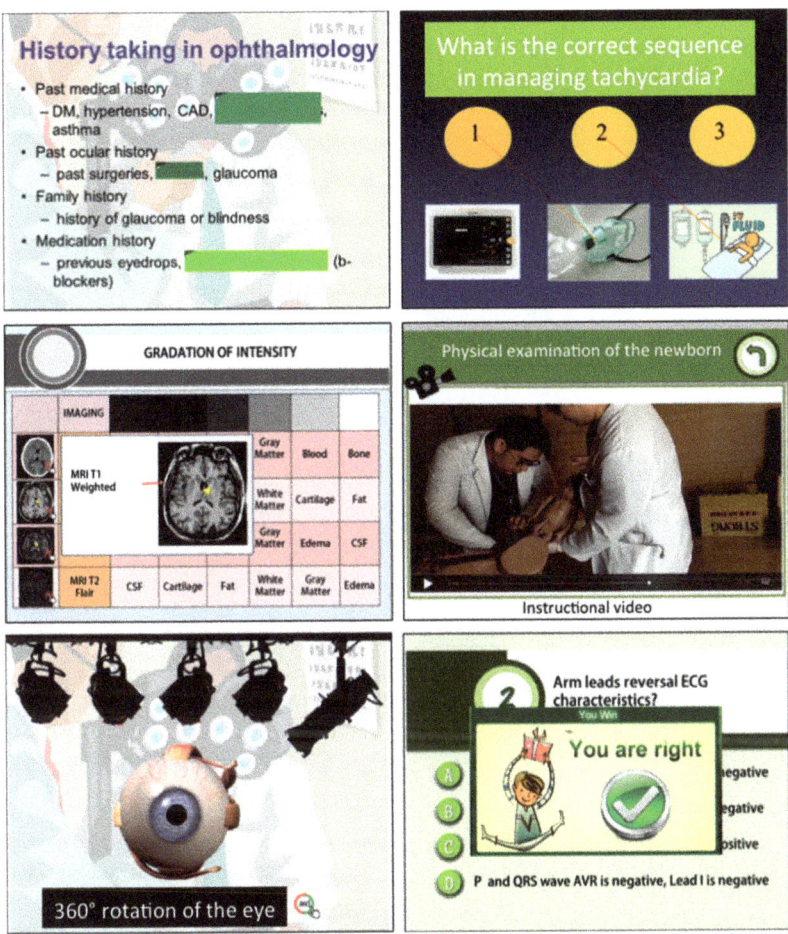

Figure 3. Interface of various interactive functions in our eBook module, including simulation models in anatomy, instructional videos, labeling exercises, comprehensive multi-page assessments, and interactive scenarios with instructive feedback.

2.2. Data Collection

We modified the Kirkpatrick model to evaluate the outcome of our interactive multimedia eBooks using two major approaches: learning outcomes and self-reported measures in confidence and dealing with problems of patients [21]. Learning outcomes were assessed by average scores of pre-test and post-test and cognitive learning gain. The short tests consisted of 5 multiple-choice questions prepared by the educator, and they were given to the students before and after participating in our eBook module. We used the pre/post-test to determine cognitive gain during eBook learning. According to Hake's criteria for effectiveness of educational intervention, absolute learning gain (%post-test score − %pre-test score) and class-average normalized gain (%post-test score − %pre-test score) / (100 − %pre-test score) were also calculated. A class-average normalized gain of 30 % was considered significant [22].

A 19-item questionnaire was designed to investigate the students' reactions to eBooks. The first part of the questionnaire consisted of 8 items regarding the quality of teaching material and their attitudes towards how helpful the eBooks were when they were performing clinical competencies in practical settings. The second part involved 5 items, which assessed the participants' perception in raising confidence during clinical practice and in developing good doctor–patient relationships. The last part of the questionnaire contained 6 items regarding the eBook platform user interface and the manner of eBook interactive content delivery. Participants rated their responses on a five-point Likert scale, with 5 being strongly agree and 1 being strongly disagree. Additional qualitative data were collected from written responses from open-ended questions on the impact of eBooks on their practice at the end of the self-assessment questionnaire.

2.3. Data Analysis

We compared the pre/post-test data and National OSCE scores using Student t-test. The ANOVA test was used to determine significant differences in mock OSCE scores, and Fisher's least significant difference (LSD) was used for post hoc comparisons. A p value of < 0.05 was considered statistically significant. All statistical analyses were conducted using SPSS version 20 (SPSS Inc., Chicago, IL, USA).

3. Results

Ninety-six medical students performing clinical rotations took part in this study. Twenty-three percent of the participants were female and 77% were male. Through the three mock OSCEs held in the study period, both groups showed significant improvement (control group, $p = 0.006$; experimental group, $p < 0.001$) (Table 1). The average scores of the 46 participants in the control group showed a significant difference when comparing the third mock OSCE to the first one ($p < 0.001$) (Figure 4). In the experimental group, a significant improvement was found between the second and first mock OSCE ($p < 0.001$), and the third and the first mock OSCE scores ($p < 0.001$) (Figure 4). Last but not least, all of the participants in our study passed the National OSCE; the average OSCE scores in the experimental group were higher than the scores in the control group (214.8 in the experimental group vs. 206.5 in the control group, $p < 0.001$) (Figure 5). In addition, in the experimental group, there was a significant difference in improvement when comparing between the pre-test and post-test scores (74.8 ± 9.87 for pre-test vs. 86.6 ± 11.49 for post-test, $p < 0.001$) (Figure 6). The absolute learning gain was 11.8, whereas the class-average normalized gain was 46.8%.

Table 1. Mock Objective Structured Clinical Examination (OSCE) mean scores of the control group and the experimental group.

	Mean Scores	p Value
Control group		0.006
First	68.26 ± 6.06	
Second	69.74 ± 4.57	
Third	71.78 ± 4.79	
Experimental group		<0.001
First	68.30 ± 6.40	
Second	74.14 ± 5.47	
Third	74.60 ± 6.99	

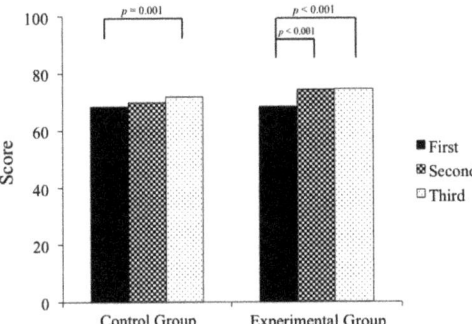

Figure 4. The average mock OSCE scores of the control group showed a significant difference when comparing the third exam to the first one ($p = 0.001$), whereas in the experimental group, there was already a significant improvement found between the second and first, and the third and the first mock OSCE scores ($p < 0.001$).

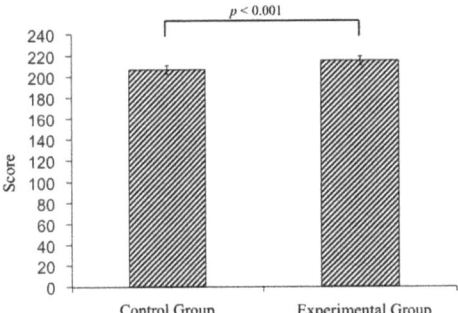

Figure 5. The average scores of National OSCE were higher in the experimental group than the scores in the control group (214.8 in the experimental group vs. 206.5 in the control group, $p < 0.001$).

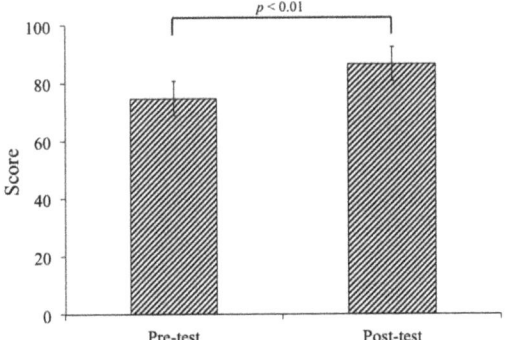

Figure 6. The students' performance score on the post-test was significantly higher than the pretest (74.8 ± 9.87 for pretest vs. 86.6 ± 11.49 for posttest, $p < 0.001$) in the experimental group. Student's t-test was used in comparison between pre-test and post-test. A p-value < 0.05 is considered statistically significant.

In the experimental group, all of the 50 participants returned the feedback questionnaire (response rate 100%). The average rating for the majority of the questions ranged between 4.0 and 4.5 (Tables 2–4), suggesting that a majority of participants perceived interactive multimedia eBooks as being useful in enhancing clinical competencies. Table 2 shows the students' response regarding the quality of teaching material and their attitudes towards how clinically relevant the eBooks were. Table 3 presents participants' responses in confidence boosting during clinical practice and in helping to develop good doctor–patient relationships after using eBooks. Table 4 shows the students' responses regarding the eBook platform user interface.

Table 2. Students' responses on the quality of teaching materials and how helpful the eBooks were when they were performing clinical competencies in practical settings. ($n = 50$).

No.	Questionnaire	Average Rating
1	Interactive materials improve my learning efficiency	4.22/agree
2	Interactive materials can improve the retention of knowledge	4.23/agree
3	Interactive materials increase my focus in learning	4.03/agree
4	Interactive materials enhance learning motivations	4.12/agree
5	Teaching materials improve my ability in solving problems	4.09/agree
6	The teaching material helps to improve my clinical skills	4.22/agree
7	The teaching material improves my ability in making appropriate treatment decisions based upon patients' needs	4.22/agree
8	eBooks increase my interest in dealing with clinical competency aspects of patient care	4.20/agree
	Overall average	4.17/agree

A five-point Likert scale was used, where rating 1: Strongly Disagree, 2: Disagree, 3: Neutral, 4: Agree, 5: Strongly Agree.

Table 3. Students' responses in raising confidence during clinical practice and in developing good doctor-patient relationships. ($n = 50$).

No.	Questionnaire	Average Rating
1	The teaching materials raise my confidence in handling difficult patient encounters	4.32/agree
2	Self-studying eBooks could enhance my skills to promote better doctor-patient relationships	4.32/agree
3	The teaching contents make it easier to understand and interpret information patients are giving me	4.31/agree
4	eBooks can allow me to obtain information from patients in a systematic way	4.32/agree
5	eBooks allow me to perform my clinical competency skills with ease, making me more aware of how patients react to me	4.29/agree
	Overall average	4.31/agree

A five-point Likert scale was used, where 1: Strongly Disagree, 2: Disagree, 3: Neutral, 4: Agree, 5: Strongly Agree.

Table 4. Students' responses regarding the eBook platform user interface. ($n = 50$).

No.	Questionnaire	Average Rating
1	Easy-to-use eBook platform user interface	4.11/agree
2	eBook platform features a variety of useful functions	4.18/agree
3	The platform enhances my learning experience	4.03/agree
4	The eBook reading interface is easy to understand	4.08/agree
5	The functions in reading interface facilitate learning	3.95/neutral
6	Using eBook platform can increase my interest in learning	4.15/agree
	Overall average	4.08/agree

A five-point Likert scale was used, where rating 1: Strongly Disagree, 2: Disagree, 3: Neutral, 4: Agree, 5: Strongly Agree.

In response to the open-ended questions, participants pointed out the benefits of eBook learning in improving their confidence in practicing clinical competencies, especially in 'difficult' patients, having more empathy by performing clinical competency skills with ease, and allowing them to be able to read subtle cues from patients, and have different solutions to different scenarios to build a stronger doctor–patient relationship (Table 5). Most of the negative aspects of the students' responses were related to the functional design of the platform. Several participants also commented on the limitation of downloading only one eBook at a time, the lack of systematic organization with which eBooks are arranged and ordered, and the need for customized labels for marking eBooks as read or unread.

Table 5. Students' open-ended responses from eBook learning.

Category	Responses
Confidence in handling difficult clinical settings	■ Helped me deal with difficult patients (e.g., difficult nasogastric tube insertion procedures) ■ Have a better understanding of what to expect of difficult patients ■ In a difficult patient setting, I could easily remember the alternative techniques and tips that were taught adequately in eBooks
More empathy towards the patient	■ To be able to perform clinical competency skills with more ease allows me to pick up on subtle cues from patients and recognize patients in distress ■ It helped me put myself in the patients' shoes and become more considerate. ■ Be more empathic and see them from the patient's point of view ■ Understand the patient's concerns
Improvement in the doctor-patient relationship	■ Have different solutions when dealing with different difficulties, which is a foundation for a stronger patient-doctor relationship ■ Helped me control my emotions and uncertainty during practice due to sufficient training of competencies from eBooks

The eBooks used in our study were accessible on mobile devices. In terms of how the participants accessed the eBooks, 46% of the participants reported that they used mobile devices as a primary device for accessing the eBooks, while 54% used a desktop computer or a laptop. Of the students who obtained eBooks from mobile devices, about 61% used tablets, 26% used smartphones with an Android system, and 13% with an iPhone.

4. Discussion

Efforts to discern patient safety and quality of care constantly push medical education into new territory [1]. As new e-learning environments are introduced into the field of medical education, there is an increasing need for establishing evaluations for these innovative e-learning systems. In concordance with other previous studies [3,23–25], the present study shows that students have positive perceptions upon integrating a new e-learning module to supplement traditional training materials. Our findings indicate that interactive multimedia eBook training offers a promising approach to enhance students' knowledge and skills on improving clinical competencies to promote safety and reliability in healthcare.

Strategic improvement in health and healthcare starts with focusing on improving medical education. In the continuum of medical education, the beginner learns by applying a defined set of rules to new unforeseen situations, and as learners acquire experience, they become more intuitive as rule-bound behaviors begin to emerge [1]. During this process of training future licensed physicians, effective and safe clinical systems are required [26]. We believe that interactive multimedia eBooks represent a novel and unique contribution in the field of e-learning in training clinical competencies. In the past, clinical competencies were taught by observations and through traditional lectures in clinical clerkship [9]. Upon clinical rotations, transitioning from clerkship observation to hands-on learning through patient care entailed challenges for medical students nearing entry to practice [10,27]. The participants in the experimental group acknowledged that interactive multimedia eBooks allowed them to be more confident and efficient in performing clinical competencies, and helped them to establish a good doctor–patient relationship during clinical practice.

The present study indicates a successful implementation of using e-learning to support clinical competency training in medical students. To our knowledge, this is the first eBook learning module in which students can acquire clinical competency skills. Our data show that integrating eBooks into clinical training could result in a more rapid significant increase in clinical skill performance upon comparing the results between the three mock OSCEs within both groups. Furthermore, our study suggests that there is a significant difference in the learning outcomes of the pre-test and post-test in the experimental group. Most training resources supporting clinical education consist of video demonstrations of clinical skills and/or mock OSCE exams [7,28]. Although the mock OSCEs show positive effects, the cost of holding formative mock OSCEs on a regular basis is high as practical considerations include training of examinees and standardized patients, test development costs, and the maintenance of facilities to administer the test [9,29].

Evidence has shown that when compared with traditional instructor-led teaching methods, e-learning can result in significant reduced costs, sometimes as much as 50% [29]. The current medical education curriculum and tuition includes clinical rotations and face-to-face teaching, especially in the final years of medical school. Defining the cost of face-to-face teaching is complex [8,9]. Our eBook module is a technology to deliver another training technique, making assessing clinical experiences simpler and more efficient, rather than replacing clinical training. Furthermore, medical educators can update the latest knowledge and skills, and add new topics any time after the original module is established. The costs of eBooks may be difficult to estimate as it may benefit several years of medical students and in different institutions. We believe our eBook module offers benefits for learners and educators, delivering cost-effective, repeatable, and standardized clinical training. Future research is recommended to inform whether eBooks can serve as an adequate supplement for other OSCE training modules on the basis of cost-effectiveness.

Our findings indicate that the mobile learning environment plays a crucial role by offering flexibility. As medical students spend a significant amount of time outside clinical training programs or classrooms, providing increased accessibility anytime and anywhere can allow them to benefit from a seamless learning environment [7,30]. Furthermore, educators can update the eBook in a timely manner to ensure delivery of the latest evidence-based medical knowledge [2]. Our eBook module can allow the creation of certain simulation curricula to meet specific needs, as teaching with real patients are limited to the disease they present with [31]. To further enhance the students' learning experience, blended learning program developments are needed on how to integrate interactive multimedia eBook resources into their teaching.

Previously, despite the many benefits of e-learning in medical education, the major barrier is a lack of interaction [7]. The keys to overcoming this challenge in our eBook module were identifying what sort of problems the students would face beforehand, providing timely and specific feedback, and setting up an online communication channel for students and educators. Besides integrating interactive multimedia designs in our eBooks, we also recruited experienced clinical educators to point out the problems that medical students often encounter or should improve on when practicing the clinical competencies in clinical scenarios. Emphasis was then given on mapping out the suitable interactive multimedia design and the responses of the automated feedback function of that particular topic. Students can use the online communication tool in the eBook platform to post questions that were still unanswered after completing the eBook to educators, enabling students to receive personalized feedback for self-improvement. After answering the students' questions, educators can not only have a better grasp of the students' training process, but also make improvements on future versions of the eBooks. Simulation with interactive virtual reality (VR) has also emerged as a new method in which we can deliver medical education. However, there are difficulties with introducing any new technology, as it requires faculty space and support [31].

An additional strength of our Bookshelf platform is that it has automated tracking functions. The tracking function can record the learners' activities and assessment outcomes during both offline and online conditions, and report them back to educators. Although several administrative functions have been facilitated, the learners have suggested some modifications in the user interface. Some participants commented on the limitation of downloading only one eBook at a time, the lack of systematic organization with which eBooks are arranged and ordered, and the need for labels marking eBooks as read or unread. These findings indicate that the user interface should be more user-friendly and updated constantly to benefit the students' learning experience.

We acknowledge some limitations in our study. First, we only conducted and evaluated the use of interactive multimedia eBooks at a single institution. Thus, our sample size was relatively small. Second, the effectiveness of interactive multimedia eBooks on OSCE scores remains modest. Although our data showed significant improvement after eBook intervention, other medical learning resources may also be involved in OSCE scores. Therefore, in future studies, the eBook learning setting could be extended to several years of medical students or to other medical curriculums or institutions to obtain generalizable results.

5. Conclusions

Application of our interactive multimedia eBook was associated with a more rapid improvement in clinical skill performance and enhanced the students' abilities and self-confidence when dealing with difficult patient encounter settings. To our knowledge, this is the first eBook in the form of interactive and multimedia design that has been established for clinical competencies. Further learning program development should be established to effectively integrate the eBooks into other areas in the medical curriculum to provide safer and better healthcare.

Author Contributions: Conceptualization, Y.-T.H. and C.-C.H.; methodology, H.-Y.L. and C.-C.H.; investigation, H.-Y.L. and C.-C.H.; data curation, Y.-T.H. and H.-Y.L.; writing—original draft preparation, Y.-T.H.; writing—review and editing, H.-Y.L. and C.-C.H. All authors have read and agreed to the published version of the manuscript.

Funding: This research was funded by Kaohsiung Chang Gung Memorial Hospital, grant number CDRPG8E0051 and CDRPG8E0052.

Acknowledgments: The authors gratefully acknowledge the time and energy contributed by participants. We would like to thank Mao-Meng, Tiao for statistical analyses.

Conflicts of Interest: The authors declare no conflict of interest.

References

1. Stevens, D.P. Finding safety in medical education. *Qual. Saf. Health Care* **2002**, *11*, 109–110. [CrossRef]
2. Ruiz, J.G.; Mintzer, M.J.; Leipzig, R.M. The impact of E-learning in medical education. *Acad. Med.* **2006**, *81*, 207–212. [CrossRef] [PubMed]
3. Warriner, D.R.; Bayley, M.; Shi, Y.; Lawford, P.V.; Narracott, A.; Fenner, J. Computer model for the cardiovascular system: Development of an e-learning tool for teaching of medical students. *BMC Med. Educ.* **2017**, *17*, 220. [CrossRef] [PubMed]
4. Fransen, F.; Martens, H.; Nagtzaam, I.; Heeneman, S. Use of e-learning in clinical clerkships: Effects on acquisition of dermatological knowledge and learning processes. *Int. J. Med. Educ.* **2018**, *9*, 11–17. [CrossRef] [PubMed]
5. Khasawneh, R.; Simonsen, K.; Snowden, J.; Higgins, J.; Beck, G. The effectiveness of e-learning in pediatric medical student education. *Med. Educ. Online* **2016**, *21*, 29516. [CrossRef]
6. Kim, K.J.; Kang, Y.; Kim, G. The gap between medical faculty's perceptions and use of e-learning resources. *Med. Educ. Online* **2017**, *22*, 1338504. [CrossRef]
7. Jang, H.W.; Kim, K.J. Use of online clinical videos for clinical skills training for medical students: Benefits and challenges. *BMC Med. Educ.* **2014**, *14*, 56. [CrossRef]

8. Liu, M.; Huang, Y.S.; Liu, K.M. Assessing core clinical competencies required of medical graduates in Taiwan. *Kaohsiung J. Med. Sci.* **2006**, *22*, 475–483. [CrossRef]
9. Wang, Y.A.; Chen, C.F.; Chen, C.H.; Wang, G.L.; Huang, A.T. A clinical clerkship collaborative program in Taiwan: Acquiring core clinical competencies through patient care responsibility. *J. Formos. Med. Assoc.* **2016**, *115*, 418–425. [CrossRef]
10. Chan, W.P.; Wu, T.Y.; Hsieh, M.S.; Chou, T.Y.; Wong, C.S.; Fang, J.T.; Chang, N.C.; Hong, C.Y.; Tzeng, C.R. Students' view upon graduation: A survey of medical education in Taiwan. *BMC Med. Educ.* **2012**, *12*, 127. [CrossRef]
11. Turner, J.L.; Dankoski, M.E. Objective structured clinical exams: A critical review. *Fam. Med.* **2008**, *40*, 574–578. [PubMed]
12. Grand'Maison, P.; Lescop, J.; Rainsberry, P.; Brailovsky, C.A. Large-scale use of an objective, structured clinical examination for licensing family physicians. *CMAJ* **1992**, *146*, 1735–1740. [PubMed]
13. Ekenze, S.O.; Okafor, C.I.; Ekenze, O.S.; Nwosu, J.N.; Ezepue, U.F. The Value of Internet Tools in Undergraduate Surgical Education: Perspective of Medical Students in a Developing Country. *World J. Surg.* **2017**, *41*, 672–680. [CrossRef] [PubMed]
14. Clark, D. Psychological myths in e-learning. *Med. Teach.* **2002**, *24*, 598–604. [CrossRef]
15. Cook, D.A.; Garside, S.; Levinson, A.J.; Dupras, D.M.; Montori, V.M. What do we mean by web-based learning? A systematic review of the variability of interventions. *Med. Educ.* **2010**, *44*, 765–774. [CrossRef]
16. Chodorow, S. Educators must take the electronic revolution seriously. *Acad. Med.* **1996**, *71*, 221–226. [CrossRef]
17. Fontaine, G.; Cossette, S.; Maheu-Cadotte, M.A.; Mailhot, T.; Deschenes, M.F.; Mathieu-Dupuis, G. Effectiveness of Adaptive E-Learning Environments on Knowledge, Competence, and Behavior in Health Professionals and Students: Protocol for a Systematic Review and Meta-Analysis. *JMIR Res. Protoc.* **2017**, *6*, e128. [CrossRef]
18. Muttappallymyalil, J.; Mendis, S.; John, L.J.; Shanthakumari, N.; Sreedharan, J.; Shaikh, R.B. Evolution of technology in teaching: Blackboard and beyond in Medical Education. *Nepal J. Epidemiol.* **2016**, *6*, 588–592. [CrossRef]
19. Choules, A.P. The use of elearning in medical education: A review of the current situation. *Postgrad. Med. J.* **2007**, *83*, 212–216. [CrossRef]
20. Hsiao, C.C.; Tiao, M.M.; Chen, C.C. Using interactive multimedia e-Books for learning blood cell morphology in pediatric hematology. *BMC Med. Educ.* **2016**, *16*, 290. [CrossRef]
21. Kirkpatrick, D.L.; Kirkpatrick, J.D. *Evaluating Training Programs: The Four Levels*, 3rd ed.; Berrett-Koehler Publishers: San Francisco, CA, USA, 2012.
22. Colt, H.G.; Davoudi, M.; Murgu, S.; Zamanian Rohani, N. Measuring learning gain during a one-day introductory bronchoscopy course. *Surg. Endosc.* **2011**, *25*, 207–216. [CrossRef] [PubMed]
23. Sinclair, P.; Kable, A.; Levett-Jones, T. The effectiveness of internet-based e-learning on clinician behavior and patient outcomes: A systematic review protocol. *JBI Database Syst. Rev. Implement. Rep.* **2015**, *13*, 52–64. [CrossRef] [PubMed]
24. Richmond, H.; Copsey, B.; Hall, A.M.; Davies, D.; Lamb, S.E. A systematic review and meta-analysis of online versus alternative methods for training licensed health care professionals to deliver clinical interventions. *BMC Med. Educ.* **2017**, *17*, 227. [CrossRef] [PubMed]
25. Singh, A.; Min, A.K. Digital lectures for learning gross anatomy: A study of their efficacy. *Korean J. Med. Educ.* **2017**, *29*, 27–32. [CrossRef] [PubMed]
26. Mohr, J.J.; Batalden, P.B. Improving safety on the front lines: The role of clinical microsystems. *Qual. Saf. Health Care* **2002**, *11*, 45–50. [CrossRef] [PubMed]
27. Lin, Y.K.; Chen, D.Y.; Lin, B.Y. Determinants and effects of medical students' core self-evaluation tendencies on clinical competence and workplace well-being in clerkship. *PLoS ONE* **2017**, *12*, e0188651. [CrossRef]
28. Lien, H.H.; Hsu, S.F.; Chen, S.C.; Yeh, J.H. Can teaching hospitals use serial formative OSCEs to improve student performance? *BMC Res. Notes* **2016**, *9*, 464. [CrossRef]
29. Gibbons, A.S.; Fairweather, P.G. Computer-based instruction. In *Training & Retraining: A Handbook for Business, Industry, Government, and the Military*; Tobias, S., Fletcher, J.D., Eds.; Macmillan Library Reference: New York, NY, USA, 2000; pp. 410–442.

30. Looi, C.-K.; Seow, P.; Zhang, B.; So, H.-J.; Chen, W.; Wong, L.-H. Leveraging mobile technology for sustainable seamless learning: A research agenda. *Br. J. Educ. Technol.* **2010**, *41*, 154–169. [CrossRef]
31. Pottle, J. Virtual reality and the transformation of medical education. *Future Healthc. J.* **2019**, *6*, 181–185. [CrossRef]

Publisher's Note: MDPI stays neutral with regard to jurisdictional claims in published maps and institutional affiliations.

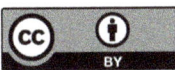
© 2020 by the authors. Licensee MDPI, Basel, Switzerland. This article is an open access article distributed under the terms and conditions of the Creative Commons Attribution (CC BY) license (http://creativecommons.org/licenses/by/4.0/).

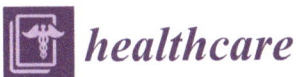

Article

To Develop Health Education Tools for Nasogastric Tube Home Caring Through Participatory Action Research

Fang-Suey Lin and Hong-Chun Shi *

Graduate School of Design, National Yunlin University of Science and Technology, Yunlin 64002, Taiwan; linfs@yuntech.edu.tw
* Correspondence: d10630019@yuntech.edu.tw

Received: 12 June 2020; Accepted: 6 August 2020; Published: 10 August 2020

Abstract: Medical institutions provide guidance on caring skills for home caregivers. Oral teaching is combined with graphical tools in a method that has been proved to be an effective way of quickly mastering home caring skills and promotes effective learning for home caregivers. The graphic design and operation contents of this method are constantly revised through interviews and observations, and by carrying out home care application graphics it forms a spiral structure of Plan–Do–Study–Act (PDSA) participatory action research (PAR). In the three cycles of the operation of PDSA PAR, the designers accurately create graphics of the caring details based on the nurses' demonstrations and develop health education tools that are suitable to provide continuous assistance and services in real-life situations. PAR combined with PDSA, in each of the three cycles of the operation—design personnel, medical personnel and home caregiver personnel, respectively—as the lead roles, guide the planning decisions for PAR. This study is a reference for the improvement and development of medical graphics for health education tools to improve accuracy.

Keywords: participatory action research; nasogastric tube; home care; medical graphics; PDSA; health education tools development

1. Introduction

Providing quality improvement training in nursing skills to home caregivers is essential for caring for patients at home, especially for those patients who require nasogastric intubation and catheterisation. Elderly or chronically ill patients are usually cared for by non-nursing professionals at home [1]. Most of the home caregivers in Taiwan are from Indonesia, Vietnam and The Philippines; how to effectively teach foreign home caregivers to take care of patients has become very important. Home caregivers have specific needs and challenges in the nursing environment, and their roles need to be recognised by the medical care system [2]. Home caregivers need to understand the symptoms and conditions of patients, soothe the patient's emotions, be able to promptly and accurately report to the nurse in charge, have basic nursing knowledge and skills, and be able to communicate effectively [3–5]. In our research study, the nurses went to the patient's home on average once a month; they replaced the patient's nasogastric tube and guided the home caregivers in operating the tube in the home environment. A nasogastric tube is a type of medical instrument that intrudes into the body of the patient [6]. It is necessary to be able to carry out standard operation procedures of feeding, routine intubation cleaning, and position inspection as part of daily care.

Long-term nasogastric tube implantation easily causes infection. In addition to the nurses' monthly professional nursing services, it can strengthen the caring procedures of home caregivers to receive relevant instruction in infection protection control, to avoid the infection of patients who are in the process of care [7]. Home caregivers should have relevant nursing knowledge and common sense when it comes to care.

The procedures of caring for a patient with a nasogastric tube are relatively complicated; nurses train home caregivers with the necessary caring skills mainly by demonstration, together with oral instruction. Due to the language barriers, the novice and foreign home caregivers are unable to communicate effectively and lack the relevant experience; these factors are likely to lead to problems occurring in the nursing process. Home caregivers who have direct contact with patients are the main providers of the patients' needs. They have a responsibility to develop a shared experience with the nurses so that they can to better perform patient care services [8]. Home caregivers with nursing knowledge can provide better care for patients. Nurses need to take into account their level of understanding when communicating with home caregivers and exchange information with home caregivers effectively [9]. It is simple and inexpensive to use an image-based training tool to assist the users' learning, which can improve their understanding and realise good learning results. Foreign home caregivers use graphical health education tools in the learning process, which is more convenient for the nurses' teaching and the learners' understanding. According to the research on the process of medical graphic intervention, the graphical operation steps can significantly improve memory and comprehension, help to correct faulty operation methods, and also avoid the boredom of traditional teaching methods [10]. The current clinical development process in graphics mostly considers the digital form but in the actual application, the final results of its use can be damaged by the lack of a corresponding evaluation process in the development process [11].

The current situation in home caregivers' quality improvement training should be regarded as a concern of public health projects, which need to attach importance to nursing knowledge education and formulate relevant policies on the operational standards of caring work at home [12]. There needs to be development of the graphic design of the nasogastric tube home care process, with the participation of the designers, nurses, and home caregivers. Based on this joint cooperation and learning, the operation and instruction of nurses played a very important role in this research process. They assisted the designers in completing the development of designing the graphics and evaluated the home caregivers' operation. The aims of this research are as follows:

- Using the participatory action research (PAR) method as the research tool, to design the graphics of procedures and considerations of nasogastric tube caring at home, explore a reasonable method of cooperation between design researchers and nurses, and develop a health education tool.
- The PAR in three cycles, in combination with the PDSA (Plan, Do, Study, Act) quality management steps and methods, continue to confirm the research objectives, repeatedly confirming and providing feedback on the contents of the graphics and texts, inspecting the quality of cooperation, and ensuring the accuracy and effectiveness of the process graphics drawing in the research process.
- The degree of participation, leadership, and knowledge exchange in each cycle by each of the participants are in different proportions; each participants' position is revisited in the different cycles by the intervention of the researchers and the research tools. The relationships between nurses and home caregivers are transformed to improve the health education tools in the spirit of cooperation.

2. Literature Review

2.1. The Present Situation of Nasogastric Tube Home Caring

Although using a nasogastric tube may produce adverse effects, most families still choose to use one because it is convenient in clinical operation, can provide patients with nutrition, and patients have a chance of returning to normal eating. For patients with nutritional supplement, nurses prefer a nasogastric tube compared with other feeding methods; however, the nasogastric tube is not easy to operate [13]. According to the nursing profession, home caring should be divided into professional nursing operations and non-professional nursing operations. The use of home care is increasing because this method of care can save public resources [14]. The placement of a nasogastric tube requires specific operation by a professional nurse [15]. The lower the caregiver's level of knowledge of the nasogastric tube care process, the higher the learning demand, and the corresponding evaluation should be included in the nasogastric tube operation process [16]. Nurses should assist home caregivers during home visits and, in general, provide intubation care manuals to improve the quality of care [17]. In addition to the guidance in intubation caring skills, nursing guidance is also required in good communication skills with which to communicate with the patients and to provide good care in terms of emotional comfort [18].

2.2. Participatory Action Research

Action research can transform knowledge into practice and then promote the formation of knowledge through practice, which is a process of continuous verification. Action research proposes changes based on the traditional collaborative approach and reflects on the whole research process, and importance is attached to the emotional feelings of all parties in the research process [19]. Action research is a process that combines theory and action to form a cycle of participation in practice. It is a process of co-creation, usually solving existing problems and then solving new ones. Different patterns and methods are adopted according to different professional studies [20]. Some action research does not presuppose the behaviour of the research object based on the theoretical framework but analyses and understands the research object by observation. Nursing is a patient-centred operation. In the context of nursing, action research can promote the coordination of the relationship between different participants [21]. Practical action research has a research cycle. To prove the validity of the theory, the practice process needs to have complete strategies and steps [22]. PAR is widely used in the field of sociological research, emphasising processes that are co-created by professional researchers and participants, including research agendas, methods, processes, and outcomes [23]. In the field of medical care, there are studies that intervene in nursing operations through PAR. Before that, nurses usually used personal experience to judge and were thought to have had communication with patients about medical behaviour. However, action studies in Intensive Care Units (ICU) have shown that encouraging nurses to be patient-centred from the perspective of patients' problems—paying close attention to patients' willingness to communicate—interferes with the communication behaviour of nurses, encouraging them to re-examine their relationship with the patient [24]. PAR often uses 'plan–action–reflection' in the process of nursing education; the adaptability and positive thinking ability of nursing students in clinical practice are thus improved [25]. The development of cross-disciplinary cooperation in the medical profession can develop common situational cognition. The action research method is the basis for this transformation, which integrates and transforms the knowledge of different specialties, changing the final practice through cooperation, communication, responsibility sharing, process improvement, and other methods [26]. PAR can promote the coordination of the interests of all the participants in the action research, give voice to patients, and take into account the equality of the interests of all parties in the research process [27].

This methodology has been applied to the knowledge to adapt the use of the PAR method to multidisciplinary cooperation, to enhance the understanding of the interdisciplinary knowledge domain, to create a knowledge spiral, and to put forward a proposal arising from the practice and put it into action such that the experts can arrive at a diagnosis [28]. However, this kind of knowledge spiral lacks the reflection process and may encourage participants to absorb knowledge in a passive state. PAR has many advantages but it can be problematic. The degree of participation of the participants varies, and the representativeness of the participants may not be widely extended to other group behaviours. This research method is considered to be unable to improve the power relationships among participants, and it is difficult to evaluate the effect of PAR on participation. Research claims are usually bold and important but avoid the negative effects and influences of excessive participation [29]. To generalise the results of the study to the benefit of other groups, communication and interaction with participants needs to be enhanced. To avoid the problem of excessive participation in PAR, selected participants have clearly defined roles to conform to the research aim and form a group of different participants, fully giving play to the role of individuals and group participants. The participants can comment at the same time, participate in the group of other individuals, give responses and supplements, and enhance participants' confidence and motivation [30].

2.3. PDSA

PDSA's approach is relatively easy to understand and its effects may be underestimated. PDSA operations with action cycles can give teams involved in an action a clearer direction [31]. PDSA can be used in a small range of operations to achieve good operational results. Service project improvement needs to be completed in different cycles [32]. PDSA should improve the problem step-by-step according to the cycles and be supported by sufficient data. Its own structure can promote the confidence of the team to deal with the problem, and the team will formulate a corresponding theory and obtain the result through appropriate observation and action [33]. Whether in the field of healthcare or other fields, the management framework using PDSA is to make planned changes and not deviate from the target in the improvement [34]. In the field of health profession education, it is believed that the application of the PDSA cycle can also promote quality learning, continuously construct the learners' knowledge systems, and promote the generation of new knowledge [35]. The PDSA method is also used in the field of healthcare, and the method can be adopted for structured problem solving, promoting quality improvement [36]. According to the research-driven results, the research should make presuppositions or assumptions; and in the process of action research introspection, the train of thought should be continuously adjusted, improving study behaviour and ultimately affecting the results of the study; these results include cost, quality of nursing, and satisfaction, and there is continuous improvement in the quality of the research [37]. Moen & Norman (2009) introduced the development course of PDCA and PDSA during the development of PDSA, and various modified versions have been produced. The Shewhart cycle, considered to be the original version in 1939, established the three steps of specification, production and inspection. In 1951 Deming proposed an improvement cycle of four parts, namely design, product, sales, and redesign, after the Japanese Ishikawa PDCA cycle of problem solving corresponding to the four parts as follows: PLAN, corresponding to design: DO, corresponding to produce; CHECK, corresponding to sales; and ACTION, corresponding to redesign. This method emphasises that standards should be established and constantly revised before PDCA is implemented, and it is also commonly used in education and training. Deming believed that CHECK means preventing doing things and should emphasise the process of introspection and correction and generate the PDSA structure in later developments [38].

Although PDSA is considered to promote standardised operations and progressive learning in the field of nursing, PDSA does not solve all the complex problems. The application of PDSA in the nursing field is considered to be simple in operation and to lack scientific rigor. The application overemphasises individual ability while ignoring systematic problems. In practice, there may be problems such as adverse execution, so a clear and reasonable process is needed to implement PDSA [39]. To avoid invalid results in the PDSA operation process, researchers need to confirm the operability of the research problem. Full exchange of views and confirmation should be conducted among the participants to ensure the accuracy of the practical results. If the practice results are not effective, the introspection process needs to be carried out until the results are recognised by the professionals.

2.4. Application of Health Education Tool Graphic in the Caring Process

The improvement of medical and disease communication through nonverbal communication in the field of medical care has gained increasing amounts of attention. Graphical tools are mostly used in areas with different ages, low levels of health literacy, or insufficient cognitive ability so as to reduce the risks caused by cognitive or educational gaps. The graphics are applied to health communication. Spoken words or graphics can enhance the accuracy of the text, and the corresponding teaching methods can result in people focusing on the health materials. Graphics are especially useful for people with a low level of literacy. When graphics are applied in the field of health care, there should be corresponding evaluation [40]. Good health education and guidance can help to improve the problems in healthcare. Oral instruction can help to connect the graphics and words and can improve the care skills and confidence of caregivers, improve patients psychologically, and improve the communication between doctors and patients [41].

During the home care use of nasogastric tubes for the elderly, the main problems are that nurses and caregivers rarely use appropriate health education tools; there is no standardised process for the design of health education tools; health education leaflets lack design and publicity, and health education tools lack evaluation. This study aims to solve the problem of providing health education tools with accompanying graphics to provide guidance on the correct steps for caregivers in the operation of nasogastric tubes. The cost of learning nasogastric tube care using dummy people is high; therefore, it is necessary to develop cheaper simple health education tools in clinical nursing practice to enhance the quality of nasogastric tube care and prevent accidents involving physical or psychological damage to both patients and caregivers [42]. In the process of home care, foreign caregivers encounter problems such as the language barrier or an inability to remember the operation steps, and some of them consider that the operation steps are not important. To solve these problems, nurses use methods such as operation videos and health education leaflets to improve the efficiency of communication [43]. In addition to these tools, the effectiveness of learning has a relationship with the frequency of the nurses visiting the home care, the operation specification, and the caregivers' health literacy. There is a need to establish a complete set of policy measures simultaneously, through different health education tools and learning methods with regard to intervention in the feeding process. Those interventions demonstrate greater accuracy in the use of the nasogastric tube in nursing care [44]. Graphical information can improve the carer's understanding of patients' medication and medical information. It is recommended that graphic designers should be included in the medical field; however, the use of graphics should be adapted and verified by users of different cultures [45].

In this study, nasogastric tube operation was taught to home caregivers at home by example. Combining the actual work needs of nurses, professional designers, and graphic designers provided research cooperation and actively assisted in the graphic recording, providing a relatively standardised development process. Home caregivers need to be able to operate independently for the majority of the time without the guidance of nurses; appropriate health education tools can help home caregivers to recall the operation process in the home caring environment to correctly perform the operation.

3. Material and Methods

3.1. Research Steps and Framework

The nurses that teach nasogastric tube home care need to spend time and energy communicating with the patient's family and home caregivers at home. When designers and researchers join in the process, they need to constantly re-examine the problems, controllable conditions, and the cycles that can be improved in the whole operation process from the viewpoint of a challenger. In the framework of action research involving people from different professional backgrounds, PDSA carries out different operational steps at each cycle according to the research time. The circular nature of the action research promotes the development of the research and deepens the cooperation of the researchers in different fields (Figure 1). With regard to the development of graphics of nasogastric tube care in PAR, recording the research process has important significance and is an important function. The execution of the first cycle of the steps can be exploratory; researchers approach the problem from the angle of the design to explore the possibility of its operation. The second cycle of the steps is to focus on improving the existing health education tools, on the basis of incorporating the nurses' professional knowledge into the design of the intervention. The third cycle of the steps is mainly based on the second cycle in the development of tools, combining this with the user suggestions and evaluations. Each cycle stakeholder's degree of participation is different; the roles and the operations are different. The overall research framework was established from the early stages of the study to develop health education tools under the condition of existing medical care with the goal of using visual graphics to communicate with the auxiliary medical care, and to provide health education tools that can be used in clinical teaching.

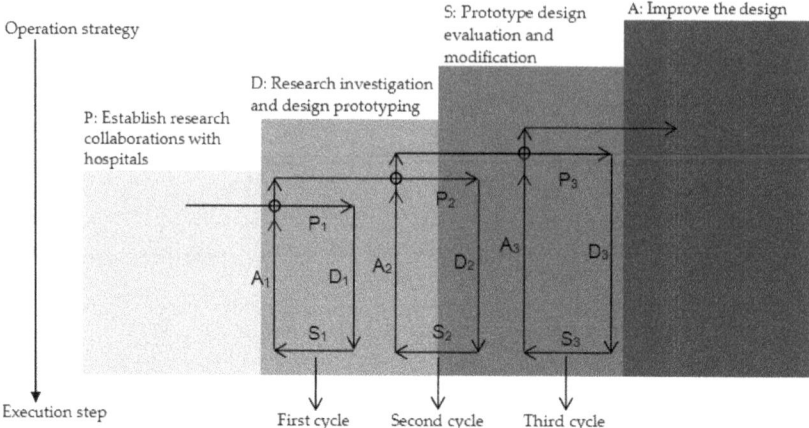

Figure 1. Participatory action research (PAR) steps and framework diagram.

In the first cycle, the researchers used the interview method, and different professionals expressed different views on the study process. The interview content was used to interpret the medical staff's attitude in the process. Problems of nasogastric tube operation in home care were discovered, and relevant suggestions were provided by hospital managers, nurse supervisors, and nurses. The researchers planned and implemented the study based on the main points and suggestions raised in the interviews.

In the second cycle, the basis of cooperation was discovered in the interviews based on the first cycle, combining the participant observation and interview and making a plan for designing the graphics of the nasogastric tube home care operation. The nurses conducted the nasogastric tube home care process. The researchers recorded the nasogastric tube home care process in the form of video audio and organised the image and text records. The professional designer made graphic designs in accordance with the recorded content. The illustrations were accompanied by bilingual text captions in Chinese/English and in Chinese/Indonesian. After completing the care process manual, the nurses reviewed the operation process, graphic content, text description, and other content, and repeatedly corrected them to improve the accuracy.

In the third cycle, nurses used the graphics developed in the second cycle to teach home caregivers. The researchers used field interviews, non-participatory observation, and final operation score statistics. After the consent of the nurses and the patient's family had been obtained, the patients were selected randomly and recruited for the clinical operation test. This study passed the National Cheng Kung University Human Research Ethics Review Committee Version (106-149). Informed consent and signatures were obtained from the subjects, and the nurses evaluated the home caregivers' operation process. According to the results presented in the first and second cycles, the nurses used an A4-size nasogastric tube graphic manual to instruct the home caregivers on the operation. Based on the feedback on the description content of the graphics, the foreign home caregivers corrected the Indonesian translation. Evaluation forms were designed according to direct observation of the procedural skills of Mackenzie Hospital. Nurses assessed the scores of the home caregivers' operations.

3.2. Participants

In total, 18 participants (Table 1) were involved in this study, including six participants with a design background (G1). Researcher R01 proposed the study based on their experience of previous studies, and the G1 team worked together to complete the study. Among the participants, R06 was a professional designer with senior experience in information graphics and graphics who could skilfully use the drawing software and accurately draw the graphics of the operation steps. There were five participants with a medical background (G2), including a nursing supervisor who conducted ethical practice and supervision of the research. Two nurses participated in the whole process from the beginning to the end of the study. There were seven home caregivers who finally used the health education tools (G3). This study did not have specific requirements with regard to the caring experience of the home caregivers. To ensure the privacy of the participants, all the participants were given codes and concealed key words such that the basic information content could not be guessed but the authenticity of the research was not affected.

In the first cycle of the PAR, the G1 group led the research for the other participants and selected an appropriate hospital for cooperation. G2 entered the phase of joint research. In the interview process, the medical personnel were equally involved in the dialogue and determined the nature of the cooperation. In the second cycle, the G2 group was the main participant. The G1 group recorded the operation of the G2 group and made graphic drawings. Both groups repeatedly confirmed the operation content and the graphic content. The G2 group asked the G3 group about its willingness to participate in the study, and G1 together with G2 invited G3 to participate in the third step. In the third cycle, the G3 group was the main participant but G1, G2, and G3 were co-participants: G3 in the role of the learner and operator; G2 in the role of teaching the nasogastric tube steps to the home caregivers, correcting action, and sorting; and finally, G1 summarised the findings and developed the graphic printing health education tools to be used in nasogastric tube home caring in the future (Figure 2).

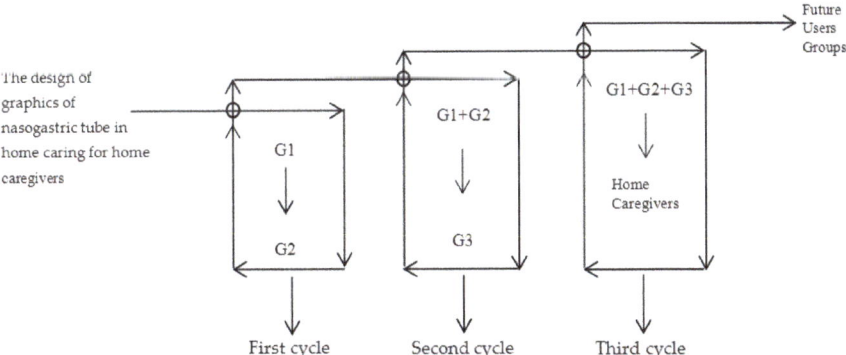

Figure 2. Target participants group structure diagram.

Table 1. Interview participants' background and research implementation.

Participant Groups	Participant Code	Gender	Age	Working Experience: Year	Participate in the Division of Labour and Work Background
Participant groups G1: design background, researcher)	Researcher-R01	Female	50–60	Design (>30)	Establish cooperation and liaison with hospitals, establish research plans, interview, observation and design guidance.
	Researcher-R02	Female	20–30	Design (>7)	Participate in interviews, records, verbatim manuscripts, home care assessment, text writing and collation, data consolidation, design graphics manual.
	Researcher-R03	Female	20–30	Design (>7)	Participate in interviews, records, verbatim manuscripts, home care assessment, text writing and collation, data consolidation, design graphics manual, graphics correction.
	Researcher-R04	Male	20–30	Design (>3)	Participate in interviews, records, verbatim manuscripts, home care assessment, text writing and collation, data consolidation, design graphics manual, graphics correction.
	Researcher-R05	Female	30–40	Design (>15)	Participate in interviews, records, verbatim manuscripts, home care assessment, text writing and collation, data consolidation, design graphics manual.
	Researcher-R06	Male	20–30	Graphic design (>10)	Draw graphics, professional graphic designer.
Participant groups G2: 6medical backgrounds	Doctor-I01	Male	50–60	Doctor/Hospital administrator (>30)	Establishment of cooperation, hospital management, participation in interviews.
	Nursing supervisor-I02	Male	30–40	Nursing supervisor (>10)	Participate in interviews and supervise the implementation of the overall research process.
	Nurse-I03	Female	30–40	Nurse (>10)	Nursing operation, participation in interviews, correction of operation graphics, home care assessment.
	Nurse-I04	Female	30–40	Nurse (>10)	Nursing operation, participation in interviews, correction of operation graphics, home care assessment.
	Nurse-I05	Female	30–40	Nurse (>10)	Participation in interviews, correction of operation graphics.

Table 1. *Cont.*

Participant Groups	Participant Code	Gender	Age	Working Experience: Year	Participate in the Division of Labour and Work Background
Participant groups G3: home caregivers	Home caregiver-FC01	Female	unknown	Foreign home caregiver (>0.2)	Participated in home caring study, interview and evaluation. New home caregivers, lack of home care experience. Nurses combined with graphics teaching; home caregiver needs to learn from the basics.
	Home caregiver-FC02	Female	unknown	Foreign home caregiver (>5)	Participated in home caring study, interview and evaluation. Experienced in home care to assist in the evaluation and revision of this study. The nurse teaches in conjunction with graphics, and the caregiver provides corrections to the graphics.
	Home caregiver-FC03	Female	unknown	Foreign home caregiver (>2)	Participated in home caring study, interview and evaluation. Has home care experience but the operational details are not in place to assist this study evaluation. The nurse corrects the details of the operation by teaching them with graphics.
	Home caregiver-FC04	Female	unknown	Foreign home caregiver (0)	Participated in home caring study, interview and evaluation. The patient had never used a nasogastric tube before and home caregiver lacked experience in nasogastric tube care.
	Home caregiver-FC05	Female	unknown	Home caregiver (>5)	Participated in home caring study, interview and evaluation. At present, the family members of the patient are taking care of the patient by themselves. When there is a foreign caregiver, the family members teach them, and the family members learn from the nurse in this study to assist the evaluation and revision. Nurses combined with graphics teaching; patients' families use the graphics teaching new home caregivers' operation steps.
	Home caregiver-FC06	Female	unknown	Foreign home caregiver (>5)	Participated in home caring study, interview and evaluation. Skilled in home-care operation, 2 weeks of training in home care, 3 weeks of adaptation in the home environment, there will be a new caregiver to take over the work in the future to assist this study evaluation and correction. After the nurse combined the graphics instruction, the caregiver provided corrections to the graphic.
	Home caregiver-FC07	Female	50–60	Foreign home caregiver (>7)	Participated in home caring study, interview and evaluation. Specific learning time of nasogastric tube operation is unknown, but relevant experience has been gained in home care, which will assist in this study to evaluate and modify. After the nurse combined the graphics instruction, the nurse provided corrections to the graphics.

3.3. Research Tools and Data Processing

Based on the differences in the participants' professional fields and the division of labour, PAR was used as a research tool. The participants clearly defined the purpose of their action, and their rights and interests were guaranteed in the process of participating in the research. The layperson has obvious limitations in participating in scientific research, and usually the participants' actions are guided towards the researcher's ideal scope. Therefore, in PAR it is necessary to combine the actions of experts and laypeople [46]. The use of PAR in this study will enable design professionals to understand the processes and methods of healthcare nurses, as well as enable nurses to better understand the professional assistance that designers can provide for them. When cooperating with the nursing community, designers need to confirm what is being designed. For home caregivers who are responsible for patients, the procedure and details of nasogastric tube operation are very important and may affect the interests of the patients. Using the PDSA quality management method can confirm each cycle of the action research: in the first cycle, the feasibility of the research problems are confirmed; in the second cycle, the health education tools' content is repeatedly confirmed; and in the third cycle, home caregivers in operation and feedback provide suggestions repeatedly. Therefore, in the three cycles of the action research framework, the operation of each cycle should be confirmed by the participants, and the processes of planning, operation, learning, introduction and implementation should be clarified by PDSA. The health education tool suitable for nasogastric tube home caring should be jointly developed for the reference of home caregivers.

3.4. Research Limitations

This research required human research ethics approval from the institute and the hospital. The research needed completion of the survey to be achieved within a specific time and also required the cooperation of the hospital nurses and the consent of the patient's family. The final evaluation process also required the consent of the home caregiver, and the nurse asked the home caregiver to give their informed consent with a signature.

After sorting out the number of nurses' individual cases, the nurses told the researcher which of their cases could participate in the evaluation of the study, which required the researcher to enter the patient's home with the nurses. In addition to giving their consent, non-nursing professionals must operate according to hospital schedules. Due to the difficulties in obtaining actual test samples, the researcher originally planned to recruit more than ten groups of participants. After on-the-spot inquiry, the researcher excluded cases such as the family members of patients who did not agree to cooperate with the study or did not use a nasogastric tube. A total of seven groups of cases participated in the survey.

4. Results

4.1. Cycle 1: Make a Plan for the Graphics Development of Home Caregivers

At the beginning of the study, the researcher proposed to solve the problems related to the process of home care by means of graphics, but the whole problem was not clear. The designers needed to find partners with a medical background, reach a consensus with the medical professional researchers (P1), and write the research plan (D1). The teams of both groups were able to accept each other's suggestions, initiate applications for in-hospital research applications and human ethics reviews (S1), and establish an agenda for the implementation of the research plan (A1).

Researcher R01 had a long-term focus on the use of graphic design to solve the problem of doctor–patient communication, discovering graphical intervention in home care and helping caregivers in their understanding and memory of the operation process. However, the quality of the graphics used as health education tools need to be improved and should include graphic accuracy and evaluation to promote learning, teaching, and memory. In discussions with nurses, the researchers found that when local home caregivers were being taught, the new foreign home caregivers had trouble communicating because of the language barrier, making it difficult to teach them complex home care work. After the theme of the plan was established, the main researcher, R01, first formed a team in the field of design, establishing a research team with researchers in the design background (R02, R03, R04, and R05) and searched for a suitable hospital to prepare their proposals and propose their intention of cooperation. After the hospital groups agreed to cooperate, five study participants I01, I02, I03, I04, and I05 participated in the cooperative discussion, forming a research group with a medical background; among these participants I01 was the main manager of the hospital and I02 was the nurse supervisor. The common characteristic of the two groups was that each participating group had a person in charge who was responsible for communication of the research issues, the meeting time, research plan, and preparation of the research materials. In the first part of the participation process, the heads of the two groups communicated with each other and with the other participants and explained the research matters. The hospital had a positive cooperative attitude. The hospital believed that the foreign caregivers experience communication problems in carrying out home care. The hospital was willing to provide assistance to those who needed the hospital's cooperation in this process. In the course of their communication, the two groups hoped that the research plan could be put into practice. As a result of past experience, the hospital had doubts about the graphic carrier and the specific application of the flowchart proposed by the researcher. As for the implementation of the study, the hospital administrator (I01) believed that:

> *During the implementation of the design, user convenience should be taken as the centre. For example, previously during the use of the hospital registration system, the registered machine was purchased but it could not be further promoted due to the problems in the operation process, resulting in the loss of the hospital after the purchase of equipment. In the process of cross-discipline cooperation, effective designs should be made to help solve the needs of patients, doctors, and nurses. Otherwise, if all the designs cannot be applied, there will be no good cooperation cases or the hospital will suffer losses.*

According to the researchers, the form of the health education tools can be adjusted according to the clinical operation needs of the medical staff. The graphics drawn to represent the home care steps should have a standard design process, and the graphics should be optimised step by step so that home caregivers can learn or recall the operation steps according to the graphics. Participant G1 proposed the study using his own speciality as the starting point and decided to develop a graphic tool for nasogastric tube home care, aimed at helping G2 and G3. G1 invited G2 to join the research and proposed the scheme of cooperative research (Figure 3). Participant G2 believed that G1 needed to address the real issues in nursing and comply with the relevant medical ethics. At the early stages of the study, the decision makers communicated repeatedly with the hospital administrators and confirmed the problems, proposed a research case whose main objective was the design and application of the graphics representing the home caring process of the nasogastric tube, and then applied for the human ethics review. After the research proposal and the application for the human ethics review were approved, the researchers communicated with the hospital to apply to execute the research case. The participants with different research backgrounds were required to communicate continuously and plan the expected research schedule of cycle 2, cycle 3 and the expected output of the research results.

4.2. Cycle 2: Design and Revision of Nasogastric Tube Home Caring Procedure Graphics

Based on the design of the nasogastric tube home caring procedure graphics plan, the nurses proposed a suggestion for the study (P2). Nasogastric tube care in home nursing is mainly divided into cleaning and feeding. The nurses believed that in the process of home caring, the caregivers mainly carry out external operation nasogastric tube inspection of the tube touching the skin, as well as carry out the specification of feeding. Preparation of the tool, inspection, implementation, and precautions should all be reflected in the graphics. In the second cycle of the PDSA implementation process, video records were made mainly for the nasogastric tube caring process, and the nasogastric tube home care process step graphics were completed (D2). Repeated revisions were made between participants

G1 and G2 (S2), and nasogastric tube home care procedure graphics were created that were fit for the nurses' use (A2).

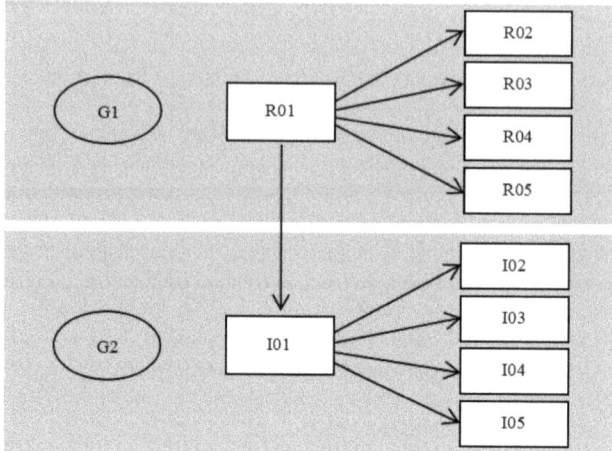

Figure 3. Participants in the first cycle.

Nurses thought that using actual patients for the operation at the early stages may raise ethical issues because of the recording and production. Therefore, it was decided to implement the step of the recording procedure using the medical dummy model. The nasogastric tube home care demonstration operation was taught by two nurses I03 and I04; a design researcher, R02, recorded the video, and four design researchers, R01, R03, R04, and R05, were participatory observers. The nurses taught the nursing procedure, the researcher continued with the operation exercise separately, and then the nurses corrected the action and the specification, revealing the unclear action procedures that needed to be confirmed with the nurses on the spot. The researchers divided the video recordings into words and captured images, and the nurses confirmed the accuracy of the content with regard to nursing materials and procedures. Three researchers, R02, R03 and R04, collected the key images and organised the operating steps into a table; these steps were mainly divided into the nasogastric tube cleaning steps and the feeding steps. After the data had been sorted out, the nurses confirmed the content, including the accuracy of the words and sentences and the image selection. The data were reviewed and classified according to their attributes. The preliminary graphic design was conducted after researcher R01 reviewed the data after it had been completed. R02, R03, R04 successively tried to use the whole-body line graphic, the simulated human graphic, different thickness line graphics, and other forms of graphic design. Too fine a line may result in the user not being able to accurately identify the graphic according to the design group discussions, and it was thought that the operation graphics should adopt line and colour in their expression, and the nasogastric tube parts and the body's performance should match the symbol. Researcher R06 carried out the complete design and drawing to ensure a uniform graphic style; researcher R01 led the team to continue when the design of the image content was confirmed. After the design draft was completed, the G1 team submitted it to the G2 team for review, adjustment, standardisation of the words, accuracy of the sentences, confirmation of the accuracy of the drawings depicting the nurses' actions, and modification of the graphics by carrying out the repeated correction process of 'Design–Fix–Redesign–Re-fix', including confirmation of the details of the graphics (such as the rotation of the nasogastric tube in graphic should be annotated; the nasogastric tube needed to show the change of the position of the gummed tape on the first and second day). The nurses thought that A4 size for the health education tools for home care would be easy to find and read, and so the designer group used this requirement for the design and the making of the prototype (Figure 4).

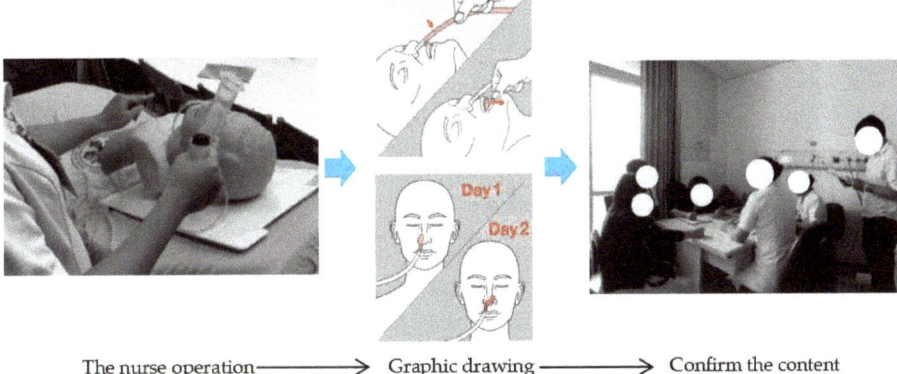

The nurse operation ⟶ Graphic drawing ⟶ Confirm the content

Figure 4. Transformation and content confirmation of nasogastric tube home caring graphics.

Researcher R01 led the G1 group, the G1 group cooperated with the G2 group, and the above research process was supervised and implemented by the nursing supervisor I02. To ensure the smooth progress of the study, the G2 group was responsible for the execution and operation of the participants during the study, and the G1 group was responsible for the steps such as the recording and learning of the operation procedure, the drawing of the graphics, the confirmation of the text details, and the selection of the graphic style and the correction. The main leader in the participant groups was responsible for monitoring and correcting the rationality of the implementation steps of the research operation (Figure 5).

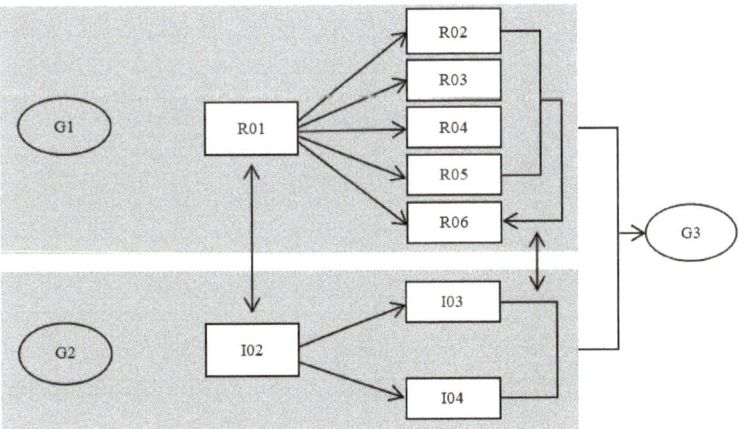

Figure 5. Participants in the second cycle.

The operation of this cycle focused on the repeated confirmation of the operation steps and the graphics to ensure the accuracy of the nursing operation content. The design group, G1, was taught by the medical group, G2, and continuously learned from and communicated with the nurses until the nurses considered that the graphic content drawn in this cycle could be used. As the dummy model was used in the demonstration operation, some real operation situations could not be represented, resulting in the loss of operation steps. The graphic correction was made based on the daily operation experience of nurses and the daily situation of cases to show the operation position more clearly.

To complete the design, communication with the nurses led to several revisions. The first amendments were: (1) add a new 'the nasogastric tube turns in half a circle' graphic and correct the 'need to change the sticking position of the nasogastric tube every day' graphic, as the designers had wrongly misunderstood the 'need to change the sticking position of the nasogastric tube every day' as the 'need to change the position of the nasogastric tube every day'. The researchers found that in the video recording the observers had no record of this part of the subtle operation; therefore, 'the nasogastric tube turns in half a circle' did not appear in the action records relating the images to the text; (2) redraw the graphic of 'after the feeding is completed, turn the tube back, then pull out the syringe to end the feeding' and add the graphic of 'cover the tube and clean the empty syringe'. The reason for the correction was that the reflection of nasogastric tube had been drawn incorrectly. Modifications were made as to the correct folding direction of the nasogastric tube and the addition of the injection tube. The nurses also suggested that the procedure of drawing out the tube core and cleaning it should be described in detail. The second correction was the addition of a graphic of 'the patient should be in a half-sitting position during the whole feeding process'. The nurses thought that the home caregivers were more likely to forget this step from the actual teaching, so the graphic was added to facilitate their review of home caring (Table 2).

Table 2. Discuss additional procedures and explanations with the nurses.

Time	Before Correction	After Correction
First correction		
Second correction		

4.3. Cycle 3: Developing Sample and Evaluation of Graphical Health Education Tools

After the nurses confirmed the operation procedure graphics of the nasogastric tube in home care, the health educational tool was output by the colour laser printer for the clinical user test, and the nurses were responsible for the user test and for the evaluation of the health education tool so that the designer could improve the final design (P3). The nurses used the graphical health education tool to teach the caregivers, and then the nurses evaluated the caregivers' operation (D3) and asked the caregivers to give feedback on the graphics and the text descriptions (S3). Finally, the researcher and the nurse discussed the content and then corrected it (A3). The process was also repeated and verified in accordance with the PDSA implementation steps to ensure that the final nasogastric tube home care operation steps, graphics, text, and translation were correct and effective.

The specific operation process of the third cycle was mainly divided into three steps: (1) the nurses found caregiver participants suitable for evaluation, and the caregivers needed to agree and sign the informed consent (Indonesian and Chinese version) to participating in instruction and evaluation of the operation graphics. The researchers were required to conduct non-participatory observation in conjunction with the nurses' visits to the patients; (2) the nurses taught the home caregivers the nasogastric tube home caring process. The operation steps and precautions were explained and demonstrated with graphics, and then the home caregivers performed the operation and the nurses checked the effectiveness after the care procedure had been completed; (3) the nurses evaluated the home caregivers, completed the final evaluation form, and asked the caregivers to give relevant suggestions on the health education tools. After the completion of the above three steps, the researchers of the study convened a meeting to revise the graphics of the final nasogastric tube home care procedure (Figure 6).

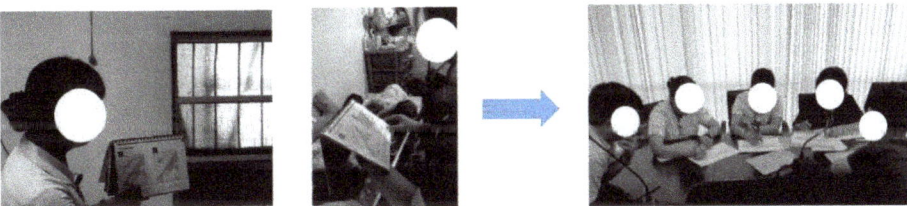

Figure 6. The nurse provides graphic evaluation for the home caregivers, and after the assessment there is a meeting to discuss the modification of the graphics.

Two nurses, I03 and I04, participated in the final application evaluation. The communication process between the G1, G2, and G3 groups was carried out under the supervision of the nurses' supervisor I02. After cases of family members' disagreement were excluded before the end of the study, seven cases (FC01–FC07) were included to form the G3 group for assessment use. Among them, six foreign home caregivers and one patient's family member attended the evaluation of this study. R01, R02, R03, R04, and R05 of the main researcher team G1 observed and recorded using a non-participatory observation method. G2 needed to repeatedly confirm G1 and G3 and was also responsible for the communication between groups G1 and G3. However, due to the long evaluation cycle, the researchers in G1 needed to repeatedly encourage evaluation. Since the graphics were still in the development stage, the daily workload of the G2 group increased. G2 was willing to continue the study in order to obtain the research results of the health education tools (Figure 7). The operational performance evaluation of the home caregivers was divided into caring preparation, nasogastric tube cleaning, and feeding procedures; nurses also conducted health education tool study effect evaluation. For this part of the evaluation, the total score was six points, scored from the average calculated in the table for each item, including 1–2 points as 'failed to meet the evaluation standard', 3 as 'close to the standard', 4 as 'reached the standard', and 5–6 as 'exceeding the standard'. In the evaluation table, the nurses and home caregivers were given satisfaction scores for this study, which ranged from 1–10, indicating satisfaction from low to high. In addition, observation time and feedback time were also recorded in the evaluation table to reflect the subjects' operational execution time and degree of proficiency (Table 3).

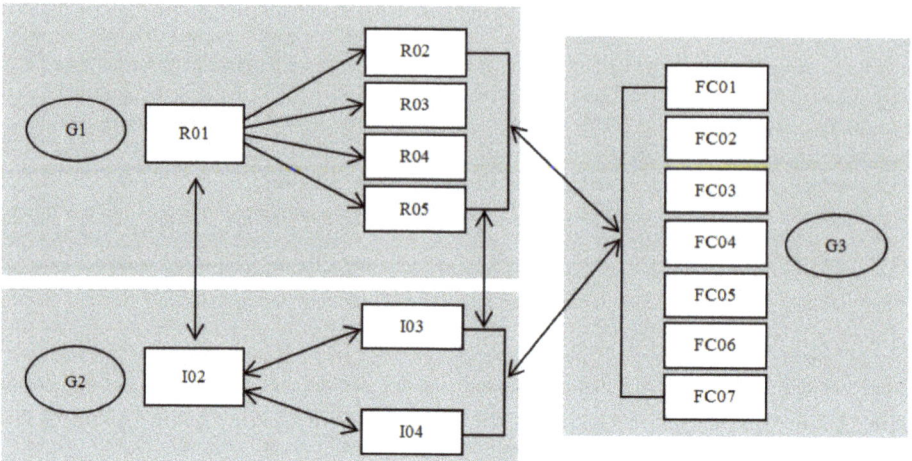

Figure 7. Participants in the third cycle.

Table 3. Assessed effectiveness of use by home caregivers.

Participants	Effectiveness	Operating Performance		Process Satisfaction		Observation Time (s)	Feedback Time(s)
		Performance (M)	Learning (M)	Nurses	Home Caregivers		
FC01	Yes	4	5	8	8	15	10
FC02	Not given	4	5	8	8	20	15
FC03	Yes	4	5	8	8	10	5
FC04	Yes	3.56	4	8	8	30	15
FC05	Yes	4.67	4	6	7	5	5
FC06	Yes	4	5	8	8	10	5
FC07	Yes	4.11	4.2	8	8	10	10

Assessment found that some caregivers had caring experience, but the operation process did not follow the normal standards of correct implementation. Since most of the home caregivers were foreigners, their communication with nurses was not smooth. In conjunction with the graphic manual, the home caregivers showed that they could understand the operation in the graphics and correct the translation of the graphics description. The nurses would use the graphics again to engender caring in the process of the operation and describe the contents and steps of the graphics in detail, so that the caregivers were clearer about the matters needing attention in the process of caring at home.

4.4. Combined with PDSA's Introspection on Participatory Action Research

In the existing cross-disciplinary cooperation, the main researcher usually takes the lead and the role of the other participants is weakened. In the PAR, participants are gradually added to each cycle of the study, and they can fully express the issues to be studied in each part of the study. The interactive roles of the participants are changed and the leadership roles are fluid. Considering the research content, G1 was the leader of the study in the first cycle, G2 was the leader of the study in the second cycle, and G3 was the leader of the study in the third cycle. Leadership awareness and teaching strategies have been proposed through cross-disciplinary cooperation. Although the researchers believe that doctors and nurses worry about novice operations as obstacles to teamwork, cross-disciplinary cooperation can strengthen their strengths and make up for their weaknesses [47]. The researchers with a design background initially played the role of organising and planning the research, and then the role of participatory operation and evaluation in the second and third cycles. Participants from a medical background initially played a role of passive cooperation, and later had important roles in strategy formulation and operation. In the second and third cycles, these participants mainly confirmed the accuracy of the professional operations. Although the home caregivers were not involved in the formulation of the strategy, in the third cycle the home caregivers could directly report on the rationality of the formulation of the PAR strategy and the effectiveness of the implementation.

The basic model of the study was the process of using the PDSA during operation after performing the first cycle, and then forming the second and the third cycle operation plan. In the structure, from planning to implementation, most of it is at the strategic level, and the decisions made are generally determined by the possessive resource owner. The difference between participatory research and traditional research lies in the power of the participants in the research process [48]. In the first cycle, researchers from a design background put forward the need for cooperation because they believed that they could help the medical side solve the corresponding problems by means of graphics. The designers thought that the graphical method was important and could play a leading role in the research, and they proposed the graphical strategy to solve the problems of the home caregivers. In the second cycle, when the nurse participants had entered the study, the design professionals and caregivers reached a consensus that the operation strategy was important. The researchers needed to obtain the nurses' professional assistance to complete the relevant design, and so the designers, in accordance with the nurses, put forward a strategy to solve the problem using video recording as a method of operation. After completion, the graphic contents needed to be confirmed by the nurses before entering the next cycle evaluation; therefore, in this part, the nurse study participants held a dominant position and had an important role. In the third cycle, the researchers and the nurses formed a joint strategy to evaluate the home caregivers; the home caregivers needed to agree to evaluate its operation. The home caregivers evaluated the health education tools and provided relevant advice according to their work experience and their number of years of experience; therefore, verification of the home caregivers location was important.

Professional respect is very important for the establishment of cross-disciplinary cooperation. In the spiral structure of PDSA PAR, the three participating groups continuously confirm the professional knowledge content transmitted to confirm the level of understanding. During the graphic design stage, it was necessary to cooperate with the medical staff who could assist the designers in revising the design drawings. The degree of cooperation and joint participation are key factors. Cross-disciplinary groups must have a deep understanding of each other's industry values and methods of solving problems, and learning from each other will become the motivation to eliminate stereotypes and cooperate with each other [49]. Implementation of PAR, on the one hand, controlled the accuracy of the graphic design and, on the other hand, the participation of the nurses, home caregivers, and researchers in the content and revision of the study to improve understanding. The home caregivers said that although some operations still needed to be memorised, the use of the graphics improved the previous situation of home caregivers having to repeatedly ask for the nurses' caring knowledge. The graphical health education tools can recall the operation process of home caregivers. The spiral structure of PAR constantly uses PDSA to correct deviations from the research goal, so as to ensure the accuracy of the research results.

5. Conclusions

This study explores the cooperation between different stakeholders under the framework of PAR and uses the form of PDSA to conduct research quality management. This research was initiated by designers, and the overall research planning was carried out on the design, production, and evaluation of the graphics. The researchers with a design background promoted the process of research design, standardised the operation cycles of the graphics development and design, and established the cross-disciplinary cooperative relationship. The spiral structure of PDSA PAR was used in the study to solve different research problems according to different research cycles and complete the final research goal. In the process of intervention in the field of nursing, design researchers are looking for a relatively universal design method to make graphical drawing more in line with the needs of healthcare users.

In the process of developing medical process graphics, it is necessary to consider the enthusiasm of the participants to cooperate with participants from different professional fields, plan clear goals in the research process, and ensure that the participants are also leaders in each cycle, jointly formulating strategies and sharing the research results. In this study, the accuracy of graphic development of the health education tools was improved, the process of learning and evaluation of the graphics was added, and the accuracy of the graphics was constantly modified in operation to ensure the quality and rationality of the graphic development. The feasibility of using graphics as a communication aid or health education tool deserves further study. Simultaneously, the scope of the results of this study needs to be promoted and compared with other forms of nasogastric tube home caring methods or tools, such as health education leaflets, oral instruction, and video operation. The clinical teaching effect tests should be statistically compared using quantitative methods. Additionally, this study is an exploratory operation into cooperation between the design field and the health care field to provide a reference for the graphical development method of medical care operation processes.

Author Contributions: Conceptualization, F.-S.L. and H.-C.S.; methodology, F.-S.L. and H.-C.S.; investigation, F.-S.L., F.-S.L.'s research group and H.-C.S.; data curation, F.-S.L.'s research group; writing—original draft preparation, H.-C.S. and F.-S.L.; writing—review and editing, F.-S.L. and H.-C.S.; visualization, F.-S.L.'s research group and H.-C.S.; funding acquisition, F.-S.L. All authors have read and agreed to the published version of the manuscript.

Funding: This research was funded by the Ministry of Science and Technology, Taiwan, grant number 106-2410-H-224-026.

Acknowledgments: Thanks to the assistance of Douliu Branch of National Cheng Kung University Hospital for the successful completion of the research. F.-S.L.'s research group gave us great assistance for the data and graphics, thanks for their help.

Conflicts of Interest: The authors declare no conflict of interest.

References

1. Cianfrocca, C.; Caponnetto, V.; Donati, D.; Lancia, L.; Tartaglini, D.; Di Stasio, E. The effects of a multidisciplinary education course on the burden, health literacy and needs of family caregivers. *Appl. Nurs. Res.* **2018**, *44*, 100–106. [CrossRef] [PubMed]
2. Akgun-Citak, E.; Attepe-Ozden, S.; Vaskelyte, A.; van Bruchem-Visser, R.L.; Pompili, S.; Kav, S.; Mattace-Raso, F.U.S. Challenges and needs of informal caregivers in elderly care: Qualitative research in four European countries, the TRACE project. *Arch. Gerontol. Geriatr.* **2020**, *87*, 103971. [CrossRef] [PubMed]
3. Richardson, T.J.; Lee, S.J.; Berg-Weger, M.; Grossberg, G.T. Caregiver Health: Health of Caregivers of Alzheimer's and Other Dementia Patients. *Curr. Psychiatry Rep.* **2013**, *15*, 367. [CrossRef] [PubMed]
4. Gitlin, L.N.; Winter, L.; Dennis, M.P.; Hodgson, N.; Hauck, W.W. Targeting and Managing Behavioral Symptoms in Individuals with Dementia: A Randomized Trial of a Nonpharmacological Intervention. *J. Am. Geriatr. Soc.* **2010**, *58*, 1465–1474. [CrossRef]
5. Nakarada-Kordic, I.; Patterson, N.; Wrapson, J.; Reay, S.D. A Systematic Review of Patient and Caregiver Experiences with a Tracheostomy. *Patient-Patient-Cent. Outcomes Res.* **2017**, *11*, 175–191. [CrossRef]
6. Schlager, A.; Metzger, Y.; Adler, S. Use of surface acoustic waves to reduce pain and discomfort related to indwelling nasogastric tube. *Endoscopy* **2010**, *42*, 1045–1048. [CrossRef]
7. Pai, S.-F.; Chang, K.-H.; Lim, S.-N.; Tsai, M.-C.; Chang, H.-J. Risk Factors Associated with Hospitalization in Elderly Patients Receiving Home Care Nursing. *J. Long-Term Care* **2017**, *21*, 53–75.

8. Kongsuwan, W.; Borvornluck, P.; Locsin, R.C. The lived experience of family caregivers caring for patients dependent on life-sustaining technologies. *Int. J. Nurs. Sci.* **2018**, *5*, 365–369. [CrossRef]
9. Hagedoorn, E.I.; Keers, J.C.; Jaarsma, T.; van der Schans, C.P.; Luttik, M.L.A.; Paans, W. The association of collaboration between family caregivers and nurses in the hospital and their preparedness for caregiving at home. *Geriatr. Nurs.* **2019**, in press. [CrossRef]
10. Almomani, B.A.; Mokhemer, E.; Al-Sawalha, N.A.; Momany, S.M. A novel approach of using educational pharmaceutical pictogram for improving inhaler techniques in patients with asthma. *Respir. Med.* **2018**, *143*, 103–108. [CrossRef]
11. Roberts, N.J.; Evans, G.; Blenkhorn, P.; Partridge, M.R. Development of an electronic pictorial asthma action plan and its use in primary care. *Patient Educ. Couns.* **2010**, *80*, 141–146. [CrossRef] [PubMed]
12. Cloyes, K.G.; Hart, S.E.; Jones, A.K.; Ellington, L. Where are the family caregivers? Finding family caregiver-related content in foundational nursing documents. *Journal of Professional Nursing.* **2020**, *36*, 76–84. [CrossRef] [PubMed]
13. Ang, S.Y.; Lim, S.H.; Lim, M.L.; Ng, X.P.; Madeleine, L.; Chan, M.M.; Lopez, V. Health care professionals' perceptions and experience of initiating different modalities for home enteral feeding. *Clin. Nutr. Espen.* **2019**, *30*, 67–72. [CrossRef] [PubMed]
14. Hsiung, H.-F. Utilization of Home Health Care among Disabled Adults. Ph.D. Thesis, National Tainan University, Taipei, Taiwan, 2010. (Unpublished).
15. Yang, F.-H.; Lin, F.-Y.; Hwu, Y.-J. Knowledge, Attitude, and Behavior of Taiwan Nurses toward Nasogastric Tube Placement Verification. *Cheng Ching Med. J.* **2017**, *13*, 55–63.
16. Ho, M.-M.; Hor, Y.-S.; Li, S.-C.; Hu, L.-H.; Hwang, P.-C.; Wang, M.-H.; Chen, M.-L. The Exploration of Home Care Patients' Unplanned Ex-tubation and the Primary Caregivers' Knowledge, and Learning Needs Related to Tubing Care. *J. Long-Term Care* **2008**, *12*, 72–90.
17. Lin, Y.-C.; Tsai, Y.-C. Home Care Experience of Assisting a Patient to Weaning NG Tube and Tracheostomy Tube. *St. Joseph's Hosp. Med. Nurs. J.* **2012**, *6*, 72–83.
18. Chen, J.-C.; Jo, L.-H.; Hu, S.-C. Using Nursing Process to Deal with Common Nursing Problems in Hospital-Based Home Nursing Program: A Study. *Nurs. Res.* **1994**, *2*, 6–16.
19. Klima Ronen, I. Action research as a methodology for professional development in leading an educational process. *Stud. Educ. Eval.* **2020**, *64*, 100826. [CrossRef]
20. Maestrini, V.; Luzzini, D.; Shani, A.B.; Canterino, F. The action research cycle reloaded: Conducting action research across buyer-supplier relationships. *J. Purch. Supply Manag.* **2016**, *22*, 289–298. [CrossRef]
21. Li, I.-C. Application of Action Research in Nursing. *Nurs. Res.* **1997**, *5*, 463–468.
22. Eden, C.; Ackermann, F. Theory into practice, practice to theory: Action research in method development. *Eur. J. Oper. Res.* **2018**, *271*, 1145–1155. [CrossRef]
23. Whyte, W.F. Participation, Action, and Research in the Classroom. *Stud. Contin. Educ.* **1997**, *1*, 1–50.
24. Noguchi, A.; Inoue, T.; Yokota, I. Promoting a nursing team's ability to notice intent to communicate in lightly sedated mechanically ventilated patients in an intensive care unit: An action research study. *Intensive Crit. Care Nurs.* **2019**, *51*, 64–72. [CrossRef] [PubMed]
25. Liang, H.-F.; Wu, K.-M.; Hung, C.-C.; Wang, Y.-H.; Peng, N.-H. Resilience enhancement among student nurses during clinical practices: A participatory action research study. *Nurse Educ. Today* **2019**, *75*, 22–27. [CrossRef]
26. Norbye, B. Healthcare students as innovative partners in the development of future healthcare services: An action research approach. *Nurse Educ. Today* **2016**, *46*, 4–9. [CrossRef]
27. Yeh, L.-L. Participatory Action Research and Its Utilization. *New Taipei J. Nurs.* **2010**, *12*, 59–68.
28. Villasante, T.R.; Garcia, F.J.G. Methodologies for the Participant Construction of Knowledge. *Syst. Pract. Action Res.* **2001**, *14*, 483–493. [CrossRef]
29. Schafft, K.A.; Greenwood, D.J. Promises and Dilemmas of Participation: Action Research, Search Conference Methodology, and Community Development. *Community Dev. Soc. J.* **2003**, *34*, 18–35. [CrossRef]
30. Ottosson, S. Participation action research-: A key to improved knowledge of management. *Technovation* **2003**, *23*, 87–94. [CrossRef]
31. Leis, J.A.; Shojania, K.G. A primer on PDSA: Executing plan–do–study–act cycles in practice, not just in name. *BMJ Qual. Saf.* **2017**, *26*, 572–577. [CrossRef]

32. Byrne, J.; Xu, G.; Carr, S. Developing an intervention to prevent acute kidney injury: Using the Plan, Do, Study, Act (PDSA) service improvement approach. *J. Ren. Care* **2015**, *41*, 3–8. [CrossRef] [PubMed]
33. Cleary, B.A. Supporting empowerment with Deming's PDSA cycle. *Empower. Organ.* **1995**, *3*, 34–39. [CrossRef]
34. Donnelly, P.; Kirk, P. Use the PDSA model for effective change management. *Educ. Prim. Care* **2015**, *26*, 279–281. [CrossRef] [PubMed]
35. Cleghorn, G.D.; Headrick, L.A. The PDSA Cycle at the Core of Learning in Health Professions Education. *Jt. Comm. J. Qual. Improv.* **1996**, *22*, 206–212. [CrossRef]
36. Walley, P.; Gowland, B. Completing the circle: From PD to PDSA. *Int. J. Health Care Qual. Assur.* **2004**, *17*, 349–358. [CrossRef]
37. Speroff, T.; Oconnor, G.T. Study designs for PDSA quality improvement research. *Qual. Manag. Health Care* **2004**, *13*, 17–32. [CrossRef]
38. Moen, R.; Norman, C. Evolution of the PDCA cycle. Available online: https://www.westga.edu/~{}dturner/PDCA.pdf (accessed on 9 August 2020).
39. Reed, J.E.; Card, A.J. The problem with Plan-Do-Study-Act cycles. *BMJ Qual. Saf.* **2016**, *25*, 147–152. [CrossRef]
40. Houts, P.S.; Doak, C.C.; Doak, L.G.; Loscalzo, M.J. The role of pictures in improving health communication: A review of research on attention, comprehension, recall, and adherence. *Patient Educ. Couns.* **2006**, *61*, 173–190. [CrossRef]
41. Lin, J.-L.; Hsieh, P.-S.; Lin, S.-H.; Song, M.-H.; Wang, S.-F. The Effectiveness of Caregiver Education for Caring Nasogastric Tube. *Tzu Chi Nurs. J.* **2005**, *4*, 49–56.
42. Chen, M.-F.; Chen, Y.-H.; Wu, R.-Y.; Yu, H.-C.; Chen, S. Naso-Gastric Tube Care Assistant: "My NG is Not NG" Model. *Qual. Mag.* **2014**, *50*, 29–32.
43. Chen, M.-J.; Lu, Y.-H.; Chen, C.-C.; Li, A.-C. A Project to Reduce the Incidence of Intubation Care Errors among Foreign Health Aides. *J. Nurs.* **2014**, *61*, 66–73.
44. Huang, S.-W.; Lee, H.-Y.; Liu, C.-Y.; Hsieh, H.-C.; Yeh, S.-H.; Chiang, S.-C.; Hsieh, C.-C.; Hsu, C.-M. Improvement of The Accuracy Rate of Correcting Nasogastric Tube Feeding Care Among Elder Family Caregivers. *Show Chwan Med. J.* **2015**, *14*, 1–11.
45. Barros, I.M.C.; Alcântara, T.S.; Mesquita, A.R.; Santos, A.C.O.; Paixão, F.P.; Lyra, D.P. The use of pictograms in the health care: A literature review. *Res. Soc. Adm. Pharm.* **2014**, *10*, 704–719. [CrossRef] [PubMed]
46. Chein, I.; Cook, S.W.; Harding, J. The field of action research. *Am. Psychol.* **1948**, *3*, 43–50. [CrossRef] [PubMed]
47. Fisher, M.; Weyant, D.; Sterrett, S.; Ambrose, H.; Apfel, A. Perceptions of interprofessional collaborative practice and patient/family satisfaction. *J. Interprofessional Educ. Pract.* **2017**, *8*, 95–102. [CrossRef]
48. Cornwall, A.; Jewkes, R. What is participatory research? *Soc. Sci. Med.* **1995**, *41*, 1667–1676. [CrossRef]
49. Ateah, C.A.; Snow, W.; Wener, P.; MacDonald, L.; Metge, C.; Davis, P.; Anderson, J. Stereotyping as a barrier to collaboration: Does interprofessional education make a difference? *Nurse Educ. Today* **2011**, *31*, 208–213. [CrossRef]

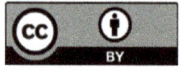

© 2020 by the authors. Licensee MDPI, Basel, Switzerland. This article is an open access article distributed under the terms and conditions of the Creative Commons Attribution (CC BY) license (http://creativecommons.org/licenses/by/4.0/).

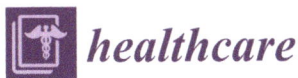

Article

Exploring Pictorial Health Education Tools for Long-Term Home Care: A Qualitative Perspective

Fang-Suey Lin [1], Hong-Chun Shi [1,*] and Kwo-Ting Fang [2]

[1] Graduate School of Design, National Yunlin University of Science and Technology, Yunlin 64002, Taiwan; linfs@yuntech.edu.tw
[2] Department of Information Management, National Yunlin University of Science and Technology, Douliu 64002, Taiwan; fangkt@yuntech.edu.tw
* Correspondence: d10630019@yuntech.edu.tw

Received: 14 June 2020; Accepted: 6 July 2020; Published: 9 July 2020

Abstract: Regarding long-term home care needs, nurses need to communicate effectively and reasonably when teaching home caregivers. Designers can assist medical staff and develop pictorial tools to enhance communication. The purpose of this study is to explore a theoretical basis from the perspective of designers, patients' home caregivers, and medical staff to construct a theoretical framework that can jointly develop pictorial health education tools and healthcare system. The qualitative methods, including in-depth interview and observation, are applied to this study; ground theory sets out to construct a framework from the verbatim transcript of the interviews. Based on interview results, six axial codes were extracted: (1) the method of interdisciplinary cooperation; (2) medical research ethics; (3) communication methods; (4) forms of health education tools; (5) development of health education tools; (6) home care intubation procedure. Eight groups of home caregivers offered suggestions from their experiences. The designers need to assist medical staff to solve real problems, pay attention to professional norms, and forms of cooperation. Health education tools need to meet the needs of medical staff and home caregivers and designers should pay attention to the processes of communication. This study can also assist in interdisciplinary cooperation to explore the theoretical basis of pictorial health education tools for nurses in the context of long term care at home.

Keywords: pictorial health education tools; long-term home care; nurses and home caregivers; communication; case study; a qualitative perspective

1. Introduction

Long-term home care is normally provided by non-professional medical staff. Nurses need to provide the necessary help to long-term home caregivers and patients, but cooperation and communication between the two can become a problem. As the elderly now live longer, the demand for improved services in long-term home care is growing [1] and, as a result, there are increasing demands on nurses' resources. With interdisciplinary collaboration needed in home care settings, designers can intervene to improve the home care system, to offer different solutions according to different home care needs, and to solve concrete operational problems [2].

To improve the service quality of long-term home care, many researchers introduced health education tools in the field of health care. This included pictorial tools for interventions, to help those with low literacy levels enhance their understanding of health knowledge [3] and improve the recall process of patients after treatment [4]. Furthermore, using images in an environment can reduce negative emotions [5]. In cooperation with designers, pictorial health education tools can be developed for long-term home care to facilitate the operation of medical staff and help patients and caregivers understand professional terminology. As a strategy to cultivate creativity, interdisciplinary cooperation is a form of teamwork to develop knowledge that can promote the integration of different fields of healthcare, and has an important impact on the overall development of learners [6]. There may be obstacles to interdisciplinary cooperation in a hospital, more so for nurses than for doctors [7].

Ageing is a relatively serious concern in the region where the researchers are located. Many elderly people need long-term home care and most of their children employ home caregivers. Most caregivers are foreigners with poor language skills and new caregivers lack relevant experience in long-term home care. Researchers have long paid attention to the skills of foreign caregivers and found that, as well as language problems and lack of nursing knowledge, they are afraid or unwilling to communicate with nurses, so mistakes may be made in the home. Based on preconceived experiences and literature, the researchers thought that pictorial health education tools could assist nurses or home caregivers. The purpose of this study is to explore a theoretical framework from the perspective of designers, home caregivers, and medical staff, and jointly develop pictorial health education tools to enhance communication and cooperation between medical and non-medical staff in the home care setting. Therefore, in this study, it is necessary to examine the following aspects in the qualitative research: (1) what is the perspective of medical staff on the use of pictorial health education tools; (2) what is the perspective of caregivers when using pictorial health education tools; (3) designers' focus on interdisciplinary cooperation in developing pictorial health education tools.

2. Literature Review

2.1. Health Literacy of Long-Term Home Caregivers

Home caregivers need to understand the expertise, procedures, and practices in the field of nursing. Knowledge of long-term home care is rooted in the health literacy of home caregivers and the application of knowledge comes from "individuals, organisations, environment and knowledge itself" [8]. Health literacy enables the public to acquire knowledge, understanding, skills, and confidence in relevant health information, which is a positive factor in nursing and needs to be considered throughout the social care system [9]. Health literacy is also defined as the relationship between patients, caregivers, and health professionals in the health care system. Health literacy involves skills that can be taught. During recent years, the relationship of nursing transformed from leader-centred to patient-centred, which changes the structure of the medical system and thus, improves patient safety and satisfaction [10]. Health literacy should be concerned, not only with operational skills, but also with changes in health behaviour, involving the development of multiple domains [11]. Health education tools to improve health literacy are not limited to development and use but should also focus on generality so that medical staff in the process of improving the health literacy of stakeholders in the family environment is similar to the development of nursing teaching tools that are suited to the medical environment [12].

Long-term caregivers only take basic training lessons and lack of medical professional background, but they play a very important role in home care. Medical terminology often confuses patients and the use of relevant strategies in nursing can reduce its negative influence on patients during a conversation. The popularity of medical vocabulary promotes understanding, enables patients to better socialise in the medical environment, considers the background of the patient's environment, explains terminology, and enables doctors to pay attention to the expressions and reflections of patients when communicating [13]. When patients think the technical terminology used in clinical diagnosis is difficult to understand, reading and understanding written text is very important. More specific information and vocabulary are needed to make it easier for patients to understand, and adding pictures to a verbal description can improve patients' comprehension. In the medical training process, the patient's ability should be taken into account, as sometimes it is better to use pictures to illustrate the information to make it easier to understand and easy to apply at home without medical staff [14].

2.2. Pictorial Health Education Tools

Medical health education tools are morphologically diverse. New technology is used to place graphic content in electronic equipment; digital technology combined with images can improve learning fluency, reduce the cognitive gap, and improve doctor–patient communication [15]. Compared with text, the images have an important influence on the effective communication of information, which can improve concentration, memory, and understanding. Images can also change the public's attitude to health education, especially for those with literacy and reading difficulties, and encourage those more willing to follow the content of image information practices [16]. The use of pictorial health education tools in medical institutions, nursing institutions, and long-term home care environments can help caregivers understand the instructions from medical staff, enhance the nursing process, and improve caregivers' health literacy and communication skills [3]. Some studies used experimental approaches to assess the influence of pictograms on people's understanding of information about health care. It was proved that when the text was accompanied by a picture, it enhanced people's recall of the text, and suggested that graphic designers and stakeholders can participate in the study and that use the reasonable way to evaluate pictorial use [17]. Pictures are also used in language training, assisting low or no speakers to acquire language skills. The use of images will help communication, making it easier to understand and remember [18]. From the perspective of auxiliary functions, for students who lack knowledge, pictures are the best way to enhance learning [19,20]. A picture can make the information interesting if features can be memorised, for example, colour, complexity, and meaning [21].

2.3. AAC Is Applied to Doctor-Patient Communication

Augmentative and Alternative Communication (AAC) along with the progress and development of technology, provide innovative solution for a wide range of users with various language barriers [22]. With technological development, AAC was more widely applied to nonverbal communication, clinical communication, and language. Pictures are an important part of AAC as it expands its application further and the conversion from language to an image requires detailed evaluation [23]. AAC's core vocabulary is suitable for improving children's oral expression and has been proved effective [24]. AAC has been used in long-term care institutions to improve the quality of care for the elderly [25]. It has also been applied in the context of intensive care unit and diversity of auxiliary communication tools. However, medical staff have little understanding of the communication board and the communication strategies used by medical staff may affect the communication ability of patients [26]. According to different needs, AAC uses high-tech, low-tech, and non-tech assistance. The emotions of stakeholders should be taken into account, which will affect their willingness to communicate [27] and the use of AAC for emotional communication between patients and caregivers can improve the patients' quality of life [28].

2.4. Grounded Theory

Grounded theory is applied by researchers who want to solve a problem in a specific environment; it provides a theoretical basis before the research is formally started. Researchers identified pre-understanding information is correct and operable in the process of practice, and in the process of concrete operation, grounded theory based on the interviews to correct the research content, according to the methods of observation, proving the problems of the research. Grounded theory is the earliest research applied in the field of nursing by Glaser and Strauss. They defined grounded theory and believed that it could be used as the basis for better theoretical construction in social research [29], to develop theories in data research and show the context of data [30]. The construction of theory needs to constantly examine the correctness of theory and the perfect nature of data, fully explain the phenomenon, and add the original theory to the new concept [31]. However, the data collection methods of grounded theory have been controversial. Researchers found that the data are objective after the data are analysed and coded by researchers to form a new framework. Glaser and Strauss thought that researchers anticipated the objective, made assumptions about scope and conditions, and interpreted and constructed study phenomenon [32]. The cooperation of people with different research backgrounds makes grounded theory a scientific qualitative research method. It holds the tradition of symbolic interaction theory and emphasis on daily life experiences and self-cognition of basic parties [33].

3. Materials and Methods

3.1. Study design and Structure

The researchers collected information about home healthcare, tracked the theme of the pictorials used by healthcare assistants, and conducted interviews and observation surveys to collect the information from the perspective of designers, patients' home caregivers, and medical staff to construct a theoretical framework, and then compared this with existing communication theories and literature. A construction framework was established that enabled the designer to attempt to develop pictorial health education tools for long-term home care (Figure 1).

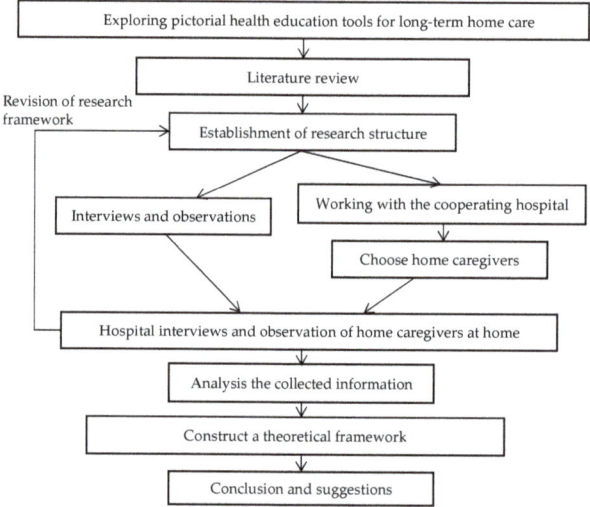

Figure 1. Exploring pictorial health education tools for long-term home care research.

3.2. In-Depth Interview and Observation Method

The researchers initially proposed to develop tools for intubation procedures, but the nurses recommend another alternative project because these procedures are performed by professional nurses and not by home caregivers. However, home caregivers could be trained in basic nursing and daily cleaning; they could also understand the routine intubation procedure, recognise if patients were in discomfort afterwards, and report this in a timely fashion to the professional nurses.

In the areas surveyed, there was a large proportion of foreign home caregivers. Long-term home care hospital nurses are responsible for training foreign home caregivers, but when there is poor verbal communication, it can lead to a decrease in overall communication and influence the learning efficiency and understanding of nursing operations. The problems faced by the researchers in determining the research content became clearer after a discussion on what images to use as communication tools in the process of teaching, how to help home caregivers, especially foreigners, with the intubation of patients, and the feasibility of developing apps for medical aid.

At the beginning of the study, interviews were conducted with hospital staffs about home caregivers' learning experiences and difficulties. These were two times semi-structured focus group interviews in the hospital. The interviewee had to consent to the recording and the interviews were adjusted according to their personal experience. A manuscript was developed to help with the questioning (Table 1). Respectively, from what the interdisciplinary cooperation norms were [6], the manner of nurses' communication [34], problems in home care procedures [35], expectations for developing health education tools [36], and nursing care for intubated patients [37]. In exploring the theoretical model, we only interviewed those working in hospitals, and the home caregivers were observed and recorded to confirm their intention of using pictorial health education tools.

Table 1. The main scope and content of the interview.

Empty Frame	Interview Questions
Interdisciplinary cooperative norms [6]	1. Introduce research directions to seek cooperation and ask if the research can be conducted in the hospital. 2. What rules need to be adhered to?
The manner of nurses' communication [34]	3. What are the basic conditions of the caregiver? 4. What cautions need to be taken when communicating with patients? 5. What are the basic communication methods between nurses and caregivers?
Problems in home care procedures [35]	6. What problems need to be solved in the process of home care? 7. What should the home caregivers do at home for intubated patients? 8. What methods does the nurse use to teach home caregivers skills?
Expectations for developing health education tools [36]	9. What specification of health education tools are more convenient to use? 10. From the nurse's perspective, what are the requirements for the design of home care tools?
Nursing care for intubated patients [37]	11. What is the key content of nursing in the home care process? 12. What matters need attention in the home care process?

3.3. Participants

The participants interviewed and observed in this study were divided into three groups, designers, medical staff, and home caregivers. In previous research, a good relationship of cooperation and participation with the hospital was established. Hospital managers were willing to assist the participants in the groups to solve specific problems and tasks. Participants described their ideas and perspectives during the team meeting. One group included five hospital participants: the hospital director, nursing supervisor, and nurses. The other group had six design participants in design research and practice, including a teacher at the school's research institute and five assistant researchers. These participants conducted a preliminary group interview to build the theoretical framework and they also participated in later research practice. Nurses from the cooperation hospital provided eight groups of cases, all of which were home caregivers of intubation patients. Operational observation and random interviews were conducted with the home caregivers when the theoretical framework of this study was established.

3.4. Content Analysis

According to interviews with the medical staff, three researchers with design backgrounds were employed to code together. The three researchers had experience in design strategy, teaching, and image design, respectively. From the perspective of the designer, the interview results with the medical staff were analysed and common words confirmed by trigonometric verification. The purpose was to reach agreement among the designers with different backgrounds to find out feasible reference suggestions and form a theoretical framework when using pictorial design to solve specific problems. The interview text was repeatedly read and confirmed. Combined with the data processing method of grounded theory, researchers conducted open coding to form a common coding book. Meanwhile, the operation method and formula of content analysis [38] were used to increase the credibility of the selection of each sentence during the interviews. This formula was used to check the degree of agreement between the interview verbatim manuscripts and the reliability of interview manuscripts. The degree of mutual agreement required the joint participation of the three coders to screen common statements and then, according to the degree of mutual agreement, encode the reliability of the three coders.

The degree of mutual agreement is as follows:

$$\text{Degree of mutual agreement} = \frac{N \times M}{N_1 + N_2 + \cdots N_n} \quad (1)$$

(M is the number of the fully agreed sentences, $N_1 \sim N_n$ are the number of participating researchers).
The content analysis reliability calculation is as follows:

$$\text{Reliability} = \frac{n \times (\text{Average mutual agreement})}{1 + [(n-1) \times \text{Average mutual agreement}]} \quad (2)$$

3.5. Research Ethics and Limitations

This study passed the National Cheng Kung University Human Research Ethics Review Committee review. The home caregivers who participated in the research signed the informed consent and agreed to be observed and interviewed. The research process was conducted with the nurse supervisor in the hospital.

This study adopts the qualitative research method and has specific research objectives for foreign caregivers who deal with home care intubation. It is only limited by the theoretical reference for developing pictorial health education tools. Due to geographical limitations, this study may not apply to other situations with home care needs as other areas may require more diversified forms of graphical tools, solicit the advice of medical staff according to different studies, and require users to have more reasonable and scientific evaluation forms.

4. Results

4.1. Open Coding and Axial Coding

This study conducted two in-depth interviews lasting about 60 min, which were sorted into verbatim drafts and coded. Based on the empty framework, open coding was conducted by the three researchers without any discussion with each other. In the first calculation of reliability, the number of keywords in the verbatim text of the interviews was 20, 26, and 21, respectively; there were too few common keywords because the reliability value was less than 0.6, so it was rejected. Before the second reliability analysis, the researchers held a meeting to analyse this and found that, in the first coding process, the reason is that the coders focused more on the researcher's problem rather than the nurse's recommendations. In the second coding process, the coders were required to find the nurses' viewpoints on the operational needs of teaching home caregivers from the perspective, the designer based on the interview results and to solve the problems of home care with the help of the design method, before coding again. After discussion, the three coders extracted the number of keywords, which were 23, 22, and 22, respectively and there were 20 common keywords. This result is shown in Table 2. The common statement calculation formula of the final triangulation test was 20 × 3 / (23 + 22 + 22) = 0.896 and the reliability value was higher than 0.6.

According to the interview results (Table 3), the interviewees of different professional respondents are different. Based on previous experience, the hospital management believed that the graphical representation should be the hospital's design of the guidance system, rather than clinical operation. While researchers raised the issue of home care, hospital administrators raised the issue of operational ethics. Therefore, when designers conduct research cooperation, according to the groups involved in the research problem, they should pay attention to the physical condition of stakeholders and the degree of physical contact in the process of research and development and abide by ethical norms. Nurses were very concerned about the operating details and thought they might occur problems in communication during the nursing process. The nurse and patient communication tools, for example, used phonetic or pinyin boards. More patients were spelling slowly, reducing communication efficiency. The researchers mentioned that in long-term home care, communication with the elderly being intubated, if there is a graphical representation, it will make it easier for home caregivers to do it.

Table 2. Interview reliability.

Times	Researcher 1	Researcher 2	Researcher 3	Common Sentence	Mutual Agreement	Reliability
1	20	26	21	2	0.090	0.228
2	23	22	22	20	0.896	0.962

Table 3. Open coding and axial coding.

Axial Coding	The Theme	Open Coding	Role	Source
Method of interdisciplinary cooperation (AC01)	Researchers and nurses need to work together	Researchers can follow them on the front line, the research topic may change, the data will be more refined.	Hospital manager	CA01-51
	Help the nurse with real difficulties	Learn as much as you can from nurses, observe their problems and help solve them. The design of the icon registration section has been developed and published before.	Hospital manager	CA01-58
	Speaking right of cooperation	So, let's start with three-tube care, which is to give you the video and paperwork. Map out the steps and bring them up when we visit the home.	Nurse	CB02-57
Medical research ethics (AC02)	Observe research ethics and avoid disputes	When doing research, patients are involved and there will be patient privacy, so relevant regulations should be adhered to.	Hospital manager	CA01-54
	Attitude of the patient and family	We need the consent of the patient and the family first.	Nurse	CB02-18
Communication methods (AC03)	Communication is important in nursing and details need to be improved	(Researcher: During direct demonstration, in which cycle did the problem appear?) The nurse replied: Communication.	Nurse	CB02-51
	How nurses teach and communicate with home caregivers	There is no video, all procedures are on-the-spot demonstrations.	Nurse	CB02-49
	The nurses explain the background of home caregivers	Indonesia predominates, as does the Philippines.	Nurse	CB02-26
	Existing communication tools are pen and paper	Written on paper, Chinese characters.	Nurse	CB02-83
	Nurses rely on personal experience to communicate and it is difficult for patients to express their true wishes	Guess with experience and then describe the meaning roughly to family members. The patient only nods and shakes their head.	Nurse	CB02-85
	There is a communication barrier between nurses and patients and it is very difficult for patients to express themselves, so nurses need to guess what patients think during communication.	He (the patient) communicated with me using his hands and feet because he can only say a few words; the patient got angry. The patient can make breathing sounds, but I can probably understand them. In terms of communication, he only listens to what he wants to hear.	Nurse	CB02-173
Health education tools form (AC04)	Nurses' expectations of health education tools	What if it's A4 size? Wall charts are not convenient in case there is no place to hang them.	Nurse	CB02-148
	Nurses use health education tools in the form of traditional printed products, but the size of the tools need to be easy to use	(We) think you can use A4 size to make a small manual and then coil it into a book, it's easy to turn pages. This will be easier than wall charts.	Nurse	CB02-150
Health education tools development (AC05)	The development of health educational tools requires recording of specific processes, but some steps may not be completed in a simulated environment	We can start with a medical dummy. But we need to know the structure of the medical dummy first. Whether the nasogastric tube can be inserted is uncertain.	Nurse	CB02-37
	Uncertainty factors in the way health education tools are developed and it is important to find an appropriate way to demonstrate an operation	We could look for a similar standard movie for your reference, or we could try to send you a video. It is mainly about the technology of placing tubes and care.	Nurse	CB02-42
Intubation home care operation (AC06)	A step-by-step demonstration of the operating process is required	That step will slowly decompose.	Nurse	CB02-15
	Difficulties in the operation of home caregivers	Most of the body cleaning is fine, only the technical aspects, such as turning the patient over and getting them in and out of bed.	Nurse	CB02-65
	The main problems considered by nurses in home care is the aseptic operation of intubated patients	In my opinion, intubation should not be the main focus of carers, but care should be mainly about disinfection and how to observe the principle of sterility.	Nurse	CB02-156
	Operational considerations and concerns	For example, matters needing attention in terms of the nasogastric tube as it is so long. We will measure and cut a suitable length and insert it. Then how to teach the family members and carers to confirm the tube is in and how to avoid it slipping.	Nurse	CB02-159
	Nurses also realised that text might not be suitable for home care, so education tools were repeatedly proposed during operation	You can't read the text directly, but we can use a medical dummy. Then provide written information while giving guidance.	Nurse	CB02-168

According to the open coding process discovered that hospital managers were concerned about the interdisciplinary cooperation method and ethical medical research, and thought that the researchers should have empathy, follow nurses in clinical operation and adjust the research direction according to the requirements of the nurses. Furthermore, research information should be as detailed as possible and research ethics in the process of cooperation was very important, especially in gaining consent from the family. If the patient or family did not give consent, the research could not go ahead.

Nurses had some doubts about whether design can actually help understanding the caring process of patients with intubation operation, they asked researchers to develop a sample of graphic tools based the videos and written materials in patients with intubation operation. This also avoided ethical issues about intubation and enabled the realisation that the placement of the tube could be difficult for non-specialists. When the researchers mentioned health education tools for learning, nurses were more inclined to use traditional textbooks. This may be associated with aseptic manipulation in the operational process as there may not be anywhere to put up wall charts in the home environment or use electronic devices, such as a mobile phone, might not be able to solve the problem of hands operation, other wearable device size is too small, not convenient to prompt operation. Therefore, finally put forward the health education tools A4 paper printed format.

Nurses believe that long-term home care should not focus on intubation but detailed care in the home environment. Although nurses consider these actions to be basic, the layman may have difficulty in the home care process. Studies have shown that nurses believe that more than half of home care infections are caused during intubation [39] and infection or cleaning in the home environment is a very important issue. Work for home caregivers, in addition to the problems of intubation care, involve physical work. When nurses described the communication behaviours of caregivers with years of nursing experience, they indicated that videos were not used for teaching, but direct demonstration was given on the spot. In terms of the number of home caregivers at present, foreign caregivers are in the majority and nurses used paper to communicate with patients.

In the process of interdisciplinary cooperation, detailed communication was required during the interviews because of the different professional backgrounds involved. Although there are many communication problems between nurses and patients or caregivers, new health education tools had not been considered to improve the current situation. Nurses' communication, especially with patients who cannot make a sound, is based on guesswork and experienced judgment; communication with foreign caregivers cannot be conducted verbally. Given these two communication issues, burses still think they can make a judgement based on previous experience and this may affect the accuracy of the communication process. From the perspective of developing pictorial health education tools, the researchers with design backgrounds believed they can effectively assist nurses in communicating and teaching; thus, improving the quality of home care operations. However, sometimes these researchers failed to pay attention to detailed operational procedures and ethical issues in the cooperation process. Despite the good intentions of the researchers, nurses were still reluctant to cooperate because their daily work is very complicated and they need to communicate with many people. Information visualisation can promote the basic knowledge of home care for the public and visual health education tools can improve doctor-patient communication and services if professional design skills are used. It is difficult for designers without a nursing background to assist nurses because they are not familiar with the professional operation of nursing. If they do not communicate in-depth with nurses, the design output may not have a practical application in the field. On the other hand, designers also need to learn about nurses' workflow and form clear steps in developing graphics. During the interviews, the researchers developed six axial coding statements, namely, the method of interdisciplinary cooperation (AC01), medical research ethics (AC02), communication methods (AC03), forms of health education tools (AC04), development of health education tools (AC05), and intubation home care operations (AC06).

4.2. The Quantities Relationship between Facts and Axial Coding in Interdisciplinary Cooperation

According to the operational steps of grounded theory, after axial coding was confirmed, the researcher selectively coded according to the context of the interviews. The selective encoding table represented the relationship between axial and interview facts and how they overlapped because it was necessary to find factual descriptions of the mutually supporting relationship between different axials in the context relationship and the specific quantitative relationships used in Table 4.

Table 4. Selective coding table: Quantitative relationship between axial coding and interview facts.

Axial Coding	AC01	AC02	AC03	AC04	AC05	AC06
AC01						
AC02	1↑ / 1←					
AC03	1↑	1←				
AC04				1←		
AC05				1↑ / 1←		
AC06	2←	1↑	2↑	1←		

Proposition 1. *Interaction between the method of interdisciplinary cooperation (AC01) and medical research ethics (AC02).*

- Researchers can follow them on the front line, the research topic may change, the data will be more refined. (Researcher: We need to come over frequently for our investigation). When doing research, patients are involved and there will be patient privacy, so relevant regulations should be adhered to (CA01-54).
- (Researcher: Let's start with the case today). Learn as much as you can from nurses, observe their problems and help solve them. The design of the icon registration section has been developed and published before (CA01-58).

Proposition 2. *The method of interdisciplinary cooperation (AC01) influences the intubation home care operation (AC06).*

- (The design background researcher explained that the ethical review of the study had been done and suggested that the study would not involve patients. In the study, the researcher showed uncertainty about the health education tools in the interdisciplinary cooperation process and asked the nurses to give relevant advice) If you want to take pictures (as the record), you may have to match our(the nurses) time and then you can take pictures beside us when we are working. That step will slowly decompose (CB02-15).
- So, let's start with three-tube care, which is to give you the video and the paperwork. Map out the steps and bring them up when we visit the home. Most of the body cleaning is fine, only the technical aspects, such as turning the patient over and getting them in and out of bed (CB02-65).

Proposition 3. *Intubation home care operation (AC06) influences medical research ethics (AC02).*

- (The nurses suggested that the intubation procedure should be photographed and the researcher confirmed if the photography and video were available). Yes, but we need the consent of the patient and the family first (CB02-18).

Proposition 4. *Communication methods (AC03) and health education tools development (AC05) influence each other and communication methods (AC03) also influence the method of interdisciplinary cooperation (AC01) and form of health education tools (AC04).*

- *(The researchers asked about the origin of the foreign caregivers). Indonesia predominates, as does the Philippines. (The researcher asked about the language of the health education tool, whether a simulation demonstration could be conducted). We can start with a medical dummy. But we need to know the structure of the medical dummy first. Whether the nasogastric tube can be inserted is uncertain (CB02-37).*
- *We could look for a similar standard movie for your reference or we could try to send you a video. It is mainly about our technology of placing tubes and care. (Researcher: We are probably going to bother you if you have to teach them what to prepare beforehand and then you have to do the homework. After all, we are non-professional majors, but we will watch relevant videos first to understand. If there are any questions, we will ask you again. Have you used videos to teach foreign caregivers in the past?) There is no video, just direct on-the-spot demonstrations (CB02-49).*
- *(Researcher: During direct demonstration, in which cycle did the problem appear?) The nurse replied: Communication. (According to the interview, the researcher further proposed drawing a step-by-step diagram after watching the video to see if a wall chart could be adopted. If there was any problem, it could be adjusted). So, let's start with three-tube care, which is to give you the video and the paperwork. Map out the steps and bring them up when we visit the home (CB02-57).*
- *What if it's A4 size? Wall charts are not convenient in case there is no place to hang them (CB02-148).*

Proposition 5. *Intubation home care operation (AC06) and medical research ethics (AC02) influence the communication method (AC03).*

- *Most of the body cleaning is fine, only the technical aspects, such as turning the patient over and getting them in and out of bed. (In terms of studying, researchers suggested there was very little data on the operation of basic nursing skills and caregivers would not buy such material. However, home caregivers' skills are important and improper operation may result in injured patients. Practical demonstration may be easier to understand, the video still has disparity compare with the fact operation, and then the researcher consulted the nurse commonly the method of communication with the intubation patient at present). Written on paper, Chinese characters (CB02-83).*
- *(The researcher asked about preparing the consent form and nurses told them to prepare it by themselves as they needed to know the language used by foreign home caregivers). Indonesia predominates, as does the Philippines (CB02-26).*
- *You can't read the text directly, but we can use a medical dummy, then provide written information while giving guidance. (Researcher: Are there any examples of how patients cannot communicate? Nurse: I have one here at the nursing home. Researcher: What do you use when you need to communicate with patients?) He (the patient) communicated with me using his hands and feet because he can only say a few words; the patient got angry. The patient can make breathing sounds, but I can probably understand them. In terms of communication, he only listens to what he wants to hear (CB02-173).*

Proposition 6. *The form of health education tools (AC04) influence intubation home care operation (AC06).*

- *(We) think you can use A4 size to make a small manual and then coil it into a book so it's easy to turn pages. This will be easier than wall charts. (The researcher proposed preparing several forms of health education tools. Only after testing can we know which pictorials can be truly understood. The nurse's assistance and modification may be needed in the drawing.) In my opinion, intubation should not be the main focus of carers, but care should be mainly about disinfection and how to observe the principle of sterility. It is mainly about the care of the tubes. We (nurses) have to change the tubes (CB02-156).*

4.3. Home Caregivers' Point of View

Through observing home caregivers, we found that their experience was valued by most families, but the initial source of nursing knowledge was diversified through either professional or non-professional channels. Most of the intubation home care was learned only by temporary learning or contact with users. Some caregivers need on-the-job training in nursing homes or are trained by nurses; they can also learn from a family member or mutual learning between home caregivers. Regardless of the stage of training or experience, home caregivers can learn from doctors or nurses, according to each patients' needs. A long period spent in home care can build a good relationship with patients.

Before intubation caring, nurses would ask the caregivers about their patients' condition. Some patients used more than one intubation method, but nurses seldom asked their families. Home caregivers undertake detailed observation of their patients in home care. The process of removing nasogastric tubes is very painful for the patient. In addition to the nurse's verbal soothing process, the caregiver must be beside the patient to comfort them. The patient cannot express his discomfort verbally, only by expression, shouting and gesturing. Although some patients are old, they are still fully conscious and they did not want to be seen by others when the tubes were replaced. Therefore, they were only observed by nurses and main researchers.

In the process of independent home care, home caregivers need to keep close contact with nurses. On the one hand, intubation needs to be performed by nurses, and on the other hand, home caregivers need to provide timely feedback about their patient's condition. It is easy for caregivers to forget the steps. Sometimes they use mobile chat software to friends or nurses about the caring details.

Home caregiver 2 indicated that the manual was effective and that bilingual text can help them understanding the care process correctly. Due to language limitations, the researcher provided home caregiver one case an intubation home care graphical manual for their reference. She pointed out the illustrated diagram and Indonesian text helped her understand how to care properly. The case of home caregiver 2 will resign her job soon and replace a new caregiver. During the transition period, home caregiver 2 will need to teach the new home caregiver using a graphic manual. In case of home caregiver 3, family members helped with teaching and supervision, indicating that having this graphic manual was helpful for their caregiver's learning and recall. Along with the graphics, corresponding native language assistance was provided. In the case of home caregiver 4, she did not learn about the procedure for nursing the nasogastric tube; therefore, the nurse had to teach her from the beginning. Home caregiver 5's patient was elderly, but was still fully conscious and could understand the intubation graphics; she found it very helpful. In the case of home caregiver 7, the caregiver can speak mandarin fluently, and her learning ability quite good; she had taken care of her particular patient for about six months and could understand the manual. The case of home caregiver 8 was quite old, and took care of the patient by herself most of the time; she took quite a long time to learn the material and had a slower recall. Nurses suggested that for new or slow learners, it was helpful for them to learn how to care for patients using graphic health education tools. First, they pointed out the steps to be done with a manual and then demonstrated the actual operation. Use a graphic manual to assist nurses in teaching process communication, and the caregivers can go over the manual by themselves. The graphic is also helpful to recall the operation process of nursing care. The caregivers cannot read Chinese, and graphics with Indonesian keywords can be understood well.

4.4. Theoretical Framework for Pictorial Processes in Long-Term Home Care and Communication Problem-Solving Strategies

The researchers put forward the case for developing a health education tool for intubation nursing. They had to respect the wishes of hospital nurses, but also make the tool convenient for home caregivers. After the tool was developed, according to the theoretical framework, it was promoted to nurses and home caregivers to improve communication in teaching and learning. The tool was based on the relationship of selective coding with facts and graphic information was added, according to an adapted AAC diamond model. The diamond model plays an important role in the problem-solving process and is also used in the teaching process of tool development in the health sector [40]. A theoretical framework similar to the diamond model was discovered after the interviews. Combining or replacing oral expression in communication, it discusses the application of the assisted oral method to communicate with home caregivers in the field of medical care and develops a communication tool for health education suitable for application (Figure 2).

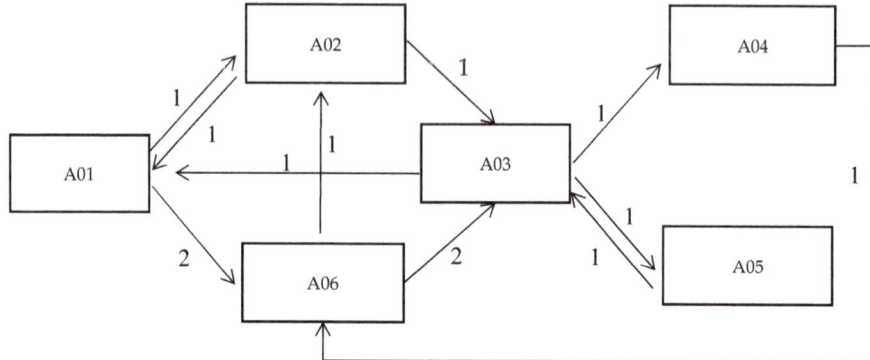

Figure 2. Theoretical framework: Augmentative and Alternative Communication (AAC) diamond model.

Communication in the medical environment is a very special social communication and the relationship between doctor–patient can affect how they interact. Regional studies suggest that many factors can cause poor communication between nurses and patients, such as language ability, nurses' workload, remuneration, and time management, all of which affect the nurses' communication behaviours and intentions [41]. Factors such as multiple uses of nursing tools, training, and clinical experience may influence nurses' willingness to use them [42]. Instrumental communication translates into tool-based teaching and learning relationships. In essence, the assistance tool transforms the communication mode between nurses and caregivers, improves the understanding of the medical process, and indirectly affects the doctor–patient relationship. However, different patients may have different standards of satisfaction, not only the satisfaction in the nursing process but also their expression, movement, tone, and environment. The emergence of communication tools and intermediaries to coordinate and communicate the needs of both sides can help the medical and the patient side to make better medical decisions and provide patient-centred services. Nurses described a home setting to the researchers:

> In the past, if a caregiver had a poor memory, you gave them a video. The average person can't remember so many steps and precautions. Nurses teach in Indonesian or Vietnamese using health education leaflets provided by existing institutions and as there are no graphics, they can only describe them orally. To see how well caregivers are learning, it would be better to have a pictorial manual.

5. Discussion

5.1. Assist Medical Staff to Solve Real Problems

During the interviews, when the researcher proposed the need for frequent communication with nurses and relevant field observations, hospital managers repeatedly stressed that researchers should work with nurses to present real data, that patients' privacy should be covered by medical research ethics and that researchers should empathise with interdisciplinary research [43]. Because there were many cases of interdisciplinary cooperation, there was a need to develop tools that helped nurses solve real practical problems. There was a concern that cooperative research did not understand the application, the hospital would lose momentum and the research would have to be applicable in practice. Nurses needed the tools to facilitate teaching carers or learning content, but in researching what was needed, the designer had to create the operation details as a beginner. The researchers wanted to choose the relevant intubation content but found that nurses who teach in the home care setting needed to teach nonprofessional carers how to avoid adverse impact on the patients. Therefore, in cooperation with the designers, nurses decided whether to use textbooks or videos and determine the most needed aspects of home care. To demonstrate the intubation procedure, the designer lacked the medical knowledge, especially in the home care setting, making it vital to cooperate with medical staff, when necessary, to understand the problems of home care in the learning process. At the same time, nurses lacked the design skills of drawing flowcharts, which is what designers are good at. However, at times, nurses did not think this part was important because of their workload. Cross-field cooperation is a process where different specialities complement each other and exchange mutual professional cognition, which may ultimately affect the form of intubation operation in a home care setting.

5.2. Professional Norms and Forms in Interprofessional Cooperation

Medical personnel have repeatedly emphasised medical ethics and believe that in the process of home care cooperation, consent should be obtained from the patient's family to avoid unnecessary disputes. It is suggested that researchers should review medical ethics, whether in the process of intubation care or the development of health education tools. Stakeholders' information should be confidential and used only in the study. The hospital should assign a supervisor to guide the entire study process during the nurse's operation and record the process. As the home caregiver is of mostly foreign nationality, the development and form of health education tools may be affected and text and image should be considered in the design. When nursing professionals and non-professionals have different levels of knowledge and communication ability, misunderstandings may occur. Interventions and tools can form the basis for effective communication [44]. Nurses believe that the biggest problem in the operation process is communication, so a schematic design of the home care intubation process should be completed and then a health education tool, applicable to the home care setting, should be developed. Nurses provide immediate on-the-spot demonstrations of the intubation process, which is the teach-back method [45]. In this study, nurses thought that the researchers should draw images from the video, which may affect the accuracy of the graphics, because of the cooperation at the beginning may increase in their workload, and it was also possible that could influence the willingness of nurses to cooperate. In the interview, nurses had expectations about the form of health education tools. The researchers proposed two different methods of communication (electronic or traditional wall chart), but the nurses thought the form of the health education tool can be an A4 size with colour printing and a Wire-O binding form, mainly related to the nurses in clinical operation convenience.

5.3. The Form of Health Education Tools Has to Meet the Needs of Medical Staff and Home Caregivers

In the process of nursing operations, non-medical professionals have some difficulty in understanding and remembering the details. There is a big difference between the hospital side and patient side in terms of medical knowledge, so hospital staff need to recognise the knowledge level of patients to help them understand the content and they should also consider using hints [46]. When the language involved is not the mother language, it affects various social and cultural relationships. To attract the attention of stakeholders, the nursing team should provide relevant solutions for the communication barriers based on medical language [47]. Additionally, foreign carers' lack of language ability further affects communication. If the family members do not agree, then new health education tools cannot be applied in the nursing process, which will continue to affect communication. Medical personnel and the design professionals were consistent in understanding research ethics and agreed that medical ethics needed to be strictly followed for the process of interdisciplinary research and cooperation to run smoothly.

Nurses thought it was more convenient to make health education tools into a manual. The intubation method was not the main concern of home care; the main focus was to follow the principles of disinfection and asepsis. The medical environment is composed of different services and professionals and effective professional collaboration is necessary to ensure the quality of care for patients and the overall medical care system [48]. The nurses' opinion on the form of health education tools was different from the designers. The designer hoped to use a more novel technical solution to help the clinical teaching process of nursing, but nurses thought that traditional printed matter was more conducive to the teaching process. At first, the design professionals wanted to draw the intubation teaching steps, but the nurses explained that professionals were still needed in the home care setting to perform the operation as home caregivers lacked the medical knowledge. They stated that home caregivers needed to concentrate on cleaning and hygiene. In terms of home care, the public wants medical institutions to provide flexible services and ensure communication is effective between nurses, home caregivers, patients and their families and that nursing is provided according to the requirements of individual patients, providing humanist care services [49].

5.4. Pay Attention to Communication Behaviour in the Nursing Process

Gerber (2016) proposed solving doctor–patient communication problems with philosophical methods. Non-traditional communication methods were applied and new tools developed that used reasonable processes in specific situations that could overcome communication barriers in diagnosis and treatment [50]. In communication theory, Habermas outlined four aspects that included tools, strategies, language and communication. Tools conveyed an object; a strategy was adopted by both sides in reaching a consensus of how to communicate, especially when there was a language difference or communication barrier. In the act of communication, clarity, truth, correctness, and appropriateness of the information was considered effective. Communication behaviours in an information system should be based on a well-structured communication path, considering the information symmetry of both parties [51]. Habermas believed that communication should be guided by mutual understanding, consensus should be reached between the two parties in the communication process and all participants in the system should be involved [52].

From the perspective of Habermas, nurses needed to face two aspects in the field of nursing. One was the responsibility they assumed for their service and the other was the obligation undertaken in operating the social system [53]. Mishler adopted Habermas' point of view in the process of medical relationships in that doctor-patient communication was very difficult to control and understand. The researchers recorded the statements about doctor–patient communication in real life, analysed the linguistics and concluded that communication behaviour should be based on ethical definitions and that technology can realise the rationality of communication so that both sides can understand and communicate [54].

Our model demonstrated that communication mode is the core of the theoretical framework and the problems encountered in the study should be clarified to improve the communication mode. Using the Johari window model to analyse the known and unknown aspects of communication between the hospital and the patient can be improved in the applied theoretical framework and later, in the development process of the graphical health education tools (Table 5). The Johari window analysis method found that the problem of communication was composed of four dimensions in a matrix of 2×2 [55]: the process of long-term home care, the problem in each region, the improvement of communication behaviour and communication tools, and changing the method of communication between the hospital and the patient.

Table 5. Johari Window analysis of communication between hospital staff and patients.

Intervention Tools: Communication Behaviours and Intervention of Communication Tools (Language, Text, Image, Body, etc.)		Hospital Staff: Doctors and Nurses	
		Known	Unknown
Patient Side: Patients, family members and home caregivers	Known	**Arena** • The patient needs home care • Existing symptoms of the patient • The physical statement of the patient	**Blindspot** • An accurate representation of a disease or symptom by the patient • The influence of mood, tone, and attitude on the other communication side • Communication in different situations
	Unknown	**Facade** • Care methods • Treatment of symptoms • Methods of home care • Steps of home care	**Unknown** • The patient's accuracy of expression • Whether caregivers and family members have adequate health literacy • Whether the patient's side has an understanding of nursing knowledge

6. Conclusions

This study can assist designers to explore the theoretical basis of pictorial health education tools for nurses in the context of long-term care at home. The communication process is a complex process involving not only the home care operation details, interdisciplinary cooperation, and medical ethics, but attention also needs to be paid to the development of communication tools and morphology. Nurses need to acknowledge the long-term home care patient's expression and the demands of home caregivers. They also need to cooperate with professional designers to develop pictorial health education tools and provide home caregivers with an easier method of understanding operational procedures and communication.

Interdisciplinary cooperation needs both groups to understand each other as much as possible without affecting each other's operating conditions. This is difficult because cooperation needs both sides to have common knowledge and experiences, or at least respect for each other's knowledge, experience, and operational methods. Cooperation in this study highlighted what both groups were good at; they had frequent question and answer sessions during the process, operational errors could be corrected and once the design professionals had developed the flowchart, it could be used for hospital nursing staff to teach home caregivers in the future.

Author Contributions: Conceptualization, F.-S.L. and H.-C.S.; methodology, K.-T.F. and H.-C.S.; investigation, F.-S.L.'s research group and H.-C.S.; data curation, F.-S.L.; writing—original draft preparation, H.-C.S. and F.-S.L.; writing—review and editing, F.-S.L. and H.-C.S.; visualization, H.-C.S.; funding acquisition, F.-S.L. All authors have read and agreed to the published version of the manuscript.

Funding: This research was funded by the Taiwan Ministry of Science and Technology, grant number 106-2410-H-224-026.

Acknowledgments: Thanks to the assistance of Douliu Branch of National Cheng Kung University Hospital for the successful completion of the research. Thanks to the other two designers who worked on the research coding, thanks for their help.

Conflicts of Interest: The authors declare no conflict of interest.

References

1. Amilon, A.; Ladenburg, J.; Siren, A.; Vernstrøm Østergaard, S. Willingness to pay for long-term home care services: Evidence from a stated preferences analysis. *J. Econ. Ageing* **2020**, *17*, 100238. [CrossRef]
2. Groop, J.; Ketokivi, M.; Gupta, M.; Holmström, J. Improving home care: Knowledge creation through engagement and design. *J. Oper. Manag.* **2017**, *53*, 9–22. [CrossRef]
3. Schubbe, D.; Scalia, P.; Yen, R.W.; Saunders, C.H.; Cohen, S.; Elwyn, G.; Muijsenbergh, M.V.D.; Durand, M.-A. Using pictures to convey health information: A systematic review and meta-analysis of the effects on patient and consumer health behaviors and outcomes. *Patient Educ. Couns.* **2020**. [CrossRef] [PubMed]
4. Wolch, G.; Ghosh, S.; Boyington, C.; Watanabe, S.M.; Fainsinger, R.; Burton-Macleod, S.; Thai, V.; Thai, J.; Fassbender, K. Impact of Adding a Pictorial Display to Enhance Recall of Cancer Patient Histories: A Randomized Trial. *J. Pain Symptom Manag.* **2017**, *53*, 109–115. [CrossRef]

5. Monti, F.; Agostini, F.; Dellabartola, S.; Neri, E.; Bozicevic, L.; Pocecco, M. Pictorial intervention in a pediatric hospital environment: Effects on parental affective perception of the unit. *J. Environ. Psychol.* **2012**, *32*, 216–224. [CrossRef]
6. Moirano, R.; Sánchez, M.A.; Štěpánek, L. Creative interdisciplinary collaboration: A systematic literature review. *Think. Ski. Creat.* **2020**, *35*, 100626. [CrossRef]
7. Yusra, R.Y.; Findyartini, A.; Soemantri, D. Healthcare professionals' perceptions regarding interprofessional collaborative practice in Indonesia. *J. Interprof. Educ. Pract.* **2019**, *15*, 24–29. [CrossRef]
8. Berta, W.; Teare, G.F.; Gilbart, E.; Ginsburg, L.S.; Lemieux-Charles, L.; Davis, D.; Rappolt, S. Spanning the know-do gap: Understanding knowledge application and capacity in long-term care homes. *Soc. Sci. Med.* **2010**, *70*, 1326–1334. [CrossRef]
9. NHS. (n.d.). Available online: http://www.healthliteracyplace.org.uk (accessed on 19 January 2020).
10. Parnell, T.A. Nursing Leadership Strategies, Health Literacy, and Patient Outcomes. *Nurse Lead.* **2014**, *12*, 49–52. [CrossRef]
11. Pleasant, A.; McKinney, J. Coming to consensus on health literacy measurement: An online discussion and consensus-gauging process. *Nurs. Outlook* **2011**, *59*, 95–106.e1. [CrossRef]
12. Taylor, L.J. Caring for your gastric tube at home. *Home Care Provid.* **1998**, *3*, 111–114. [CrossRef]
13. Roter, D. Oral literacy demand of health care communication: Challenges and solutions. *Nurs. Outlook* **2011**, *59*, 79–84. [CrossRef] [PubMed]
14. Wittink, H.; Oosterhaven, J. Patient education and health literacy. *Musculoskelet. Sci. Pract.* **2018**, *38*, 120–127. [CrossRef] [PubMed]
15. Lin, F.S.; Lin, C.Y.; Hsueh, Y.J.; Lee, C.Y.; Hsieh, C.P. Graphical Tools for Doctor-Patient Communication: An App Prototype Design in Children's Pain Management. In *HCI International 2016—Posters' Extended Abstracts*; Springer International Publishing: Berlin/Heidelberg, Germany, 2016; Volume 618.
16. Houts, P.S.; Shankar, S.; Klassen, A.C.; Robinson, E.B. Use of Pictures to Facilitate Nutrition Education for Low-income African American Women. *J. Nutr. Educ. Behav.* **2006**, *38*, 317–318. [CrossRef]
17. Barros, I.M.; Alcântara, T.S.; Mesquita, A.R.; Santos, A.C.O.; Paixão, F.P.; Lyra, D.P. The use of pictograms in the health care: A literature review. *Res. Soc. Adm. Pharm.* **2014**, *10*, 704–719. [CrossRef]
18. Bondy, A.S.; Frost, L.A. The Picture Exchange Communication System. *Focus Autistic Behav.* **1994**, *9*, 1–19. [CrossRef]
19. Filippatou, D.; Pumfrey, P.D. Pictures, Titles, Reading Accuracy and Reading Comprehension: A research review (1973–1995). *Educ. Res.* **1996**, *38*, 259–291. [CrossRef]
20. Carney, R.N.; Levin, J.R. Pictorial Illustrations Still Improve Students' Learning from Text. *Educ. Psychol. Rev.* **2002**, *14*, 5–26. [CrossRef]
21. Levin, J.R.; Anglin, G.J.; Carney, R.N. On Empirically Validating Functions of Pictures in Prose. *Psychol. Illus.* **1987**, *1*, 51–85. [CrossRef]
22. Light, J.; McNaughton, D. The changing face of augmentative and alternative communication: Past, present, and future challenges. *Augment. Altern. Commun.* **2012**, *28*, 197–204. [CrossRef]
23. Radici, E. Augmentative and Alternative Communication: The role of Communication Partners. Ph.D. Thesis, Università degli Studi di Milano-Bicocca, Milan, Italy, 2017.
24. Meinzen-Derr, J.; Sheldon, R.M.; Henry, S.; Grether, S.M.; Smith, L.E.; Mays, L.; Riddle, I.; Altaye, M.; Wiley, S. Enhancing language in children who are deaf/hard-of-hearing using augmentative and alternative communication technology strategies. *Int. J. Pediatr. Otorhinolaryngol.* **2019**, *125*, 23–31. [CrossRef]
25. Comiotto, G.S.; Kappaun, S.; Cesa, C.C. The knowledge of healthcare professionals about augmentative and alternative communication in the long term care institutions for the elderly. *Rev. CEFAC* **2016**, *18*, 1161–1168. [CrossRef]
26. Jansson, S.; Martin, T.R.S.; Johnson, E.; Nilsson, S. Healthcare professionals' use of augmentative and alternative communication in an intensive care unit: A survey study. *Intensive Crit. Care Nurs.* **2019**, *54*, 64–70. [CrossRef] [PubMed]
27. Istanboulian, L.; Rose, L.; Gorospe, F.; Yunusova, Y.; Dale, C.M. Barriers to and facilitators for the use of augmentative and alternative communication and voice restorative strategies for adults with an advanced airway in the intensive care unit: A scoping review. *J. Crit. Care* **2020**, *57*, 168–176. [CrossRef]

28. Corallo, F.; Bonanno, L.; Buono, V.L.; De Salvo, S.; Rifici, C.; Pollicino, P.; Allone, C.; Palmeri, R.; Todaro, A.; Alagna, A.; et al. Augmentative and Alternative Communication Effects on Quality of Life in Patients with Locked-in Syndrome and Their Caregivers. *J. Stroke Cerebrovasc. Dis.* **2017**, *26*, 1929–1933. [CrossRef]
29. Glaser, B.G.; Strauss, A.L. *The Discovery of Grounded Theory: Strategies for Qualitative Research*; Aldine Transaction: Chicago, IL, USA, 1967.
30. Charmaz, K.C. *Constructing Grounded Theory: A Practical Guide through Qualitative Analysis*; Chongqing University Press: Chongqing, China, 2009.
31. Ozanne, J.L.; Strauss, A.; Corbin, J. Basics of Qualitative Research. *J. Mark. Res.* **1992**, *29*, 382. [CrossRef]
32. Denzin, N.K.; Lincoln, Y.S. *Handbook of Qualitative Research*; Chongqing University Press: Chongqing, China, 2013; pp. 550–551.
33. Zhai, H.Y.; Bih, H.D.; Liou, C.X.; Yang, K.S. *Research Methods in Social and Behavior Science: Qualitative Methods*; Social Science Academic Press: Beijing, China, 2013; pp. 59–75.
34. Romagnoli, K.M.; Handler, S.; Hochheiser, H. Home care: More than just a visiting nurse. *BMJ Qual. Saf.* **2013**, *22*, 972–974. [CrossRef]
35. Cissé, M.; Yalçındağ, S.; Kergosien, Y.; Şahin, E.; Lenté, C.; Matta, A. OR problems related to Home Health Care: A review of relevant routing and scheduling problems. *Oper. Res. Health Care* **2017**, 1–22. [CrossRef]
36. Baron-Epel, O.; Levin-Zamir, D.; Satran-Argaman, C.; Livny, N.; Amit, N. A participatory process for developing quality assurance tools for health education programs. *Patient Educ. Couns.* **2004**, *54*, 213–219. [CrossRef]
37. Otuzoğlu, M.; Karahan, A. Determining the effectiveness of illustrated communication material for communication with intubated patients at an intensive care unit. *Int. J. Nurs. Pract.* **2013**, *20*, 490–498. [CrossRef]
38. Yang, G.S.; Wen, C.Y.; Wu, C.X.; Li, Y.Y. *Social and Behavioral Science Research*; Tung Hua Book Co., Ltd.: Taipei, Taiwan, 2002.
39. Russell, D.; Dowding, D.; McDonald, M.V.; Adams, V.; Rosati, R.J.; Larson, E.L.; Shang, J. Factors for compliance with infection control practices in home healthcare: Findings from a survey of nurses' knowledge and attitudes toward infection control. *Am. J. Infect. Control* **2018**, *46*, 1211–1217. [CrossRef] [PubMed]
40. Ferreira, F.K.; Song, E.H.; Gomes, H.; Garcia, E.B.; Ferreira, L.M. New mindset in scientific method in the health field: Design Thinking. *Clinics* **2015**, *70*, 770 772. [CrossRef]
41. Wune, G.; Ayalew, Y.; Hailu, A.; Gebretensaye, T. Nurses to patients communication and barriers perceived by nurses at Tikur Anbessa Specilized Hospital, Addis Ababa, Ethiopia 2018. *Int. J. Afr. Nurs. Sci.* **2020**, *12*, 100197. [CrossRef]
42. Ballard, S.A.; Peretti, M.; Lungu, O.; Voyer, P.; Tabamo, F.; Alfonso, L.; Cetin-Sahin, D.; Johnson, S.M.; Wilchesky, M. Factors affecting nursing staff use of a communication tool to reduce potentially preventable acute care transfers in long-term care. *Geriatr. Nurs.* **2017**, *38*, 505–509. [CrossRef]
43. Rova, M. Embodying kinaesthetic empathy through interdisciplinary practice-based research. *Arts Psychother.* **2017**, *55*, 164–173. [CrossRef]
44. Crawford, T.; Candlin, S.; Roger, P. New perspectives on understanding cultural diversity in nurse–patient communication. *Collegian* **2017**, *24*, 63–69. [CrossRef]
45. Nickles, D.; Dolansky, M.; Marek, J.; Burke, K. Nursing students use of teach-back to improve patients' knowledge and satisfaction: A quality improvement project. *J. Prof. Nurs.* **2019**, *36*, 70–76. [CrossRef]
46. Jucks, R.; Paus, E.; Bromme, R. Patients' medical knowledge and health counseling: What kind of information helps to make communication patient-centered? *Patient Educ. Couns.* **2012**, *88*, 177–183. [CrossRef] [PubMed]
47. Hull, M. Medical language proficiency: A discussion of interprofessional language competencies and potential for patient risk. *Int. J. Nurs. Stud.* **2016**, *54*, 158–172. [CrossRef] [PubMed]
48. Wei, H.; Watson, J. Healthcare interprofessional team members' perspectives on human caring: A directed content analysis study. *Int. J. Nurs. Sci.* **2018**, *6*, 17–23. [CrossRef]
49. Walsh, S.; O'Shea, E.; Pierse, T.; Kennelly, B.; Keogh, F.; Doherty, E. Public preferences for home care services for people with dementia: A discrete choice experiment on personhood. *Soc. Sci. Med.* **2020**, *245*, 112675. [CrossRef] [PubMed]
50. Gerber, B. Should we use philosophy to teach clinical communication skills? *Afr. J. Prim. Health Care Fam. Med.* **2016**, *8*, 2–4. [CrossRef] [PubMed]

51. Lyytinen, K.; Hirschheim, R. Information systems as rational discourse: An application of Habermas's theory of communicative action. *Scand. J. Manag.* **1988**, *4*, 19–30. [CrossRef]
52. Ross, A.; Chiasson, M. Habermas and information systems research: New directions. *Inf. Organ.* **2011**, *21*, 123–141. [CrossRef]
53. Stewart, L.; Holmes, C.; Usher, K. Reclaiming caring in nursing leadership: A deconstruction of leadership using a Habermasian lens. *Collegian* **2012**, *19*, 223–229. [CrossRef]
54. Barry, C.A.; Stevenson, F.A.; Britten, N.; Barber, N.; Bradley, C.P. Giving voice to the lifeworld. More humane, more effective medical care? A qualitative study of doctor–patient communication in general practice. *Soc. Sci. Med.* **2001**, *53*, 487–505. [CrossRef]
55. Hamzah, M.I.; Othman, A.K.; Hassan, F.; Razak, N.A.; Yunus, N.A.M. Conceptualizing a Schematic Grid View of Customer Knowledge from the Johari Window's Perspective. *Procedia Econ. Financ.* **2016**, *37*, 471–479. [CrossRef]

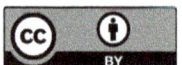

© 2020 by the authors. Licensee MDPI, Basel, Switzerland. This article is an open access article distributed under the terms and conditions of the Creative Commons Attribution (CC BY) license (http://creativecommons.org/licenses/by/4.0/).

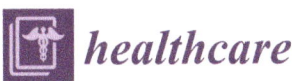

Study Protocol

Knowledge Retention of the NIH Stroke Scale among Stroke Unit Health Care Workers Using Video vs. E-Learning: Protocol for a Web-Based, Randomized Controlled Trial

Avinash Koka [1,*], Mélanie Suppan [2], Emmanuel Carrera [3], Paula Fraga-Freijeiro [4], Kiril Massuk [4], Marie-Eve Imbeault [4], Nathalie Missilier Perruzzo [3], Sophia Achab [5,6], Alexander Salerno [4], Davide Strambo [4], Patrik Michel [4], Loric Stuby [7] and Laurent Suppan [1,*]

1. Division of Emergency Medicine, Department of Anesthesiology, Clinical Pharmacology, Intensive Care and Emergency Medicine, University of Geneva Hospitals and Faculty of Medicine, 1211 Geneva, Switzerland
2. Division of Anesthesiology, Department of Anesthesiology, Clinical Pharmacology, Intensive Care and Emergency Medicine, University of Geneva Hospitals and Faculty of Medicine, 1211 Geneva, Switzerland; melanie.suppan@hcuge.ch
3. Stroke Center, Department of Neurology, Geneva University Hospitals and Faculty of Medicine University of Geneva, 1211 Geneva, Switzerland; emmanuel.carrera@hcuge.ch (E.C.); Nathalie.Peruzzo-Missillier@hcuge.ch (N.M.P.)
4. Stroke Center, Neurology Service, Department of Clinical Neurosciences, Lausanne University Hospital, 1011 Lausanne, Switzerland; Paula.Fraga-Freijeiro@chuv.ch (P.F.-F.); Kiril.Massuk@chuv.ch (K.M.); Marie-Eve.Imbeault@chuv.ch (M.-E.I.); Alexander.Salerno@chuv.ch (A.S.); Davide.Strambo@chuv.ch (D.S.); patrik.michel@chuv.ch (P.M.)
5. Specialized Facility in Behavioral Addictions ReConnecte HUG, 1211 Geneva, Switzerland; sophia.achab@hcuge.ch
6. WHO Collaborating Center in Training and Research in Mental Health, UniGe, 1211 Geneva, Switzerland
7. Genève TEAM Ambulances, Emergency Medical Services, 1201 Geneva, Switzerland; l.stuby@gt-ambulances.ch
* Correspondence: avinash.koka@hcuge.ch (A.K.); laurent.suppan@hcuge.ch (L.S.)

Citation: Koka, A.; Suppan, M.; Carrera, E.; Fraga-Freijeiro, P.; Massuk, K.; Imbeault, M.-E.; Missilier Perruzzo, N.; Achab, S.; Salerno, A.; Strambo, D.; et al. Knowledge Retention of the NIH Stroke Scale among Stroke Unit Health Care Workers Using Video vs. E-Learning: Protocol for a Web-Based, Randomized Controlled Trial. *Healthcare* 2021, *9*, 1460. https://doi.org/10.3390/healthcare9111460

Academic Editors: José João Mendes, Vanessa Machado, João Botelho and Luís Proença

Received: 22 September 2021
Accepted: 25 October 2021
Published: 28 October 2021

Publisher's Note: MDPI stays neutral with regard to jurisdictional claims in published maps and institutional affiliations.

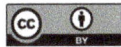

Copyright: © 2021 by the authors. Licensee MDPI, Basel, Switzerland. This article is an open access article distributed under the terms and conditions of the Creative Commons Attribution (CC BY) license (https://creativecommons.org/licenses/by/4.0/).

Abstract: The National Institutes of Health Stroke Scale (NIHSS) is commonly used to triage and monitor the evolution of stroke victims. Data regarding NIHSS knowledge in nurses and physicians working with stroke patients are scarce, and a progressive decline in specific knowledge regarding this challenging scale is to be expected even among NIHSS certified personnel. This protocol was designed according to the CONSORT-eHealth (Consolidated Standards of Reporting Trials) guidelines. It describes the design of a randomized controlled trial whose primary objective is to determine if nurses and physicians who work in stroke units improve their NIHSS knowledge more significantly after following a highly interactive e-learning module than after following the traditional didactic video. Univariate and multivariable linear regression will be used to analyze the primary outcome, which will be the difference between the score on a 50-question quiz answered before and immediately after following the allocated learning material. Secondary outcomes will include knowledge retention at one month, assessed using the same 50-question quiz, user satisfaction, user course duration perception, and probability of recommending the allocated learning method. The study is scheduled to begin during the first semester of 2022.

Keywords: NIHSS; e-learning; video; NIHSS certification; stroke; stroke unit; medical education; continuous education

1. Introduction

1.1. Background

Stroke is a frequent and time-critical emergency associated with significant morbidity and mortality [1,2]. Even though relative stroke incidence and mortality have declined since 1990, the expansion of the global population has resulted in an overall increase in the absolute number of strokes [3]. In the context of the COVID-19 pandemic, an association between SARS-CoV-2 infection and stroke has been described, with infected patients being at higher risk of worse functional outcomes and even death [4]. Efficiently assessing stroke victims is therefore more important than ever to limit the high morbidity burden associated with this pathology. Indeed, some interventions, such as intravenous thrombolysis and thrombectomy, improve functional and survival prognosis after stroke [1]. As these treatments are more effective when performed rapidly, cerebral imagery must be promptly obtained after patient admission. Scanners and Magnetic Resonance Imaging units are, however, often overloaded and overbooked [5,6], and delays in obtaining cerebral imagery are associated with worse functional and survival outcomes [7]. Adequate and timely triage is therefore mandatory, and most guidelines recommend using the National Institutes of Health Stroke Scale (NIHSS) to triage stroke victims for revascularization treatments [5,8]. Both patients with very mild [9] and very severe stroke [10] have their particularities of presentations, causes, and outcomes. Moreover, the NIHSS is also used in many stroke units to monitor the patients' evolution [11,12], with neurological monitoring every 6 h being mandatory in Swiss stroke units in the initial surveillance phase after stroke [13]. It is therefore critical that stroke unit personnel master the application of this scale, as interpersonal variability in its interpretation can lead to inappropriate diagnostic or therapeutic procedures [14].

Digital learning resources play an important role in education today [15]. Over the last decade, e-learning modules have become popular in health professional education [16,17]. Medical and paramedical personnel often work in shift patterns, thus greatly limiting their availability for traditional teaching sessions. E-learning modules are very helpful in this setting, as the content can be viewed without time constraints, can be interrupted and resumed as needed, and can be highly interactive. Self-paced highly interactive e-learning modules have been shown to improve user satisfaction [18,19].

Traditionally, the NIHSS has been taught using a didactic video created by Dr. P. Lyden [20], which is freely available on the internet [21]. Although usually effective in teaching medical procedures [22], videos lack interactivity, making them less engaging than interactive learning materials. However, engagement has been shown to improve knowledge acquisition [23,24].

To enhance learner engagement, we have created a highly interactive electronic learning (e-learning) module using Storyline (Articulate Global, Inc., New York, NY, USA). This module was shown to be more effective than the traditional didactic video in paramedics [18] and in medical students [19]. However, the two prior studies assessing the impact of this e-learning module were carried out in populations naïve to the use of this scale. Moreover, these studies were not designed to determine an effect on knowledge retention.

With time, nurses and physicians working in a stroke unit might have forgotten or overlooked certain key aspects of the application of the NIHSS. We hypothesize that our e-learning module might be more effective in reminding them of the principles underlying the application of the NIHSS than the traditional didactic video. We furthermore hypothesize that knowledge retention at one month should be higher after following this module.

1.2. Objectives

Our primary objective is to determine if healthcare workers belonging to a stroke unit improve their NIHSS knowledge more significantly after following a highly interactive e-learning module than after following the traditional didactic video.

The secondary objectives are to perform a cross-sectional description of actual NIHSS knowledge in these specific wards and to determine whether following either training material allows better retention of knowledge at one month.

2. Materials and Methods

2.1. Study Design and Setting

A prospective, multi-centric, web-based, triple-blind (participants, investigators, data analyst) randomized controlled trial will be carried out following the CONSORT-eHealth guidelines [25] and integrating elements from the Checklist for Reporting Results of Internet E-Surveys (CHERRIES) (Figure 1) [26].

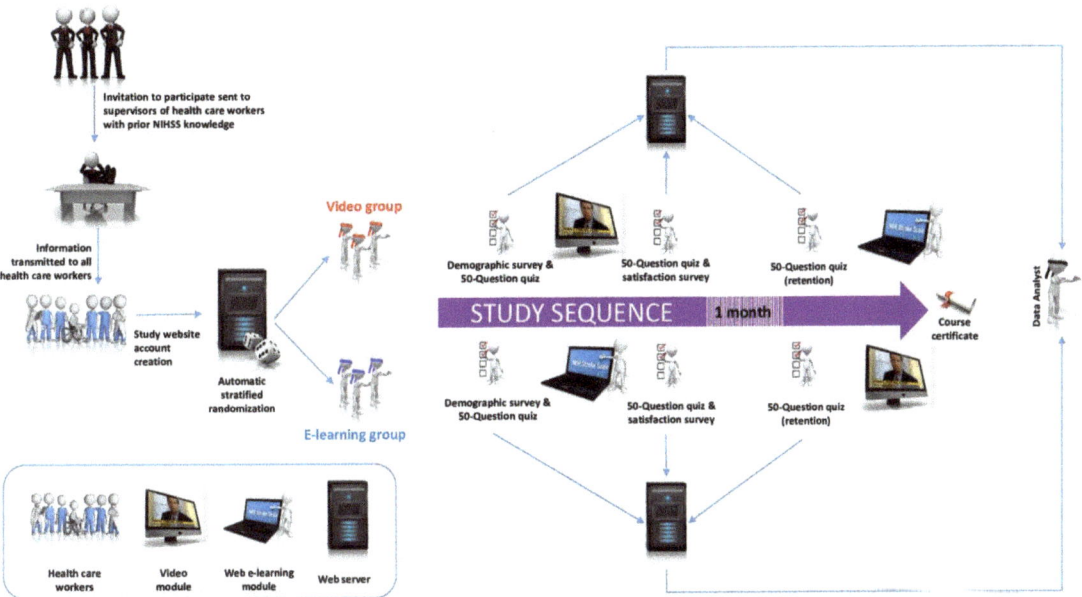

Figure 1. Study design.

2.2. Online Platform

An internet-based and GDPR (General Data Protection Regulation)-compliant study platform will be created using the Joomla 3.9 content management system (Open Source Matters, Inc., New York, NY, USA) [27]. Randomization will be stratified according to professional status (nurse or resident physician), prior NIHSS knowledge (limited, moderate, or extended), and institution by virtue of specific links displayed on the front page. Clicking on the appropriate link will automatically randomize the participant into one of two groups (video or e-learning) through the use of Gegabyte's Random Article module [28]. A specific and straightforward registration form (Membership Pro, Joomdonation [29]) will then be displayed. Participants will have to enter and confirm a valid e-mail address, choose a secure password, and validate a captcha field. After clicking on the "Register" button, a generic email containing a data policy statement will be sent to the email address entered by the participant. Simultaneously, the participant will be automatically logged in and a first questionnaire will be displayed.

2.3. First Questionnaire

This questionnaire (Table 1) is designed to gather all relevant demographic information regarding the participant and to obtain data regarding their prior NIHSS training and knowledge. It will be administered using the Community Surveys 5.6 component (CoreJoomla) [30].

Table 1. First questionnaire.

Page	Field	Original Question	English Translation
1	Demographics	Age	Age [a]
		Genre	Gender [b]
		Années d'expérience clinique au total	Number of years of total clinical experience [a]
		Années d'expérience clinique dans un service de neurologie et/ou de neurochirurgie	Number of years of clinical experience in a neurology and/or neurosurgery ward [a]
		Maîtrise du Français	French proficiency [c]
		Maîtrise de l'Anglais	English proficiency [c]
		Dans quel service travaillez-vous principalement: • Unité Cérébrovasculaire—surveillance continue • Unité Cérébrovasculaire-étage • Etage de neurologie • Soins intermédiaires de neurologie • Etage de neurochirurgie • Soins intermédiaires de neurochirurgie • Autre	In which ward do you most frequently work: [b] • Stroke unit-surveillance unit • Stroke unit-regular ward • Neurology ward • Neurology intermediate care unit • Neurosurgical ward • Neurosurgical intermediate care unit • Other
2	Prior NIHSS knowledge	Avez-vous effectué une formation interne du service pour apprendre à faire une évaluation NIHSS?	Have you completed an in house NIHSS training? [b]
		Avez-vous complété une formation certifiante officielle NIHSS?	Have you completed the official NIHSS certification course? [b]
		Nombre d'années de pratique avec l'échelle NIHSS	Number of years of clinical experience with the NIHSS scale [a]
		Fréquence d'application du NIHSS: • Plusieurs fois par jour • Environ 1 fois par jour • Environ 1 fois par semaine • Environ 1 fois par mois • Très rarement ou jamais	NIHSS use frequency: [b] • Many times per day • Circa once a day • Circa once a week • Circa once per month • Almost never or never
		Je me sens à l'aise par rapport à l'application du NIHSS	I feel comfortable using the NIHSS [c]

[a] Regex: regular expression validation. [b] MCQ: multiple-choice question (only one answer accepted). [c] 5-point Likert scale.

Regular expression (Regex) rules will be used to avoid invalid data entry. A 5-point Likert scale (very low/not at all to very high/very much) will be used to record appropriate data.

After completing this first questionnaire, participants will be redirected to a first 50-question quiz designed to assess their baseline knowledge. This quiz is identical to the one used in our previous studies [18,19]. After completing this quiz, participants will be shown the training material they have been allocated to.

2.4. Learning Material

The control group will follow the traditional didactic video created by Dr. P. Lyden [20], USA, which we have subtitled in French [31]. Meanwhile, the e-learning group will be presented with version 21c of our e-learning module [32]. This module was created using Storyline 3 (Articulate Global Inc., New York, NY, USA) and contains 184 interactive slides. Its structure follows the logic supporting the NIHSS (Figure 2).

Participants are required to go through all 12 chapters before reaching the final chapter, which summarizes the entire NIHSS score. Video extracts taken from the original didactic video have been embedded in each chapter (Figure 3), as their presence has been shown to improve knowledge acquisition [19].

In this module, quizzes and feedback [33,34] are used extensively to enhance learner engagement and promote knowledge acquisition (Figure 4). Whenever the learner gives a wrong answer, the feedback message includes the possibility to review the scoring logic related to the specific NIHSS item being tested.

Depending on the complexity of the item, specific animations or interactions are used to facilitate knowledge acquisition. This is for example the case for visual fields (Figure 5) and for extinction/inattention (Figure 6).

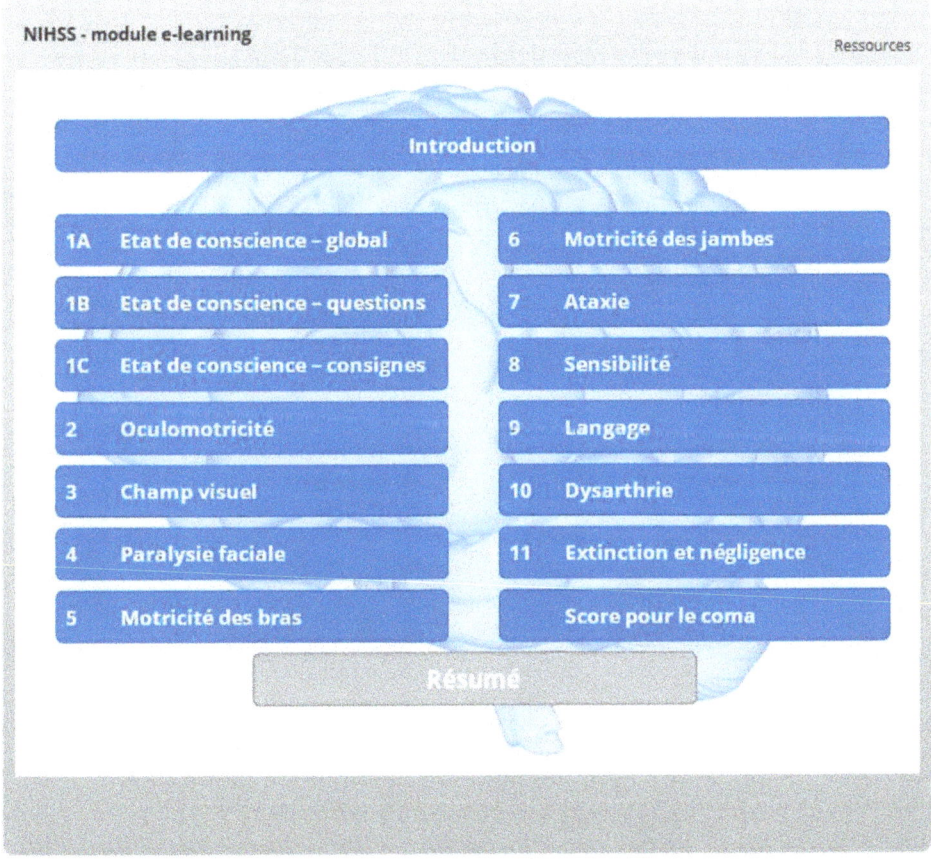

Figure 2. Table of contents of the interactive e-learning module.

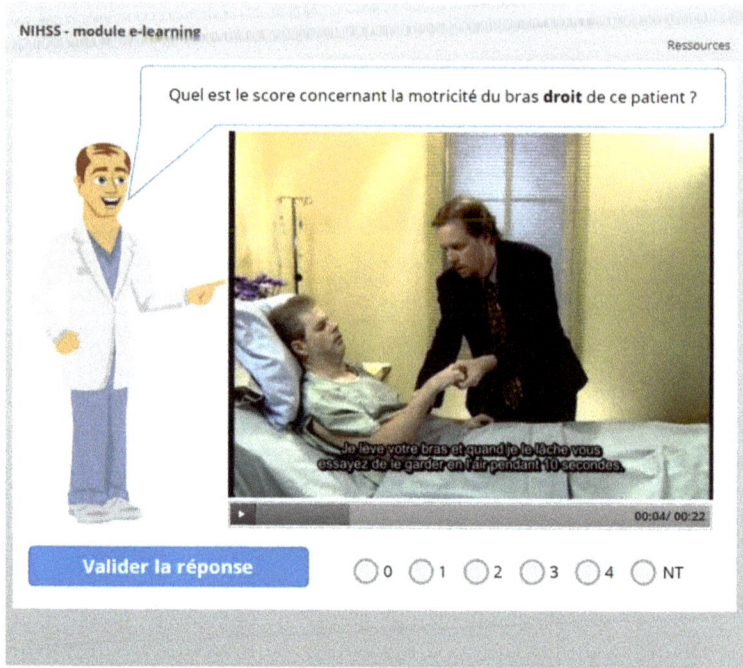

Figure 3. Embedded video and quiz interaction.

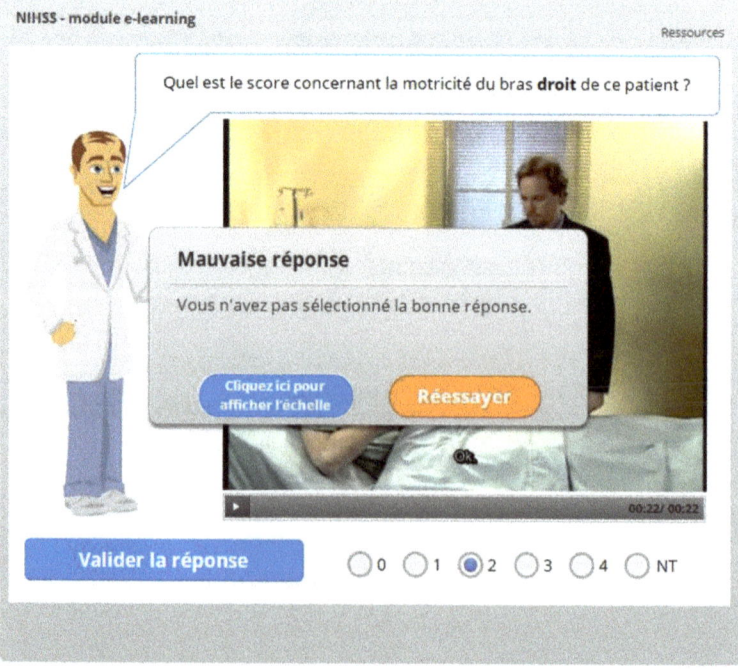

Figure 4. Feedback displayed after a wrong answer.

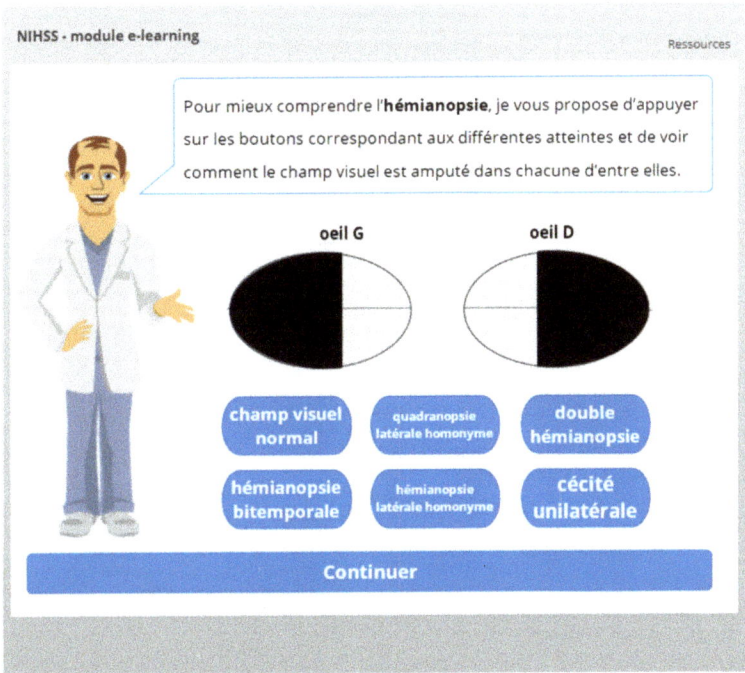

Figure 5. Interactive slide used to remind or teach visual fields.

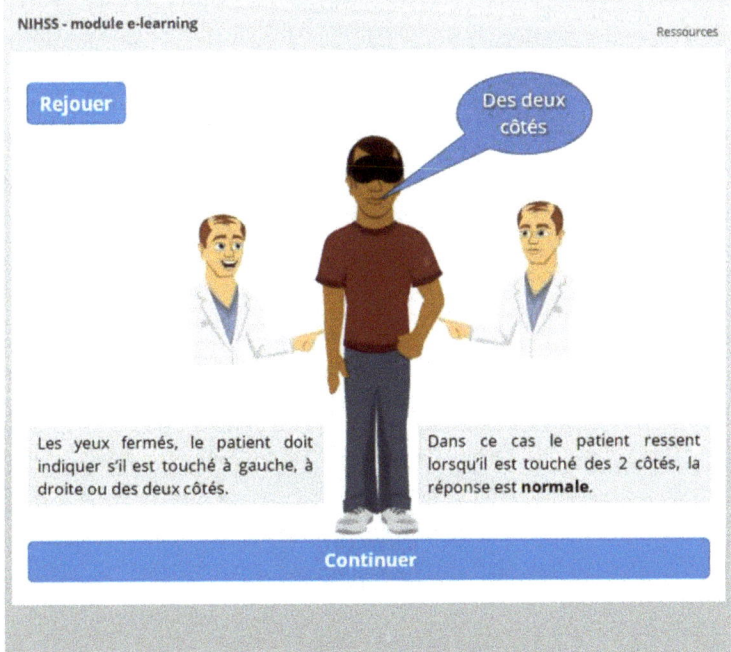

Figure 6. Interactive slide used to remind or teach the concept of extinction.

After completing the learning material, participants will be asked to answer the same 50-question quiz to determine their knowledge acquisition. At the end of this quiz, a post-course satisfaction questionnaire will be displayed (Table 2).

Table 2. Post-course questionnaire.

Page	Field	Original Question	English Translation
1	Prior NIHSS learning method exposition	Aviez-vous déjà suivi cette méthode de formation au NIHSS?	Had you already been exposed to this NIHSS learning method in the past? [a]
		Quand avez-vous suivi cette formation? • Il y a moins d'un mois • Il y a moins de 6 mois • Il y a moins d'un an • Il y a plus d'un an • Je ne me souviens pas	When did you undergo this training? • Less than a month ago • Less than 6 months ago • Less than one year ago • More than one year ago • I do not remember
	Current training-context	Dans quel cadre avez-vous suivi cette formation? • Demandée par mon service • Trouvée cette formation sur internet par hazard • Information recue par email	In which context did you undergo this training? • Required by my employers • Found it online by chance • Information received via email
	Current training-satisfaction	Comment évaluez-vous le niveau de difficulté global de cette formation?	How would you access the overall difficulty level of this training? [b]
		Que pensez-vous de la durée de cette méthode de formation?	What do you think about the duration of this training? [b]
		Quel est votre niveau de satisfaction concernant la méthode de formation?	What is your level of satisfaction regarding the learning method? [b]
		Recommanderiez-vous cette méthode de formation à vos collègues?	Would you recommend this training method to your colleagues? [b]
		Avez-vous des commentaires supplémentaires?	Do you have any additional comments?

[a] MCQ: multiple choice question (only one answer accepted). [b] 5-point Likert scale.

2.5. Knowledge Retention

One month (28 days) after completing the second 50-question quiz, participants will receive an email inviting them to test their knowledge retention. After completing this last questionnaire, they will be awarded a course completion certificate. There will be no other incentive to promote their participation.

2.6. Outcomes

The primary outcome will be the difference between the score on the 50-question quiz answered before and after following the allocated learning material. Secondary outcomes will be the overall performance in the pre-course 50-question quiz according to profession and prior NIHSS experience, performance in the same quiz undertaken one month after completion of the learning material (knowledge retention), time to course and quiz completion, user satisfaction with the learning method, user perception of the duration of the course, and probability that the user would recommend the learning material they have been allocated to a colleague.

2.7. Participants and Sample Size

Seventy-two participants are required to have 80% chance of detecting a difference of 2 points in the post-course 50-question quiz between groups at the 5% significance level. A total of 120 invitations should be sent, and a participation rate of 60% will therefore be required.

Disclaimers and data policy statements will be displayed on the front page and on the registration page (through a link that will open these statements in a modal).

2.8. Data Curation and Statistical Analysis

Stata 16 (StataCorp LLC, College Station, TX, USA) will be used for data curation and statistical analysis. Data will be curated by one author L.S. (Laurent Suppan), who will assign neutral names randomly to the e-learning group and the video group. The curated DTA file will then be transferred to another author L.S. (Loric Stuby) for data analysis.

A univariate linear regression will be used to analyze the primary outcome. Then, a multivariable linear regression model will be generated with profession, prior NIHSS knowledge, and work center as adjustment variables. The conditions of application will be checked, i.e., the residues distributions normality assessed graphically on a histogram and the homoscedasticity using the residual-versus-fitted plot function in Stata.

The analysis of the same quiz undertaken one month later (knowledge retention) will follow the same procedure as the primary outcome.

The assessment of the distribution of the other continuous variables, i.e., time for course completion and time for quiz completion, will be done graphically and using the Shapiro–Wilk test in case of doubt. Data will be described as means (95%CI) or median (Q1–Q3) depending on what is applied. Then, a Student's unpaired t-test or the Mann–Whitney U test will be applied.

The cross-sectional assessment of the performance in the pre-course 50-question quiz will be described overall and according to profession and prior NIHSS experience.

A sensitivity analysis will be performed by excluding those who have previously followed either the e-learning module or the video from Patrick Lyden [20].

User satisfaction, user course duration perception, and probability of recommendation will be assessed using a 5-point Likert scale and analyzed graphically, then using the Fisher's exact test.

The data file will be uploaded to the Mendeley Data repository.

2.9. Ethical Considerations

The study protocol was submitted to the regional ethics committees of both university hospitals (Req-2021-00543), which waived the need for ethical approval as this study falls outside of the scope of the Swiss Human Research Act from 2011.

The study is scheduled to begin during the first semester of 2022.

3. Discussion

3.1. Main Considerations

This prospective, multi-centric, web-based, triple-blind (participants, investigators, data analyst) randomized controlled study comparing video-based and e-learning should help determine if a highly interactive e-learning module improves NIHSS knowledge and skills more efficiently than the traditional didactic video amongst a mixed population of stroke unit, neurology and neurosurgery ward nurses, and physicians with different levels of experience and expertise.

Results of previous studies have shown that knowledge acquisition was higher in medical students than in paramedics [19]. This is probably due to a better understanding of the neurological system and of clinical testing, even though participants within both groups had no prior NIHSS knowledge. The current study is the first to test the impact of the e-learning module on a population with pre-existing NIHSS knowledge.

Further, we should also be able to determine the impact of these learning modalities on knowledge retention at one month. The decline in performance has been shown to be nonlinear; among participants displaying a significant decline in knowledge retention at 3 months, half of them present a significant decline already after 4 weeks [35]. This time interval has been recently used [36]. Electronic health (e-health) literacy was already high in some countries prior to the COVID-19 pandemic [37] and should have considerably increased in the wake of this crisis. Therefore, determining the most efficient asynchronous distance learning modality to help health care workers improve their NIHSS knowledge is both timely and relevant.

Given the importance the NIHSS score plays in the diagnosis, treatment decisions, and follow-up of stroke patients [1], it is essential to ensure that the NIHSS application skills are maintained at a high level. The study design should also help us gain knowledge of the current performance of neurology and neurosurgery nurses and physicians, prior to any teaching intervention, by virtue of the first (baseline) quiz. This could help determine the necessity of recurrent training in these highly specialized wards to maintain high performance in NIHSS application. There is little reason to believe that the potential decline in NIHSS application knowledge this study could reveal would be different in other settings or countries, and the results obtained should therefore be generalizable.

3.2. Strengths and Limitations

Both pathways of the study require approximately two to four hours to be completed, and participants will be asked to repeat the 50-question quiz after one month. There is currently a high level of fatigue amongst hospital staff related to the COVID-19 pandemic [38]. Even though the personnel and the different hierarchies express a high level of enthusiasm for this type of study, uncertainty remains regarding the number of participants who will engage in this study, and attrition might be high [39]. Furthermore, even though each participant will have their own login and password, we will not have any way to ascertain that the quizzes will be completed by one person and not a group of colleagues. However, we will emphasize the single-person performance aspect of this study in the instruction page, and believe that the risk of such bias is low. Although we will specify that no external resources are allowed, we will have no way to verify that these have not been used (e.g., detailed NIHSS form or internet page with explanations). The temptation to do so can be important, especially when study subjects desire to prove that their baseline NIHSS knowledge is high. This could bias the results with an over-assessment of baseline knowledge. The heterogeneity of English and French proficiency among nurses and physicians of both hospitals could have an impact on the results of the study. The e-learning is entirely in French, and Dr. P. Lyden's [20] original video is in English. To minimize this effect, the entire video (be it the extracts in the e-learning or the full video) has been subtitled in French. Further, participants will also be asked about their language proficiency in the initial demographic questionnaire, and the distribution assessed among groups. Finally, using a 50-question quiz to determine NIHSS knowledge cannot be considered as entirely representative of the actual clinical application of this scale. The video vignettes have, however, been validated in prior studies and should therefore represent an acceptable surrogate outcome [18,19]. Moreover, reusing the same 50-question quiz could lead to an improvement from one time to another due to a "priming effect" of the first questionnaire. However, this effect should be smoothed out given the randomization as it should occur similarly in both groups.

Author Contributions: Conceptualization, L.S. (Laurent Suppan), M.S., E.C., P.M. and A.K.; methodology, L.S. (Laurent Suppan), L.S. (Loric Stuby), M.S., E.C., P.M. and A.K.; software, M.S., L.S. (Laurent Suppan), L.S. (Loric Stuby) and A.K.; investigation, A.K., M.S., E.C., P.F.-F., K.M., M.-E.I., N.M.P., S.A., A.S., D.S., P.M., L.S. (Laurent Suppan), L.S. (Loric Stuby); writing—original draft preparation, A.K. and L.S. (Laurent Suppan); writing—review and editing, A.K., M.S., E.C., P.F.-F., K.M., M.-E.I., N.M.P., S.A., A.S., D.S., P.M., L.S. (Laurent Suppan), L.S. (Loric Stuby); supervision, L.S. (Laurent Suppan); project administration, M.S., L.S. (Laurent Suppan), L.S. (Loric Stuby) and A.K. All authors have read and agreed to the published version of the manuscript.

Funding: This research received no external funding.

Institutional Review Board Statement: Ethical review and approval were waived for this study, as this study was considered as falling outside of the scope of the Swiss legislation regulating research on human subjects.

Informed Consent Statement: Not applicable.

Data Availability Statement: Not applicable.

Conflicts of Interest: The authors declare no conflict of interest.

References

1. Powers, W.J.; Rabinstein, A.A.; Ackerson, T.; Adeoye, O.M.; Bambakidis, N.C.; Becker, K.; Biller, J.; Brown, M.; Demaerschalk, B.M.; Hoh, B.; et al. 2018 Guidelines for the Early Management of Patients With Acute Ischemic Stroke: A Guideline for Healthcare Professionals From the American Heart Association/American Stroke Association. *Stroke* **2018**, *49*, e46–e110. [CrossRef]
2. Katan, M.; Luft, A. Global Burden of Stroke. *Semin. Neurol.* **2018**, *38*, 208–211. [CrossRef] [PubMed]
3. Feigin, V.L.; Stark, B.A.; Johnson, C.O.; Roth, G.A.; Bisignano, C.; Abady, G.G.; Abbasifard, M.; Abbasi-Kangevari, M.; Abd-Allah, F.; Abedi, V.; et al. Global, regional, and national burden of stroke and its risk factors, 1990–2019: A systematic analysis for the Global Burden of Disease Study 2019. *Lancet Neurol.* **2021**, *20*, 795–820. [CrossRef]
4. Ntaios, G.; Michel, P.; Georgiopoulos, G.; Guo, Y.; Li, W.; Xiong, J.; Calleja, P.; Ostos, F.; González-Ortega, G.; Fuentes, B.; et al. Characteristics and Outcomes in Patients With COVID-19 and Acute Ischemic Stroke. *Stroke* **2020**, *51*, e254–e258. [CrossRef]
5. Mowla, A.; Doyle, J.; Lail, N.S.; Rajabzadeh-Oghaz, H.; Deline, C.; Shirania, P.; Ching, M.; Crumlish, A.; Steck, D.A.; Janicke, D.; et al. Delays in door-to-needle time for acute ischemic stroke in the emergency department: A comprehensive stroke center experience. *J. Neurol. Sci.* **2017**, *376*, 102–105. [CrossRef]
6. Perotte, R.; Lewin, G.O.; Tambe, U.; Galorenzo, J.B.; Vawdrey, D.K.; Akala, O.O.; Makkar, J.S.; Lin, D.J.; Mainieri, L.; Chang, B.C. Improving Emergency Department Flow: Reducing Turnaround Time for Emergent CT Scans. *AMIA Annu. Symp. Proc.* **2018**, *2018*, 897–906.
7. Wardlaw, J.M.; Seymour, J.; Cairns, J.; Keir, S.; Lewis, S.; Sandercock, P. Immediate Computed Tomography Scanning of Acute Stroke Is Cost-Effective and Improves Quality of Life. *Stroke* **2004**, *35*, 2477–2483. [CrossRef] [PubMed]
8. Lyden, P. Using the National Institutes of Health Stroke Scale. *Stroke* **2017**, *48*, 513–519. [CrossRef]
9. Eskioglou, E.; Huchmandzadeh Millotte, M.; Amiguet, M.; Michel, P. National Institutes of Health Stroke Scale Zero Strokes. *Stroke* **2018**, *49*, 3057–3059. [CrossRef]
10. Bill, O.; Zufferey, P.; Faouzi, M.; Michel, P. Severe stroke: Patient profile and predictors of favorable outcome. *J. Thromb. Haemost.* **2013**, *11*, 92–99. [CrossRef]
11. Delgado, M.G.; Michel, P.; Naves, M.; Maeder, P.; Reichhart, M.; Wintermark, M.; Bogousslavsky, J. Early profiles of clinical evolution after intravenous thrombolysis in an unselected stroke population. *J. Neurol. Neurosurg. Psychiatry* **2010**, *81*, 282–285. [CrossRef] [PubMed]
12. Wee, C.-K.; McAuliffe, W.; Phatouros, C.C.; Phillips, T.J.; Blacker, D.; Singh, T.P.; Baker, E.; Hankey, G.J. Outcomes of Endovascular Thrombectomy with and without Thrombolysis for Acute Large Artery Ischaemic Stroke at a Tertiary Stroke Centre. *Cerebrovasc. Dis. Extra* **2017**, *7*, 95–102. [CrossRef] [PubMed]
13. CHOP 2021 MG. Traitement Neurologique Complexe de l'AVC Aigu en Stroke Unit (SU), Selon la Durée de Traitement en Heures. Available online: https://medcode.ch/ch/fr/chops/CHOP%202021/99.BA.2 (accessed on 14 June 2021).
14. Josephson, S.A.; Hills, N.K.; Johnston, S.C. NIH Stroke Scale Reliability in Ratings from a Large Sample of Clinicians. *Cerebrovasc. Dis.* **2006**, *22*, 389–395. [CrossRef]
15. Scott, K.; Morris, A.; Marais, B. Medical student use of digital learning resources. *Clin. Teach.* **2018**, *15*, 29–33. [CrossRef] [PubMed]
16. Kim, K.-J.; Kim, G. Development of e-learning in medical education: 10 years' experience of Korean medical schools. *Korean J. Med. Educ.* **2019**, *31*, 205–214. [CrossRef]
17. Rouleau, G.; Gagnon, M.-P.; Côté, J.; Payne-Gagnon, J.; Hudson, E.; Dubois, C.-A.; Bouix-Picasso, J. Effects of E-Learning in a Continuing Education Context on Nursing Care: Systematic Review of Systematic Qualitative, Quantitative, and Mixed-Studies Reviews. *J. Med. Internet Res.* **2019**, *21*, e15118. [CrossRef]
18. Koka, A.; Suppan, L.; Cottet, P.; Carrera, E.; Stuby, L.; Suppan, M. Teaching NIHSS to Paramedics, E-learning vs Video: A Randomized Controlled Trial (Preprint). *J. Med. Internet Res.* **2020**, *22*, e18358. [CrossRef] [PubMed]
19. Suppan, M.; Stuby, L.; Carrera, E.; Cottet, P.; Koka, A.; Assal, F.; Savoldelli, G.L.; Suppan, L. Asynchronous Distance Learning of the National Institutes of Health Stroke Scale During the COVID-19 Pandemic (E-Learning vs Video): Randomized Controlled Trial. *J. Med. Internet Res.* **2021**, *23*, e23594. [CrossRef]
20. Lyden, P.; Brott, T.; Tilley, B.; Welch, K.M.; Mascha, E.J.; Levine, S.; Haley, E.C.; Grotta, J.; Marler, J. Improved reliability of the NIH Stroke Scale using video training. NINDS TPA Stroke Study Group. *Stroke* **1994**, *25*, 2220–2226. [CrossRef]
21. Lyden, P. NIH Stroke Scale Training—Part 2—Basic Instruction. Available online: https://www.youtube.com/watch?v=gzHuNvDhVwE (accessed on 14 June 2021).
22. Bochenska, K.; Milad, M.P.; DeLancey, J.O.; Lewicky-Gaupp, C. Instructional Video and Medical Student Surgical Knot-Tying Proficiency: Randomized Controlled Trial. *JMIR Med. Educ.* **2018**, *4*, e9. [CrossRef]
23. Wade, S.W.T.; Moscova, M.; Tedla, N.; Moses, D.A.; Young, N.; Kyaw, M.; Velan, G.M. Adaptive Tutorials Versus Web-Based Resources in Radiology: A Mixed Methods Analysis of Efficacy and Engagement in Senior Medical Students. *Acad. Radiol.* **2019**, *26*, 1421–1431. [CrossRef]
24. Croxton, R.A. The Role of Interactivity in Student Satisfaction and Persistence in Online Learning. *J. Online Learn. Teach.* **2014**, *10*, 314–325.

25. Eysenbach, G. CONSORT-EHEALTH Group CONSORT-EHEALTH: Improving and standardizing evaluation reports of Web-based and mobile health interventions. *J. Med. Internet Res.* **2011**, *13*, e126. [CrossRef]
26. Eysenbach, G. Improving the quality of Web surveys: The Checklist for Reporting Results of Internet E-Surveys (CHERRIES). *J. Med. Internet Res.* **2004**, *6*, e34. [CrossRef] [PubMed]
27. Open Source Matters Joomla Content Management System. Available online: https://www.joomla.org/ (accessed on 30 September 2020).
28. Gegabyte Technology. Random Article. Available online: https://www.gegabyte.org/downloads/joomla-extensions/joomla3/modules/291-random-article (accessed on 30 September 2020).
29. Joomdonation Membership Pro. Available online: https://joomdonation.com/joomla-extensions/membership-pro-joomla-membership-subscription.html (accessed on 30 September 2020).
30. Corejoomla Community Surveys Pro. Available online: https://www.corejoomla.com/products/community-surveys.html (accessed on 30 September 2020).
31. Suppan, M.; Stuby, L.; Koka, A.; Suppan, L. NIHSS Video Subtitled in French. Available online: https://nihss-study.ch/video (accessed on 30 September 2021).
32. Stuby, L.; Suppan, L.; Koka, A.; Suppan, M. NIHSS—e-Learning Module in French. Available online: https://nihss-study.ch/nihss-e-learning/21c/story_html5.html (accessed on 30 September 2021).
33. Kopp, V.; Stark, R.; Fischer, M.R. Fostering diagnostic knowledge through computer-supported, case-based worked examples: Effects of erroneous examples and feedback. *Med. Educ.* **2008**, *42*, 823–829. [CrossRef] [PubMed]
34. Latimier, A.; Riegert, A.; Peyre, H.; Ly, S.T.; Casati, R.; Ramus, F. Does pre-testing promote better retention than post-testing? *Npj Sci. Learn.* **2019**, *4*, 1–7. [CrossRef] [PubMed]
35. Stuby, L.; Currat, L.; Gartner, B.; Mayoraz, M.; Harbarth, S.; Suppan, L.; Suppan, M. Impact of face-to-face teaching in addition to electronic learning on personal protective equipment doffing proficiency in student paramedics: Protocol for a randomized controlled trial. *JMIR Res. Protoc.* **2021**, *10*, e26927. [CrossRef] [PubMed]
36. Kamuche, F.U.; Ledman, R.E. Relationship of Time and Learning Retention. *J. Coll. Teach. Learn.* **2005**, *2*, 25. [CrossRef]
37. Kirchberg, J.; Fritzmann, J.; Weitz, J.; Bork, U. eHealth Literacy of German Physicians in the Pre–COVID-19 Era: Questionnaire Study. *JMIR mHealth uHealth* **2020**, *8*, e20099. [CrossRef] [PubMed]
38. Zou, X.; Liu, S.; Li, J.; Chen, W.; Ye, J.; Yang, Y.; Zhou, F.; Ling, L. Factors Associated With Healthcare Workers' Insomnia Symptoms and Fatigue in the Fight Against COVID-19, and the Role of Organizational Support. *Front. Psychiatry* **2021**, *12*, 652717. [CrossRef]
39. Eysenbach, G. The law of attrition. *J. Med. Internet Res.* **2005**, *7*, e11. [CrossRef] [PubMed]

MDPI
St. Alban-Anlage 66
4052 Basel
Switzerland
Tel. +41 61 683 77 34
Fax +41 61 302 89 18
www.mdpi.com

Healthcare Editorial Office
E-mail: healthcare@mdpi.com
www.mdpi.com/journal/healthcare

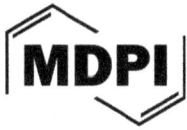